HUMAN RESOURCES IN HEALTHCARE

HUMAN RESOURCES IN HEALTHCARE

Managing for Success

FOURTH EDITION

Bruce J. Fried and
Myron D. Fottler, Editors

AUPHA

Health Administration Press, Chicago, Illinois

Association of University Programs in Health Administration, Arlington, Virginia

Your board, staff, or clients may also benefit from this book's insight. For more information on quantity discounts, contact the Health Administration Press Marketing Manager at (312) 424-9470.

19   18   5   4

Library of Congress Cataloging-in-Publication Data

Human resources in healthcare : managing for success / Bruce J. Fried and Myron D. Fottler, editors.—Fourth edition.
     p. ; cm.
  Includes bibliographical references and index.
  ISBN 978-1-56793-708-4 (alk. paper)
  I. Fried, Bruce, 1952– , editor. II. Fottler, Myron D., editor. III. Association of University Programs in Health Administration, publisher.
  [DNLM: 1. Personnel Management—methods. WX 159]
  RA971.35
  362.1068'3—dc23
                    2015004329

The paper used in this publication meets the minimum requirements of American National Standard for Information Sciences—Permanence of Paper for Printed Library Materials, ANSI Z39.48-1984. ∞ ™

Acquisitions editor: Tulie O'Connor; Project manager: Andrew Baumann; Manuscript editor: Karin Horler; Cover designer: Carla Nessa; Layout: Cepheus Edmondson

Found an error or a typo? We want to know! Please e-mail it to hapbooks@ache.org, and put "Book Error" in the subject line.

For photocopying and copyright information, please contact Copyright Clearance Center at www.copyright.com or at (978) 750-8400.

Health Administration Press
A division of the Foundation of the American
   College of Healthcare Executives
One North Franklin Street, Suite 1700
Chicago, IL 60606-3529
(312) 424-2800

Association of University Programs
   in Health Administration
2000 North 14th Street
Suite 780
Arlington, VA 22201
(703) 894-0940

BRIEF CONTENTS

DETAILED CONTENTS

PREFACE

This book is the fourth edition of *Human Resources in Healthcare: Managing for Success.* The first edition was published in 2001, an infamous year that brought issues of globalization to the forefront in the United States. Economic vulnerability had been present for some time, notably in the loss of dominance of the United States as a manufacturing economy dating to the 1970s. For Americans born after World War II, we experienced—many for the first time—a vulnerability that extended beyond economics, politics, and changes in social structure. We learned in a brutal manner that our sense of personal safety was illusional and that globalization was more than an abstract concept. The lessons of the Vietnam War, notably that US military dominance had disintegrated, were reinforced by two arguably inconclusive wars. US vulnerability extended from personal safety concerns to cyber-security threats and the global emergence and reemergence of diseases. From within, we saw the disintegration of confidence in our economic structures, culminating in the 2008 economic collapse spurred by a deregulated banking sector.

Technologically, the changes have been monumental, leading to extraordinary progress in communication, medicine, and countless other areas of life but also posing very significant threats. Socially, the demographics of the US population came to encompass increasing diversity in both numbers and types, viewed by many as a validation of the American dream and by others as a threat to the American identity. Election of the first African-American president was seen by many as a victory for hope, upward mobility, and profound cultural change, but by many others as a threat to the social order. With few exceptions, the political environment in Washington, DC, was characterized by unprecedented polarization and outright hatred.

Healthcare, of course, has not stood still since 2001. It has undergone tremendous changes, many of which were affected by larger economic, political, technological, and social factors. Economic constraints and the unconstrained increase in the cost of healthcare fed into demands for "bending the cost curve," leading to changes in incentive structures in the US healthcare system and its payment mechanisms. Politically, even in the midst of congressional gridlock, passage of the Affordable Care Act in 2010 represented the most important federal legislation since the enactment of Medicare in 1965.

As of this writing, the law continues to be under attack, and the eventual state of the law is uncertain.

Whatever the eventual outcome, more people are likely to have access to healthcare services, placing additional pressures on the healthcare system for effectiveness and efficiency. Socially, the aging of the baby boomers has, as predicted, placed increasing pressures on the healthcare system. The increasing diversity of the population has reinforced the need for cultural competence and systems of care that are responsive to social and cultural differences. In the workforce, generational diversity has created the need to consider reward and motivational structures that are generationally appropriate.

Healthcare systems continue to be under pressure to meet three aims: quality, cost containment, and access to care. Attention to quality has become increasingly acute as incentive structures focus on rewarding quality and in effect have begun to place sanctions on organizations, in some cases arguably, for substandard care. Quality improvement processes are a mainstay of organizations, requiring the active engagement and participation of employees.

Enter healthcare human resources management (HRM). Despite the changes of the past 15 years, people continue to play a critical and central role in providing health services. While automation and other technological advances have allowed other industries to downsize, technological changes in the healthcare industry generate the need for trained and well-managed health professionals. While other industries have outsourced an incalculable number of jobs, healthcare services cannot be significantly outsourced, with the exception of medical tourism, which operates on the margins of US healthcare.

Moreover, the healthcare workforce is under increasing pressure. Incentive structures have led to increased severity among hospitalized patients, and cost containment pressures have led in some instances to decreases in staffing with the remaining workers facing an increased workload. Managers are being asked to manage and retain a workforce that is in many cases highly stressed and mobile. Millennials, in contrast to earlier generations, tend to have a high need for personal development but only limited attachment to the organization. Further, jobs are changing as the healthcare system creates demands for new competencies. Effective job design, training, and performance management mechanisms need to be well developed and executed effectively.

We could go on documenting changes in the healthcare system, but instead we will describe the current edition of *Human Resources in Healthcare* and how each chapter in this edition addresses key realities and changes in healthcare. Undoubtedly, we will have overlooked some changes, and future changes are difficult to predict with confidence. Therefore, we offer this volume under the assumption that readers consider the content of this book in the spirit of continuous lifetime learning. Change is a given, but recognizing change and adapting effectively do not necessarily follow. In the words of Albert Einstein: "As far as the laws of mathematics refer to reality, they are not certain; and as far as they are certain, they do not refer to reality." We could say the same about healthcare and healthcare management.

Effective HRM is a product of at least three elements: cognitive knowledge, affective competencies, and experience. This book addresses domains of cognitive knowledge, including the idea of organizational strategy and HRM; the larger environment within which HRM occurs, including the legal environment and health workforce labor markets; and the multiple processes and systems involved in managing the healthcare workforce. For this knowledge (and, for that matter, any management knowledge) to be applied effectively, managers need to possess a variety of effective characteristics including competencies in such areas as emotional intelligence, interviewing, conflict management, and problem solving. Mastery of HRM, like virtually every other aspect of life, requires experience, practice, and learning from successes and failures through self-insight, reflection, and mentoring. The topics in this book are a starting point for developing mastery in working effectively with people in healthcare organizations.

In Chapter 1, Myron D. Fottler establishes the framework for this book: strategic HRM. An overall theme is that HRM is a responsibility of all people in the organization and certainly is not limited to the formal human resources (HR) department. The basic premise of strategic HRM is that HR practices and processes need to support the mission and strategies of the organization. This situation is far from a given. We have found repeatedly in the classroom that when we query a group of experienced managers, we are far more likely to find examples of poor HR practices than effective ones. Similarly, HR departments, which should be a key part of the senior management team, are very often viewed as operating in opposition to the interests of employees and the organization as a whole.

All organizations operate within a legal environment, and in Chapter 2, Drake Maynard provides foundational knowledge in the multitude of laws, regulations, and court decisions affecting HRM. Like other aspects of the law, the legal framework for HRM is in a constant state of flux with changing legislation at multiple levels, new interpretations resulting from court decisions, and changing regulations. Among the many areas of law covered are the Americans with Disabilities Act as amended, Title VII of the Civil Rights Act, the Fair Labor Standards Act, and the Family and Medical Leave Act. The chapter discusses the legal issues surrounding sexual harassment, the forms of sexual harassment, and how managers can avoid as well as respond to charges of sexual harassment. Written by a legal expert in employment law and containing many references to landmark legal cases, the chapter is nevertheless remarkably accessible to the nonlawyer. While most managers need not have a thorough knowledge of all aspects of employment law, they need to know the boundaries of the law and realize when their practices may be testing the boundaries of legality. This chapter effectively provides this foundation.

Healthcare organizations likely employ a broader range of professionals than do any other type of organization. The role of health professionals continues to evolve as a result of changes in technology, health services, and competency requirements. In Chapter 3, Kenneth R. White and Dolores G. Clement provide essential information on the distinction between professions and occupations, the process of becoming a professional, licensure and regulation, scope of practice, and the changing role of professionals. They also provide background information on factors associated with supply and demand for health professionals, including changes in technology, changes in payment mechanisms, and the increasing diversity of the settings in which healthcare services are provided.

John C. Hyde II authors a new chapter in this book on the credentialing of healthcare providers. Physicians have a complex relationship with many healthcare organizations yet play a central role in determining the quality of health services. In Chapter 4, Hyde discusses the legal framework and key court cases related to credentialing and privileging. He details the Joint Commission requirements to ensure high-quality and safe patient care and describes the processes that organizations should follow in ensuring a competent workforce. Hyde acknowledges the uncertainties and risks in credentialing and the difficulties faced, for example, when a surgeon requests privileges for a new procedure despite having limited experience with the procedure.

The issue of diversity is perhaps the most misunderstood aspect of management, yet its importance is integral to employee satisfaction and effectiveness as well as the quality of patient care. In Chapter 5, Rupert M. Evans Sr. stresses the importance of understanding the impact of diversity among patients and healthcare workers. He provides an expansive definition of diversity, characterizing diversity as falling into the three categories of human diversity, cultural diversity, and systems diversity. Using this framework, he makes the important distinction between diversity and the idea of inclusion. Taking a positive approach, he cites the business case for diversity and the potential for effectively managing diversity to positively affect patient outcomes and reduce disparities.

An employee's actual job is a central part of HRM. As described by Myron D. Fottler in Chapter 6, jobs continue to change in their competency requirements, how they are designed, and how they interact with other jobs in an organization. Jobs also are the foundation for other HR practices. For example, without a clear understanding of job requirements, establishing selection criteria for new employees is not possible. Nor is it possible to effectively coach individuals on their performance.

In Chapter 7, Bruce J. Fried and Michael Gates address the interrelated topics of recruitment, selection, and retention. In a rapidly changing healthcare system, finding and selecting the right people for the job is critical. However, selecting the best people for the job does not mean that prospective employees will choose to work for the organization, and it certainly does not ensure that they will stay with the organization. Fried and Gates describe alternative modes of employee recruitment as well as effective techniques for distinguishing between job applicants with similar skill sets and backgrounds. They address the controversial area of organizational fit and analyze its role in the selection process. Employee retention is of paramount importance in healthcare, and the authors provide evidence to support the importance of retention and evidence-based practices that organizations can use to maximize the likelihood of retaining the right people.

Part of keeping people in the organization is working with them to continually improve their performance. In Chapter 8, Bruce Fried addresses the topics of measuring employee performance and using this information to help employees develop their skills. This process, known as *performance management*, also includes ensuring a work environment where people are respected and valued. In this edition of the book, we have added a section on an unfortunate but highly prevalent aspect of organizational life: the bully. We describe the phenomenon of bullying, how to prevent it from occurring, and how to respond once it comes to light.

Reward systems are central to employee motivation, satisfaction, and performance. Noting that people work for both intrinsic and extrinsic rewards, Chapter 9 focuses on extrinsic rewards, namely compensation. In this chapter, Bruce J. Fried and Howard L. Smith address the role of compensation within the overall reward structure of the organization. They address the key topic of how jobs are valued in monetary terms and how objective job evaluation processes often need to be tempered by labor market considerations. In light of the current emphasis on individual and organization-wide pay for performance, they describe the strengths and drawbacks of different forms of incentive compensation, as well as considerations and trends in physician compensation.

Financial compensation is but one part of the total compensation that an employee receives. Employee benefits play a critical role in employees' decision to join an organization, their satisfaction, and their likelihood of staying with the organization. Dolores G. Clement, Maria A. Curran, and Sharon L. Jahn devote a chapter to the highly significant role played by employee benefits, in terms of both the cost to the organization and the motivational potential of these benefits. They provide a road map of employee benefits ranging from mandatory benefits, such as Social Security contributions and workers' compensation, to an array of voluntary benefits including health insurance, life insurance, and leave. Of particular importance is the attention to benefits plan design and how different employees value various benefits. Among the benefits design issues addressed are the inclusion of domestic partners in benefits, budget concerns, and related information about self-insurance and stop-loss insurance.

Performance improvement is a critical function in all organizations and is particularly important in healthcare, where technologies and methods of providing care are in a state of continuous change. In Chapter 11, Donna L. Kaye and Myron D. Fottler address performance improvement from both organizational and individual perspectives. They note that performance improvement initiatives are typically based on enhancing individual skills and expanding an employee's skill set. Training activities typically focus on the individual employee's current job and on remediating particular skill-set deficits. While these activities are important, when conducted alone they ignore the impact of organizational factors on individual performance. By contrast, organizational development is centered on enhancing both current and future jobs, improving the work group or organization over the long term, and attending to future work demands. Organizational development interventions are broad and include such activities as organizational diagnosis, succession planning, and communication. Kaye and Fottler describe a broad array of key organizational development processes and provide guidance on implementation.

Among the many sectors of the economy, healthcare organizations and public-sector organizations hold the greatest potential for increased unionization. Laws and rules governing unionization in healthcare are somewhat different from those in other sectors. In Chapter 12, Donna Malvey and Amanda Raffenaud summarize the legislative framework and judicial rulings governing healthcare unionization, describe the evolving role of unions in healthcare, and provide a description of the unionization and labor relations process in healthcare organizations. They describe all phases of the labor relations process, from the union recognition phase through contract administration. The specific requirements and obligations of management and unions in healthcare organizations, based largely on the 1974 amendments to the National Labor Relations Act, are described. The chapter also addresses the controversial area of physician unionization and the potential impact of the Affordable Care Act on unions. Given the likelihood of increased unionization in healthcare, the authors provide guidance on working effectively in a unionized environment.

Among the most difficult tasks in the healthcare system is projecting health workforce needs and matching these needs with supply. While most of the chapters in this book approach workforce issues from an organizational perspective, Erin P. Fraher and Marisa Morrison address workforce planning from a broader macro policy perspective. They discuss and assess methods used to ensure that the United States, or, for that matter, any country or jurisdiction, has the needed workforce in place, now and into the future. They examine workforce planning not in a vacuum, but cognizant of changes throughout the healthcare system that may affect workforce needs as well as new skill requirements. They address multiple related topics, including the distinction between "demand" and "need," the nature of oversupply and shortages, and alternative methods of assessing projected supply of and demand for health workers, as well as the lasting problem of uncertainty in making accurate projections.

The nursing profession is critical to the functioning of the healthcare system. In the hospital sector, nurses are the only professional group present 24 hours a day and every day of the year. Nurses are highly skilled, indispensable, and central to patient care and quality. In Chapter 14, Cheryl B. Jones, George H. Pink, and Lindsay T. Munn begin with a description of the types of nursing personnel, their education, competency requirements, and scope of practice. Understanding nursing roles is essential to understanding the critical factors involved in nurse staffing and deployment. They then discuss the substance of nurses' work, staffing and alternative methods of measuring nursing workload, and issues such as the role of nurses in unionized and nonunionized settings, nurse–physician relationships, and stress and burnout. They also address the key influence nurses have in value-based purchasing, being heavily involved, for example, in care coordination and in ensuring a patient- and caregiver-centered experience.

The quality improvement movement has finally achieved its migration from manufacturing and service industries to healthcare. Given incentive schemes that link reimbursement to quality indicators, and the availability of information on quality to payers and consumers, quality and patient safety are clearly hallmarks of healthcare organizations. Quality improvement is based on a synthesis of process analysis, measurement, and human creativity. In Chapter 15, Jordan Albritton and Bruce J. Fried provide a review of the quality improvement approach and summarize its forms (e.g., Lean). They take the view that a great deal of attention has been given to the mechanics of quality improvement, namely, the use of such quality improvement tools as run charts and Pareto diagrams. However, the human element, which is necessary to interpret data and devise creative and effective solutions to quality problems, has received less attention. In this chapter, Albritton and Fried identify the HR requirements, such as the development of effective quality improvement teams, that are essential to effectively apply quality improvement tools, interpret data, and develop effective and sustainable quality improvement changes.

The two appendixes are new to this book. Appendix A discusses HR metrics. Evaluation has become increasingly important in all aspects of organizational life, including HR functions. Appendix A provides background information on the need for and use of HR metrics, and offers examples of HR metrics. Appendix B includes six problem-based learning (PBL) cases. PBL is a student-centered learning methodology requiring the student, along with team members, to research a complex problem and design an evidence-based and feasible solution to the issue. As described in Appendix B, student teams read the case problem and identify what they need to learn in order to respond to the problem. These learning objectives form the basis for independent research and eventual collaboration of team members in writing the case response. The PBL method has a motivational element in that students themselves define their learning needs. Substantively, this approach provides the opportunity for students to delve into specific HR issues in greater depth and to use the most current research and writing on the topics presented in the cases.

This textbook and the accompanying instructor resources are designed to facilitate discussion and learning. The instructor resources include Power-Point slides for each chapter and key teaching points. For access information, e-mail hapbooks@ache.org.

ACKNOWLEDGMENTS

We are first and foremost very grateful to our colleagues who participated in writing this book. They are all very busy and successful people who generously gave of their time and expertise to write creative and interesting chapters, and were enormously responsive to our comments and suggestions. Thank you so much to all contributing authors.

Next, our colleagues at Health Administration Press provided extraordinary guidance from the overall book concept to the finest editing details. In fact, as one chapter author indicated in an e-mail to a Health Administration Press editor, "I wish you could edit all my manuscripts!" So we offer special thanks to Andrew Baumann, Janet Davis, Cepheus Edmondson, Karin Horler, and Tulie O'Connor.

Bruce J. Fried and Myron D. Fottler

Thanks to my wife, Nancy, for her limitless emotional and intellectual support, and for, to the extent humanly possible, keeping me grounded in reality. For continuously keeping me motivated, challenged, and inspired, credit most certainly goes to Aaron, Shoshana, Noah, Kit, and Scout. I am also thankful for the opportunity over the past 23 years to have taught and learned from the enormously talented students at the University of North Carolina at Chapel Hill.

Bruce J. Fried

Thanks to Alicia Beardsley-Pigon, my student assistant and health services administration graduate student at the University of Central Florida. Her assistance and patience with typing versions of my chapters, facilitating communications with editorial colleagues and other authors, and finding appropriate and relevant materials to update the chapters were invaluable and very much appreciated. My gratitude also goes to my wife, Carol, for her support on this and other projects over the years. Finally, I thank Reid Oetjen, chair of the Department of Health Management and Informatics at the University of Central Florida, for his support of this project.

Myron D. Fottler

STRATEGIC HUMAN RESOURCES MANAGEMENT

Myron D. Fottler

Learning Objectives

After completing this chapter, the reader should be able to

- define strategic human resources management,
- outline key human resources functions,
- discuss the significance of human resources management to present and future healthcare executives, and
- describe the organizational and human resources systems that affect organizational outcomes.

Introduction

Like most other service industries, the healthcare industry is labor intensive. One reason for healthcare's reliance on an extensive workforce is that producing a service and then storing it for later consumption is not possible.

In healthcare, the production of the service that is purchased and the consumption of that service occur simultaneously. Thus, the interaction between healthcare consumers and healthcare providers is an integral part of the delivery of health services. Given the dependence on healthcare professionals to deliver services, the possibility of heterogeneity of service quality must be recognized within an employee (as skills and competencies change over time) and among employees (as different individuals or representatives of various professions provide a service).

Human resources are all of the people who currently contribute to the work of the organization as well as those who might contribute in the future and those who have contributed in the recent past. The term *human resources* also refers to the management of these people's contributions and in this sense is often abbreviated *HR*.

The intensive use of labor for service delivery and the possibility of variability in professional practice require that leaders in the industry direct their attention toward managing the performance of the people involved in the delivery of services. The effective management of people requires that healthcare executives understand the factors that influence the performance of individuals employed in their organizations. These factors include not only the traditional *human resources management* (HRM) activities (i.e., recruitment and selection, training and development, appraisal, compensation, and employee relations) but also the environmental and other organizational aspects that impinge on human resources' activities.

Strategic human resources management (SHRM) is the process of formulating HR strategies and implementation tactics that are aligned and reinforce the organization's business strategy. It requires development of a comprehensive set of managerial activities and tasks related to developing and maintaining a qualified workforce. This workforce, in turn, contributes to organizational effectiveness, as defined by the organization's strategic goals. SHRM occurs in a complex and dynamic milieu of forces within the organizational context. A significant trend within the last decade is for HR managers to adopt a strategic perspective in their job and to recognize critical linkages between organizational strategy and HR strategies.

This book explains and illustrates the methods and practices for increasing the probability that competent personnel will be available to provide the services delivered by the organization and the probability that these employees will appropriately perform the necessary tasks. Implementing these methods and practices means that requirements for positions must be determined, qualified persons must be recruited and selected, employees must be trained and developed to meet future organizational needs, job performance must be evaluated, and adequate rewards must be provided to attract and retain top performers.

All of these functions must be managed within the legal constraints imposed by society (i.e., legislation, regulation, and court decisions). This chapter emphasizes that HR functions are performed within the context of the overall activities of the organization. These functions are influenced or constrained by the environment, the organizational mission and strategies that are being pursued, and the systems indigenous to the organization.

Why study SHRM? How does this topic relate to the career interests or aspirations of present or future healthcare executives? Staffing the organization, designing jobs, building teams, developing employee skills, identifying approaches to improve performance and customer service, and rewarding employee success are as relevant to line managers as they are to HR managers. A successful healthcare executive needs to understand human behavior, work with employees effectively, and be knowledgeable about the numerous systems and practices available to put together a skilled and motivated workforce. The executive also has to be aware of economic, technological, social, and legal issues that facilitate or constrain efforts to attain strategic objectives.

Healthcare executives do not want to hire the wrong person, experience high turnover, manage unmotivated employees, be taken to court for discrimination actions, be cited for unsafe practices, have poorly trained staff undermine patient satisfaction, or engage in unfair labor practices. Despite their best efforts, executives often fail at HRM because they hire the wrong people or they do not motivate or develop their staff. The material in this book can help executives avoid mistakes and achieve great results with their workforce.

Healthcare organizations can gain a competitive advantage over competitors by effectively managing their human resources. This competitive advantage may include cost leadership (i.e., being a low-cost provider) and product differentiation (i.e., having high levels of service quality). A 1994 study examined the HR practices and productivity levels of 968 organizations across 35 industries (Huselid 1994). The effectiveness of each organization's HR practices was rated based on the presence of such benefits as incentive plans, employee grievance systems, formal performance appraisal systems, and employee participation in decision making. The study found that organizations with high HRM effectiveness ratings clearly outperformed those with low HRM rankings. A similar study of 293 publicly held companies reported that productivity was highly correlated with effective HR practices (Huselid, Jackson, and Schuler 1997).

Several more recent studies have also shown that effective management of human resources can increase profitability, annual sales per employee, productivity, market value, and growth and earnings per share (Kaufman 2010; Messersmith and Guthrie 2010). In these studies, surveys were used to study the sophistication of the organization's HR practices, and responses created a score from 0 to 100, where high scores represented state-of-the-art practices. Performance was measured using accounting financial data. Results indicated that organizations with better HR practices experienced greater increases in financial performance relative to others. In addition, a survey of 200 chief financial officers (CFOs) revealed that 92 percent believed that effective management of employees improves customer satisfaction (Mayer, Ehrhart, and Schneider 2009). Customers also report more satisfaction when the climate of the organization is more positive, employees generally get along well, and turnover is low (Nishii, Lepak, and Schneider 2008).

Exhibit 1.1 summarizes HR practices that appear to enhance the effectiveness and outcomes of organizations. These practices are often present in organizations that are effective in managing their human resources, and they recur repeatedly in studies of high-performing organizations. In addition, these practices are interrelated and mutually reinforcing; achieving a positive result by implementing just one practice on its own is difficult. Recent research in healthcare suggests that innovative and sophisticated HR practices are becoming more prevalent and enhance an organization's overall performance (Platonova and Hernandez 2013).

While these HR practices generally have a positive impact on organizational performance, their relative effectiveness may vary depending on their alignment (or lack thereof) among themselves and with the organization's

EXHIBIT 1.1
Effective HR
Practices for
Healthcare
Organizations

Category	Practices
HR planning/job analysis	• Encourage employee involvement so that HR practices and managerial initiatives have strong buy-in. • Encourage teamwork to make employees more willing to collaborate. • Use self-managed teams and decentralization as basic elements of organizational design to minimize management layers. • Develop strategies to enhance employee work/life balance.
Staffing	• Be proactive in identifying and attracting talent. • In selecting new employees, use additional criteria beyond basic skills (i.e., attitudes, customer focus, and cultural fit). • Provide opportunities for employee growth so that employees are stretched to enhance their skills.
Training/organizational development	• Invest in training and organizational programs to enhance employee skills related to organizational goals. • Provide employees with future career opportunities by giving promotional priority to internal candidates. • Include customer service in new employee onboarding and skill development.
Performance management and compensation	• Recognize employees by providing monetary and nonmonetary rewards. • Offer high compensation contingent on organizational performance to reduce employee turnover and increase attraction to high-quality employees. • Reduce status distinction and barriers such as dress, language, office arrangement, parking, and wage differentials. • Base individual and team compensation on goal-oriented results.

(continued)

Employee rights	• Communicate effectively with employees to keep them informed of major issues and initiatives. • Share financial, salary, and performance information to develop a high-trust organization. • Provide employment security for employees who perform well so that they are not down-sized because of economic downturns or strategic errors by senior management.

EXHIBIT 1.1
Effective HR Practices for Healthcare Organizations *(continued from previous page)*

Sources: Chuang and Liao (2010); Gomez-Mejia and Balkin (2011); Pfeffer (1995, 1998); Wright et al. (2005).

mission, values, culture, strategies, goals, and objectives (Ford et al. 2006). These HR practices may vary in their impact on healthcare organizations depending on how well each one is aligned with and reinforces the others as well as how well it is aligned with the overall business strategy.

No HR practices, even those identified in Exhibit 1.1, are "good" in and of themselves. Rather, their impact is always dependent on how well the process fits with the factors noted previously. Fit, or alignment, leads to better performance, while its lack creates inconsistencies (Ulrich, Younger, and Brockband 2008). In general, organizational performance is enhanced when HR practices are aligned with business strategy, are attuned to the external environment, enable the organization to capitalize on its distinctive capabilities, and reinforce one another. Even though proving a causal relationship between HR practices and organizational performance is extremely difficult, it is reasonable for healthcare organizations to consider implementation of the practices associated with high-performing organizations.

The bad news is that achieving competitive advantage through HRM inevitably takes time to accomplish (Pfeffer 1998). The good news is that, once achieved, this type of competitive advantage is likely to be enduring and difficult for competitors to duplicate. Measurement is crucial in implementing these HR practices. Failure to evaluate the impact of HR practices dooms these practices to second-class status, neglect, and potential breakdown. Feedback from measurement is essential for further development of HR practices as a whole as well as for monitoring how well each practice is achieving its intended outcomes.

Wolf (2012) notes seven characteristics of high-performing healthcare organizations:

1. Visionary leadership
2. Consistent and effective communication
3. Selecting for fit and ongoing development of staff

4. Agile and open culture
5. Central focus on service
6. Constant recognition and broad community outreach
7. Solid physician/clinical relationships

It is the combination of these characteristics that helps healthcare organizations drive exceptional outcomes in patient experience, engagement, quality, and financial outcomes.

Most of these HR practices are described in more detail throughout the book. Although the evidence presented in the literature shows that effective HR practices can strongly enhance an organization's competitive advantage, it fails to indicate *why* these practices have such an influence. In this chapter, we describe a model—the SHRM model—that attempts to explain this phenomenon. First, however, a discussion of environmental trends is in order.

Environmental Trends

Major environmental trends affecting healthcare institutions include changing private and government reimbursement (i.e., the Affordable Care Act), emergence of new competitors, advent of new technology, low or declining inpatient occupancy rates, changes in physician–organization relationships, transformation of the demography and increase in diversity of the workforce, shortage of capital, increasing market penetration by managed care, heightened pressures to contain costs, and greater expectations of patients. These trends have resulted in increased competition, the need for higher levels of performance, and concern for institutional survival. Many healthcare organizations are closing facilities; undergoing corporate reorganization; instituting staffing freezes and/or reductions in workforce; allowing greater flexibility in work scheduling; providing services despite fewer resources; restructuring and/or redesigning jobs; outsourcing many functions; and developing leaner management structures, with fewer levels and wider spans of control.

The Society for Human Resource Management (2014) regularly surveys expert panels to review recent and future trends in HRM. Broader trends identified include the following:

- The continuing impact of the US economy has created challenges that have affected budgets, hiring, and capital HR strategies.
- The need for skilled and educated workers is creating competition for those in highest demand, which influences all areas of HR.

- Ongoing developments in information and communication technologies (i.e., social media) have influenced recruiting and selection.
- Demographic changes have increased the percentage of aging employees and have increased diversity, affecting all aspects of HR practice.
- These demographic changes have caused employers to emphasize flexible and effective work/life strategies.
- Metrics and more in-depth data analysis are being required to demonstrate the return on investment of HR expenditures.
- The increase in uncertainty and market volatility have made uncertainty the new normal.
- Implementation of the Affordable Care Act, as well as the need to ensure compliance with a wide variety of federal and state laws, has created continuing challenges for HR managers.

Most of the growth in the capital HR function over the past few decades has been attributed to its crucial role in keeping organizations in compliance with HR laws and regulations produced by federal, state, and local governments (Equal Employment Opportunity Commission 2014).

Gomez-Mejia, Balkin, and Cardy (2012) identified the eight most significant HR environmental challenges as rapid change, the rise of the Internet, workforce diversity, globalization, legislation, evolving work and family roles, skill shortages, and the rise of the service sector. In addition, the Society for Human Resource Management (2012) has projected that three major challenges in HR over the next ten years will be retaining and rewarding the best employees, developing the next generation of corporate leaders, and creating an organizational culture that attracts the best employees. To survive and prosper, healthcare organizations need to continuously and rapidly adapt to change. HR is almost always at the heart of an effective response system (Ulrich, Younger, and Brockband 2008).

Organizations are pursuing major competitive strategies to respond to the turbulent healthcare environment, including offering low-cost healthcare services, providing superior patient service through high-quality technical capability and customer service, specializing in key clinical areas (e.g., becoming centers of excellence), and diversifying within or outside healthcare. In addition, organizations are entering into strategic alliances and restructuring themselves to "do more with less" (i.e., to provide high clinical and service quality while containing costs). Regardless of which specific strategies are pursued (e.g., inpatient hospital services), healthcare organizations are experiencing a decrease in staffing levels in many traditional service areas and an increase in staffing in new ventures, medical informatics, specialized clinical areas, and related support services.

The HR strategies that experts believe will be most effective in managing employees in the next ten years include the following (Society for Human Resource Management 2012):

- Providing flexible worker arrangements
- Creating an organizational culture where trust, open communication, and fairness are emphasized and demonstrated
- Providing employees with opportunities for career advancement
- Offering a higher total rewards package than other organizations that compete for the same talent

Staffing profiles in healthcare are characterized by a limited number of highly skilled and well-compensated professionals. Healthcare organizations are no longer employers of last resort for the unskilled. At the same time, however, most organizations are experiencing shortages of nursing and allied health personnel.

The development of appropriate responses to the ever-changing healthcare environment has received so much attention that the concept of HRM planning is now well accepted in healthcare organizations. However, implementation of such plans has often been problematic. Often the process ends with the development of goals and objectives and does not include strategies or methods of implementation and ways to monitor results. Implementation appears to be the major difficulty in the overall management process (Porter 1980).

A major reason for this lack of implementation has been the failure of healthcare executives to assess and manage the external, interface, and internal stakeholders whose cooperation and support are necessary to successfully implement any business strategy (i.e., corporate, business, or functional). Successful strategy implementation requires healthcare executives to identify, diagnose, and manage key stakeholders (Blair and Fottler 1990).

A stakeholder is any individual or group with a stake in the organization. External stakeholders include patients and their families, public and private regulatory agencies, and third-party payers. Interface stakeholders operate in both the internal and external environments; these stakeholders may include members of the medical staff who have admitting privileges or who are board members at several institutions. Internal stakeholders operate within the organization, such as managers, professionals, and nonprofessional employees.

Involving supportive stakeholders, such as employees and HR managers, is crucial to the success of any HRM plan. If HR executives are not actively involved, then the employee planning, recruitment, selection, development, appraisal, and compensation necessary for successful plan implementation are not likely to occur.

The SHRM Model

A strategic approach to HRM includes the following (Fottler et al. 1990):

- Assessing the organization's environment and mission
- Formulating the organization's business strategy
- Identifying HR requirements based on the business strategy
- Comparing the current HR inventory—in terms of numbers, characteristics, and practices—with future strategic requirements
- Developing an HR strategy based on the differences between the current inventory and future requirements
- Implementing the appropriate HR practices to reinforce the business strategy and to attain competitive advantage

Exhibit 1.2 provides some examples of possible linkages between strategic decisions and HR practices.

SHRM has not been given as high a priority in healthcare as it has received in many other industries. This neglect is particularly surprising in a labor-intensive industry that requires the right people in the right jobs at the right times and that often undergoes shortages in some occupations. In addition, the literature in the field offers evidence that organizations that use more progressive HR approaches achieve significantly better financial results than comparable, although less progressive, organizations do (see Exhibit 1.1) (Huselid 1994; Huselid, Jackson, and Schuler 1997).

Exhibit 1.3 illustrates some strategic HR trends that affect job analysis and planning, staffing, training and development, performance appraisal, compensation, employee rights and discipline, and employee and labor relations. These trends are discussed in more detail in later chapters of this book. The bottom line of Exhibit 1.3 is that organizations are moving to higher levels of flexibility, collaboration, decentralization, and team orientation. This transformation is driven by the environmental changes and the organizational responses to those changes discussed earlier. However, few healthcare organizations facilitate these advanced options.

The benefits of SHRM to both the organization and its stakeholders have been identified as management of positive rather than negative behavior, explicit communication of organization goals, stimulation of critical thinking and continual examination of assumptions, identification of gaps between the

EXHIBIT 1.2
Implications
of Strategic
Decisions on HR
Practices

Strategic Decision	Implications on HR Practices
Pursue low-cost competitive strategy	Provide lower compensation Negotiate give-backs in labor relations Provide training to improve efficiency
Pursue service quality differentiation competitive strategy	Provide high compensation Recruit top-quality candidates Evaluate performance on the basis of patient satisfaction Provide training in guest relations
Pursue growth through acquisition	Adjust compensation Select candidates from acquired organization Outplace redundant workers Provide training to new employees
Pursue growth through development of new markets	Promote existing employees on the basis of an objective performance-appraisal system
Purchase new technology	Provide training in using and maintaining the technology
Offer new service/product line	Recruit and select physicians and other personnel
Increase productivity and cost effectiveness through process improvement	Encourage work teams to be innovative Take risks Assume a long-term perspective

current situation and future vision, engagement of line managers, identification of HR constraints and opportunities, and creation of common bonds (Gomez-Mejia, Balkin, and Cardy 2012).

The SHRM Process

As illustrated in Exhibit 1.4, a healthcare organization is made up of systems that require constant interaction within the environment. To remain viable, an organization must adapt its strategic planning and thinking to extend to

EXHIBIT 1.3
Strategic HR
Trends

Old HR Practices	Current HR Practices

Job Analysis/Planning

Explicit job descriptions	⟶	Broad job classes
Detailed HR planning	⟶	Loose work planning
Detailed controls	⟶	Flexibility
Efficiency	⟶	Innovation

Staffing

Supervisors make hiring decisions	⟶	Team makes hiring decisions
Emphasis on candidate's technical qualifications	⟶	Emphasis on "fit" of applicant within the culture
Layoffs	⟶	Voluntary incentives to retire
Letting laid-off workers fend for themselves	⟶	Providing continued support to terminated employees

Training and Development

Individual training	⟶	Team-based training
Job-specific training	⟶	Generic training emphasizing flexibility
"Buy" skills by hiring experienced workers	⟶	"Make" skills by training less-skilled workers
Organization responsible for career development	⟶	Employee responsible for career development

Performance Appraisal

Uniform appraisal procedures	⟶	Customized appraisals
Control-oriented appraisals	⟶	Developmental appraisals
Supervisor inputs only	⟶	Appraisals with multiple inputs

Compensation

Seniority	⟶	Performance-based pay
Centralized pay decisions	⟶	Decentralized pay decisions
Fixed fringe benefits	⟶	Flexible fringe benefits (i.e., cafeteria approach)

Employee Rights and Discipline

Emphasis on employer protection	⟶	Emphasis on employee protection
Informal ethical standards	⟶	Explicit ethical codes and enforcement procedures
Emphasis on discipline to reduce mistakes	⟶	Emphasis on prevention to reduce mistakes

Employee and Labor Relations

Top-down communication	⟶	Bottom-up communication and feedback
Adversarial approach	⟶	Collaboration approach
Preventive labor relations	⟶	Employee freedom of choice

external changes. The internal components of the organization are affected by these changes, so the organization's plans may necessitate modifications in the internal systems and HR process systems. Harmony among these systems is necessary. The characteristics, performance levels, and amount of coherence in operating practices among these systems influence the outcomes achieved in terms of organizational and employee-level measures of performance. HR goals, objectives, process systems, culture, technology, and workforce must be aligned with each other (i.e., internal alignment) and with organizational strategies (i.e., external alignment) (Ford et al. 2006).

HR systems are also significantly affected by forces in the external environment as well as factors within the organization (Lengnick-Hall et al. 2009). When a healthcare organization systematically understands, creates, coordinates, aligns, and integrates all of its policies and practices, it creates an HRM system. Many HR policies and practices working together are necessary to get best results (Subramony 2009).

Internal and External Environmental Assessment

Environmental assessment is a crucial element of SHRM. As a result of changes in the legal/regulatory climate, economic conditions, and labor-market realities, healthcare organizations face constantly changing opportunities and threats. These opportunities and threats make particular services or markets more or less attractive in the organization's perspective.

Healthcare executives need to assess not only their organizational strengths and weaknesses but also their internal systems; their human resources' skills, knowledge, and abilities; and their portfolio of service markets. HRM involves paying attention to the effect of environmental and internal components on the HR process. Because of the critical role of healthcare professionals in delivering services, managers should develop HR policies and practices that are closely related to, influenced by, and supportive of the strategic goals and plans of their organization.

Organizations, either explicitly or implicitly, pursue a strategy in their operations. Deciding on a strategy means determining the products or services that will be created and the markets to which the chosen services will be offered. Once the selection is made, the methods to be used to compete in the chosen market must be identified. The methods adopted are based on internal resources available, or potentially available, for use by managers.

As shown in Exhibit 1.4, strategies should consider environmental conditions and organizational capabilities. To be in a position to take advantage of opportunities that are anticipated to occur, as well as to parry potential threats from changed conditions or competitor initiatives, managers must have detailed knowledge of the current and future operating environment. Cognizance of internal strengths and weaknesses allows managers to develop plans based on an accurate assessment of the organization's ability to perform in the marketplace at the desired level.

EXHIBIT 1.4
SHRM Model

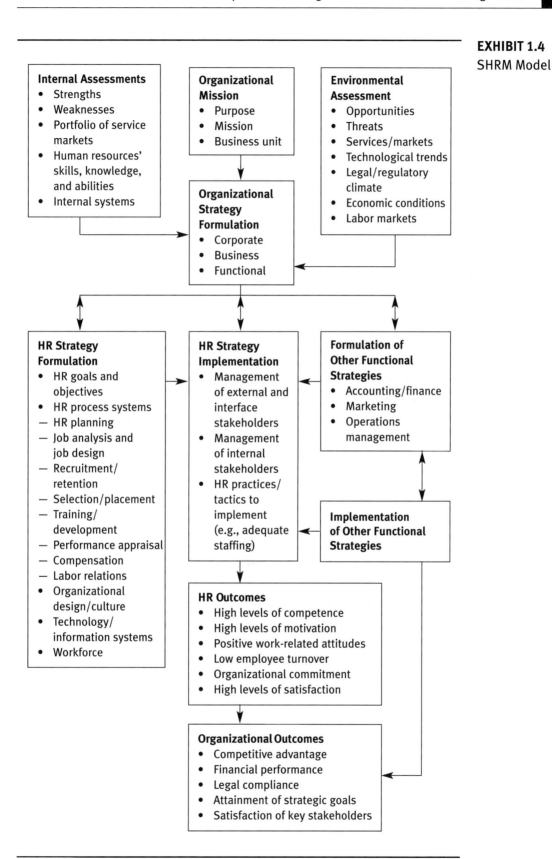

SHRM does not occur in a vacuum; rather, it occurs in a complex and dynamic constellation of forces in the organizational context. One significant trend has been for HR managers to adopt a strategic perspective and to recognize the critical links between HR and organizational goals. As seen in Exhibit 1.4, the SHRM process starts with the identification of the organization's purpose, mission, and business unit, as defined by the board of directors and the senior management team. The process ends with the HR function serving as a strategic partner to the operating departments. Under this new view of HRM, the HR manager's job is to help operating managers achieve their strategic goals by serving as the expert in employment-related activities and issues.

The implementation of an organization's strategy through HR has become more and more dependent on technology. Today, most Americans use mobile phones, many of which have thousands of applications that make the phones "smart." Healthcare organizations have quickly realized that HR applications can help them manage their employees more effectively by increasing operational efficiency and meeting expectations of different generations in the workforce. Mobile devices make it easier to deliver services, provide information to job applicants, offer training modules, manage interview skills, and coordinate work arrangements (Rafter 2010).

When HR is viewed as a strategic partner, talking about the single best way to do anything makes no sense. Instead, the organization must adopt HR practices that are consistent with its strategic mission, goals, and objectives. In addition, all healthcare executives are HR managers. Proper management of employees entails having effective supervisors and line managers throughout the organization.

Organizational Mission and Corporate Strategy

An organization's purpose is its basic reason for existence. The purpose of a hospital may be to deliver high-quality clinical care to the population in a given service area. An organization's mission, created by its board and senior managers, specifies how the organization intends to manage itself to most effectively fulfill its purpose. The mission statement often provides subtle clues on the importance the organization places on its human resources. The purpose and mission affect HR practices in obvious ways. A nursing home, for example, must employ nursing personnel, nurse aides, and food service workers to meet the needs of its patients.

The first step in formulating a corporate and business strategy is doing a *SWOT* (strengths, weaknesses, opportunities, and threats) *analysis*. The managers then attempt to use the organization's strengths to capitalize on environmental opportunities and to cope with environmental threats. Human resources play a fundamental role in SWOT analysis because the nature and type of people who work within an organization and the organization's ability to attract new talent represent significant strengths and weaknesses.

Most organizations formulate strategy at three basic levels: the corporate level, the business level, and functional levels. Corporate strategy is a set of strategic alternatives that an organization chooses from as it manages its operations simultaneously across several industries and markets. Business strategy is a set of strategic alternatives that an organization chooses from to most effectively compete in a particular industry or market. Functional strategies consider how the organization will manage each of its major functions (i.e., marketing, finance, and HR).

A key challenge for HR managers when the organization is using a corporate growth strategy is recruiting and training the large numbers of qualified employees who are needed to provide services in added operations. New-hire training programs may also be needed to orient and update the skills of incoming employees. In Exhibit 1.4, the two-way arrows connecting "Organizational Strategy Formulation" with "HR Strategy Formulation" and "HR Strategy Implementation" indicate that the impact of the HR function should be considered in the development of organizational strategy. When HR is a true strategic partner, all organizational parties consult with and support one another. Consequently, the two-way arrows from "Organizational Strategy Formation" indicate the parties that should also be considered in formulating an organizational strategy.

HR Strategy Formulation and Implementation

Once the organization's corporate and business strategies have been determined, managers can then develop an HR strategy. This strategy commonly includes a staffing strategy (planning, recruitment, selection, placement), a developmental strategy (performance management, training, development, career planning), and a compensation strategy (salary structure, employee incentives).

A *staffing strategy* refers to a set of activities used by the organization to determine its future HR needs, recruit qualified applicants with an interest in the organization, and select the best of those applicants as new employees. This strategy should be undertaken only after a careful and systematic development of the corporate and business strategies so that staffing activities mesh with other strategic elements of the organization. For example, if retrenchment is part of the business strategy, the staffing strategy will focus on determining which employees to retain and what process to use in termination.

A *developmental strategy* helps the organization enhance the quality of its human resources. This strategy must also be consistent with the corporate and business strategies. For example, if the organization wishes to follow a strategy of differentiating itself from competitors through customer focus and service quality, it will need to invest heavily in training its employees to provide the highest-quality service and to ensure that performance management focuses on measuring, recognizing, and rewarding performance—all of which lead to high levels of service quality. Alternatively, if the business strategy is to be a leader in providing low-cost services, the developmental strategy may focus on training to enhance productivity to keep overall costs low.

A *compensation strategy* must also complement the organization's other strategies. For example, if the organization is pursuing a strategy of related diversification, its compensation strategy must be geared toward rewarding employees whose skills allow them to move from the original business to related businesses (i.e., inpatient care to home health care). The organization may choose to pay a premium to highly talented individuals who have skills that are relevant to one of its new businesses. When formulating and implementing an HR strategy and the basic HR components discussed earlier, managers must account for other key parts of the organization, such as organizational design, corporate culture, technology, and the workforce.

Organizational design refers to the framework of jobs, positions, groups of positions, and reporting relationships among positions. Most healthcare organizations use a functional design whereby members of a specific occupation or role are grouped into functional departments such as OB-GYN, surgery, and emergency services. Management roles are also divided into functional areas such as marketing, finance, and HR. The top of the organizational chart is likely to reflect positions such as chief executive officer (CEO) and vice presidents of marketing, finance, and HR.

To operate efficiently and allow for seamless service, an organization with a functional design requires considerable coordination across its departments. Many healthcare organizations have been moving toward a flat organizational structure or horizontal corporation. Such an organization is created by eliminating levels of management, reducing bureaucracy, using wide spans of control, and relying heavily on teamwork and coordination to get work accomplished. These horizontal corporations are designed to be highly flexible, adaptable, streamlined, and empowered. The HR function in such organizations is typically diffused throughout the system so that operating managers take on more of the responsibility for HR activities and the HR staff play a consultative role.

Corporate culture refers to the set of values that help members of that culture understand what they stand for, how they do things, and what they consider important. Because culture is the foundation of the organization's internal environment, it plays a major role in shaping the management of human resources, determining how well organizational members will function together and how well the organization will be able to achieve its goals. There is no ideal culture for all organizations, but a strong and well-articulated culture enables employees to know what the organization stands for, what it values, and how to behave. A number of forces shape an organization's culture, including the founder or founders, institutional affiliations, shared experiences, symbols, stories, slogans, heroes, and ceremonies.

Managers must recognize the importance of culture and take appropriate care to transmit that culture to others in the organization. Culture can be transmitted through orientation, training, consistent behavior (i.e., walking the talk), corporate history, and telling and retelling of stories. Culture may facilitate the work of either HR managers or line managers. If the organization has a strong, well-understood, and attractive culture, attracting and retaining qualified employees become easier. If the culture is perceived as weak or unattractive, recruitment and retention become problematic. Likewise, the HR function can reinforce an existing culture by selecting new employees who have values that are consistent with that culture.

Technology also plays a role in the formulation and implementation of an HR strategy. The HR activities of healthcare organizations are different from those in the manufacturing industry. In healthcare, different criteria for hiring and methods of training are used. In addition, healthcare organizations typically emphasize educational credentials. Many aspects of technology play a role in HR in all healthcare settings. For example, automation of certain routine functions may reduce demand for certain HR activities but may increase it for others. Computers, robotics, and social media are important technological elements that affect HRM, and rapid changes in technology affect employee selection, training, compensation, and other areas.

Appropriately designed management information systems provide data to support planning and management decision making. HR information is a crucial element of such a system because this information can be used for both planning and operational purposes. For example, strategic planning efforts may require data on the number of professionals in various positions who will be available to fill future needs. Internal planning may require HR data in categories such as productivity trends, employee skills, work demands, and employee turnover rates. The use of an intranet (an internal Internet that is available to members of an organization) can improve service to all employees, help the HR department, and reduce many routine administrative costs.

Finally, *workforce* composition and trends also affect HR strategy formulation and implementation. The American workforce has become increasingly diverse in numerous ways. It has seen growth in the number of older employees, women, Latinos, Asian Americans, African Americans, foreign-born workers, individuals with disabilities, single parents, gays, lesbians, and people with special dietary preferences.

In 2012, approximately 34 percent of the US workforce were minorities, including African Americans (12 percent), Asian Americans (5 percent), Hispanics (15 percent), and other minorities (2 percent) (Bureau of Labor

Statistics 2012). In some sectors of healthcare (e.g., nursing homes), minorities compose more than half of the labor force. Women with children younger than age six are now the fastest-growing workforce component (Bureau of Labor Statistics 2012). These trends are likely to accelerate in the future.

Previously, most employers observed a fairly predictable employee pattern: People entered the workforce at a young age, maintained stable employment for many years, and retired at the usual age—on or around age 65. This pattern has changed and continues to evolve as a result of demographic factors, improved health, and the abolition of mandatory retirement.

Most companies today have workforce populations that fall into four generations: traditionalists, baby boomers, Generation X, and millennials (also known as Generation Y) (Twenge et al. 2010). Each generation has grown up in different environments that have shaped its members' attitudes and values toward work. HR professionals must therefore be aware of such values and attitudes and their possible impact in shaping HR policies and practices. While not everyone within each generation shares the same values and attitudes, the generations do tend to have distinctive characteristics (Pew Research Center 2010) (Exhibit 1.5).

A common guideline for HR professionals in dealing with a multigenerational workforce is to assume both similarities and differences exist, seek to understand them, and develop appropriate programs. Most HR policies should be formulated to appeal to a wide variety of employees.

As mentioned earlier, the successful implementation of an HR strategy generally requires identifying and managing key stakeholders (Blair and Fottler 1990, 1998). These stakeholders may be internal (i.e., employees), interface (i.e., physicians who are not employees), or external (i.e., third-party payers). The HR strategy, as well as all other strategies, can only be implemented through people; therefore, implementation requires motivational and communication processes, goal setting, and leadership. Specific practices or tactics are also necessary to implement the HR strategy. For example, if a healthcare organization's business strategy is to differentiate itself from competitors through its high-level focus on meeting customer (patient) needs, then the organization may formulate an HR strategy to provide all employees with training in guest relations.

However, that training strategy alone will not accomplish the business objective. Methods for implementation also need to be decided. For example, should the training be provided in-house or externally through programs such as those run by the Disney Institute? How will each employee's success in applying the principles be measured and rewarded? The answers to such questions provide the specific tactics needed to implement the HR strategy associated with the business goal of differentiation through customer service. Obviously, the organization will also develop and implement other

Generation	Values and Attitudes
Traditionalists (born 1929–1945)	• Disciplined • Hardworking • Sense of obligation • Saving • Need for respect • Respecting chain of command • Loyal • Comfortable with stability • Uncomfortable with conflict
Baby boomers (born 1946–1964)	• Developed a sense of capability of changing the world • Believe hard work and sacrifice are the price to pay for success • Strong sense of entitlement • Not as loyal as traditionalists • Value health, wellness, personal growth, and diversity
Generation X (born 1965–1981)	• First generation predicted to earn less than their parents • Value work–life balance • Not overly loyal to their employers • Value continuous learning and skill development • Some level of comfort with change and computer technology • Value individualism, flexibility • Do not favor micromanaging
Millennials (born 1982–1999)	• Grew up with the most technological changes and advances • Tend to exhibit high levels of self-esteem and confidence • Accustomed to instant feedback from playing computer and video games • Comfortable with multitasking, change, and innovation • Willing to work in and are effective working in teams • Social media is integral to everyday life and is responsible for their need to be in constant connection with others

EXHIBIT 1.5
Values and Attitudes of Four Generations

Source: Pew Research Center (2010).

functional strategies in accounting/finance, marketing, operations management, and other areas. Positive or negative organizational outcomes are determined by how well these functional strategies are formulated, aligned, and implemented.

Outcomes and Performance

The outcomes achieved by a healthcare organization depend on its environment, its mission, its strategies, its HR process systems, its internal systems and the consistency with which the operating practices are followed across these systems, and its capability to execute all of these factors. The appropriate methods for organizing and relating these factors are determined by the outcomes desired by managers and other major stakeholders, and numerous methods exist for conceptualizing organizational performance and outcomes (Gallery and Carey 2014; Lowe 2010). For this discussion, the specific outcomes are HR outcomes and organizational outcomes (see the two bottom boxes in Exhibit 1.4).

HR Outcomes and Performance

Numerous HR outcomes are associated with HR practices. An organization should provide its workforce with job security, meaningful work, safe conditions of employment, equitable financial compensation, and a satisfactory quality of work life. Organizations will not be able to attract and retain the number, type, and quality of professionals required to deliver quality health services if the internal work environment is unsuitable. In addition, employees are a valuable stakeholder group whose concerns are important because of the complexity of the service they provide. Job satisfaction, commitment to the organization, motivation, levels of job stress, and other constructs can be used as measures of employee attitude and psychological condition.

HR metrics are measures of HR outcomes and performance. Part of HR's role as a strategic business partner is to measure the effectiveness of the HR function as a whole as well as to perform specific HR tasks. HR has come under scrutiny as management and other areas of the organization inquire how HR activities contribute to performance outcomes (*HR Focus* 2005a). Specifically, the questions often focus on the return on investment (ROI) of HR activities.

Human capital metrics have been developed to determine how HR activities contribute to the organization's bottom line. Some employers gather data on the ROI of recruitment sources, such as print advertising, Internet advertising, college recruitment, internal transfers, and career fairs (Garvey 2005). Other employers track productivity using cost metrics, such as the time to fill positions, the percentage of diverse candidates hired, interview-to-offer ratios, offer-to-acceptance ratios, hiring manager satisfaction, new-hire satisfaction, cost per hire, headcount ratios, turnover costs, financial benefits of employee retention, and the ROI of training (Garvey 2005; Schneider 2006). Such metrics relate to specific HR activities, but the overall contribution of the HR function to organizational performance and outcomes also needs to be measured (Lawler, Levenson, and Boudreau 2004).

The *HR scorecard* is one method to measure this contribution. This tool is basically a modified version of the balanced scorecard, which is a measurement and control system that looks at a mix of quantitative and qualitative factors to evaluate organizational performance (Kaplan and Norton 1996). The "balance" reflects the need for short-term and long-term objectives, financial and nonfinancial metrics, lagging and leading indicators, and internal and external performance perspectives. A book titled *The Workforce Scorecard* extends research on the balanced scorecard to maximize workforce potential (Huselid, Becker, and Beatty 2005). The authors show that traditional financial performance measures are "lagging" performance indicators that can be predicted by the way organizations manage their human resources. HR practices are the "leading" indicators, predicting subsequent financial performance.

The Mayo Clinic has developed its own HR balanced scorecard that allows the HR function to become more involved in the organization's strategic planning (Fottler, Erickson, and Rivers 2006). Based on the assumption "what gets measured gets managed," the Mayo Clinic's HR balanced scorecard measures and monitors a large number of input and output HR indicators that are aligned with the organization's mission and strategic goals. This HR scorecard measures financial (i.e., staff retention savings), customer (i.e., employee retention, patient satisfaction), internal (i.e., time to fill positions), and learning (i.e., staff satisfaction, perceived training participation) areas.

Organizational Outcomes and Performance

For long-term survival, a healthcare organization must have a balanced exchange relationship with the environment. This equitable relationship is mutually beneficial to the organization and to the environment with which it interacts. A number of outcome measures, such as growth, profitability, ROI, competitive advantage, legal compliance, strategic objectives attainment, and key stakeholder satisfaction, can be used to determine how well the organization is performing in the marketplace and producing a service that will be valued by consumers. Stakeholder satisfaction measures may include such indexes as patient satisfaction, cost per patient day, and community perception.

The mission and objectives of the organization are reflected in the outcomes stressed by management and in the strategies, general tactics, and HR practices that are chosen. Management makes decisions that, in combination with the level of fit achieved among the internal systems, determine the outcomes the institution can achieve. For example, almost all healthcare organizations need to earn some profit for continued viability. However, some organizations refrain from initiating new ventures that may be highly profitable if the ventures do not fit their overall mission of providing quality services needed by a defined population group.

Conversely, some organizations may start services that are break-even propositions at best because those services are viewed as critical to their mission and the needs of their target market. The concerns of such an organization are reflected not only in the choice of services it offers but also in the HR approaches it uses and the outcome measures it views as important. This organization likely places more emphasis on assessment criteria for employee performance and nursing unit operations that stress the provision of quality care than on criteria concerned with efficient use of supplies and the maintenance of staffing ratios. This selection of priorities does not mean that the organization is ignoring efficiency of operations; it just signals that the organization places greater weight on the former criteria. The outcome measures used to judge the institution should reflect its priorities.

Another institution may place greater emphasis on economic return, profitability, and efficiency of operations. Quality of care is also important to that organization, but the driving force for becoming a low-cost provider causes the organization to make decisions that reflect its business strategy; therefore, it stresses maintenance or reduction of staffing levels and strictly prohibits overtime. Its recruitment and selection criteria stress identification and selection of employees who will meet minimum job requirements and expectations and, possibly, will accept lower pay levels. In an organization that strives to be efficient, less energy may be spent on "social maintenance" activities designed to meet employee needs and to keep them from leaving or unionizing. The outcomes in this situation will reflect, at least in the short run, higher economic return and lower measures of quality of work life.

The HR Brand

Regardless of their specific outcome objectives, most healthcare organizations seek competitive advantage over their competitors. The ultimate goal of the HR function should be to develop a distinctive brand so that employees, potential employees, and the general public view that particular organization as the preferred choice rather than as the last resort.

In HR, *branding* refers to the organization's corporate image or culture (Johnson and Roberts 2006). Because organizations are constantly competing for the best talent, developing an attractive HR brand is extremely important. A brand embodies the values and standards that guide employee behavior. It indicates the purpose of the organization, the types of people it hires, and the results it recognizes and rewards (Barker 2005). If an organization can convey that it is a great place to work, it can attract the "right" people (Snell and Bohlander 2013). Being acknowledged by an external source is a good way to create a recognized HR brand. Inclusion on national, published "best" lists, such as the following, helps an organization build a base of followers and enhances its recruitment and retention programs:

- *Fortune*'s 100 Best Companies to Work For
- *Fortune*'s 50 Best Companies for Asians, Blacks, and Hispanics
- *Working Mother*'s 100 Best Companies
- *Computerworld*'s Best Places to Work in IT

Being selected for *Fortune*'s 100 Best Companies list is so desirable that some organizations try to change their culture, philosophy, and brand just to be included (Phillips 2005). Research shows that organizations that are more attractive to employees also tend to perform better financially (Paauwe 2009). Such organizations appear to be able to simultaneously satisfy both investors and employees.

Southern Ohio Medicine Center (SOMC) in Portsmouth, Ohio, which ranked 18th on *Fortune*'s 100 Best Companies list in 2014, is a nonprofit, 233-bed hospital that was founded in 1907 and lies along the border of Ohio and Kentucky. SOMC is known to provide a friendly culture and high employee satisfaction rates, with 93 percent of employees saying management is approachable and 95 percent stating that they were made to feel welcome upon joining the company. Part of this hospital's success in employee satisfaction is a result of the personal interest that its CEO and president, Randy Arnett, takes in his employees' personal and work experiences. He has been noted to take the time to make rounds and chat with his employees. Overall, 96 percent of SOMC employees are proud to tell people where they work (Great Rated! 2014).

The immediate goal of building a strong HR brand is to attract and retain the best employees. However, the ultimate goal is to enhance the organization's outcomes and performance—that is, to achieve competitive advantage.

Human Resources and The Joint Commission

The Joint Commission requires healthcare organizations to assess their staffing effectiveness by continually screening for issues that can potentially arise as a result of inadequate staffing. *Staffing effectiveness* is defined as the number, competency, and skill mix of staff related to the provision of needed care, treatment, and services. The Joint Commission's focus is on the link between HR strategy implementation (i.e., adequate staffing) and organizational outcomes (i.e., clinical outcomes); see these two boxes in Exhibit 1.4.

Under The Joint Commission's Standard HR 1.30, a healthcare facility selects a minimum of four screening indicators—two for clinical/service issues and two for HR. The idea behind using two sets of indicators is to understand their relationship with one another; it also emphasizes that no indicator, in and of itself, can directly demonstrate staffing effectiveness. An example of a clinical/service screening indicator is an adverse drug event, and examples of HR screening indicators are overtime and staff vacancy rates. Staffing inefficiencies may be revealed by examining multiple screening indicators related to patient outcomes.

A facility has to choose at least one indicator for each clinical/service and HR category from The Joint Commission's list, and additional screening indicators can be selected on the basis of the facility's unique characteristics, specialties, and services. This selection also defines the expected impact that the absence of direct and indirect caregivers may have on patient outcomes. The data collected on these indicators are analyzed to identify potential staffing-effectiveness issues when performance varies from expected targets—that is, ranges of performance are evaluated, external comparisons are made, and improvement goals are assessed. The data are analyzed over time against the screening indicators to identify trends, patterns, or the stability of a process. At least once a year, managers report to the senior management team regarding the aggregation and analysis of data related to staffing effectiveness and regarding any actions taken to improve staffing.

HR screening indicators include the following:

- Overtime
- Staff vacancy rates
- Staff turnover rates
- Understaffing, as compared to the facility's staffing plan
- Nursing hours per patient day
- Staff injuries on the job
- On-call per diem use
- Sick time

Clinical/service screening indicators include the following:

- Patient readmission rates
- Patient infection rates
- Patient clinical outcomes by diagnostic category

The healthcare organization is expected to drill down to determine the causes when data vary from what is expected. The organization then undertakes steps leading to appropriate actions that are likely to remedy identified problems. For example, analysis of the data may indicate the need for evaluation of the organization's staffing practices. If so, the organization takes specific actions to improve its performance.

Examples of strategies that may be used to address identified staffing issues include the following:

- Staff recruitment
- Education/training
- Service curtailment
- Increased technology support
- Reorganization of work flow
- Provision of additional ancillary or support staff
- Adjustment of skill base

A Strategic Perspective on Human Resources

Managers at all levels are becoming increasingly aware that critical sources of competitive advantage include appropriate systems for attracting, motivating, and managing the organization's human resources. Adopting a strategic view of human resources involves considering employees as human "assets" and developing appropriate policies and programs to increase the value of these assets to the organization and the marketplace. Effective organizations realize that their employees have value, much as the organization's physical and capital assets have value.

Viewing human resources from an investment perspective, rather than as variable costs of production, allows the organization to determine how to best invest in its people. This perspective leads to a dilemma. An organization that does not invest in its employees may be less attractive to both current and prospective employees, which causes inefficiency and weakens the organization's competitive position. However, an organization that does invest in its people needs to ensure that these investments are not lost. Consequently, an organization needs to develop strategies to ensure that its employees stay long enough that it can realize an acceptable return on its investment in employee skills and knowledge.

Not all organizations realize that human assets can be strategically managed from an investment perspective. Management may or may not have an appreciation of the value of the organization's human assets relative to its other assets, such as brand names, distribution channels, real estate, and facilities and equipment. Organizations may be characterized as human resources oriented or not on the basis of their answers to the following:

- Does the organization see its people as central to its missions and strategy?
- Do the organization's mission statement and strategy objectives mention or espouse the value of human assets?
- Does the organization's management philosophy encourage the development of any strategy that prevents the depreciation of its human assets, or does the organization view its human assets as a cost to be minimized?

Often, an HR investment perspective is not adopted because it involves making a longer-term commitment to employees. Because employees can leave and most organizations are infused with short-term measures of performance, investments in human assets are often ignored. Organizations that are performing well may see no need to change their HR strategies. Those that are not doing well usually need a quick fix to turn things around and therefore ignore longer-term investments in people. However, although investment in human resources does not yield immediate results, it yields positive outcomes that are likely to last longer and are more difficult to duplicate by competitors.

Who Performs HR Tasks?

The person or unit that performs HR tasks has changed drastically. In many companies, the traditional HR department no longer exists, and no particular unit or individual is charged with performing HR tasks (Schramm 2011). Internal restructuring has often resulted in a shift as to who carries out HR tasks, but it has not eliminated the functions identified in Exhibit 1.4. In fact, in some healthcare organizations, the HR department continues to perform the majority of HR functions. However, questions are being raised: "Can some HR tasks be performed more efficiently by line managers or by outside vendors?" "Can some HR tasks be centralized or eliminated altogether?" "Can technology perform HR tasks that were once previously done by HR staff?" (Rison and Tower 2005).

Over time, the number of HR staff has declined, and continues to decline, as others have assumed responsibility for certain HR functions. Outsourcing, shared service centers, and line managers assist in performing many HR functions and activities. While most organizations are expected to outsource more HR tasks in the future, the strategic components of HR will likely remain within the organization itself (Mathis, Jackson, and Valentine 2014; Wright 2008). HR managers will continue to be involved with strategic HR matters and other key functions, including performance management and compensation management (Mathis, Jackson, and Valentine 2014; Schramm 2011).

The shift toward strategic HR is beginning to permit the HR function to shed its administrative image and to focus on more mission-oriented activities, as noted earlier (*HR Focus* 2006). This shift also means that *all* healthcare executives need to become skilled managers of their human resources. More HR professionals are assuming a strategic perspective when it comes to managing HR-related issues (*HR Focus* 2005b; Meisinger 2005). As they do so, they are continually upgrading and enhancing their professional capabilities (Khatri 2006). This evolution means that HR professionals must be given a seat at the board of directors' table to help the chief officers, senior management, and board members make appropriate decisions concerning HR matters. The best-run healthcare organizations, such as the Mayo Clinic, have used HR professionals on their board of directors and in their strategic planning process (Fottler, Erickson, and Rivers 2006).

The critical HR issues to which an HR professional can lend expertise and therefore help organizational governance include selecting the incoming CEO, tying the CEO's compensation to performance, and identifying and developing optimum business and HR strategies (Kenney 2005). In addition, the HR professional can contribute to leveraging HR's role in major change strategies (e.g., mergers and acquisitions), developing and implementing HR metrics that are aligned with business strategies, and helping line managers achieve their unit goals (Pinola 2002).

In 2009 the Cornell University Center for Advanced Human Resource Studies (CAHRS 2010) conducted its first Chief Human Resource Officer (CHRO) Survey, which focused on the roles and relationships of CHROs. Of the 148 CHROs polled, 54 respondents (39 percent) completed the survey. Almost 80 percent of the CHROs surveyed indicated three roles in which they had the greatest impact: strategic adviser, confidant/coach, and talent architect. They spent almost equal time in these roles (21 percent, 15 percent, and 17 percent, respectively). Although they spent the most time (22 percent) as functional leaders, they did not consider the role to have a great impact on the organization. They spent almost three-fourths of their time (72 percent) with senior leaders (45 percent) or HR team members (27 percent), with the remaining time allocated to other constituents. Moreover, they spent other time with CEOs, other executives, and the HR team (about 15 percent each). Of their executive colleagues, they spent the most time with the CEO (30 percent), business unit presidents (19 percent), and the CFO (16 percent). The chief HR officer in most of these organizations is clearly a member of the executive team. Of course, these data are not necessarily representative of the healthcare industry. If such data were available for the healthcare industry, the results might indicate lower levels of HR function influence.

Summary

In healthcare, the intensive reliance on professionals to deliver high-quality services requires organizations and their leaders to focus attention on the strategic management of their human resources and to be aware of the factors that influence the performance of all their employees. To assist healthcare executives in understanding this dynamic, this chapter presents a model that explains the interrelationship among corporate strategy, selected organizational design features, HRM activities, employee outcomes, and organizational outcomes.

The outcomes achieved by the organization are influenced by numerous HR and non-HR factors. The mission determines the direction that the organization takes and the goals it desires to achieve. The amount of integration or alignment of mission, strategy, HR functions, behavioral components, and non-HR strategies defines the level of achievement that is possible.

Healthcare organizations are increasingly striving to impress a distinctive HR brand image upon employees, potential employees, and the general public. To do this, they are modifying their cultures and working to be included on national lists of best companies. Successful branding results in competitive advantage in both labor and service markets. Organizations are also increasing the volume and quality of HR metrics they collect and use in an effort to better align their HR strategies with their business strategies. Finally, the locus of HRM is shifting, as HR professionals retain strategic functions within the organization while administrative tasks are outsourced or are delegated to line managers.

Discussion Questions

1. Distinguish among corporate, business, and functional strategies. How does each strategy relate to HRM? Why?

2. How may an organization's human resources be viewed as either a strength or a weakness when doing a SWOT analysis? What could be done to strengthen human resources in the event that it is seen as a weakness?

3. List factors under the control of healthcare managers that contribute to the decrease in the number of people applying to health professions schools. Describe the steps that healthcare organizations can take to improve this situation.

4. What are the organizational advantages of integrating strategic management and HRM? What are the steps involved in such an integration?

5. One healthcare organization is pursuing a business strategy of differentiating its service product through providing excellent customer service. What HR metrics do you recommend to reinforce this business strategy? Why?

6. In what sense are all healthcare executives HR managers? How can executives best prepare to perform well in this HR function?

Experiential Exercises

Exercise 1   Before class, obtain the annual report of any healthcare organization of your choice. Review the material presented and the language used. Write a one-page memo that assesses the organization's philosophy regarding its human resources. In class, form a group of four or five students. As a group, compare and contrast the organizations that the group members investigated. Discuss the following:

1. How can you differentiate organizations that merely "talk the talk" from those that also "walk the walk"?
2. What factors influence how an organization perceives its human resources?
3. How do "better" organizations perceive their human resources?
4. What did you learn from this exercise?

Exercise 2   Before class, review the HR practices shown in Exhibit 1.1. Consider how your current or most recent employer follows any three of these practices. Write a 1- to 2-page summary that lists the three practices you selected and their compatibilities (or incompatibilities) with your employer's HR practices. In class, form a group of four or five students and share your perceptions. Discuss the following:

1. What similarities and differences arise among the practices in your organization and those in your group members' employers?
2. Which of the practices seem to be least followed by these organizations, and why?

Exercise 3   Each year, *Fortune* magazine publishes its "100 Best Companies to Work For" list. Editors of the list base their selection on an extensive review of the HR practices of many organizations as well as on surveys of those organizations' current and former employees.

Use the Internet to identify three healthcare organizations on the latest *Fortune* "best companies" list. Next, visit the websites of these organizations, and review the posted information from the perspective of a prospective job applicant. Then, as a potential employee, answer the following:

1. What information on the websites most interested you, and why?
2. Which organization's website scored best with you, and why?
3. What implications do these websites have for you as a future healthcare executive who will be planning and implementing HR practices? What information will you include on your organization's website that will attract and retain employees?

References

Barker, J. 2005. "How to Pick the Best People (and Keep Them)." *Potentials* 38 (4): 33–36.

Blair, J., and M. Fottler. 1998. *Strategic Leadership for Medical Groups: Navigating Your Strategic Web*. San Francisco: Jossey-Bass.

———. 1990. *Challenges in Health Care Management: Strategic Perspectives for Managing Key Stakeholders*. San Francisco: Jossey-Bass.

Bureau of Labor Statistics. 2012. *Labor Force Characteristics by Race and Ethnicity, 2011*. Published August. www.bls.gov/cps/cpsrace2011.pdf.

Chuang, C. H., and H. Liao. 2010. "Strategic Human Resource Management in Service Context: Taking Care of Business by Taking Care of Employees and Customers." *Personnel Psychology* 63 (1): 153–96.

Cornell University Center for Advanced Human Resource Studies (CAHRS). 2010. *The Chief Human Resource Officer: Shifting Roles & Challenges*. Accessed December 16, 2014. www.ilr.cornell.edu/cahrs/news/upload/CAHRS_09CHROSurvey_Summary.pdf.

Equal Employment Opportunity Commission. 2014. "Title VII of the Civil Rights Act of 1964." Accessed February 14. www.eeoc.gov/laws/statutes/titlevii.cfm.

Ford, R. C., S. A. Sivo, M. D. Fottler, D. Dickson, K. Bradley, and L. Johnson. 2006. "Aligning Internal Organizational Factors with a Service Excellence Mission: An Exploratory Investigation in Healthcare." *Health Care Management Review* 31 (4): 259–69.

Fottler, M. D., J. D. Blair, R. L. Phillips, and C. A. Duran. 1990. "Achieving Competitive Advantage Through Strategic Human Resource Management." *Hospital & Health Services Administration* 35 (3): 341–63.

Fottler, M. D., E. Erickson, and P. A. Rivers. 2006. "Bringing Human Resources to the Table: Utilization of an HR Balanced Scorecard at Mayo Clinic." *Healthcare Management Review* 31 (1): 64–72.

Gallery, M. E., and S. C. Carey. 2014. *Outcomes, Performance, Structure (OPS): Three Keys to Organizational Excellence*. Milwaukee, WI: ASQ Quality Press.

Garvey, C. 2005. "New Generation Hiring Metrics." *HR Magazine* 50 (4): 70–76.

Gomez-Mejia, L. R., and D. B. Balkin. 2011. *Management: People, Performance, Change*. Upper Saddle River, NJ: Prentice Hall.

Gomez-Mejia, L. R., D. B. Balkin, and R. L. Cardy. 2012. *Managing Human Resources*, seventh edition. Upper Saddle River, NJ: Pearson Education.

Great Rated! 2014. "Southern Ohio Medical Center." Accessed December 16. http://us.greatrated.com/southern-ohio-medical-center.

HR Focus. 2006. "HR Departments Struggle to Move Up from Administrative to Strategic Status." *HR Focus* 83 (3): 8.

———. 2005a. "Getting Real and Specific with Measurement." *HR Focus* 82 (1): 11–13.

———. 2005b. "HR's Growing Role in M&A." *HR Focus* 82 (8): 1–15.

Huselid, M. A. 1994. "Documenting HR's Effect on Company Performance." *HR Magazine* 39 (1): 79–85.

Huselid, M. A., B. E. Becker, and R. W. Beatty. 2005. *The Workforce Scorecard.* Boston: Harvard Business School Press.

Huselid, M. A., S. E. Jackson, and R. S. Schuler. 1997. "Technical and Strategic Human Resources Management Effectiveness as Determinants of Firm Performance." *Academy of Management Journal* 40 (1): 171–88.

Johnson, M., and P. Roberts. 2006. "Rules of Attraction." *Marketing Health Services* 26 (1): 38–40.

Kaplan, R. S., and D. P. Norton. 1996. *The Balanced Scorecard.* Boston: Harvard Business School Press.

Kaufman, B. E. 2010. "SHRM Theory in the Post-Huselid Era: Why It Is Fundamentally Misspecified." *Industrial Relations* 49 (2): 286–313.

Kenney, R. 2005. "The Boardroom Role of Human Resources." *Corporate Board* 26 (1): 12–16.

Khatri, N. 2006. "Building HR Capability in HR Organizations." *Healthcare Management Review* 31 (1): 45–54.

Lawler, E. E., A. Levenson, and J. W. Boudreau. 2004. "HR Metrics and Analytics: Use and Impact." *Human Resources Planning* 27 (1): 27–35.

Lengnick-Hall, M. L., C. A. Lengnick-Hall, L. S. Andrade, and B. Drake. 2009. "Strategic Human Resource Management: Evolution of the Field." *Human Resource Management Review* 19 (2): 68–85.

Lowe, G. 2010. *Creating Healthy Organizations.* Toronto, Canada: University of Toronto Press.

Mathis, R. L., J. H. Jackson, and S. R. Valentine. 2014. *Human Resource Management*, fourteenth edition. Stanford, CT: Cengage Learning.

Mayer, D., M. G. Ehrhart, and B. Schneider. 2009. "Service Attribute Boundary Conditions of the Service Climate–Customer Satisfaction Link." *Academy of Management Journal* 52 (5): 1034–50.

Meisinger, S. 2005. "Fast Company: Do They Really 'Hate' HR?" *HR Magazine* 50 (9): 12.

Messersmith, J. G., and J. P. Guthrie. 2010. "High Performance Work Systems in Emergent Organizations: Implications for Firm Performance." *Human Resource Management* 49 (2): 241–64.

Nishii, L. H., D. P. Lepak, and B. Schneider. 2008. "Employee Attributions of the 'Why' of HR Practices: Their Effects on Employee Attitudes and Behaviors, and Customer Satisfaction." *Personnel Psychology* 61 (3): 503–45.

Paauwe, J. 2009. "HRM and Performance: Achievements, Methodological Issues, and Prospects." *Journal of Management Studies* 46 (1): 130–42.

Pew Research Center. 2010. *Millennials: A Portrait of Generation Next.* Published February. www.pewsocialtrends.org/files/2010/10/millennials-confident-connected-open-to-change.pdf.

Pfeffer, J. 1998. *The Human Equation: Building Profits by Putting People First.* Boston: Harvard Business School Press.

———. 1995. "Producing Sustainable Competitive Advantage Through the Effective Management of People." *Academy of Management Perspectives* 9 (1): 55–69.

Phillips, J. J. 2005. "The Value of Human Capital: What Logic and Intuition Are Telling Us." *Chief Learning Officer* 4 (8): 50–52.

Pinola, R. 2002. "What CFOs Want from HR." *HR Focus* 79 (9): 1.

Platonova, E. A., and S. R. Hernandez. 2013. "Innovative Human Resource Practices in U.S. Hospitals: An Empirical Study." *Journal of Healthcare Management* 58 (4): 290–301.

Porter, M. E. 1980. *Competitive Strategy.* New York: The Free Press.

Rafter, M. 2010. "Happy Days." *Workforce Management*, October, 21–26.

Rison, R. P., and J. Tower. 2005. "How to Reduce the Cost of HR and Continue to Provide Value." *Human Resource Planning* 28 (1): 14–19.

Schneider, C. 2006. "The New Human Capital Metrics." *CFO* 22 (2): 22–27.

Schramm, J. 2011. "Under Pressure." *HR Magazine* 56 (4): 104.

Snell, S., and G. Bohlander. 2013. *Managing Human Resources,* sixteenth edition. Mason, OH: South-Western Cengage Learning.

Society for Human Resource Management. 2014. "Future Insights: The Top Trends for 2014 According to SHRM's HR Subject Matter Expert Panels." Published January 22. www.shrm.org/research/futureworkplacetrends/pages/toptrendsfor2014.aspx.

———. 2012. "Challenges Facing HR over the Next 10 Years." Published November 1. www.shrm.org/research/surveyfindings/articles/pages/challengesfacing hroverthenext10years.aspx.

Subramony, M. 2009. "Meta-Analytic Investigation of the Relationship Between HRM Bundles and Firm Performance." *Human Resource Management* 48 (5): 745–68.

Twenge, J., S. Campbell, B. Hoffman, and C. Lance. 2010. "Generational Differences in Work Values: Leisure and Extrinsic Values Increasing Social and Intrinsic Values Decreasing." *Journal of Management* 36 (5): 1117–42.

Ulrich, D., J. Younger, and W. Brockband. 2008. "The Twenty-First Century HR Organizations." *Human Resource Management* 47 (4): 829–49.

Wolf, J. A. 2012. "Organizational Culture: A Critical Choice at the Heart of an Exceptional Patient Experience." The Beryl Institute. Published September 3. www.theberylinstitute.org/blogpost/593434/148723/Organizational-Culture-A-Critical-Choice-at-the-Heart-of-an-Exceptional-Patient-Experience.

Wright, P. M. 2008. *Human Resource Strategy: Adapting to the Age of Globalization.* Society for Human Resource Management Foundation practice guideline.

Accessed December 16, 2014. www.shrm.org/india/hr-topics-and-strategy/strategic-hrm/documents/hr%20strategy%20epg-%20final%20online.pdf.

Wright, P. M., T. M. Gardner, L. M. Moynihan, and M. R. Allen. 2005. "The Relationship between HR Practices and Firm Performance: Examining Causal Order." *Personnel Psychology* 58 (2): 409–46.

2

EMPLOYMENT LAW, EMPLOYEE RELATIONS, AND HEALTHCARE

Drake Maynard

Learning Objectives

After completing this chapter, the reader should be able to

- understand the impact of legal considerations on key human resources activities and functions;
- define and understand the distinctions between employment at will, contract employment, and employment with a property interest protected by due process;
- know the major federal statutes of employment law, including those that prohibit discrimination;
- understand the concepts of reasonable accommodation and undue hardship;
- discuss the reasons for the changes made by Congress in Title VII of the 1964 Civil Rights Act and in the Americans with Disabilities Act;
- discuss the history and development of employment law in the United States;
- understand the distinction between statutory law and case law, and how one influences the other;
- describe the development of the US Supreme Court's views on retaliation and how that influences strategic human resources management;
- describe strategies that organizations use to prevent and remedy discrimination in the workplace;
- recognize the legal background for a variety of employee rights and responsibilities in the field of healthcare;
- understand the importance of periodic reviews of human resources practices and processes for compliance purposes;
- discuss serious disciplinary actions, the bases for taking them, and basic due process;

- discuss the development of the legal concept of sexual harassment and the two varieties of sexual harassment;
- explain how an employer can minimize legal liability from sexual harassment;
- discuss how technology has affected employment law and human resources management; and
- discuss strategic and operational approaches to resolving complex employee relations issues.

Introduction

How does employment law affect and regulate human resources (HR) management today? Consider the breadth of Title VII of the 1964 Civil Rights Act: It prohibits discrimination in any "terms, conditions, or privileges of employment." In 50 years of litigation, no court has found an aspect of employment that is not covered by this prohibition. All aspects of HR activity are covered by this prohibition and by several other statutes as well. The reach of prohibited discrimination is similarly broad for persons with disabilities (the Americans with Disabilities Act Amendments Act [ADAAA]; also covered are persons *regarded* as disabled) and for persons aged 40 years or older (the Age Discrimination in Employment Act [ADEA]). Hiring, promotions, transfers, opportunities for training, leave, payment of employees, discipline, termination, allegations of sexual harassment and retaliation—all these HR activities are regulated by these statutes as well as by the Fair Labor Standards Act (FLSA), the Family and Medical Leave Act (FMLA), the Genetic Information Nondiscrimination Act (GINA), and others.

Imagine this scenario: You've achieved the next step on your career ladder and now are the deputy director for administration in one of the larger clinical divisions in your healthcare system. You've put in your time working in other, lower-level roles in the field. You have your eye on the big office and the reserved parking space.

Then, your HR administrator, Bette, walks in. She looks worried, which is never a good thing. Before she sits down, she starts talking.

"We have a problem in our walk-in clinic. Sandy, one of the nurses assigned to that clinic, has been out for nearly three months on FMLA leave caring for her mother, who is dying of cancer. Her mother has rallied, and Sandy has asked for additional time off. She says that several other employees are willing to help her through our leave donation program. Initially, the supervisor, on my advice, denied her request and told Sandy to return to work next week; her FMLA leave runs out then. Then this morning we got a fax from a therapist saying that Sandy is clinically depressed because her mother is dying and we won't let her stay at home. The therapist says that Sandy is too depressed to work and needs at least six to eight more weeks of leave, or until her mother dies. That might be any day now, or it might be six months from now."

She pauses to take a breath. You respond, "So, is that the whole situation?"

"Actually, no," she says. "Because of Sandy's absence, we've had to work some of our clinic nurses overtime. Now the clinic manager says we don't have any more budget to pay for overtime. She asked if we could just give the nurses hour-for-hour paid time off. I told her the FLSA wouldn't allow that."

"So what are our options here?" you ask.

"Pay them overtime. Period. Hire temporaries, which will likely cost even more than overtime. Cut back on clinic hours, which will affect revenue. But that's not all."

Not all? This is beginning to sound like a late-night TV commercial. "What else could be going on here?" you choke out.

"Well, the legal department tells me they've been contacted by an attorney who says she represents Sandy. The attorney says that Sandy believes we've violated her rights under GINA by asking about her family history of cancer. And she says that Sandy has a disabling condition—her depression— under the ADAAA and needs a reasonable accommodation, which would be to grant her an indefinite leave of absence, preferably with pay under our leave donation program, until her depression improves. Oh, and the attorney says that Sandy believes she is being discriminated against because a male employee—one of the assistant directors of the healthcare system—was given an indefinite leave of absence with pay when his wife had a terminal illness. The attorney also says that denying Sandy further extended leave because of her mother's terminal illness is retaliation under the FMLA for Sandy's asking for FMLA leave in the first place."

You close your eyes and bow your head. Behind your eyelids you see explosions—possibly your weekends for the next six months exploding under the pressure of handling this situation. "Give me the bottom line here," you say.

"Okay. Sandy's running out of FMLA leave this week. We denied her request for further leave because we can't afford to have her out of the rotation any longer. Her leave has caused fiscal problems because we've paid overtime pay—that's time and a half—to nurses working overtime covering for her. I'm fighting off our clinic manager, who wants to violate the FLSA by not paying overtime from this point forward. Sandy's attorney says we're discriminating against her on the basis of her sex by denying her leave, that we're violating the ADAAA by not giving her indefinite leave as a reasonable accommodation, that we've violated GINA when Sandy's supervisor asked her if cancer ran in her mother's family, and, finally, that we're retaliating against Sandy for requesting and using FMLA leave by denying her the indefinite leave she's requested. Those are the issues we have right now. Oh, I did check, and Sandy's 42 years old—her attorney may try to throw in an ADEA allegation."

Your head begins spinning rapidly. ADAAA? FLSA? GINA? ADEA? FMLA? Overtime pay? Retaliation? Reasonable accommodation? Can you find any way out of this? All you want to do is provide excellent patient care at an affordable cost to the people in your community. If you had wanted to be a lawyer, you would have gone to law school. Now it feels like you are being thrown into the shark pool. What are you going to do?

Perhaps this scenario is somewhat involved, but it is not necessarily fantastic, as any reading of recent court cases or other current employment law materials will show. Do such situations occur regularly? Most likely not, for most employers. But even one such event has the potential to cause significant damage. Employees now have a wide array of legal protections and entitlements, and laws and regulations often strictly regulate employers' responses to the brandishing of those protections and entitlements. This chapter discusses how these laws arose, what restrictions they place on employer activity, and how to address those restrictions in both an operational and a strategic fashion.

History of Employment Law in the United States

Prior to 1938, few, if any, laws regulated employment conditions or the behavior of employers in the United States. Attempts to rein in or prohibit child labor or to establish a minimum wage were thwarted by US Supreme Court decisions that upheld the rights of women and children to perform dangerous and dirty work for long hours and little pay (for example, *Hammer v. Dagenhart*, 247 U.S. 251 [1918]). But in 1938, President Franklin D. Roosevelt pushed the FLSA through Congress. This law was a part of Roosevelt's New Deal legislative program. It set a minimum wage of 25 cents an hour and a standard workweek of 44 hours. The FLSA also called for a premium wage of one-half of the usual hourly rate to be added on to pay for all hours worked beyond 44. And, for the first time, child labor was prohibited.

The FLSA applied only to a few private-sector employers, primarily industrial concerns, and did not apply to the still-small public sector.

US employers remained free to refuse to hire female employees for work deemed too dangerous for women. And they were free to post signs saying "No Irish need apply" and to exclude other ethnic and racial groups from the workforce. The concept of employment discrimination did not exist at this time simply because no laws prohibited such activity. And little in the way of societal pressure existed to remedy this situation.

The next steps in US employment law began in the 1960s. This decade saw the passage of the Equal Pay Act (an amendment to the FLSA) in 1963, Title VII of the Civil Rights Act in 1964, and the ADEA in 1967. Thus, by the end of the 1960s, most employers were barred from discrimination in wages paid to men and women; discrimination in employment based on race, sex, religion, color, or national origin; and discrimination against persons aged 40 years or older.

The Civil Rights Act of 1964 contained the most far-reaching prohibitions on employment discrimination. Whereas the Equal Pay Act only prohibited discrimination in pay between men and women, and the ADEA only protected persons aged 40 years or older, the Civil Rights Act protected women, minorities, persons of various ethnicities, and the religious practices and beliefs of all employees. It even protected against discrimination among persons of color based on the darkness or lightness of their skin color (through the prohibition against discrimination based on color). For the first time, the vast majority of private-sector American employers (any employer with 15 or more employees who worked more than 20 weeks in the current or previous year) were prohibited from discriminating against employees and applicants. Public-sector employers were still not covered (this coverage would come in the 1972 amendments to this law). The Civil Rights Act also created the Equal Employment Opportunity Commission (EEOC), a federal agency designed to enforce the provisions of the act through investigations and, where necessary, court action.

Title VII, as this legislation came to be known (because the provisions prohibiting discrimination in employment were found in Title VII of the law; the whole act covered a variety of nondiscriminatory activity, including housing and public accommodations), incorporated two important concepts that would help to shape the future of employment law in the United States.

First, the language of Title VII that defined the limits of prohibited discriminatory acts was masterfully crafted. Since its inception, courts have interpreted this language, "terms, conditions, or privileges of employment" (42 U.S.C. § 2000e-2(a)(1)), to cover any act or failure to act in every possible aspect of employment. The value of this broad approach has been proven over the years as creative employers have come up with new and innovative ways to justify old practices of employment discrimination, only to have these practices struck down by the courts. This approach also has the merit of not being bound by technology, so that employment discrimination in social media is still prohibited, just as it was when print media was king.

Second, the provision found in Title VII (§ 2000e(j)) that requires an employer to "reasonably accommodate to an employee's or prospective

employee's religious observance or practice" introduced the concept of reasonable accommodation to US employment law. As discussed later in this
chapter, reasonable accommodation is central to the Americans with Disabilities Act (ADA) and the later ADAAA. This provision created an additional
responsibility for employers. Simply avoiding discrimination based on an
employee or applicant's religious beliefs and practices was not enough; the
employer had to make advertent efforts to accommodate such practices in the
workplace. This requirement led to a number of lawsuits involving aspects of
religious belief, such as the following: on facial hair in the workplace, *Fra-
ternal Order of Police Newark Lodge No. 12 v. City of Newark*, 170 F.3d 359
(3d Cir., 1999), *EEOC v. Federal Express Corp.*, No. CV-100-50 (S.D. Ga.,
2001), and *Booth v. Maryland* (4th Cir., 2003); on clothing, *U.S. v. New York
City Transit Authority* (E.D. N.Y., 2010), *EEOC v. Blockbuster, Inc.* (D.Ariz.,
2005), and *Draper v. Logan County* (W.D. Ky., 2003); on hours of work and
scheduling, *Harrell v. Donahue* (8th Cir., 2011), *EEOC v. Mesaba Airlines*
(D.Minn., 2009); and on work assignments, *Slater v. Douglas County* (D.Or.,
2010), *EEOC v. Chi Chi's Restaurant* (D.C. Md. 1996), and *Rodriguez v.
City of Chicago*, 156 F.3d 771, 776–77 (7th Cir. 1998), *cert. denied*, 119 S.
Ct. 1038 (1999).

While the 1960s saw explosive growth in both the number of laws
affecting employment and the types of practices that were prohibited or
permitted, the 1970s and 1980s were relatively fallow periods for legislative
activity on the employment law front. The 1970s saw the passage of the
Rehabilitation Act of 1973 (29 U.S.C. § 701), a weak foreshadowing of the
ADA. The Rehabilitation Act was also limited in coverage; it reached only
federal agencies of the executive branch and federal contractors and subcontractors whose contracts exceeded $10,000. It did contain the concept of
"reasonable accommodation" to achieve its goal of nondiscrimination.

While the legislative side of employment law was relatively quiet in the
1970s and 1980s, the courts were very active in interpreting the implications
of the laws enacted in the 1960s. The US Supreme Court established the
concept of disparate impact in the landmark case of *Griggs v. Duke Power Co.*,
401 U.S. 424 (1971). In this case, a power company had implemented promotional qualifications that included a requirement of a high school diploma,
and in the process had ended up with many African-American employees who
were barred from upward mobility to better-paying jobs. The court found
that while this requirement was not discriminatory on its face (any person
with a high school diploma could qualify for promotion), the fact that the
company's workforce was drawn from an area with segregated schools that
graduated significantly fewer African Americans than whites meant that such
a "facially neutral" requirement had an adverse impact on the ability of African Americans to move into higher-paying jobs. The decision established that

such requirements or tests had to have a business necessity, rather than just be a preference of the employer. Disparate impact theory did away with the necessity for the employee to prove any discriminatory intent on the part of the employer.

In 1975, in *Albemarle Paper Co. v. Moody*, 422 U.S. 405 (1975), the Supreme Court went even further and held that employee plaintiffs could rebut an employer's defense of business necessity by showing that another, nondiscriminatory practice was just as effective as the employer's discriminatory practice.

In *Griggs v. Duke Power Co.*, the Supreme Court held that employers were responsible in court for establishing and proving the business necessity of a test. Some years later, in *Wards Cove Packing Co. v. Antonio*, 490 U.S. 642 (1989), the court took a step back from the *Griggs* decision, holding, among other things, that the employer's only burden in a disparate impact case was to produce a business necessity for the employment practice in question. The repercussions of the *Wards Cove* decision were far-reaching and are discussed later in this chapter.

The courts also began to recognize that sexual harassment represented a violation of Title VII's prohibition against discrimination on the basis of sex. Cases involving what is now recognized as sexual harassment had been filed as far back as 1974, the year of *Barnes v. Train*, Civ. No. 1828-73 (D.D.C.) (order of August 9, 1974). Initially, the courts focused on what is now known as *quid pro quo* sexual harassment, in which the employer conditioned some aspect of employment (pay increases, promotions, keeping one's job) on compliance with the sexual demands of the supervisor or employer. Many courts found that such activity, while deplorable, did not represent a violation of Title VII. In *Corne v. Bausch and Lomb, Inc.*, 390 F.Supp. 161 (1975), in which the plaintiffs argued that their rights under Title VII had been violated by the repeated "verbal and physical sexual advances of the Defendant Price" (the supervisor of the plaintiffs), the court found:

> In the present case, Mr. Price's conduct appears to be nothing more than a personal proclivity, peculiarity or mannerism. By his alleged sexual advances, Mr. Price was satisfying a personal urge. Certainly no employer policy is here involved; rather than the company being benefited in any way by the conduct of Price, it is obvious it can only be damaged by the very nature of the acts complained of.

In 1986, the US Supreme Court, in *Meritor Savings Bank v. Vinson*, 477 U.S. 57 (1986), relying on EEOC guidelines on sexual harassment (Guidelines on Discrimination Because of Sex, 29 C.F.R. § 1604.11), found that the creation of a hostile work environment through overt acts of sexual harassment or through "discriminatory intimidation, ridicule, and insult whether based on sex, race, religion, or national origin" violated Title VII. The *Meritor* case established the "hostile work environment" theory of sexual harassment; it also laid the groundwork for later decisions establishing the liability of employers for the actions of supervisors and other employees.

While the 1980s were primarily a time of judicial interpretation of existing employment law, the 1990s saw extensive legislative and judicial activity in this area. Congress enacted the ADA (42 U.S.C. chapter 126) in 1990, substituting its provisions for the relatively toothless Rehabilitation Act of 1973. The thrust of the ADA in the area of employment was twofold: It prohibited discrimination in employment against those defined as "disabled" under the law, and it required that employers take advertent steps through the concept of reasonable accommodation to eradicate barriers against applicants and current employees who were defined as disabled under the law.

In 1993, Congress passed the FMLA (29 U.S.C. § 2601). Unlike other laws discussed in this chapter, this law was not designed to remedy existing or historic discrimination, but rather to provide a new entitlement for employees. For eligible employees of covered employers, the FMLA provided three new entitlements: up to 12 weeks of unpaid leave for a variety of reasons, a guarantee of continuation of employer-paid health insurance during the period of leave, and a guarantee of a return to the same or similar position as the employee had left. The act also contained a provision that has bedeviled managers and HR professionals ever since—intermittent leave.

Intermittent leave allows an employee to take the unpaid leave in increments; the concept was that some situations covered by the act (such as chemotherapy for cancer) do not require leave to be used all at once, but in small amounts over time. The concept is consistent with the overall purpose of the act in providing (unpaid) leave for employees with serious health conditions. However, as employers have discovered since 1993, this provision of the FMLA is unusually susceptible to abuse and can be difficult to administer, despite the US Department of Labor's protestations to the contrary (US Department of Labor, Wage and Hour Division 2013b). In February 2013 the Wage and Hour Division of the Department of Labor released a survey conducted in 2012, which concluded that "most employers" (85 percent) had no difficulty in complying with the FMLA (US Department of Labor, Wage and Hour Division 2013b).

In response to a series of US Supreme Court decisions (*Wards Cove*, discussed previously, as well as *Price Waterhouse v. Hopkins*, 490 U.S. 228 [1989], and *Patterson v. McLean Credit Union*, 491 U.S. 164 [1989]) that were seen as whittling away at the protections afforded by Title VII, Congress passed the Civil Rights Act of 1991. The 1991 act amended Title VII by allowing the use of juries for the first time, and permitting plaintiffs to sue for and recover punitive and compensatory damages under both the ADA and Title VII. Congress specifically overturned the Supreme Court's decision in *Wards Cove* by enshrining in statute the judicial theory of disparate impact as it had been prior to that decision; Congress further neutered the *Price Waterhouse* decision by allowing plaintiffs to recover when an employer's decision is shown to be discriminatory even where the employer shows that it would have made the same decision absent discrimination. The 1991 act also incorporated a prohibition against both quid pro quo and hostile work environment sexual harassment.

The year 1998 was particularly productive for the Supreme Court in terms of decisions on employment law. That year saw the Court's ground-breaking decisions in *Burlington Industries, Inc. v. Ellerth*, 524 U.S. 724, 118 S Ct., and *Faragher v. City of Boca Raton*, 524 U.S. 775, 118 S. Ct. *Ellerth* and *Faragher* both dealt with employer liability for harassment by supervisors. The court provided an avenue for employers to avoid liability for the (unauthorized) actions of supervisors in committing sexual harassment. The court held that where a "tangible employment action" (*Ellerth*, 2270) was not present, employers who tried to prevent and correct such harassment (usually through the mechanism of a sexual harassment policy and a complaint procedure) and whose complaining party did not use the complaint procedure would be able to affirmatively defend against liability for a supervisor's actions. (This principle also applies to other forms of harassment prohibited by Title VII, such as racial harassment.) However, if a "tangible employment action" such as dismissal or loss of income was taken, employers would be unable to raise the affirmative defense to liability.

That same year, the court also took on the issue of same-sex sexual harassment. In *Oncale v. Sundowner Offshore Services, Inc.*, 523 U.S. 75 (1998), the court held that "Title VII's prohibition of discrimination 'because of . . . sex' protects men as well as women" (*Oncale*, 80).

A look back over the changes in the field of US employment law in the twentieth century would reveal that the nation went from having few, if any, legal prohibitions against employment discrimination (and perhaps not even a concept of employment discrimination) to establishing statutorily and judicially enforced prohibitions against discrimination in nearly every aspect of employment on the basis of race, sex, religion, national origin, color, age (40 years or older), and disability covering most employers in the United States. And the United States went from having no legal restrictions on the employer–employee relationship to imposing significant legal obligations on employers prohibiting child labor and requiring employers to pay employees at least a minimum wage, to affirmatively assist the disabled in employment, to accommodate in employment the religious beliefs and practices of a diverse workforce, and to provide support for persons taking care of the health needs of family members and themselves.

The National Labor Relations Act and the National Labor Relations Board: The Split Between Public and Private Employers

Despite the declining levels of union membership among American workers (2013 figures from the Bureau of Labor Statistics show a decline in union membership from 1983 to 2013 of nearly 9 percent, representing a drop of more than 3 million employees [Bureau of Labor Statistics 2014]), the National Labor Relations Act (NLRA) and its enforcement body, the National Labor Relations Board (NLRB), remain a potent force in employment law and the regulation of the working relationship in the United States.

The influence of the NLRA and the NLRB can be seen in the ongoing controversy over social media in the workplace (see the section "Employment Law in the Twenty-First Century" later in this chapter). The NLRB, in *Hispanics United of Buffalo, Inc.*, 359 NLRB No. 37 (December 14, 2012), found that the employer had violated section 8(a)(1) of the NLRA by terminating five employees for making comments on Facebook in regard to a coworker's criticism of their work performance. This section of the NLRA is as follows:

> *Any prohibited interference by an employer with the rights of employees to organize, to form, join, or assist a labor organization, to bargain collectively, to engage in other concerted activities for mutual aid or protection, or to refrain from any or all of these activities, constitutes a violation of this section. (National Labor Relations Board 1997, 14)*

However, the authority of the NLRB is limited by its enabling legislation, the NLRA. In section 2, the term *employer* excludes the United States, the states, and any political subdivision of a state.[1] This definition prohibits the exercise of jurisdiction by the NLRB over state or federal agencies (or agencies of political subdivisions of a state). The NLRB does have authority over nonprofit and for-profit private employers. However, state law may regulate collective bargaining and other rights typically associated with unions for public employers.

Varieties of Employment Status in the United States

In the United States, employment typically consists of one of three primary statuses: at-will employment, employment under a contract, and, in the public sector, a property interest in employment protected by due process.

Among all the states, only Montana does not recognize the common-law principle of at-will employment. Montana has statutorily amended the concept of employment at will for all employers in the state by allowing employers in the state to discharge employees only for "good cause," meaning "reasonable job-related grounds for dismissal based on a failure to satisfactorily perform job duties, disruption of the employer's operation, or other legitimate business reason" (Mont. Code Ann. § 39-2-903(5)). In the remaining 49 states, employers may dismiss an employee at any time for a good reason, a bad reason, or no reason at all. (Under the "at-will" doctrine, employees enjoy a somewhat corresponding right to leave employment at any time without notice or reason.)

This status provides wide-ranging freedom for employers to dismiss employees. However, even under at-will employment, employers face restrictions on how freely and for what reasons they may dismiss employees. For example, states have restricted the freedom of employers to regulate legal, off-duty conduct such as smoking. Colorado, Indiana, New Jersey, Oregon, and South Dakota all prohibit employer action against smokers (Co. Rev. Stat. Ann § 24-34-402.5; Ind. Code §§ 22-5-4-1 et seq.; N.J. Stat. Ann. §§ 34:6B-1 et seq.; Or. Rev. Stat. §§ 659A.315 and 659A.885; S.D. Codified Laws § 60-4-11).

Many states also provide public policy exceptions to employment at will. For example, the North Carolina Court of Appeals, in *Sides v. Duke University*, 74 N.C. App. 331, 342, 328 S.E. 2d 818, 826 (1985) (later adopted by the North Carolina Supreme Court in *Coman v. Thomas Manufacturing Co.*, 325 N.C. 172, 381 S.E. 2d 445 [1989]), held that terminating an employee for refusing to commit perjury violated the public policy of having all persons speak truthfully in court. Similarly, some states provide protection for persons reporting violations of law (whistle-blowing) or reporting for jury duty.

The "at-will" doctrine also has statutory exceptions that vary from state to state. The primary statutory restriction on at-will employment comes from federal employment laws such as the Civil Rights Act of 1991 (Title VII), the ADEA, and the ADAAA. All of these statutes expressly prohibit an employer's ability to dismiss employees on the basis of sex, race, religion, national origin, color, age, or disability. In addition, the FLSA and the FMLA prohibit dismissing an employee in retaliation for exercising his or her rights under those laws.

Some employers regulate the employment relationship through employment contracts. These contracts typically involve basic aspects of employment such as salary, benefits, and work to be performed; often contracts are for a fixed period. Most employment contracts provide for dismissal of the person before the end of the contract for reasons such as misconduct. Depending on the industry, employment contracts may regulate activities beyond the period of the contract through noncompetition clauses that limit the person's ability to work in the same or a similar field of work.

The final type of employment status is primarily limited to the public sector. States and political subdivisions of states may guarantee employment to eligible employees until "just cause," "good cause," or "cause" for dismissal occurs, at which point employees may be dismissed provided certain processes are followed. This guarantee creates what is known as a "property interest." In 1972, the US Supreme Court's decision in *Board of Regents v. Roth*, 408 U.S. 564 (1972), brought this concept forward. In *Roth*, the court held that under the Fourteenth Amendment to the US Constitution (which provides that the states may not deprive a person of life, liberty, or property without due process of law), when an employee has a property interest the public employer may only remove or alter that property interest through due process. (See the section "The Constitution, Employers, and Employees" in this chapter for a discussion of due process.)

Property interests are generally created by state legislatures, or by bodies of political subdivisions that have quasi-legislative authority. Removing a property interest requires a pre- or post-termination hearing. Such hearings, to constitute due process, must include timely notice of the hearing, an opportunity to provide information (evidence), an impartial finder of fact, the right to counsel, and the right to cross-examine witnesses put forward by the employer.

The Constitution, Employers, and Employees

For many employers (specifically, private-sector and not-for-profit employers), constitutional protections such as freedom of speech or the prohibition against unreasonable search and seizure are not HR management issues. But in the public sector, constitutional protections are a significant aspect of effective employee relations. This difference results from both the nature of the employer and the Constitution itself. Among its purposes, the Constitution serves as an *über* law regulating relations among the federal government, the states (and their subdivisions), and the people of the United States. While the body of the Constitution primarily regulates federal–state government relationships, the amendments focus primarily on the relationship between government (federal and state) and the people.

Thus, government employers (at all levels) have a dual role that private or not-for-profit employers do not share: They are the government while at the same time they are employers. Employees of the government have a dual role also; they are employees and they are the people for whom the Constitution was established to regulate government behavior.

So, while private employers can conduct random drug tests of their employees as frequently as they wish, the Fourth Amendment's prohibition against unlawful search and seizure strictly regulates how public employers can require drug tests of employees. And while private or not-for-profit employers can rummage through an employee's locked desk drawers, search employees' secured lockers, or even go into employees' locked cars, the Fourth Amendment requires public employers to get a search warrant before engaging in similar behavior.

The Fourteenth Amendment has a particular impact on public employers. This amendment, which states in part, "nor shall any state deprive any person of life, liberty, or property, without due process of law," is integral to the creation of the property interest, and the regulation of how states (and their subdivisions) may alter or remove a property interest from employees. (See the section "Varieties of Employment Status in the United States" earlier in this chapter.)

Constitutional protections for government employers (search warrants, random drug testing only for safety-sensitive positions, due process in altering or terminating an employee's property interest) add an additional layer of complexity (and potential liability) to effective employee relations in the public sector.

Disparate Treatment and Disparate Impact Theories in Discrimination Law

Discrimination law in the United States began with the passage of the Civil Rights Act of 1964. Title VII of this act defined *disparate treatment* as failing or refusing "to hire or to discharge any individual, or otherwise to discriminate against any individual with respect to his compensation, terms, conditions, or privileges of employment, because of such individual's race, color, religion, sex, or national origin." This initial statement of nondiscrimination in employment was intended to address what was perceived to be a singularly egregious societal issue—deliberate, intentional discrimination in employment based on an individual's race, sex, religion, color, or national origin. Disparate treatment was therefore the thrust of employment law decisions for nearly a decade until the US Supreme Court decision in *Griggs v. Duke Power*. In *Griggs*, the US Supreme Court defined the second conceptual basis for prohibited discrimination—disparate impact.

Disparate treatment is intentional discrimination. Examples of such discrimination include statements such as "We will only hire Asians as waitpersons in our Chinese restaurant, to provide an authentic dining experience" (prohibited by Title VII, 2000e-2(e)(1)), "This job is too dangerous for women" (*Dothard v. Rawlinson*, 433 U.S. 321 [1977]), and "We're only auditioning black actors and actresses for this play because that's part of the director's artistic vision" (Title VII, 2000e-2(e)(1)).

On the other hand, disparate impact discrimination is (possibly) unintentional discrimination by policy, by process, or by tests. In *Griggs*, a requirement of a high school diploma that screened out a disproportionate number of African-American applicants resulted in racial discrimination in promotion. In *United States v. North Carolina*, 512 F.Supp. 968 (E.D. N.C. 1981), *aff'd without opinion*, 679 F.2d 980 (4th Cir. 1982), *cert. denied*, 459 U.S. 1103 (1983), a requirement of the North Carolina State Highway Patrol that applicants be at least 5 feet 8 inches tall screened out a disproportionate number of female applicants, resulting in sex discrimination in hiring. A physical abilities test used by the Massachusetts Department of Corrections screened out twice as many female applicants as male applicants. In a subsequent lawsuit filed because of that practice, the Department of Justice reached a settlement with the state, which agreed to discontinue the use of the test.

None of these cases involved allegations of intentional (disparate treatment) discrimination. Instead, the route to proving discrimination rested on statistical information about black and white high school graduates (*Griggs*), the average height of men and women (*United States v. North Carolina*) and the job-related physical abilities of men and women (*U.S. v. Commonwealth of Massachusetts*), along with the defendants' failure to show that these practices were job related and consistent with business necessity under the Civil Rights Act of 1991, 42 U.S.C. §2000e-2(k)(1)(A)(i).

An employer can defend against claims of disparate treatment discrimination by showing that it treated similarly situated employees in similar ways. Other defense factors include the race of the person making the contested decision; the racial, sexual, or national origin makeup of the workforce; and lack of evidence of any ethnic or racial slurs by persons involved in the decision.

The primary defense for employers against a claim of disparate impact is the argument that the practice in question is job related and consistent with business necessity. However, employee plaintiffs can trump this claim with evidence showing that another practice that is less discriminatory would achieve the same business goal.

Employment Law in the Twenty-First Century

In the twenty-first century, employment law (and the corresponding practice of HR management) has become even more complex than before.

Technology in both society and the workplace accounts for some of this increase in complexity. Toward the end of the twentieth century, the use of computers (especially personal computers, laptops, and smartphones) and the Internet became more prevalent, giving rise to concerns about inappropriate and unauthorized use of computers for personal activities, as well as inappropriate use of the Internet (excessive personal e-mails, accessing the Internet for activities such as viewing pornography and Web-based gambling). Just as statutory and case law began to catch up with the technological changes from the last quarter of the twentieth century (decisions and laws dealing with employer monitoring of employees, some fledgling steps toward reconciling the First Amendment with the new devices and programs), technology continued to pull the workplace ahead of developing law. Social media—Facebook, Twitter, Instagram, blogging, and so forth—fueled this latest leap forward.

Statutory law did not stand still in the early years of the twenty-first century. Congress revised the ADA in 2008 in an action similar to its rewriting of the Civil Rights Act in 1991 to remedy or nullify Supreme Court decisions. And the ongoing conflict in the Middle East and Afghanistan fueled changes to the FMLA allowing additional unpaid leave for the family members of military service members.

The EEOC, not to be outdone, continued to press the boundaries of employment law further by supporting (through official pronouncements, policies, and legal action) nondiscrimination against lesbian, gay, bisexual, and transgender employees; adding obesity to the list of disabilities; and seeking nondiscriminatory policies and practices in the workplace for caregivers.

The Supreme Court embarked on a series of decisions first increasing the ability of employees to file lawsuits alleging retaliation and then later circumscribing that ability.

Technology and the Twenty-First Century Workplace

The prevalence of cell phones with Internet access (smartphones) has helped to promote the spread of social media. CBS News reported in October 2012 that worldwide users of smartphones topped 1 billion (Dover 2012).

The beginning of the rise of social media may be traced to the development of the Web-based application Facebook. Facebook began in 2004 as a way for college students to connect on the Internet. It rapidly grew to include anyone who claimed to be at least 13 years old. According to a study in 2011 by Neilsen Media Research, Facebook is the second most accessed website in the United States (Fernandes 2011). In October 2012, Facebook CEO Mark Zuckerberg (appropriately via a Facebook post) claimed that Facebook had passed the 1 billion user mark (note that this same month also marked the 1 billion user mark for smartphones) (Lee 2012).

A 2011 study by the Society of Corporate Compliance and Ethics showed that an increasing number of employers (42 percent in 2011) punished employees for social media activity (Guerrero 2013). What do employees do with Facebook, Twitter, and YouTube at work to get into trouble with employers? One answer is the infamous video posted to YouTube by two Domino's Pizza employees in North Carolina, showing an employee sneezing onto food, sticking cheese up his nose and placing it on a sandwich, and other non-health-department-approved activities. Domino's corporate response was telling: "Anyone with a camera and an Internet link can cause a lot of damage" (*Today Show* 2009). The employees were fired and also charged with health code violations.

More commonly, problem situations involve employees using Facebook or blogs to provide critical information or assessments about employers. In the nonprofit and private sectors the NLRB has come out strongly protecting employees who, through blogging, engage in "concerted activity," which is protected by the NLRA.

The NLRB issued General Counsel memos on this topic in 2011 and 2012. In *Karl Knauz Motors, Inc. d/b/a Knauz BMW and Robert Becker*, Case 13–CA–046452 (2012), the NLRB required a car dealership to remove the "Courtesy" provision in its employee handbook, which had been allegedly used to terminate a salesman because of his derogatory comments on Facebook about serving hot dogs at an event designed to sell luxury automobiles (BMWs), because it violated section 8(a)(1) of the NLRA.[2] In *Design Technology Group, LLC d/b/a Bettie Page Clothing and DTG California Management, LLC d/b/a Bettie Page Clothing, a Single Employer and Vanessa Morris*, Case 20–CA–035511, the NLRB found, as in the *Becker* case, that postings on Facebook constituted protected "concerted activity" and that a company rule prohibiting this also violated section 8(a)(1); it ordered the removal of the offending rule in the company's employee handbook.

In *Hispanics United of Buffalo, Inc.*, 359 NLRB No. 37 (December 14, 2012), as described previously, an employer dismissed five nonunion employees for posting comments on Facebook regarding a coworker's criticism of their work performance. The NLRB found that the Facebook comments of the five dismissed employees constituted "concerted activity" protected by section 8(a)(1) of the NLRA.

In May 2012 the NLRB General Counsel issued a report on social media cases (Purcell 2012). The report analyzed seven NLRB decisions and concluded that many employer policies on social media either violate or potentially violate the protections found in section 8(a)(1) of the NLRA. The report noted that employer policies restricting the communication of confidential information, prohibiting the revelation of nonpublic company information on public sites, prohibiting the use of offensive or demeaning language, and advising employees not to "pick fights" online violated section 8(a)(1) of the NLRA. The General Counsel did find, however, that a company social media policy that prohibited online bullying, harassment, discrimination, or retaliation did not violate the act.

The NLRB appears determined to address how social media and the NLRA interact. It seems to favor the view that the vast majority of employment-related Facebook postings, tweets (Twitter messages), and blog postings are protected as "concerted activity" by the NLRA.

Beyond the NLRB, a number of state legislatures are trying to fill an ever-widening gap between speeding technological advances and the plodding law. At least 26 states have active legislation on social media issues. The main thrust of most legislation is to prohibit employers from requiring applicants or employees to grant the employer access to the applicants' or employees' social media sites, usually by providing a username and password. Such legislation is most likely the fallout from a 2011 incident in which a Maryland correctional officer was asked by his employer for his social media account username and password (Protalinski 2011).

Interestingly, little if any statutory law (and even less case law) provides guidance on what employers may legitimately regulate regarding employees' use of social media (whether on company equipment or on the employee's own devices) or the extent to which employers' use of public social media content may be a legitimate tool to scrutinize potential employees.

HR professionals can assist their organizations by carefully reviewing any existing or proposed social media policies to try to eliminate provisions that are or may be found to violate the NLRA's protection of "concerted activity" or any state statute. Further, HR professionals may help their organizations by strongly recommending scrutiny of any adverse employment action based in whole or in part on an employee's or applicant's social media activity.

The Law Does Not Stand Still

In an action similar to its earlier revisiting and revision of the 1964 Civil Rights Act, Congress returned to the ADA in 2008. Congress and many advocates for the disabled had become increasingly unhappy over the Supreme Court's restrictions of the ADA. In a series of cases in 1999 the Supreme Court ruled that corrective measures (such as eyeglasses, *Sutton v. United Airlines, Inc.*, 527 U.S. 471 [1999], and blood pressure medication, *Murphy v. United Parcel Service, Inc.*, 527 U.S. 516 [1999]) could remedy an individual's disability and remove the individual from the coverage and protection of the act. Then in 2002, in *Toyota Motor Manufacturing, Kentucky, Inc. v. Williams*, 534 U.S. 184 (2002), the court again narrowed the availability of coverage under the ADA by further restricting the interpretation of "major life activities."

In 2008 Congress moved to overturn the Supreme Court decisions that were felt to be unduly restrictive of the act's remedial purpose. In the ADAAA, Congress specifically overturned the court's decision in *Toyota v. Williams* and wrote into the statute definitions and interpretations specifically designed to address what were considered to be too-restrictive judicial interpretations in case law. The ADAAA included clarification that corrective devices or drug treatments that remedied a particular condition did not remove an individual from coverage under the act; it also specifically stated that episodic conditions, such as epilepsy or migraine headaches, were considered disabling conditions even when the disease or its symptoms were in remission. (The passage of the ADAAA represented an affirmation of the doctrine of the separation of powers that is fundamental to the American system of government. Congress passed a law [the ADA], the Supreme Court interpreted it, and because Congress disagreed with the court's interpretations, it overturned a series of Supreme Court decisions by rewriting the laws. In an unusual move, Congress made the ADAAA retroactive to the day the Supreme Court issued the *Toyota* decision, thereby officially invalidating that decision.)

In amending the ADA to overturn Supreme Court decisions, Congress made three significant changes. First, it significantly expanded the interpretation of "substantially limits" so that conditions with a lesser impact now qualify as disabling conditions. Second, it enlarged the definition of "major life activities" so that more conditions now qualify as disabling conditions. Under the ADA the following activities were considered "major life activities": manual tasks, walking, talking, seeing, hearing, breathing, learning, and speaking. Under the ADAAA, additional activities were added: sleeping, lifting, bending, concentration, thinking, communicating, reading, working, immunity, digestion, cell growth, bladder function, neurological system function, brain function, respiratory function, endocrine system function, circulatory system function, and reproduction. Finally, the new ADAAA made episodic conditions, even in remission, disabling conditions. The result of these changes was to shift the question in disability situations from "Are you disabled?" to "What sort of accommodation do you need?" The net effect has been to increase the number of individuals able to claim a disabling condition and thus be entitled to reasonable accommodation.

Also in 2008, Congress also amended the FMLA, although not in as fundamental a fashion as it had with the ADA. Because of ongoing military conflicts in the Middle East and Afghanistan, additional resources were needed to support the families of military members facing dislocation caused by military service and also coping with family members returning home wounded, sick, or disabled.

These changes introduced two new concepts to the FMLA: exigency leave and military caregiver leave. Exigency leave (up to 12 weeks of unpaid leave) is available to family members of military members on active duty. This provision does not provide 12 additional weeks of unpaid leave; combined regular family/medical leave and exigency leave cannot exceed 12 weeks in a 12-month period (US Department of Labor, Wage and Hour Division 2014).

Military caregiver leave is available to employees to care for a military service member with a serious injury or illness. This leave is for up to 26 weeks and is also unpaid. Like exigency leave, military caregiver leave is not an additional 26 weeks of leave added on to the 12 weeks of regular family/ medical leave. In a single 12-month period an employee who is eligible for both military caregiver leave and family/medical leave cannot take more than 26 weeks combined for both leaves (US Department of Labor, Wage and Hour Division 2013a).

The Equal Employment Opportunity Commission Strides Confidently into the Future

The EEOC has become an activist organization. With nearly two-thirds of charges resolved in favor of employers (EEOC 2014a) and with a relatively steady, if not slightly declining, number of charges filed (EEOC 2014b), the EEOC has found the energy and the will to venture into areas not yet dealt with by statutory and (in some areas) case law.

For many years, plaintiffs have brought into court the proposition that employer discrimination against lesbian, gay, or bisexual employees and applicants violates Title VII's prohibition against discrimination based on sex. The courts have uniformly ruled against this proposition. Notwithstanding the overwhelming lack of success this proposition has had in courts across the United States, the EEOC embarked on a course to establish through case law that such discrimination is indeed prohibited sex discrimination under Title VII. In 2011 the EEOC found that claims by lesbian, gay, and bisexual employees were legitimate claims of sex discrimination under Title VII. Similarly, the EEOC has found that discrimination against transgender individuals also is prohibited sex discrimination.

Employers may feel that this effort by the EEOC is overreaching, and may feel confident that the courts will continue to find that Title VII does not prohibit this form of discrimination. However, with a 2013 Gallup poll showing national support for same-sex marriage reaching majority levels (Jones 2013) and given that courts found sex discrimination in sexual harassment without statutory support (until 1991), such confidence may well be misplaced.

The EEOC has also broken new ground by defining obesity (as opposed to morbid obesity, defined clinically as being more than 100 pounds overweight [US National Library of Medicine, National Institutes of Health 2014]) as a disability under the ADAAA. The EEOC filed suit in 2010 against an employer that had fired an employee because of her "severe" obesity, even though the employee remained able to perform her job duties (*EEOC v. Resources for Human Development*, E.D. La. 2010). Prior to this suit, case law under the ADA generally held that obesity was not a disability

(*EEOC v. Watkins Motor Lines Inc.*, 463 F.3d 436 [6th Cir. 2006]). The EEOC's position in the *Resources for Human Development* case that the 2009 rewriting of the ADA into the ADAAA, with the consequent expansion of the definitions of *major life activity* and *major body functions*, had transformed obesity into a disability apparently convinced the court. Although the court did not provide a decision (the defendant settled with the EEOC rather than go to trial), the EEOC will undoubtedly use the same logic in other courts.

Seemingly out of nowhere, in 2007 the EEOC took up the cause of caregivers in the workplace. The EEOC circularly defines *caregiver* as "a worker with caregiving responsibilities," which can include caring for children, caring for elderly family members, or caring for individuals with disabilities (EEOC 2007). The legal underpinning of the EEOC's concept is fairly straightforward; caregiver discrimination is couched in terms of practices that violate Title VII's prohibition against discrimination on the basis of sex. These practices include failing to approve leave requests from women with children but approving similar requests from male employees, hiring or promoting men with children but failing to hire or promote similarly situated women, and taking adverse action against formerly well-regarded female employees after they become pregnant. The careful observer will note that these actions could easily have been characterized as sex discrimination without resorting to creating a new category of discrimination.

This chapter previously discussed the possibility that the courts would adopt the EEOC's position on discrimination against lesbian, gay, bisexual, and transgender individuals, analogizing this situation to the efforts in the 1970s and 1980s to have the courts recognize sexual harassment as sex discrimination. The EEOC also appears to have had some early success with advocating for obesity as a disability. However, caregiver discrimination may face a steeper slope of acceptance. The fact that many employees in the workplace now are caregivers to children, the elderly, and individuals with disabilities may not translate into judicial empathy.

HR professionals may assist their organizations by bringing awareness of the EEOC's efforts in these areas to the attention of the organization, and by urging closer scrutiny of actions that, in whole or in part, may rest on the employee's obesity; the employee's identification as lesbian, gay, bisexual, or transgender; or the employee's actual or perceived responsibilities as a caregiver.

Retaliation: Is It or Isn't It?

In 2006, the US Supreme Court took an unexpectedly employee-friendly tone. In *Burlington Northern & Santa Fe (BNSF) Railway Co. v. White*, 548 U.S. 53 (2006), the court set out a new, lower standard defining "adverse action" in the context of Title VII retaliation claims. The court applied a "reasonable person" standard whereby any action taken by an employer that a reasonable person would consider adverse triggers Title VII's retaliation protections. This decision was generally felt to increase the possibility that employees would file retaliation claims. And perhaps it did. According to EEOC statistics (EEOC 2014b), Title VII retaliation charges increased from 19,560 charges in 2006 (the year of *Burlington Northern*) to 31,429 charges five years later.

In 2011 the court again addressed the question of retaliation, but from a different angle. Eric Thompson, an employee of North American Stainless, filed a retaliation charge against his former employer alleging that he was fired because his fiancé at the time (also employed by North American Stainless) had filed a sex discrimination charge with the EEOC. In *Thompson v. North American Stainless*, No. 09-921 (January 24, 2011), the court found that North American Stainless did indeed discharge Thompson in retaliation for his fiancé's EEOC charges. However, the court declined to give any standards beyond the facts of the case as to how close or distant a relation would have to be to invoke the retaliation protection of Title VII.

EEOC charge statistics show that Title VII retaliation charges increased slightly from 31,429 in 2011 to 31,478 in 2013 (EEOC 2014b). However, in the wake of the *Burlington Northern* and *North American Stainless* decisions, Title VII retaliation charges filed with EEOC nearly doubled from 2006 (the date of the *Burlington Northern* decision) to 2013. EEOC charge statistics for 2013 show that retaliation charges for all statutes (including the ADEA, ADAAA, Equal Pay Act, and GINA) were the largest number of charges filed on any issue (EEOC 2014b).

The Supreme Court took a step back in 2013 with its decision in *University of Texas Southwestern Medical Center v. Nassar*, 133 S.Ct. 2517 (2013), holding that retaliation claims required a higher standard of proof than other types of Title VII discrimination complaints.

Protection against retaliation is not limited to Title VII. The FMLA (29 U.S.C. § 2615) prohibits retaliation against anyone seeking to exercise rights under that law. The FLSA, in section 15(a)(3), prohibits retaliation against any person making a complaint, either oral or written, under that act. Section 12203 of the ADAAA continues the ADA's prohibition against retaliation. The ADEA prohibits retaliation as well (29 U.S.C. § 623(d)).

So, what is the impact of retaliation and employment law on employers? The Supreme Court has defined what retaliation is (*Burlington Northern*), it has given some guidance on how far retaliation may reach (fiancés in *North American Stainless*), and it has provided direction on the standard of proof for retaliation (*Nassar*). Many of the federal nondiscrimination statutes (Title VII, ADAAA) specifically prohibit retaliation, as do some of the employment laws (FLSA, FMLA). And since 2006 (*Burlington Northern*), retaliation charges filed with the EEOC have nearly doubled.

Although employees may not be prevailing in any greater numbers despite the increase in charges filed, the goal, as any HR professional or any manager knows, is to avoid having charges filed, as opposed to succeeding once a charge or lawsuit has been filed.

How Employment Law and Employee Relations Can Promote Strategic Human Resources Management

How can managers, executives, and HR professionals use their knowledge of employment law to navigate successfully through the deep and difficult waters of employee relations in the twenty-first century? How can this knowledge inform and shape effective strategic HR management?

The Impact of Legal Issues on Human Resources Management

HR management and the law: Some people would say this combination is more like oil and water than like chocolate and peanut butter. HR management, dealing with people, their personalities, and their idiosyncrasies, is complex enough without having to factor in concepts and realities like reasonable accommodation or intermittent leave with a guaranteed job.

But look back at the scenario that opened this chapter. Although the scenario is more complex than reality usually is, a review of court decisions will show that at least parts of this hypothetical situation have occurred, some of them over and over again. Employees do take FMLA leave but are unable to return to work exactly at the end of 12 weeks. Supervisors do, either intentionally or unwittingly, enforce policies or practices that are in violation of federal laws such as the FLSA. Supervisors and employees say and do things that are prone to incite other employees to go to court.

When these things happen (or, in the best-case scenario, are foreseen to potentially happen in the future), HR managers are often the organization's first line of defense against expensive (and potentially unnecessary) legal liability.

Employee Relations

Employee relations work (like most other aspects of HR management) has evolved over the years. Although the field of employee relations began with duties that resembled those of recreation directors more than anything else, HR professionals handling employee relations now need a firm knowledge of both state and federal employment laws, the organization's own policies and practices, and precedential HR management decisions in the organization. Employee relations activities are potentially a part of every HR decision or plan an organization engages in. Employment specialists know where to go for the best recruits, but they may not be aware of the EEOC's efforts to reduce reliance on the use of criminal convictions to thin out large applicant pools. Classification and compensation specialists know how to structure job families and control how employees move up through classes; they may not be familiar with the disparate impact teachings of *Griggs*. Employee relations is where the HR management disciplines come together, usually at the juncture of a messy, difficult, and potentially legally dangerous situation.

The View from 25,000 Feet: Where the Problems Are

From the perspective of employee relations, organizational difficulties can be found in three areas: decisions involving recruitment, selection, or job advancement; decisions involving discipline, termination, or both; and the need to ensure organizational compliance with federal employment laws such as the FLSA or the FMLA—or, more colloquially, hiring, firing, and paying.

In the recruitment, selection, and advancement area, potential problems could include situations such as these:

- An interview panel member asks a female applicant if she is pregnant or thinking about becoming pregnant because the job has been vacant for a while and they need somebody who will be there.

- During an interview with an African-American applicant, the interviewer says, "We really have enough blacks working here now. We're hoping to hire a Hispanic or perhaps a Native American."

- During a reference check for a current employee, one employee says to the outside recruiter, "We'll be glad to see him go; he's a troublemaker and he has already filed two discrimination complaints in our grievance system."

- Despite diverse applicant pools, one of your divisions seems to hire predominantly white females who are recent college graduates.

Of course, these problems are not the only ones. Others to watch out for include these:

- Despite a policy requiring reference checking, one of your department heads hires someone who turns out to have been terminated from his last two jobs because he falsified his resume.

- Promotional opportunities in one of your clinics are not advertised (which is required by your organization's policy) and seem to be awarded to "friends" of the supervisor, many of whom are white males, just like the supervisor.

- Behind the scenes, a hiring supervisor tells certain employees to apply for vacant positions while trying to discourage other employees from applying. The first group is all male; the second group, all female.

Do these things really happen anymore? Of course they do. How does knowledge of employment law and good employee relations practices help prevent or resolve such problems? One way is that these problems, and similar ones, are old news—that is, they have been occurring since before the rise of employment law in the 1960s. Take, for example, an area in which promotional opportunities are not advertised or are only selectively advertised. This old practice is now seen as an indication of intent to discriminate. One possible resolution is to revise the organization's HR policies and practices, train supervisors and hiring officials in those policies and practices, and then monitor hiring and promotional activity. Too often, however, the response to a problem is to create a policy to "fix" the problem, and then walk away. This approach is the HR equivalent of putting a Band-Aid on a tumor. More effective than just policymaking is the practice of consistently training supervisors and reinforcing that training through monitoring of activity and feedback.

One area of continuing difficulty is in the selection process, principally in face-to-face interviews. HR management, like any other human activity, has its myths and tall tales. One of the most predominant of these misconceptions is the "legal/illegal" interview question dichotomy. (See the "Web Resources" section at the end of this chapter.) A review of employment laws shows that despite the existence of collections and lists of "legal" and "illegal" questions, only one question is truly illegal (that is, specifically prohibited) under federal employment law. That question is "Are you disabled?" The ADAAA specifically prohibits asking applicants whether they have a disability or not. Otherwise, an interviewer or interview panel is legally free to ask questions such as "Are you pregnant?" "Do you plan on having children?" "What religious holidays do you observe?" or even "How old are you?"

Why aren't these questions illegal? Don't the pregnancy/children questions violate Title VII? Doesn't the age question violate the ADEA? And that question about religious holidays—doesn't it violate the Constitution?

None of these questions violate any specific provision of law. However, these questions are all high-risk questions for several reasons. First, such questions may well propel an unsuccessful applicant to file a charge with the EEOC or a state human rights agency. Second, none of these questions are job related or consistent with business necessity. That is, these questions may indicate an intent to discriminate (for instance, "How old are you?" could be evidence of intentional age discrimination). The questions may be evidence that the policies and practices of the organization, while neutral on their face, could mask systemic discrimination against a protected class. Finally, the question about having children may invoke EEOC scrutiny (see the discussion of caregiver discrimination earlier in this chapter).

Discipline and termination are emotionally difficult events for everyone. Some supervisors tend to avoid these actions, even when justified and necessary, to avoid an unpleasant interaction with a subordinate. Sometimes, supervisors and management just want to get these events over with as quickly as possible, so they avoid involving the HR department until after the event is over. These missteps can lead to an action that is contrary to previous decisions in similar situations, a decision that appears to be discriminatory in some fashion, or a decision that is not in compliance with the organization's own policy and procedures.

Can HR managers proactively attempt to prevent these things from happening? One element of strategic HR management in employee relations is to find a way to have human resources (usually the employee relations component) be a part, from the beginning, of all situations that have the potential for disciplinary action, termination, or both. This requirement helps to make sure that decisions are consistent with the way similar situations have been handled in the past, that the organization's HR policies and procedures are followed, and that snap decisions based on emotion are avoided. From the legal perspective, following established policies and procedures, or even just following the same practices consistently, is a significant way to reduce potential legal liability. Not following policy and procedures, or ignoring established practices or procedure, is one indicator (to third-party reviewers such as outside investigators or juries) of a discriminatory practice or intent.

In addition to the challenges of hiring and firing, what pitfalls await the unwary organization in the simple acts of compliance with well-regulated and enforced federal employment laws?

While the goals of the FLSA are simple, the rules implementing those goals are not. With an anticipated review and potential revision of the regulations on eligibility for overtime set for 2015, these rules may well get more complex and most assuredly will generate more litigation. Some broad-stroke issues to be aware of in dealing with FLSA include the concept that a position must be considered exempt (not eligible for overtime compensation) because the organization "can't afford to pay for overtime"; for public employers who can compensate overtime work with paid time off, the concept that if this "compensatory time off" is not used, then it is lost; and for private-sector employers, the concept that interns are volunteers and do not have to be compensated.

A strategic approach to dealing with these and other FLSA issues involves two parts: first, a comprehensive training program, repeated at appropriate intervals, presenting the basics of wage and hour concepts and introducing the people or departments in the organization that are available to help with these kinds of issues; and, second, periodic monitoring of wage and hour practices to detect and remedy any failures in compliance. This approach will not catch every problem (willful noncompliance with FLSA rules often means a great savings to the unit or the organization, and thus managers face an incentive to cut corners in compliance), but it should minimize significant compliance failures.

How difficult is compliance with the FMLA? A Society for Human Resource Management survey in 2007 showed that many HR professionals have difficulty with three areas of FMLA compliance: dealing with episodic health incidents (such as migraines or back pain), dealing with intermittent FMLA requests (and their timing), and the granting of FMLA requests thought to be illegitimate because of the complexity of Department of Labor regulations (Society for Human Resource Management 2007). The survey indicated that, contrary to Department of Labor statements, many organizations, especially large ones, have significant difficulty in administering the FMLA.

One area of significant confusion and difficulty is the return to work of an employee who has been out on FMLA leave. A recurring situation in healthcare (with its many physically strenuous activities) is that the employee has exhausted his or her 12 weeks of leave but is not ready to return to work. That particular situation will be dealt with in the next section. Another possible difficulty concerns the employee's fitness (or lack thereof) to return to work at the conclusion of FMLA leave. In jobs that require physical effort and ability (which includes many job classifications in the healthcare field), a returning employee needs to be able to perform all the essential tasks of the job. Section 104(a)(4) of the FMLA permits an employer to require a "fitness for duty" test, providing it is uniformly applied and is specifically targeted at the health condition that caused the employee to take FMLA leave. To avoid multiple problems with this seemingly simple action, a strategic HR management approach is to have clear, specific policies on return to work from any medical absence, to train supervisors and managers on how these situations are to be handled, and to require the participation of the HR component of the organization whenever a situation arises. Even this in-depth approach does not guarantee a lack of problems, but it does put the organization in the best position when problems (or complaints or investigations) occur.

Multiple-Issue Problems: Using the Cost–Benefit Approach

The last section discussed what appeared to be a simple FMLA situation: a return to work by an employee. That section noted how to approach a return-to-work situation that involved fitness for duty but did not examine all the potential aspects of this situation.

For example, the FMLA, like most other federal employment laws, prohibits retaliation for requesting or taking FMLA leave. What if the employee felt that the organization's efforts to ensure his or her fitness to return to work were in retaliation for requesting and taking FMLA leave? That question is the first issue. What if the employee is not able (or has not been medically released) to return to work at the exhaustion of the FMLA leave? That is the second issue. What if the employee still has accumulated paid time off at the end of the FMLA leave that he or she wishes to use? That is yet another issue, this one involving the organization's policies and practices. What if the employee comes forward and says that his or her reason for taking FMLA leave is a disability, and requests an extension of leave as a reasonable accommodation? Yet another issue emerges.

Here, one situation—an employee at the end of 12 weeks of FMLA leave—presents at least three legal issues—alleged retaliation, the possible need for reasonable accommodation under the ADAAA, and the inability to return to work when FMLA leave is exhausted. An additional issue is the organization's practice or policies regarding use of accumulated paid time off. How can such a tangled skein of employee needs, employer needs, and legal requirements be untangled? Is the Gordian knot approach the best method?

Cutting through the issues and making a quick, decisive judgment is always attractive. However, it may not be the most effective method. Another approach that can be more effective is to separate the issues into either operational or legal/policy issues. Using this technique, the operational issues are the employer's need to have the employee return to work, the employer's need to ensure that the returning employee is fit for duty, the employee's need for more time for recovery, the employee's desire to not return to work until he or she is fit for duty, and the employee's reliance on the organization's policies regarding use of leave time. The legal/policy issues are the employer's desire to avoid or diminish any potential legal liability resulting from its decisions, the employer's responsibility to consistently administer its policies on leave usage, the employee's desire to be able to use accumulated leave in the manner that the employer's policies permit, and the employee's desire not to be retaliated against for asserting his or her legal rights.

How does this separation technique help to resolve this situation? The organization is most likely to focus on the operational issues: returning a fit employee to duty as quickly as possible. Avoiding or diminishing legal liability may not be on the horizon unless HR or legal personnel raise these issues. The employee is also focused on operational issues: getting back to work once he or she is fit for duty. However, the employee may be more focused on legal/policy issues, at least initially, than the organization: using accumulated paid leave per the organization's policies and avoiding retaliation.

Can a single path to resolution that is satisfactory to everyone be found? Often, the answer is no. But the separation of issues may aid resolution by focusing on common desires: Both the organization and the employee want the employee to return to work fit for duty. And while the organization wishes to diminish or avoid legal liability arising out of this situation, the employee wishes to avoid retaliation. Differences come in these areas: The organization wishes for this resolution to happen sooner rather than later; the employee is willing for it to happen later, especially with the ability to use accumulated paid leave. By concentrating on establishing what both sides agree on, and working to reduce the differences between their positions, the experienced employee relations professional may be able to craft a resolution that is at least minimally acceptable to both sides.

Sometimes, however, this resolution is difficult, if not impossible, to achieve. Sometimes resolution comes down to putting a price on what the organization wants or needs, and determining if its cost is worth the benefit of having it.

Take these work situations. An employee requests an extension of FMLA leave and threatens to file an EEOC charge if it is not granted. Employees' concerns about the organization's wage and hour practices raise the possibility of an audit by investigators from the Department of Labor's Wage and Hour Division. A former employee has retained an attorney and is threatening to go to court with the allegation that the organization terminated her because of her age and her disability unless she is given her job back.

How can a cost be assigned to these events? How can the value of resolving these events quickly and definitively be evaluated? A good place to start is to look at who will be involved in an EEOC charge or a wage and hour investigation. How much time will be spent responding to requests for information (locating it, compiling it, reviewing it to make sure that no confidential information is provided)? How will this time affect the mission of the organization? Will critical persons be required to participate in responding to the charge, providing information for the wage and hour investigation, working with the lawyers, providing depositions, or testifying in court, as opposed to doing the critical work of the organization?

This type of analysis provides greater understanding and information about the big question: What is the value to the organization of not having to contest an EEOC charge, not having to endure a wage and hour investigation, or not having to defend a lawsuit? If the answer is (and it almost always is) that the organization will find more value in resolving the issue sooner rather than later, resolving it quickly rather than in a lingering manner, or resolving it less expensively than waiting for a regulatory award or a jury decision, then methods for resolution are available.

One such method is mediation. EEOC offers mediation services when charges are filed (EEOC 2014c). Mediation offers both sides a low-risk, low-cost method of finding resolution. In many states, the judicial system either offers or requires mediation. And even when mediation does not result in resolution, it offers each side an opportunity to hear and consider the factors motivating the other side.

But what if the organization does not wish to settle or to accept a compromise resolution? What if the organization wishes to contest the EEOC charge vigorously or wishes to take the lawsuit to a jury? Clearly, in these situations the organization has done at least a basic cost–benefit analysis and determined that the benefit of being vindicated by a "no cause" determination by the EEOC or an appropriate court decision is worth the time and expense involved.

Why would an organization want to go to these time-consuming and expensive lengths? It may wish to obtain a public decision declaring that it did not discriminate, that it pays employees appropriately and legally, or that it complies with federal law and regulations in the employment side of its operations. The organization may wish to make a statement through its defense of its actions: We didn't discriminate or violate federal law, and we will fight to establish that. The organization may believe strongly that its actions were appropriate and wishes to have that position vindicated in the legal system.

But, at the end of the process, whether an organization chooses to attempt to resolve employee relations issues informally, through nonjudicial means, or whether it chooses to defend itself in the regulatory or judicial arenas, it has made, however roughly, a cost–benefit analysis indicating that its path is the one of more value to the organization.

Strategic Tools for Operational Employee Relations

A great deal of employee relations work is, by the nature of employee relations, reactive. This work includes such activities as investigating complaints or grievances, reacting to and attempting to resolve workplace issues and situations, counseling employees, and providing technical advice and assistance to supervisors and managers who are dealing with a work issue. These issues, and others like them, are the operational side of employee relations, dealing with current, real-time issues.

The most effective employee relations programs also have a proactive or strategic side. This strategic approach takes advantage of the information that employee relations collects from its operational activities, information such as which work unit is filing an unusually high rate of grievances, which supervisors are prompting employees to come in for counseling, or which work units seem to have a high rate of turnover and other similar information. Analysis of this information can yield significant value to the organization.

What can be done with this information? How can an organization use the data strategically to head off employee unrest, keep morale from dropping, alleviate the reasons for turnover, and calm negative energy in a work unit? One effective tool for good management is ongoing supervisory training. In many cases, a supervisor's reluctance to take action or failure to act positively is a result of a lack of information. A program of regularly scheduled training for supervisors and managers on the organization's policies and processes is particularly useful, especially in a situation in which real-life examples and possible approaches to resolution can be discussed. Such training and communication are useful even when the only information that supervisors and managers take away is who to contact when a problem or a potential problem arises.

What should supervisors and managers be trained on? The organization will be helped by having clearly written policies and procedures that have been developed with an understanding of how the organization is structured and the work needs of the organization. These policies need to address common situations, yet be written to provide flexibility in unusual or unanticipated instances. Useful and effective policies are reviewed on a regular basis and revised as needed. Input from groups in the organization, including employees, can be extremely helpful in making the changes effective and meaningful.

Regular review of HR policies is another strategic tool. Laws change, organizational goals change, and the work environment changes. To have strategic value, HR policies need to be reviewed at regular intervals to make sure that the policies still serve the goals of the organization.

Policies that are difficult to locate are much less effective. In today's environment of total access to information, policies need to be in a variety of forms and open to access in a variety of locations. Unlike in the past, a paper copy of a policy is not very useful; it may, in fact, be unhelpful. Changes in policies can be easily made in electronic documents or formats; changes to paper policies require getting rid of the old and putting in the new policy. Because making these changes is not necessarily a top priority, policies that are old, outdated, and potentially dangerous may hang around in a hard-copy format.

Elsewhere in this book is an entire chapter on performance management and performance evaluations. Performance evaluations, or at least the concept that evaluations should be honestly done and factually based, are a key component of strategic employee relations. A big knock on performance evaluations is that they are often neither honest nor factually based. According to many performance evaluation programs, all the employees, like the children of Lake Wobegon, are above average. The "advantage" of this lack of honesty in evaluations is that no one contests an Above Average or Outstanding evaluation. Harmony and happiness reign—until a supervisor comes forward and wants to begin disciplinary proceedings (or even termination), and human resources asks the fateful question: "So, what do the last few performance evaluations look like?" And then the supervisor reluctantly brings forward a sheaf of Above Average or Outstanding ratings and proceeds to explain that they are not really accurate, the employee has never really done a satisfactory job, and it's time to do something about it. At this point, the whole process breaks down.

A performance evaluation process that is honest and accurate provides a multitude of benefits, not the least of which is identifying above-average and below-average performers. The identification of above-average performers helps the organization to target them for career advancement opportunities and other retention-enhancing practices. The value of identifying below-average employees is obvious. But none of these positive processes can go forward without an accurate and honest performance evaluation process.

One way that human resources can help move the organization forward is to have a programmatic performance evaluation process (also known as an HR audit) in place. Just as performance evaluations identify for employees what is going well, what is good enough, and what needs improvement, so an HR audit provides the organization with the same data about its HR programs. An audit of the organization's HR policies and processes every few years is a good way to monitor how current these policies and processes are and how they are meeting (or not meeting) the needs of the organization. Such an audit, done at the organization's pace and for the organization's purposes, will nearly always be more productive and less costly than having an audit conducted by regulatory agency investigators following up a complaint of potential rule or law violations.

This approach leads to the last strategic point here. Reviews of and changes to HR policies and processes are more productively conducted when no crisis exists. That is, a review of the disciplinary process is easier to do and can be conducted with less effort when the organization is facing no current grievances, EEOC charges, or lawsuits. Such a crisis-free review also avoids allegations that the changes were made to cover up or remove old, noncompliant (or even illegal) policies and procedures.

Dealing with Unsatisfactory Performance and Detrimental Personal Conduct Discipline

Literally hundreds of books, articles, blogs, videos, and other material on employee disciplinary practices are available. (A quick search of Amazon.com turned up more than 100 books dealing with this topic—including the third edition of this book. A similar search on YouTube had nearly 8,000 hits.) Clearly, much research and discussion has addressed (and continues to address) the topic of employee discipline.

Employee discipline in healthcare may have more strategic weight than it does in other work environments. Unlike in many other fields of work, sloppy, careless, or negligent work or work habits can have a significant impact on patient care, even to the point of fatality. Poor customer service can have a significant impact on revenue and an organization's reputation, both locally and, in some cases, globally. Therefore, how a healthcare organization handles employee discipline can be critical to its success and its standing in the community it serves.

However they might be dressed up, most disciplinary practices incorporate the time-honored concepts of discipline based on job performance and discipline based on an employee's behavior and ability to conform that behavior to the norms of the organization. Most organizations boil these down to job performance and personal conduct.

These divisions recognize that discipline has several goals. In discipline focused on job performance, the first goal is to have the employee perform at least at an acceptable level. Other goals of this type of discipline are to motivate the employee to perform at a satisfactory level; to make sure the employee has all the tools, knowledge, and skills necessary to perform at a satisfactory level; and to make the employee aware of negative consequences for less-than-satisfactory performance. The reasons for these goals are not too difficult to grasp. Whether dealing with a new employee having difficulty or a seasoned employee whose performance has become noticeably less satisfactory, the organization has devoted significant time, effort, and funds to recruiting, selecting, and training the employee. Any organization not willing to devote a little more effort to increasing employee performance in these cases would be a poor steward of its funds. And in today's workplace, with fewer employees doing more work, obtaining at least satisfactory performance from all employees is critical.

The purposes of discipline based on poor behavior (the traditional phrase is "detrimental conduct") are simple and straightforward: if necessary, remove the employee from the workforce to avoid further problems, and clarify for all employees what behaviors are not accepted and not tolerated. This type of discipline, unlike job performance discipline, is not about training. In most cases the unacceptable conduct is behavior that is not tolerated in most contexts. This behavior would include stealing from the employer, violence in the workplace (both physical and verbal) against colleagues or supervisors, falsifying records, and similar behaviors. While telling an employee that a particular aspect of his or her job performance is less than standard and informing the employee of the standard makes sense, telling an employee that stealing from the employer or falsifying records is unacceptable and that further disciplinary action may be taken should the action occur again seems nonsensical and slightly humorous.

How are these two disparate bases for discipline defined? Capturing the essence of the actions for which job performance discipline may be imposed is relatively easy. Aspects of performance, such as the quality of work, the quantity of work, the timeliness of work, and the accuracy of work, help set the parameters of job performance. Some behavioral aspects should be included as well. These aspects include regular attendance (a Google search for "absenteeism problem" brings up about 3.5 million hits), customer service, and teamwork.

Discipline based on detrimental conduct is less easy to define. Looking at aspects of such behavior may be more helpful in understanding what type of problem is represented by unacceptable conduct. One such aspect is that the behavior is intentional. While some performance issues may be characterized as accidental or negligent, no one accidentally steals from the employer. No one accidentally hits another employee in the face or uses a racial or sexual epithet. This type of employee behavior, in addition to being intentional, may be a violation of criminal law.

Some employers attempt to set out all the reasons that an employee may be disciplined on any basis. This attempt is at best a poor use of time, and at worst, counterproductive. If the performance standards are general enough to be applicable to everyone, then they are too general to enforce. And delimiting the human activities that represent detrimental conduct is simply impossible. Even doing so under the guise of providing examples can backfire when supervisors try to make a particular situation fit an example.

The two bases for discipline also take different procedural routes based on the different goals. Discipline based on job performance should involve multiple steps because the organization (as well as the employee) benefits from giving an employee several opportunities to correct substandard performance. The use of multiple disciplinary steps also helps reinforce the standards of the work unit and provides numerous opportunities for employee and supervisor feedback. Discipline for unacceptable conduct, on the other hand, usually involves one step—termination of the employee.

For either form of disciplinary action, documentation is important. HR departments, especially in the employee relations function, have been chided about a perceived overemphasis on documentation. Indeed, documenting a performance issue or the beginning of a behavior issue as it is occurring is often impossible. But even documentation developed later has benefits. Third-party reviewers (regulatory agencies such as the EEOC and the Department of Labor, as well as arbitrators and courts) rely on documentation to support live testimony. In many situations, if an event or issue is not documented, then "it didn't happen." The results of a lack of documentation are not always that stark, but documentation can help keep a situation from devolving into a "swearing contest." (Note that documentation is not always helpful. If the documentation contradicts the verbal reports, such as in a situation in which the supervisor is attempting to discipline an employee for poor performance, while stacks of Good or Above Average performance evaluations exist, then the proposed discipline may fail or be seen as discriminatory. See the "Strategic Tools for Operational Employee Relations" section earlier in this chapter.)

Avoiding the Land Mines

Certain typical or recurring employee discipline situations can easily be avoided. The fact that these kinds of problems continue to occur is evidence of a lack of supervisory training and an ongoing failure to involve employee relations professionals at an early stage.

One such typical occurrence is often referred to as "the straw that broke the camel's back." This situation occurs when an employee's poor performance (often poor quality of work, or work that is frequently untimely) is allowed to continue through supervisory neglect or a lack of willingness to address the issue. The poor performance goes on (often accompanied by dishonestly high performance ratings) until someone farther up the chain decides that enough is enough and wants the offending employee gone immediately.

If the organization is one that divides discipline into performance and conduct bases, and differentiates the process used for each, then such clearly performance-based issues should not (and perhaps cannot) be addressed by immediate termination.

This situation embodies three of the most frequently encountered "land mines" for effective disciplinary action: failure to take action on a timely basis, dishonest and inaccurate performance ratings, and failure to follow the organization's established policies and procedures. Other variations on this theme include inconsistently applying policies or discipline (leading in some cases to EEOC charges and lawsuits), and choosing not to follow policies or employment statutes because noncompliance is easier, less time-consuming, and cheaper.

Effective strategic employee relations relies on a three-pronged effort to prevent or ameliorate these tendencies. The first is conducting regular and ongoing supervisory training (including the right people in human resources to contact, and how to do so) about the organization's policies and how to comply with employment laws. The second consists of monitoring HR activities, analyzing the data collected, and providing feedback in a useful time frame to managers and supervisors. Finally, employee relations needs to be a presence in the work units without the necessity of a crisis. Through a combination of operational and strategic efforts, human resources and employee relations provide value to the organization.

Other Employment Law and Employee Relations Issues

Healthcare managers should be aware of the following additional employment law and employee relations issues that are not covered in detail in this chapter:

- Dual employee/patient status—In the world of healthcare, having employees as patients is not uncommon. Such a dual status raises legal and ethical issues.
- Romance in the workplace—With longer working hours, many employees today do not have the time or opportunity to meet other persons outside

the workplace. Office romance is an issue that has provoked extreme HR action at both ends of the spectrum: "love contracts" in which employees agree not to date colleagues or subordinates, and employers' encouragement of romance between coworkers.

- Employee privacy, the Health Insurance Portability and Accountability Act (HIPAA), and other confidentiality issues—A variety of laws, regulations, and individual employer policies regulate all aspects of employee privacy.

- Impact of state employment and nondiscrimination laws on the workplace—Employment laws, some with greater protections for employees or restrictions on employers than comparable federal laws, vary from state to state. An entire book would be needed (and several have been written) to set out these individual differences.

- Effect of US laws on overseas employment—As globalization increases, the question of whose employment laws apply is significant. Some US employment laws (such as Title VII) apply to US citizens working outside the country; others do not.

- Equal pay for equal work—This early nondiscrimination law waxes and wanes in the amount of attention it receives.

- Pregnancy discrimination (including lactation discrimination)—Awareness of this issue, addressed in another early nondiscrimination law, was given new impetus by the lactation provisions in the Affordable Care Act.

- Discrimination under the Genetic Information Nondiscrimination Act (GINA)—This law, passed in 2008, prohibits discrimination on the basis of genetic information. Its impact is primarily limited to access to employer group health and life insurance.

- Drug testing for applicants and employees—This topic not only involves constitutional restrictions in some cases but also varies from state to state.

- Pre-employment medical testing or "fitness for duty" testing for employees—This important aspect of the ADAAA has had significant impact in a variety of situations for employers, especially in healthcare.

- Freedom of speech issues for public employees and employers—The US Supreme Court has significantly narrowed any expectation of free speech for public employees, to the benefit of public employers.

- Searching employee spaces; "expectation of privacy" issues—These issues have both a constitutional aspect (for public employers) and a state law aspect in a number of jurisdictions.

- Workers' compensation laws—These laws are generally state-specific.

- Domestic violence in (and out) of the workplace—Heightened awareness of this problem has led to a variety of state law treatments of it, including protection for victims and prohibition against discrimination.

- Safety and health issues—This category includes the laws and regulations enforced by the Occupational Safety and Health Administration (OSHA).

Summary

Employment law has changed and evolved since the enactment of the FLSA in 1938. The American workplace has gone from being a place where stereotypes were accepted, and even enforced, to a place where considering race, sex, age, or disability is prohibited and employees have statutory protections against harassment, retaliation, and even unintentional discrimination. Effective HR and employee relations professionals use their knowledge of these laws and regulations (see Exhibit 2.1) to enable their organizations to strategically deal with the age-old problems of poor performance, irregular attendance, and detrimental personal conduct, while working with supervisors and managers to improve their skills to prevent or reduce the recurrence of such situations.

EXHIBIT 2.1
Employment
Laws in the
United States

Civil Rights Act of 1991 (Title VII)—42 U.S.C. § 1981a and 42 U.S.C. §§ 2000e-2(k)–(n)

Pregnancy Discrimination Act—42 U.S.C. § 2000(e)

Genetic Information Nondiscrimination Act (GINA)—P.L. 110-233, 122 Stat. 881

Equal Pay Act—29 U.S.C. § 206(d)

Health Insurance Portability and Accountability Act (HIPAA)—P.L. 104-191

US Constitution

– First Amendment

– Fourth Amendment

– Fifth Amendment

– Fourteenth Amendment

Americans with Disabilities Act Amendments Act (ADAAA)—P.L. 110-325

Fair Labor Standards Act (FLSA)—29 U.S.C. § 201 et seq.

Age Discrimination in Employment Act (ADEA)—29 U.S.C. chapter 14

Family and Medical Leave Act (FMLA)—29 U.S.C. § 2601, et seq.

Uniformed Services Employment Reemployment Rights Act of 1994 (USERRA)—38 U.S.C. § 4311

(continued)

EXHIBIT 2.1
Employment
Laws in the
United States
*(continued from
previous page)*

Immigration Reform and Control Act of 1986 (IRCA)—P.L. 99-603, 100 Stat. 3359 (1986)

Employee Polygraph Protection Act—P.L. 100-347

Section 1981 of the Civil Rights Act of 1866—42 U.S.C. §1981

Fair Credit Reporting Act (FCRA)—15 USC § 1681 et seq.

Employee Retirement Income Security Act (ERISA)—29 U.S.C. chapter 18

National Labor Relations Act (NLRA)—29 U.S.C. §§ 151–169

Occupational Safety and Health Act (OSHA)—29 U.S.C. title 29, chapter 15

Consumer Credit Protection Act—15 U.S.C. § 1671 et seq.

Uniform Guidelines on Employee Selection Procedures—29 C.F.R. part 1607

Fair and Accurate Credit Transactions Act (FACTA)—5 U.S.C. 1681 et seq.

Consolidated Omnibus Budget Reconciliation Act (COBRA)—P.L. 99-272

Worker Adjustment and Retraining Notification Act (WARN)

(Federal contractors > $50,000) EEO-1 Report

(Federal contractors > $50,000) Executive Orders 11246, 11375, and 11478—dealing with equal employment opportunity for federal contractors with more than $50,000 in federal contracts

(Federal contractors > $10,000) Vocational Rehabilitation Act—equal employment opportunity requirements that apply to federal contractors with more than $10,000 in federal contracts

(Federal contractors) Drug-Free Workplace Act of 1988—drug-free workplace requirements for federal contractors with more than $100,000 in federal contracts

(Federal contractors) Davis-Bacon Act—applies to federal contractors (above $2,000) repairing, altering, or constructing public buildings/works; implements local wage rate requirement and time and one half for all work done over 40 hours in a workweek

(Federal contractors) Copeland Act—amendment to Davis-Bacon Act that prohibits an employer from requiring an employee to "kick back" any portion of compensation

(Federal contractors > $2,500) McNamara-O'Hara Service Contract Act—requires contractors and subcontractors performing services on prime contracts in excess of $2,500 to pay service employees in various classes no less than the wage rates and fringe benefits found prevailing in the locality

(Federal contractors > $10,000) Walsh-Healey Public Contracts Act—requires contractors engaged in the manufacturing or furnishing of materials, supplies, articles, or equipment to the US government or the District of Columbia to pay employees who produce, assemble, handle, or ship goods under contracts exceeding $10,000, the federal minimum wage for all hours worked and time and one half their regular rate of pay for all hours worked over 40 in a workweek

Discussion Questions

1. Why should an employer with at-will employees be interested in providing due process?

2. What effect should conduct that occurs outside the workplace and outside working hours have on an employee's continued employment? How much control and regulation should an employer attempt to have over nonwork or nonworkplace conduct?

3. Why are retaliation issues the most numerous charges that the EEOC receives? Is it because court decisions have made it too easy to raise this issue? Is it because employers in the United States are unusually vengeful? Or are other reasons involved?

4. Why is the EEOC going beyond its statutory authority by focusing on issues that are not found in the law, such as caregiver discrimination and discrimination against lesbian, gay, bisexual, and transgender individuals? Is racial or sexual discrimination no longer an employment issue in the United States?

5. If people are careless enough to post information about themselves (e.g., pictures, stories, blogs) that is of an unflattering or negative nature on public Internet sites, why shouldn't employers be able to access that information and use it in making selection and advancement decisions?

6. Have Congress and the courts made it too difficult for employers to manage their human resources effectively? Do employees now have so many rights that employers cannot get services delivered?

7. Is sexual harassment or office romance more of a problem in the workplace? Why? Are sexual harassment and office romance greater problems in healthcare than in other industries? Why or why not?

8. From your own experience, discuss the accuracy of this statement: "No good deed goes unpunished."

9. A supervisor's preference for her paramour creates tension and dissension in workplace. What are the legal implications of supervisor–employee romance?

Experiential Exercises

Case 1   A series of thefts from your pharmacy area have occurred in the last six weeks. The director of security and the head of pharmacy services now require all persons working in the pharmacy department with access to drugs to clock out after their shifts and then go through a security check before leaving the building. Several employees have complained that they should be paid for this time because the security check is for the employer's benefit. The director of security and the head of pharmacy services have responded that this security check is for the benefit of the employees to ensure that no one is unjustly accused.

Issues for Discussion

1. Is either party correct?
2. If so, which one and why?

Case 2 Your director of nursing has terminated Bobbi for excessive absenteeism in violation of the Nursing Department's policy. Bobbi shows up in the HR department to complain to you that she has been the victim of retaliation and wants to file an internal complaint. In discussing the allegation of retaliation, you find out that Bobbi's first cousin, Shawna, has filed two EEOC charges against the Nursing Department alleging that she did not receive reasonable accommodation for her disability and that she was retaliated against after she filed the first EEOC charge. Bobbi says her dismissal was in retaliation for Shawna's filing of the two EEOC charges.

Issues for Discussion
1. What elements of retaliation are present here?
2. Is a cousin a close enough relationship that retaliation is possible?

Case 3 Shaunte comes into your office in the HR department one morning and tells a sad story. Her supervisor, Henry, has forced an intimate relationship on her, which has lasted for six months. Now she is coming forward to complain because she cannot take this harassment any longer and wants it stopped. She also asks that you keep her name out of the investigation.

In talking with Henry, you get a very different story. He and Shaunte have been dating for six months. It was mutual and consensual, and he made every effort to keep their personal relationship separate from their work relationship.

Issues for Discussion
1. Who do you believe? Why? Who else will you talk with?
2. Does it make any difference whom you find more credible?
3. Is it possible to keep Shaunte's name out of this investigation?
4. If you find Shaunte more credible, what are your recommendations to management?
5. If you find Henry more credible, what are your recommendations to management?

Case 4 You are the director of an outpatient facility that offers a variety of medical and counseling services in Montana. An office support employee in the substance abuse counseling clinic has been arrested for driving under the influence. Management comes to HR to seek your advice on how to manage this situation.

Issues for Discussion
1. How significant is the fact that the employee has been arrested rather than convicted?
2. Does a connection exist between this employee's job and the offense she has been charged with?
3. What should happen between now and the time this charge is resolved in the judicial system?
4. Would you handle this matter differently if this facility were located somewhere other than Montana?

Case 5   During a selection procedure for a vacancy in your Accounts Receivable department, the hiring manager asks Applicant A for her username and password for her accounts on Facebook, Twitter, and Instagram. Applicant A refuses to provide them. Later, Applicant B, who provided his username and passwords for these social media sites to the supervisor, is hired. Applicant A comes in to HR to complain.

Issues for Discussion

1. What state is your facility located in? Does it matter?
2. Why is the hiring manager asking for this information?
3. What relevant information might the hiring manager be looking for?
4. Is this inquiry job-related and consistent with business necessity?

Case 6   Your clinic, in an effort to be family friendly and also to improve recruitment of persons with caregiving responsibilities, has offered more than is required under the FMLA. The clinic extends up to 12 weeks of unpaid leave to employees who have completed six months of full-time service or nine months of part-time service. One of your employees, who has completed seven months of full-time service, requests six weeks of this leave for recovery after surgery to remove her gallbladder. Her manager recommends not granting this request because the employee, for reasons that do not appear to be related to her gallbladder condition, has used all her accrued leave and has a zero balance of paid time off.

Issues for Discussion

1. Would denial of this request possibly represent a violation of Title VII? The FMLA? The ADAAA?
2. How might you go about determining if this denial is or is not discriminatory?
3. Could this condition qualify as a disability?
4. If this condition were a disability, would unpaid leave represent a reasonable accommodation?

Case 7(a)   One of your nurses (Sandy) in a large clinic is nearing the end of her FMLA leave; she went out on leave to take care of her mother, who is terminally ill with cancer. She has now requested an additional six to eight weeks of leave. The clinic manager's response was that she had requested and been granted 12 weeks of FMLA leave, but she was needed back in the clinic when that leave was concluded.

Sandy contacts the HR office and says that she has several fellow employees who are willing to donate additional leave to help cover her further absence. She also tells HR that she believes her manager's denial of further leave is in retaliation for her request for FMLA leave in the first place.

Issues for Discussion

1. Could the denial of additional leave be considered retaliation under the FMLA?
2. Does the availability of donated leave from other employees help or hinder this situation? Why?
3. How might this situation be resolved?

Case 7(b) During the discussion about additional leave in case 7(a), HR receives a fax from a therapist saying that Sandy is clinically depressed because her mother is dying and she has been denied further leave. The therapist says that Sandy is too depressed to work and needs at least six to eight more weeks of leave, or until her mother dies, which might be any day now or might be six months from now.

Issues for Discussion

1. Does this development bring into play any other employment laws?
2. What responsibility does the clinic have now to discuss leave with the employee?
3. Would the clinic face any consequences for not engaging in a discussion about this situation and the possibility of leave for the employee?
4. Would indefinite leave for the nurse be a reasonable accommodation? How could you determine if it were unreasonable?

Case 7(c) Because of Sandy's absence in cases 7(a) and 7(b), some of the clinic nurses have worked significant amounts of overtime. The clinic's budget does not have the funding to pay for all the overtime, so the clinic manager has suggested to HR that the clinic give the nurses hour-for-hour paid time off.

Issues for Discussion

1. What are the potential problems if the clinic manager's suggestion is implemented?
2. Does the clinic have alternatives to paying for the overtime the nurses have accrued?

Issues for Discussion for Cases 7(a) to 7(c)

1. What are the legal/policy issues and what are the operational issues in these cases?
2. What are the primary interests of the employee and the primary interests of the organization?
3. What might a possible resolution of these situations include?

Notes

1. "When used in this Act . . . The term 'employer' includes any person acting as an agent of an employer, directly or indirectly, but shall not include the United States or any wholly owned Government corporation, or any Federal Reserve Bank, or any State or political subdivision thereof, or any person subject to the Railway Labor Act, as amended from time to time, or any labor organization (other than when acting as an employer), or anyone acting in the capacity of officer or agent of such labor organization." 29 U.S.C. § 152(2).
2. "(a) It shall be an unfair labor practice for an employer— (1) to interfere with, restrain, or coerce employees in the exercise of the rights guaranteed in this title." Section 8(a)(1) of the NLRA.

References

Bureau of Labor Statistics. 2014. "Union Members—2013." News Release USDL-14-0095. Issued January 24. www.bls.gov/news.release/pdf/union2.pdf.

Dover, S. 2012. "Study: Number of Smartphone Users Tops 1 Billion." CBS News. Published October 17. www.cbsnews.com/news/study-number-of-smartphone-users-tops-1-billion/.

Equal Employment Opportunity Commission (EEOC). 2014a. "Americans with Disabilities Act of 1990 (ADA) Charges (Includes Concurrent Charges with Title VII, ADEA, and EPA) FY 1997–FY 2013." Accessed October 21. www.eeoc.gov/eeoc/statistics/enforcement/ada-charges.cfm.

———. 2014b. "Charge Statistics FY 1997 Through FY 2013." Accessed October 21. www.eeoc.gov/eeoc/statistics/enforcement/charges.cfm.

———. 2014c. "Mediation." Accessed October 21. www.eeoc.gov/federal/adr/mediation.cfm.

———. 2007. "Enforcement Guidance: Unlawful Disparate Treatment of Workers with Caregiving Responsibilities." EEOC Notice 915.002. Published May 23. www.eeoc.gov/policy/docs/caregiving.html.

Fernandes, R. 2011. "Facebook Second Most Accessed Site, Behind Google in the US." Tech2. Published December 31. http://tech.firstpost.com/news-analysis/facebook-second-most-accessed-site-behind-google-in-the-us-24393.html.

Guerrero, A. 2013. "7 Tips for Checking Facebook at Work." *U.S. News & World Report*. Published May 29. http://money.usnews.com/money/careers/articles/2013/05/29/7-tips-for-checking-facebook-at-work.

Jones, J. M. 2013. "Same-Sex Marriage Support Solidifies Above 50% in U.S." Gallup. Published May 13. www.gallup.com/poll/162398/sex-marriage-support-solidifies-above.aspx.

Lee, D. 2012. "Facebook Surpasses One Billion Users as It Tempts New Markets." BBC News. Published October 5. www.bbc.com/news/technology-19816709.

National Labor Relations Board. 1997. "Basic Guide to the National Labor Relations Act." Accessed December 23, 2014. www.nlrb.gov/sites/default/files/attachments/basic-page/node-3024/basicguide.pdf.

Protalinski, E. 2011. "Employer Demands Facebook Login Credentials During Interview." ZDNet. Published February 20. www.zdnet.com/blog/facebook/employer-demands-facebook-login-credentials-during-interview/327.

Purcell, A. 2012. "Report of the Acting General Counsel Concerning Social Media Cases." National Labor Relations Board Memorandum OM 12-59. Published May 30. http://mynlrb.nlrb.gov/link/document.aspx/09031d4580a375cd.

Society for Human Resource Management. 2007. *FMLA and Its Impact on Organizations*. Published July. www.shrm.org/research/surveyfindings/documents/fmla%20and%20its%20impact%20on%20organizations%20survey%20report.pdf.

Today Show. 2009. "Dominos Pizza on the Today Show—Workers Fired for Dominos Prank Video." YouTube video from a show televised by NBC. Posted April 17 by "nautques4ever." www.youtube.com/watch?v=xaNuE3DsJHM.

US Department of Labor, Wage and Hour Division. 2014. "Military Family Leave Provisions of the FMLA (Family and Medical Leave Act) Frequently Asked Questions and Answers." Accessed October 21. www.dol.gov/whd/fmla/finalrule/MilitaryFAQs.pdf.

———. 2013a. "The Military Family Leave Provisions Under the Family and Medical Leave Act." Fact Sheet #28M. Revised February. www.dol.gov/whd/regs/compliance/whdfs28m.htm.

———. 2013b. "Family and Medical Leave Act Benefits Workers and Their Families, Employers: US Labor Department Releases Key Findings on Act's 20th Anniversary." News Release 13-0175-NAT. Issued February 4. www.dol.gov/opa/media/press/whd/WHD20130175.htm.

US National Library of Medicine, National Institutes of Health. 2014. "Overweight." MedlinePlus. Updated October 9. www.nlm.nih.gov/medlineplus/ency/article/003101.htm.

Web Resources

- Job Accommodation Network (job accommodation/ADAAA issues): http://askjan.org
- Equal Employment Opportunity Commission: Home, www.eeoc.gov; publications, www.eeoc.gov/eeoc/publications/
- Legal and illegal questions: www.workforce.com/articles/interview-questions-legal-or-illegal
- US Department of Labor Wage and Hour Division: www.dol.gov/whd/
- Strategic HR Inc.'s listing of employment laws broken down by number of employees: http://strategichrinc.com/library/hr-links/

HEALTHCARE PROFESSIONALS

Kenneth R. White and Dolores G. Clement

Learning Objectives

After completing this chapter, the reader should be able to

- understand the role of healthcare professionals in the human resources management function of healthcare organizations;
- define the elements of a profession, with an understanding of the theoretical underpinnings of the healthcare professions in particular;
- describe the healthcare professions, which include the majority of healthcare workers, and the required educational levels, scopes of practice, and licensure issues for each;
- relate knowledge of the healthcare professions to selected human resources management issues and systems development; and
- comprehend the changing nature of the existing and emerging healthcare professions in the healthcare workforce, particularly the impact of managed care.

Introduction

Healthcare professionals are central to the delivery of high-quality healthcare services. Extensive training, education, and skills are essential in meeting the needs and demands of the population for safe, competent healthcare. Healthcare professionals acquire these specialized techniques and skills through systematic programs of intellectual study that are the basis for socialization into their profession. Additionally, the healthcare industry is labor intensive and is distinguished from other service industries by the number of licensed and registered personnel that it employs and the variety of healthcare fields that it encompasses. These healthcare fields have emerged as a result of the specialization of medicine, the increased scope of advanced practice nursing, the development of public health, an increased emphasis on health promotion and prevention, and technological advances and growth.

Because of the division of labor within medical and health services delivery, many tasks that were once the responsibility of physicians are now shared with other healthcare professionals. Healthcare is delivered by interprofessional teams with the physician at the helm, with a greater emphasis on patient- and family-centered care. The collaboration of healthcare delivery teams raises important questions for the industry: What healthcare professions are involved in patient- and family-centered care collaboration? What is the extent of their scope of practice?

This chapter responds to the aforementioned questions by defining key terms, describing the healthcare professions and labor force, explaining the role of human resources (HR) in healthcare, and discussing key HR issues that affect the delivery of healthcare.

Professionalization

Although the terms *occupation* and *profession* often are used interchangeably, they can be differentiated.

An *occupation* enables workers to provide services and is the principal activity that supports one's livelihood. However, it is different from a profession in several ways. An occupation typically does not require higher skill specialization. An individual in an occupation is usually supervised, adheres to a defined work schedule, and earns an hourly wage rate. An individual in an occupation may be trained for a specific job or function and, as a result, is less able to move from one organization to another.

A *profession* requires specialized knowledge and training that enable professionals to gain more authority and responsibility and to provide service that adheres to a code of ethics. A professional usually has more autonomy in determining the content of the service he or she provides and in monitoring the workload needed to do so. A professional generally earns a salary, requires higher education, and works with more independence and mobility than nonprofessionals do.

The distinction between an occupation and a profession is important because the evolving process of healthcare delivery requires professionals who are empowered to make decisions in the absence of direct supervision. The proliferation of knowledge and skills needed in the prevention, diagnosis, and treatment of disease has required increasing levels of education. Undergraduate- or graduate-level degrees are now required for entry into virtually every professional field. Some professions, such as pharmacy, physical therapy, and nursing, are moving toward professional doctorates (i.e., Doctor of Pharmacy [PharmD], Doctor of Physical Therapy [DPT], and Doctor of Nursing Practice [DNP], respectively) for practice.

A countervailing force against the increasing educational requirements of the healthcare professions is ongoing change in the mechanisms for delivery and payment of services. With consolidation of the healthcare system and the rise of managed care, along with its demands for efficiency, fewer financial resources are available. As a result, healthcare organizations are pressured to replace highly trained—and therefore more expensive—healthcare professionals with unlicensed support personnel. Fewer professionals are being asked to do more, and those with advanced degrees are required to supervise more assistants who are functionally trained for specified organizational roles.

Functional training produces personnel who can perform tasks but who may not know the theory behind the practice; understanding theory is essential to becoming fully skilled and being able to make complex management and patient care decisions. Conversely, knowing the theory without having the experience also makes competent practice difficult. When educating potential healthcare professionals, on-the-job training or a period of apprenticeship is needed in addition to basic coursework. Dreyfus and Dreyfus (2009) contend that both theoretical knowledge and practiced response are needed in the acquisition of skill in a profession. These authors lay out five stages of abilities that an individual passes through as he or she develops a skill:

1. *Novice.* At this stage, the novice learns tasks and skills that enable him or her to determine actions based on recognized situations. Rules and guidelines direct the novice's energy and action at this stage.
2. *Advanced beginner.* At this stage, the advanced beginner has gained enough experience and knowledge that certain behaviors become automatic, and he or she can begin to learn when tasks should be addressed.
3. *Competent.* At this stage, the competent individual has mastered the practiced response of definable tasks and processes and has acquired the ability to deal with the unexpected events that may not conform to plans.
4. *Proficient.* At this stage, the proficient individual has developed the ability to discern a situation, intuitively assess it, plan what needs to be done, decide on an action, and perform the action with less effort than in the earlier stages.
5. *Expert.* At this stage, the expert can accomplish the goals without realizing that rules are being followed because the skill and knowledge required to reach the goal have become second nature.

Theoretical understanding is melded with practice in each progressive stage. Functional training can help an individual progress through the first three stages and can provide the individual with the calculative rationality or inferential reasoning ability to be able to apply and improve theories and rules learned. For skill development at the proficient and expert levels, deliberative rationality or the ability to challenge and improve theories and rules learned is required. Healthcare professionals need to become experts in fields where self-direction, autonomy, and decision making for patient care may be required (Dreyfus and Dreyfus 2009).

Healthcare Professionals

The healthcare industry is the largest and most powerful industry in the United States. It constitutes nearly 9 percent of the country's total labor force and 17.9 percent of the gross domestic product (Bureau of Labor Statistics 2013). Healthcare professionals include physicians, nurses, dentists, pharmacists, optometrists, psychologists, nonphysician practitioners such as physician assistants and nurse practitioners, healthcare managers, and allied health professionals. Allied health professionals are a huge group that consists of therapists, medical and radiologic technologists, social workers, health educators, and other ancillary personnel. Healthcare professionals are represented by professional associations. Exhibit 3.1 provides a sample of professional associations in healthcare.

EXHIBIT 3.1
Resource Guide for the Healthcare Professional

Organization	Target Audience	Website
Accrediting Organizations		
Accreditation Association for Ambulatory Health Care	Ambulatory health-care facilities	www.aaahc.org
Accreditation Council for Graduate Medical Education	Graduate medical education programs	www.acgme.org
American Osteopathic Association	Osteopathic hospitals and health systems	www.osteopathic.org
CARF International (formerly Commission on Accreditation of Rehabilitation Facilities)	Rehabilitation facilities	www.carf.org
The Joint Commission	Hospitals and health systems	www.jointcommission.org
National Committee for Quality Assurance	Health plans	www.ncqa.org

(continued)

American Association of Blood Banks	Blood banks	www.aabb.org
American College of Surgeons	Surgeons	www.facs.org
American College of Surgeons: Cancer Programs	Cancer programs	www.facs.org/cancer
College of American Pathologists	Clinical laboratories	www.cap.org
American College of Radiology	Diagnostic imaging	www.acr.org
Professional Associations		
American College of Healthcare Executives	Healthcare executives	www.ache.org http://healthmanagementcareers.org
National Association of Health Services Executives	African-American healthcare executives	www.nahse.org
Medical Group Management Association	Physician practice managers and executives	www.mgma.com
Center for the Health Professions	Health professionals	http://futurehealth.ucsf.edu
American Society for Healthcare Human Resources Administration	Healthcare HR professionals	www.ashhra.org
American Association for Physician Leadership	Physician executives	www.physicianleaders.org
American College of Health Care Administrators	Long-term care administrators	www.achca.org
Association for Healthcare Documentation Integrity	Medical transcriptionists	www.ahdionline.org
American Association of Nurse Anesthetists	Nurse anesthetists	www.aana.com
American Association for Respiratory Care	Respiratory therapists	www.aarc.org
American Health Information Management Association	Medical records and information management professionals	www.ahima.org

EXHIBIT 3.1
Resource Guide for the Healthcare Professional *(continued from previous page)*

(continued)

American Medical Technologists	Medical technologists	www.american medtech.org
American Nurses Association	Registered nurses	www.ana.org
American Association for Homecare	Home health care administrators	www.aahomecare.org
American Occupational Therapy Association, Inc.	Occupational therapists	www.aota.org
American Organization of Nurse Executives	Nurse executives	www.aone.org
National League for Nursing	Nurse faculty and educators	www.nln.org
American Physical Therapy Association	Physical therapists	www.apta.org
American Society for Clinical Pathology	Pathologists and laboratory professionals	www.ascp.org
American Society of Health-System Pharmacists	Health system pharmacists	www.ashp.org
American Society of Radiologic Technologists	Radiologic technologists	www.asrt.org
American Speech-Language-Hearing Association	Speech-language pathologists; audiologists; and speech, language, and hearing scientists	www.asha.org
Healthcare Financial Management Association	Controllers, chief financial officers, and accountants	www.hfma.org
Healthcare Information and Management Systems Society	Health information and technology	www.himss.org
National Cancer Registrars Association	Cancer registry professionals	www.ncra-usa.org
Trade Associations		
American Hospital Association	Hospitals, health systems, and personal membership groups	www.aha.org

(continued)

Federation of American Hospitals	Investor-owned hospitals and health systems	www.fah.org
Association of American Medical Colleges	Teaching hospitals and health systems	www.aamc.org
Catholic Health Association of the United States	Catholic hospitals and health systems	www.chausa.org
America's Health Insurance Plans	Health insurers	www.ahip.org

EXHIBIT 3.1
Resource Guide for the Healthcare Professional
(continued from previous page)

Healthcare professionals work in a variety of settings, including hospitals; ambulatory care centers; managed care organizations; long-term care organizations; mental health organizations; pharmaceutical companies; community health centers; physician offices; laboratories; research institutions; and schools of medicine, nursing, and allied health professions. According to the Bureau of Labor Statistics (2013), healthcare professionals are employed by the following:

- Hospitals (31 percent)
- Nursing and personal and residential care facilities (14 percent)
- Physician offices and clinics (12 percent)
- Home health care services (6 percent)
- Dentist offices and clinics (5 percent)
- Other health service sites (32 percent)

The US Department of Labor recognizes about 400 different job titles in the healthcare sector; however, many of these job titles are not included in the definition of healthcare professionals used in this chapter. For example, almost one-third of those employed in the healthcare sector probably belong in the support staff category—that is, employees who are not part of the patient care team or involved in delivering health services directly. These approximately 2.3 million nursing aides, home health aides, and personal attendants are critical to the delivery of healthcare services (Bureau of Labor Statistics 2013).

The primary reasons for the increased supply of and demand for healthcare professionals include the following interrelated forces:

- Technological growth
- Specialization
- Changes in third-party coverage

- The aging of the population
- The proliferation of new and diverse healthcare delivery settings

This chapter focuses primarily on nurses, pharmacists, selected allied health professionals, and healthcare administrators.

Nurses

The art of caring, combined with the science of healthcare delivery, is the essence of nursing. The common theme that unites different types of nurses who work in varied areas is the nursing process, which is the essential core of practice for delivering holistic, patient-focused care. The nursing process has five components (American Nurses Association 2014b):

1. *Assessment.* This involves collecting and analyzing physical, psychological, sociocultural, spiritual, economic, and lifestyle factors about a patient.
2. *Diagnosis.* The nursing diagnosis is the nurse's clinical judgment about the client's response to actual or potential health conditions or needs.
3. *Outcomes/planning.* Based on the assessment and diagnosis, an individualized care plan is written in the patient's record so that nurses as well as other members of the interprofessional team have access to it.
4. *Implementation.* This includes supervising or carrying out the actual treatment plan and documenting it in the patient's record.
5. *Evaluation.* This focuses on continuous assessment of the plan and modifications, as needed.

Nurses also serve as patient advocates, interprofessional team members, managers, executives, consultants, researchers, and entrepreneurs.

Nurses make up the largest group of licensed healthcare professionals in the United States. According to the National Sample Survey of Registered Nurses (NSSRN), the United States has 3.1 million licensed registered nurses (RNs), of whom more than 2.5 million (84.8 percent) are employed in healthcare organizations (Health Resources and Services Administration [HRSA] 2010). Approximately 62 percent of employed RNs, or 1.6 million, work in hospitals, while more than 18 percent work in ambulatory settings. Complementing this workforce in 2012 were jobs for 738,400 licensed practical nurses (LPNs), or licensed vocational nurses (LVNs) as they are known in some states (Bureau of Labor Statistics 2014b). The projected increase in demand for LPNs/LVNs is expected to be 25 percent by the year 2022, which is faster than average (Bureau of Labor Statistics 2014b).

According to the demographic profiles from the NSSRN (HRSA 2010), most nurses are women. In 2008, the average age of a nurse was 46 years, although a slowdown in the aging trend resulted from an increase in employed RNs younger than 30 years of age—the first increase in this age group since 1977. The number of men in nursing is on the rise, with men accounting for 6.2 percent of employed RNs who were licensed before 2000 and 9.6 percent of those licensed since 2000. Nurses who are from ethnic/racial minority backgrounds represent 16.8 percent of nurses (this figure is up from 11 percent in 2004) (HRSA 2010). Although significant gains have occurred in recruiting underrepresented minorities into nursing, more work is needed to increase the numbers of men and persons from racial/ethnic backgrounds.

Registered Nurses and Licensed Practical Nurses

All US states require nurses to be licensed to practice. The licensure requirements include graduation from an approved nursing program and successful completion of a national examination. Educational preparation distinguishes the two levels of nurses.

RNs must complete an associate degree in nursing, a diploma program, or a baccalaureate degree in nursing (BSN) to qualify for the licensure examination. Associate degree programs generally take two years to complete and are offered by community and junior colleges, and hospital-based diploma programs can be completed in about three years. The fastest growing avenue for nursing education is the baccalaureate preparation, which typically can be completed in four years and is offered by colleges and universities. LPNs, on the other hand, must complete a state-approved program in practical nursing and must achieve a passing score on a national examination. Each state maintains regulations and practice acts that delineate the scope of nursing practice for RNs and LPNs.

An Institute of Medicine (2010) report titled *The Future of Nursing: Leading Change, Advancing Health* recommended higher levels of education in the nursing profession. The purpose of this recommendation was to prepare nurses for the more complex care needs of sicker patients and the sophisticated technologies available for providing care. This report was followed with a specific goal to increase the proportion of baccalaureate-prepared nurses to 80 percent by 2020. As of 2013, 55 percent of the RN workforce held a baccalaureate degree or higher (HRSA 2013). Nurse executives have indicated they have a preference in hiring baccalaureate-prepared nurses, and many organizations have tuition assistance programs to facilitate baccalaureate degree attainment (Pittman et al. 2013).

In addition to licensure and educational achievements, some nurses obtain certification in nursing specialty areas such as acute and critical care, infection control, trauma/emergency, acute care surgery, or obstetrics. The nursing field comprises many specialties and subspecialties; certification in these areas requires specialty education, practical experience, and successful completion of a national examination. Some nurses obtain certification in these specialty areas because certification helps them maintain their competence and membership in professional associations. To remain certified, continued employment, continuing education units, or reexamination may be required.

Advanced Practice Registered Nurses

An advanced practice registered nurse (APRN) is a nurse

1. who has completed an accredited graduate-level education program preparing him/her for one of the four recognized APRN roles;
2. who has passed a national certification examination that measures APRN role and population-focused competencies and who maintains continued competence as evidenced by recertification in the role and population through the national certification program;
3. who has acquired advanced clinical knowledge and skills preparing him/her to provide direct care to patients;
4. whose practice builds on the competencies of registered nurses (RNs) by demonstrating a greater depth and breadth of knowledge, a greater synthesis of data, increased complexity of skills and interventions, and greater role autonomy;
5. who is educationally prepared to assume responsibility and accountability for health promotion and/or maintenance as well as the assessment, diagnosis, and management of patient problems, which includes the use and prescription of pharmacologic and non-pharmacologic interventions; and
6. who has obtained a license to practice as an APRN in one of the four APRN roles: certified registered nurse anesthetist (CRNA), certified nurse midwife (CNM), clinical nurse specialist (CNS), or certified nurse practitioner (CNP). (National Council of State Boards of Nursing 2008, 7)

The Affordable Care Act (Public Law 111-148) includes several sections that specifically address the role of the APRN. It provides federal support for Title VIII of the Public Health Service Act to recruit new nurses into the profession in an attempt to promote career advancement within nursing to improve care delivery and safety. Section 5309 of the Affordable Care Act includes specific funding to promote nurse retention and career advancement. In addition, several sections of the new law provide specific reimbursement or loan forgiveness to nurses who establish careers in public health or nursing research and education (American Nurses Association 2014a).

The APRN role is defined by seven core competencies or skillful performance areas. The first core competency of direct clinical practice is central to and informs all of the other areas, as follows (Hamric 2014):

1. Direct clinical practice (central)
2. Expert coaching and guidance of patients, families, and other care providers
3. Consultation
4. Research and evidence-based practice
5. Clinical, professional, and systems leadership
6. Collaboration
7. Ethical decision making

Additional core competencies may be needed in each specialty area that an APRN pursues. The largest subset of APRNs is made up of nurse practitioners (NPs), who may further specialize in primary or acute care of families or individuals across the life span, adult care or gerontology, neonatology or pediatrics, women's health, or psychiatric and mental health.

Each state maintains its own laws and regulations regarding recognition of an APRN, but the general requirements in all states include licensure as an RN and successful completion of a national specialty examination that measures APRN role and population-focused competencies and includes continued competence renewal. Some states permit certain categories of APRNs to write prescriptions for certain classes of drugs. This prescribing authority varies from one state to another and may be regulated by boards of medicine, nursing, pharmacy, or allied health. Some states require practice agreements for physician supervision or collaboration of APRN practice, although some managed care plans now include APRNs on their lists of primary care providers.

Some APRNs specialize in certain areas of practice. Certified nurse midwives (CNMs) specialize in low-risk obstetric care, including all aspects of the prenatal, labor and delivery, and postnatal processes. Certified registered nurse anesthetists (CRNAs) complete additional education to specialize in the administration of anesthesia and analgesia to patients and clients. Often, nurse anesthetists work collaboratively with surgeons and anesthesiologists as part of the perioperative care team. Clinical nurse specialists (CNSs) hold master's degrees, have successfully completed a specialty certification examination, and are generally employed by hospitals as nursing experts in particular specialties. The scope of the CNS is not as broad as that of the NP; CNSs work with a specialty population under a somewhat circumscribed set of conditions, and the patient management authority still rests with physicians. In contrast, NPs have developed an autonomous role in which their collaboration is encouraged, and they generally have the legal authority to implement management actions. Advanced practice nurses are generally board certified in the practice specialty.

Pharmacists

Up to the latter part of the twentieth century, pharmacists performed the traditional role of preparing drug products and filling prescriptions. Pharmacists now are also key members of healthcare teams and experts for clients and patients on the effects of specific drugs, drug interactions, and generic drug substitutions for brand-name drugs.

To be eligible for licensure, pharmacists must graduate from an accredited bachelor's degree program in pharmacy, successfully complete a state board examination, and obtain practical experience or complete a supervised internship. After passing a national examination, a registered pharmacist (RPh) is permitted to carry out the scope of practice outlined by state regulations. Since 2000, most schools of pharmacy have begun offering only the six-year Doctor of Pharmacy (PharmD) degree. The extensive training of doctorally prepared pharmacists allows them to pursue careers in research, education, healthcare management and leadership, or clinical pharmacy, as a member of interprofessional patient care teams. This educational preparation also requires successful completion of a state board examination and other practical clinical experience, as outlined by state laws.

Allied Health Professionals

Allied health professionals work collaboratively with physicians, nurses, pharmacists, and other healthcare providers (Association of Schools of Allied Health Professions 2014), although an allied health professional may also be a direct provider of health services. The US Public Health Service defines an allied health professional as follows (Health Professions Education Extension Amendments of 1992, Public Health Service Act § 701):

> a health professional (other than a registered nurse or a physician assistant) who has received a certificate, an associate's degree, a bachelor's degree, a master's degree, a doctoral degree, or post-baccalaureate training in a science related to health care; who shares in the responsibility for the delivery of health care services or related services, including (1) services relating to the identification, evaluation and prevention of disease and disorders, (2) dietary and nutrition services, (3) health promotion services, (4) rehabilitation services, or (5) health systems management services; and who has not received a degree of doctor of medicine, a degree of doctor of osteopathy, a degree of doctor of veterinary medicine or equivalent degree, a degree of doctor of optometry or equivalent degree, a degree of doctor of podiatric medicine or equivalent degree, a degree of bachelor of science in pharmacy or equivalent degree, a graduate degree in public health or equivalent degree, a degree of doctor of chiropractic or equivalent degree, a graduate degree in health administration or equivalent degree, a degree of doctor of clinical psychology or equivalent degree, or a degree in social work or equivalent degree.

A debate on the exclusiveness and inclusiveness of this definition continues. Some healthcare observers consider nursing, public health, and social work to fall under the umbrella of allied health, but these professions are often categorized as separate groups. Exhibit 3.2 lists the major categories that compose the allied health profession and the job titles and a sample of positions that normally fall under each category.

EXHIBIT 3.2
Major Categories of the Allied Health Profession and Professional Titles

Behavioral Health Services

- Substance abuse counselor
- Home health aide
- Mental health aide
- Community health worker
- Mental health assistant

Clinical Laboratory Sciences

- Laboratory associate
- Laboratory technician
- Laboratory microbiologist
- Chemist (biochemist)
- Microbiologist
- Associate laboratory microbiologist

Dental Services

- Dental assistant
- Dental laboratory technologist
- Dental hygienist

Dietetic Services

- Dietitian
- Dietary assistant
- Assistant director of food service
- Associate supervising dietitian

Emergency Medical Services

- Ambulance technician
- Emergency medical technician

Health Information Management Services

- Director of medical records
- Assistant director of medical records
- Medical record specialist
- Coder
- Senior analyst of medical records
- Health information manager
- Data analyst

Medical and Surgical Services

- Electroencephalograph technician
- Electroencephalograph technologist
- Operating room technician
- Biomedical equipment technician
- Biomedical engineer
- Cardiovascular technologist
- Medical equipment specialist
- Electrocardiograph technician
- Dialysis technologist
- Surgical assistant
- Ambulatory care technician

(continued)

EXHIBIT 3.2
Major
Categories
of the Allied
Health
Profession and
Professional
Titles
*(continued from
previous page)*

Occupational Therapy

- Occupational therapist
- Occupational therapy assistant
- Occupational therapy aide

Ophthalmology

- Ophthalmic technician
- Optometric aide
- Optician

Orthotics/Prosthetics

- Orthopedic assistant

Physical Therapy

- Physical therapist
- Physical therapy assistant

Radiological Services

- Nuclear medicine technician
- Radiation technician
- Ultrasound technician
- Medical radiation dosimetrist
- Nuclear medicine technologist
- Diagnostic medical sonographer
- Radiologic (medical) technologist

Rehabilitation Services

- Art therapist
- Exercise physiologist
- Recreational therapist
- Recreation therapy assistant
- Addiction counselor
- Addiction specialist
- Psychiatric social health technician
- Music therapist
- Dance therapist
- Rehabilitation counselor
- Rehabilitation technician
- Sign-language interpreter

Respiratory Therapy Services

- Respiratory therapist
- Respiratory therapy assistant
- Respiratory therapy technician

Speech-Language Pathology/Audiology Services

- Audiology clinician
- Staff speech pathologist
- Staff audiologist
- Speech clinician

Other Allied Health Services

- Central supply technician
- Podiatric assistant
- Health unit coordinator
- Home health aide
- Medical illustrator
- Veterinary assistant
- Chiropractic assistant

According to the 2012 National Occupational and Wage Estimates, the allied health professions and occupations (licensed and unlicensed) constitute 52.8 percent of the healthcare workforce in the United States (Bureau of Labor Statistics 2013). This number excludes physicians, nurses, dentists, pharmacists, veterinarians, chiropractors, optometrists, and podiatrists. The allied health profession is the most heterogeneous of the personnel groupings in healthcare, and its members are integral to interprofessional teams.

The Institute of Medicine (2011) acknowledges that no single definition of allied health or list of allied health professionals exists. Collectively putting the variety of professions together to constitute one large group is somewhat arbitrary, yet the roles and responsibilities are critical to health services delivery. Allied health professionals can be divided generally into two subcategories of personnel: (1) therapists/ technologists and (2) technicians/assistants. Some of the job titles presented in Exhibit 3.2 may not fit into these two categories. In general, the therapist/technologist category represents those who have higher-level professional training and who are often responsible for supervising those in the technician/assistant category.

Therapists/technologists usually hold a bachelor's or higher-level degree, and they are trained to evaluate patients, understand diagnoses, and develop treatment plans in their area of expertise. On the other hand, technicians/assistants are most likely to have two years of postsecondary education or less, and they are functionally trained with procedural skills for specified tasks.

Educational and training programs for the allied health profession are sponsored by a variety of organizations in different academic and clinical settings. They range from degree offerings at colleges and universities to clinical programs in hospitals and other health facilities. The Association of Schools of Allied Health Professions (2013) membership includes 119 academic institutions, two accreditation agencies, and individual members. In addition to four-year academic institutions, community colleges, vocational or technical schools, and academic health centers can all sponsor allied health programs. These programs can also be stand-alone when aligned with an academic health center, or they can be under the auspices of the school of medicine or nursing if a specific school of allied health professions does not exist. Dental and pharmacy technicians/assistants may be trained in their respective schools or in a school of allied health professions.

A vast number of undergraduate allied health programs are accredited by the Commission on Accreditation of Allied Health Education Programs (CAAHEP), a freestanding agency that in 1994 replaced the American Medical Association's Committee on Allied Health Education and Accreditation. The formation of CAAHEP was intended to simplify the accrediting process, to be more inclusive of allied health programs that provide entry-level education, and to serve as an initiator of more far-reaching change. Some key allied health graduate programs, such as physical therapy and occupational therapy, are accredited through specialty professional accreditation organizations.

Healthcare Managers

Healthcare managers organize, coordinate, and manage the delivery of health services; provide leadership; and guide the strategic direction of healthcare organizations. The variety and numbers of healthcare professionals they employ, the complexity of healthcare delivery, and environmental pressures to provide access, quality, and efficient services make healthcare institutions among the most complex organizations to manage.

Healthcare management is taught at the undergraduate and graduate levels in a variety of settings, and these programs lead to a number of different degrees. The settings include schools of medicine, public health, healthcare business, and allied health professions. A bachelor's degree in health administration allows individuals to pursue positions such as nursing home administrator, supervisor, or middle manager in healthcare organizations. Most students who aspire to have a career in healthcare management go on to receive a master's degree.

Graduate education programs in healthcare management are accredited by the Commission on Accreditation of Healthcare Management Education. The most common degrees include the master of health administration (MHA), master of business administration (MBA) with a healthcare emphasis, master of public health (MPH), or master of public administration (MPA). However, the MHA degree, or its equivalent, has been the accepted training model for entry-level managers in the healthcare industry. The MHA program, in contrast to the MPH program, offers core courses that focus on building business management (theory and applied management), quantitative, and analytical skills and that emphasize experiential training. In addition, some MHA programs require students to complete three-month internships or 12-month residencies as part of their two- or three-year curricula. Some graduates elect to complete postgraduate fellowships that are available in selected hospitals, health systems, managed care organizations, consulting firms, and other health-related organizations.

A growing number of healthcare managers are physicians and other clinicians. As evidence, membership in the American Association for Physician Leadership (formerly the American College of Physician Executives) has increased to more than 11,000 in 2014, more than double the number in 1990 (American Association for Physician Leadership 2014). Physicians, nurses, and other clinicians refocus their careers on the business side of the enterprise, getting involved in the strategy, decision making, resource allocation, and operations of healthcare organizations. A traditional management role for physician executives is the chief medical officer (or a similar position) in a hospital, overseeing the medical staff and serving as a liaison between clinical care and administration. Likewise, a typical management career path for nurses is to become the chief nursing officer, with responsibility for the clinical care provided by employed professional staff.

Typically, chief medical officers begin their careers practicing medicine, then slowly transition into the operations side of healthcare. However, physician executives work at every level and in every setting in healthcare. Many physician executives earn a graduate degree such as an MHA or an MBA if they are interested in pursuing a formal educational program in healthcare management. As of 2015, 75 medical schools offer a combined MD/MBA program (Association of American Medical Colleges 2014), and MD/MHA degrees have also proliferated. Whether physician executives start as managers or later shift to become executives after clinical practice, they represent an alternative way to make an impact on healthcare delivery.

Nursing home administrator programs require students to pass a national examination administered by the National Association of Long Term Care Administrator Boards. Passing this examination is a standard requirement in all states, but the educational preparation needed to qualify for this exam varies from state to state. Although more than one-third of states still allow less than a bachelor's degree as the minimum academic preparation, approximately 70 percent of practicing nursing home administrators have, at a minimum, a bachelor's degree. As the population continues to live longer, the demand and educational requirements for long-term care administrators are predicted to increase, along with the growth of educational programs targeted to this sector.

Considerations for Human Resources Management

The role of HR management in healthcare organizations is to develop and implement systems, in accordance with regulatory guidelines and licensure laws, for selection, evaluation, and retention of healthcare professionals. In light of this role, HR personnel should be aware that each of the healthcare professions, and often the subspecialties within those professions, has specific requirements that allow an individual to qualify for an entry-level job in his or her chosen profession. The requirements of national accrediting organizations (e.g., The Joint Commission), regulatory bodies (e.g., the Centers for Medicare & Medicaid Services), and licensure authorities (e.g., state licensure boards) should be considered in all aspects of HR management. This section briefly discusses some of the issues that a healthcare organization's HR department must consider when dealing with healthcare professionals.

Qualifications
In developing a comprehensive employee-compensation program, HR personnel must include the specific skill and knowledge required for each job in the organization. Those qualifications must be determined and stated in writing for each job. The job description usually contains the level of education,

experience, judgment ability, accountability, physical skills, responsibilities, communication skills, and any special certification or licensure requirements. HR personnel need to be aware of all specifications for all job titles within the organization. This knowledge of healthcare professionals is necessary to ensure that essential qualifications of individuals coincide with job specifications, and it is also necessary for determining wage and salary ranges (see Chapter 6).

Licensure and Certification

An HR department must have policies and procedures that describe the way in which licensure is verified on initial employment. Also, HR must have a system in place for tracking the expiration dates of licenses and for ensuring licensure renewal. Therefore, HR employees must be conscious of whether the information received is a *primary verification* (in which the information directly comes from the licensing authority) or a *secondary verification* (in which a candidate submits a document copy that indicates licensure has been granted, including the expiration date). Certifications must be verified during the selection process, although certifications and licenses are generally not statutory requirements. Many healthcare organizations accept a copy of a certification document as verification. If the certification is a job requirement, systems must be in place to track expiration dates and to access new certification documents.

Career Ladders

In selecting healthcare professionals, HR personnel must consider past employment history, including the explanation of gaps in employment. To assess the amount of individual experience, evaluating the candidate's breadth and depth of responsibility in previous jobs is essential. Many healthcare organizations have career ladders, which are mechanisms that advance a healthcare professional within the organization. Career ladders are based on the Dreyfus and Dreyfus model of novice to expert (explained earlier in the chapter), and experience may be used as a criterion for assignment of an individual to a particular job category. In addition, healthcare organizations may conduct annual reviews of employees who have leadership and management potential. This review entails HR working with senior management to assess the competency, ability, and career progression of employees on an ongoing basis.

Educational Services

Healthcare professionals require continuous, lifelong learning. Healthcare organizations must have in-house training and development plans to ensure that their healthcare professionals achieve competency in new technologies, programs, and equipment and are aware of policy and procedure changes.

Certain competencies must be renewed annually in areas such as cardiopulmonary resuscitation, safety and infection control, and disaster planning.

In addition to developing specific training programs, healthcare organizations should provide orientation for all new employees and interprofessional team training programs. Such organization-specific training enables the leadership to share the values, mission, goals, and policies of the institution. Such clear communication often serves as a retention tool that enables employees to better understand how the organization works and how to be successful in that organization. Similarly, some professions and licensing jurisdictions may require continuing education that is profession specific.

A healthcare organization can provide training and development in a variety of ways. On one end of the spectrum, training and development can be outsourced to a firm that specializes in conducting educational programs. Conversely, another option is to consolidate all training and development in-house, typically managed by the HR department. Regardless of how each healthcare organization provides continuing education, training and development should be a priority. Strong programs can be viewed as recruitment and retention tools. Therefore, healthcare organizations must be cognizant of fiscal resources necessary to support these educational requirements.

Practitioner Impairment

Healthcare professionals are accountable to the public for maintaining high professional standards, and the governing body of a healthcare organization is, by statute, responsible for the quality of care rendered in the organization. This quality is easily jeopardized by an impaired practitioner. An *impaired practitioner* is a healthcare professional who is unable to carry out his or her professional duties with reasonable skill and safety because of a physical or mental illness, including deterioration through aging, loss of motor skill, or excessive use of drugs and alcohol.

The HR department must periodically evaluate the performance of all healthcare professionals in the organization to ensure their competence (i.e., the basic education and training necessary for the job) and proficiency (i.e., the demonstrated ability to perform job tasks). Mechanisms to identify and deal with the impaired practitioner, such as policies and procedures that describe how the organization will handle investigations, subsequent recommendations for treatment, monitoring, and employment restrictions or separation, must be in place. Hospitals, for instance, usually have a process in place for the governing board (which has the ultimate responsibility for the quality of care delivered in the organization) to review provider credentials and performance and to oversee any employment actions. Each national or state licensing authority maintains legal requirements for reporting impaired practitioners.

As a result of ever-increasing changes in the health professions, new challenges and opportunities, such as the issues described in this section, will face the HR department of every healthcare organization in the foreseeable future.

Changing Nature of the Health Professions

Changes in the organization and financing of healthcare services have shifted delivery from the hospital to outpatient facilities, the home, long-term care facilities, and the community. This trend is largely the result of three major forces: (1) a shift in managed care reimbursement to outpatient settings and a focus on cost containment; (2) technological advances, such as telemedicine and the electronic health record; and (3) medical innovation—specifically, the fact that the science of medicine has progressed to the point that complicated procedures that once required several nights of stay can now be treated with a simple procedure or even solely with medication. These changes are intended to improve the delivery of healthcare while reducing cost and increasing access for patients.

As the setting for the delivery of care continued to change, so did arrangements between physicians and healthcare organizations. For instance, physicians can function as individual providers (in either solo or group practice) and refer patients to the hospital. Typically, these private-practice doctors have admitting privileges to the hospital but are not governed by the hospital, do not serve as attending physicians, and infrequently participate on hospital committees. Physicians considered "on staff" at any hospital refer and treat patients at that hospital. They are credentialed by the hospital credentialing committee (usually managed by the chief of staff office) and are governed by the medical staff bylaws. This scenario is a common type of hospital–physician arrangement.

However, a trend toward employment of physicians by hospitals has been growing. In this arrangement, physicians are on staff, referring to and treating at only the hospital that employs them. Because they are considered employees, physicians not only are held to the HR policies of the healthcare organization but also are governed by the medical staff bylaws. Physicians who are employed by a hospital can also maintain a private practice.

Finally, the field of hospitalists is also growing. Typically, these physicians do not run their own practice aside from their hospital employment. Hospitalists work full time for the hospital and are trained in delivering specialized inpatient care. Regardless of the type of arrangement, most hospitals have a chief medical officer, or a similar position, who oversees the roles and responsibilities of the hospitalist as a member of the medical staff; the hospitalist's employee issues and responsibilities are typically managed by the HR department. These hospital–physician arrangements get more complex in academic medical centers, which must integrate the roles and responsibilities of the physicians, the hospital, and the medical school.

As a result of the changing environment and declining reimbursement, more primary care physicians are joining or forming group practices. Large physician-owned group practices offer several advantages to physicians, including competitive advantage with vendors and manufacturers, improved negotiating power with managed care organizations, shared risk and decision making, and improved flexibility and choice for patients. Physicians usually own or share ownership in the group practice and therefore are responsible for the business operations. Typically, group practices employ an office manager who works closely with the physicians to manage the day-to-day operations. Often, a full-time administrator is on staff not only to manage everyday issues but also to formulate strategies and oversee personnel, billing and collection, purchasing, patient flow, and other functions. Many group practices opt to outsource their business functions, including HR, to specialized firms. For complete details on medical practice management, go to www.mgma.com.

These shifts in healthcare settings and arrangements have changed the roles, functions, and expectations of the healthcare workforce and have led to the emergence of the following issues.

Supply and Demand

Over time, the nursing labor market has cycled through periods of shortages and surpluses (Auerbach, Buerhaus, and Staiger 2011). Indicators of demand include numbers of vacancies, turnover rates, and an increase in salaries. To fill positions, hospitals—the largest employers of nurses and allied health professionals—have raised salaries, provided scholarships, and given other incentives such as sign-on bonuses and tuition reimbursement.

The supply of nurses and allied health professionals is reflected in the number of students in educational programs and those available for the healthcare workforce. The future supply of such professionals continues to be threatened by the following factors:

- *The aging of the nursing workforce.* According to the results of the 2010 National Sample Survey of Registered Nurses (HRSA 2010), 55 to 67 percent of nurse faculty are aged 46–60, while only 25 to 34 percent are aged 30–45. Only 1 to 2 percent are under 30 years. In 2012, 40 percent of associate degree nurse faculty, 53 percent of baccalaureate nurse faculty, and 58 percent of both master's and doctoral faculty positions remained unfilled. Additionally, from 2003 to 2009 the percentage of students who are older than 30 years increased from 41 percent to 49 percent in associate degree nursing programs, while the percentage dropped from 21 percent to 14 percent in baccalaureate nursing programs. The lack of younger nurses in faculty positions is apparent.

- *The barriers to available educational resources.* In an American Association of Colleges of Nursing (2014) faculty vacancy survey, the 680 schools of nursing that responded had an average of 2.0 full-time faculty vacancies per school and a range of 1 to 29. According to the National League for Nursing's (2013) annual survey of schools of nursing, three factors were cited as the main contributors to inhibiting basic RN educational opportunities: lack of clinical placements (44 percent), lack of faculty (30 percent), and lack of classroom space (10 percent). By contrast, graduate programs consistently cite a lack of faculty as the primary obstacle to increasing enrollments.

- *The lack of capacity to accept qualified applicants.* The number of basic RN programs grew throughout the mid-2000s, and admissions statistics indicate that capacity shortages began to ease (National League for Nursing 2013). However, in 2012, 28 percent of qualified applicants were turned away from basic nursing programs (associate degree, diploma, baccalaureate) (National League for Nursing 2013).

As a result, recruitment of nursing and allied health profession students has become a major focus of practitioners, professional associations, and academic institutions. In response, healthcare organizations (in addition to increasing salaries) are developing innovative ways to recruit and retain nurses and allied health professionals. Such developments include opening or sponsoring new schools, offering shorter and more flexible shifts, and providing child care.

Complementary and Alternative Medicine Therapies

Complementary and alternative medicine (CAM) therapies have gained more popularity, judging by the growing number of publications on this topic in the lay press and in academic literature. A turning point in this acceptance and increased respectability was the seminal study of the prevalence of the use of alternative or unconventional therapies (Eisenberg et al. 1993). In the study, Eisenberg and colleagues concluded that one in three adults relied on treatments and interventions that are not widely taught at medical schools in the United States; examples of these alternative interventions included acupuncture, chiropractic, and massage therapies. Consumers (Laiyemo et al. 2014) and healthcare workers (Johnson et al. 2012) are using more CAM therapies—often without informing their doctors. In recognizing the growing demand for CAM therapies, health systems are pursuing integration of conventional medical care with CAM therapies, often referred to as "integrative health" (Knutson et al. 2013). Integrative health as a specialty area may be increasingly considered an emerging healthcare profession.

Nonphysician Licensed Independent Practitioners

With the Affordable Care Act, greater reliance has been placed on nonphysician licensed independent practitioners (LIPs). Collaborative practice models with nurse practitioners, physician assistants, pharmacists, and other therapists are appropriate in both acute and long-term healthcare delivery. Strides have been made in the direct reimbursement for some LIP services, which is an impetus for further collaboration in practice.

Recruitment and Retention

Recruitment and retention of healthcare professionals are important in the face of continuing shortages in key healthcare professions, including nursing and allied health professions. In October 2014, the Bureau of Labor Statistics (2014a) released a report indicating that job growth in the healthcare sector was responsible for 20 percent of the new jobs created. With this growing demand, a significant RN workforce shortage is projected to spread across the country in the next two decades, with more shortage intensity in the South and the West (Juraschek et al. 2012). These shortages require current professionals to treat more patients and to work longer hours. Such conditions can contribute to individual moral distress and burnout, emergency department diversions, increased patient wait times, threatened patient safety, and unfavorable patient outcomes (Blegen et al. 2011; Tubbs-Cooley et al. 2013).

In response, healthcare organizations need to develop and execute recruitment and retention programs. These programs require senior management support and dedicated financial and human resources. Such programs should focus on building a culture of employee engagement and retention, attracting the new generation of workers, and redesigning work processes (American Hospital Association 2010). While salary is an important aspect of employee recruitment and retention, other aspects of work are also influential, such as leadership support, ability to contribute to the organization and provide quality care to patients, degree of autonomy, positive relationships with direct supervisors and peers, good working conditions, and ability to maintain work/life balance. Additional tools for retaining employees include conducting employee-engagement surveys, providing mentoring, and making training programs available.

One innovative way to differentiate a hospital from its competitors, which helps in recruitment and retention, is to achieve Magnet status. The American Nurses Credentialing Center's Magnet Recognition Program was developed in 1993 as a way to specifically recognize excellence in nursing services at the institutional level and to benchmark best practices to be disseminated throughout the industry. Hospitals that apply for and achieve Magnet status have created and demonstrated a professional practice environment that ensures quality outcomes. These hospitals are recognized for their best practices in nursing care, improved patient outcomes, and increased workplace satisfaction. The actual evaluation process is based on five model components: transformational leadership; structural empowerment; exemplary professional practice; new knowledge, innovation, and improvements; and empirical quality results. For more information on Magnet status, see www.nursecredentialing.org/Magnet/ProgramOverview.

Entrepreneurship

Given the bureaucratic nature of organizations, the regulation of the healthcare industry, and additional constraints by payers and managed care, many healthcare professionals are choosing to pursue opportunities on their own. The service economy coupled with knowledge-based professions may encourage pursuit of new and different ventures for individuals who have the personality, skills, and tenacity to go into business for themselves. An entrepreneur must have a mix of management skills and the means to depart from a traditional career path to practice on one's own.

White and Begun (1998) characterize the entrepreneurial personality traits of a profession in terms of the willingness to take the risks associated with undertaking new ventures. Each profession may be categorized either as defending the status quo, which therefore entails little risk (defender professions), or as looking for new and different opportunities with greater risk (prospector professions). White and Begun view the more entrepreneurial professions as more diversified in terms of processes and services delivered. The accrediting bodies of such entrepreneurial professions encourage educational innovation that may extend to nontraditional careers. Each of the healthcare professions has, to greater or lesser extents, defender and prospector aspects.

Workforce Diversity

Each of the healthcare professions must continue to monitor and encourage diversity in its membership because the demographic shifts occurring in the United States will have an impact on the workforce composition in the coming decades. Although workforce diversity is a broad concept, it focuses on differences in gender, age, race, and sexual orientation; these aspects reflect not only the population that healthcare serves but also the people who provide the services. Some professions are dominated by one gender or the other, which is illustrated by the predominantly female field of nursing or the historically predominantly male field of healthcare management. The healthcare management profession, however, has made strides as more female managers have entered the field. Labor shortages and employee turnover are common in the healthcare professions. Consequently, healthcare executives must balance the needs of new entrants into the profession and those already in the profession. The diversity of the members of a profession should reflect the diversity of the members of the population being served.

Summary

Healthcare professionals are a large segment of the US labor force. Historically, the development of healthcare professionals is related to the following trends:

- Supply and demand
- Increased use of technology
- Changes in disease and illness
- The impact of healthcare financing and delivery

The healthcare workforce is widely diverse. The different levels of education, scopes of practice, and practice settings contribute to the complexity of managing this workforce. The coming decades will be characterized by some reforms within the healthcare professions because of increasing pressures to finance and deliver healthcare with higher-quality, lower-cost, and measurable outcomes.

Discussion Questions

1. Describe the process of professionalization. What is the difference between a profession and an occupation?

2. Describe the major types of healthcare professionals (excluding physicians and dentists) and their roles, training, licensure requirements, and practice settings.

3. Describe and apply the issues of HR management and systems development to healthcare professionals.

4. How has managed care affected the healthcare professions?

5. Which nonphysician practitioners provide primary care? What is their role in the delivery of health services?

Experiential Exercise

The purpose of this exercise is to give you an opportunity to explore one healthcare profession in detail. From all of the healthcare professions, select one for analysis. Exhibit 3.1 provides a starting point for selection. Describe the following characteristics of the profession you selected:

- Knowledge base
- Collective goals
- Training
- Licensure (this varies by state)
- Number of professionals in practice, categorized according to
  - Vertical differentiation (position, experience, education level)
  - Horizontal differentiation (geography, practice setting, specialty)
- History and evolution of the profession
- Professional associations and their roles
- Competitor professions
- Strategic issues that face the profession and the profession's position on these issues

To get started on this exercise, you may wish to go to the websites of professional organizations and state licensing boards. You may also interview members of the profession as well as leaders in the field.

References

American Association of Colleges of Nursing. 2014. *Special Survey on Vacant Faculty Positions for Academic Year 2013–2014.* Accessed December 16. www.aacn. nche.edu/leading-initiatives/research-data/vacancy13.pdf.

American Association for Physician Leadership. 2014. "Introducing: American Association for Physician Leadership." Published September 22. www. physicianleaders.org/news/press-releases/2014/09/22/introducing-american-association-for-physician-leadership.

American Hospital Association. 2010. *Workforce 2015: Strategy Trumps Shortage.* Published January. www.aha.org/advocacy-issues/workforce/workforce2015. shtml.

American Nurses Association (ANA). 2014a. "Health Care Reform and the APRN." Accessed December 31. www.nursingworld.org/EspeciallyForYou/Advanced PracticeNurses/Health-Care-Reform-and-the-APRN.

———. 2014b. "The Nursing Process." Accessed December 31. www.nursingworld. org/EspeciallyForYou/What-is-Nursing/Tools-You-Need/Thenursing process.html.

Association of American Medical Colleges. 2014. "MD/MBA Programs." Accessed December 16. http://services.aamc.org/30/msar/home.

Association of Schools of Allied Health Professions. 2014. "Allied Health Professionals." Accessed December 16. www.asahp.org/wp-content/uploads/2014/08/Health-Professions-Facts.pdf.

————. 2013. *Annual Report*. Accessed December 16. www.asahp.org/wp-content/uploads/2014/01/2013-Annual-Report.pdf.

Auerbach, D. I., P. I. Buerhaus, and D. O. Staiger. 2011. "Registered Nurse Supply Grows Faster Than Projected Amid Surge in New Entrants Ages 23–26." *Health Affairs* 30 (12): 2286–92.

Blegen, M. A., C. J. Goode, J. Spetz, T. Vaughn, and S. H. Park. 2011. "Nurse Staffing Effects on Patient Outcomes: Safety-Net and Non-Safety-Net Hospitals." *Medical Care* 49 (4): 406–14.

Bureau of Labor Statistics. 2014a. *Current Employment Statistics Highlights*. Published November. www.bls.gov/web/empsit/ceshighlights.pdf.

————. 2014b. *Occupational Outlook Handbook, 2014–15 Edition: Licensed Practical and Licensed Vocational Nurses*. Accessed December 16. www.bls.gov/ooh/healthcare/licensed-practical-and-licensed-vocational-nurses.htm.

————. 2013. "May 2012 National Occupational Employment and Wage Estimates United States." Accessed September 11. www.bls.gov/oes/current/oes_nat.htm#29-0000.

Dreyfus, H. L., and S. E. Dreyfus. 2009. "The Relationship of Theory and Practice in the Acquisition of Skill." In *Expertise in Nursing Practice: Caring, Clinical Judgment, and Ethics*, second edition, edited by P. Benner, C. A. Tanner, and C. A. Chesla, 1–24. New York: Springer.

Eisenberg, D. M., R. D. Kessler, C. Foster, R. E. Norlock, D. R. Calkins, and T. L. Delbanco. 1993. "Unconventional Medicine in the United States." *New England Journal of Medicine* 328 (24): 246–52.

Hamric, A. B. 2014. "Hamric's Integrated Model of Advanced Practice Nursing." In *Advanced Practice Nursing: An Integrative Approach*, fifth edition, edited by A. B. Hamric, C. M. Hanson, M. F. Tracy, and E. T. O'Grady, 44–45. St. Louis, MO: Elsevier Saunders.

Health Professions Education Extension Amendments of 1992, Public Health Service Act § 701. Washington, DC: Government Printing Office.

Health Resources and Services Administration (HRSA). 2013. *The U.S. Nursing Workforce: Trends in Supply and Education*. Published April. http://bhpr.hrsa.gov/healthworkforce/reports/nursingworkforce/nursingworkforcefullreport.pdf.

————. 2010. *The Registered Nurse Population: Findings from the 2008 National Sample Survey of Registered Nurses*. Published September. http://bhpr.hrsa.gov/healthworkforce/supplydemand/nursing/rnsamplesurvey/rnsurveyfinal.pdf.

Institute of Medicine. 2011. *Allied Health Workforce and Services: Workshop Summary*. Washington, DC: National Academies Press.

————. 2010. *The Future of Nursing: Leading Change, Advancing Health*. Washington, DC: National Academies Press.

Johnson, P. J., A. Ward, L. Knutson, and S. Sendelbach. 2012. "Personal Use of Complementary and Alternative Medicine (CAM) by U.S. Health Care Workers." *Health Services Research* 47 (1, pt. 1): 211–27.

Juraschek, S. P., X. Zhang, V. Ranganathan, and V. W. Lin. 2012. "United States Registered Nurse Workforce Report Card and Shortage Forecast." *American Journal of Medical Quality* 27 (3): 241–49.

Knutson, L., P. J. Johnson, A. Sidebottom, and A. Fyfe-Johnson. 2013. "Development of a Hospital-Based Integrative Healthcare Program." *Journal of Nursing Administration* 43 (2): 101–7.

Laiyemo, M. A., G. Nunlee-Bland, F. A. Lombardo, R. G. Adams, and A. O. Laiyemo. 2014. "Characteristics and Health Perceptions of Complementary and Alternative Medicine Users in the United States." *American Journal of the Medical Sciences*. Published November 6. doi: 10.1097/MAJ.0000000000000363.

National Council of State Boards of Nursing. 2008. *Consensus Model for APRN Regulation: Licensure, Accreditation, Certification & Education*. Report of the APRN Consensus Work Group and the National Council of State Boards of Nursing APRN Advisory Committee. Published July 7. www.ncsbn.org/Consensus_Model_for_APRN_Regulation_July_2008.pdf.

National League for Nursing. 2013. *Annual Survey of Schools of Nursing, Fall 2012*. Accessed December 19. www.nln.org/researchgrants/slides/index.htm.

Pittman, P., C. N. Herrera, K. Horton, P. A. Thompson, J. M. Ware, and M. Terry. 2013. "Healthcare Employers' Policies on Nurse Education." *Journal of Health Administration* 58 (6): 399–411.

Tubbs-Cooley, H. L., J. P. Cimiotti, J. H. Silber, D. M. Sloane, and L. H. Aiken. 2013. "An Observational Study of Nurse Staffing Ratios and Hospital Readmission Among Children Admitted for Common Conditions." *BMJ Quality & Safety* 22 (9): 735–42.

White, K. R., and J. W. Begun. 1998. "Nursing Entrepreneurship in an Era of Chaos and Complexity." *Nursing Administration Quarterly* 22 (2): 40–47.

CREDENTIALING OF HEALTHCARE PROVIDERS

John C. Hyde II

Learning Objectives

After completing this chapter, the reader should be able to

- understand the overall need for credentialing and privileging,
- define the steps and elements of the credentialing and privileging process,
- discuss the relationships between quality outcomes and credentialing and privileging, and
- discuss future issues related to credentialing and privileging.

Introduction

From a conceptual perspective, the healthcare facility is charged by federal and state governments and by accrediting bodies, such as The Joint Commission, with ensuring that its medical staff possess the requisite licensure, training, experience, certifications, and health status necessary to provide patient care in a safe and effective manner. With increasing public awareness of the movement for healthcare quality and increasing public access to provider outcome measures, the healthcare facility is bound to undertake a credentialing and privileging process that meets these requirements and serves to assure the public that all providers will be fully vetted under the prevailing standards of healthcare administration. Credentialing "involves the collection, verification, and assessment of information regarding three critical parameters: current licensure; education and relevant training; and experience, ability, and current competence to perform the requested privilege(s)" (Joint Commission 2014, MS-24–MS-25). *Privileging* in this context refers to the demonstrated and verifiable ability and subsequent approval to perform specific elements of a practitioner's specialty (such as heart valve replacement surgery by a cardiothoracic or cardiovascular surgeon).

According to The Joint Commission (2014, MS-15),

> The organized medical staff is structured such that it has the ability to function in guiding and governing its members. The primary function of the organized medical staff is to approve and amend medical staff bylaws and to provide oversight for the quality of care, treatment, and services provided by practitioners with privileges.

Given the expectation of oversight and primary responsibility for ensuring that the hospital's medical staff performs at the prevailing standard of care, more than 30 states have adopted a legal cause of action, or the right of the patient to sue the healthcare facility, over negligent credentialing or privileging and lack of administrative oversight to protect the public from improperly credentialed and privileged physicians and other nonemployee healthcare providers. Although this chapter focuses on the physician members of the medical staff, identical issues are subsumed in the credentialing and privileges of independent practitioners or those who practice in hospitals under the guidance or supervision of physicians, including dentists, podiatrists, psychologists, certified registered nurse anesthetists, midwives, physician assistants, and advanced practice nurse practitioners. This category varies among states, and specific requirements are spelled out in each state's practice regulations for a given type of practitioner.

Healthcare management literature (Hyde 2003; Rolph, Adams, and McGuigan 2007; Williams et al. 2005) has established that quality outcomes are tied to adherence to prevailing standards established through mandates such as Medicare's Conditions of Participation, which requires that a hospital "have an organized medical staff that operates under bylaws approved by the governing body and is responsible for the quality of medical care provided to patients by the hospital" and specifies that "the medical staff must examine the credentials of candidates for medical staff membership and make recommendations to the governing body on appointment" (42 C.F.R. § 482.22). This mandate clearly specifies that while the medical staff examines and recommends medical staff on the basis of credentials and privileges, the governing body, or the hospital in this instance, is ultimately responsible for the medical care delivered by these credentialed and privileged physicians.

These administrative mandates require the facility's management to provide oversight and leadership in the credentialing/privileging process. This level of involvement is obviously tied to the organization's financial and long-term viability. No healthcare facility can survive while providing a substandard level of care given the increasing competition and the public's demand for not only affordable but also high-quality care. Further, the hospital's failure to provide sufficient oversight and not simply rubber-stamp the medical staff's recommendations for privileges becomes the basis for hospital culpability in credentialing and privileging decisions. Therefore, healthcare managers must treat this obligation as such and ensure that their participation is active and thorough. No longer can the credentialing/privileging process be left to administrative clerks, because the failure to properly credential and privilege medical staff members has the potential to catastrophically harm the institution.

Historical Background

The idea that patient quality outcomes are linked to provider ability is not new. The origins of medical and surgical educational standards can be traced to the American College of Surgeons (founded in 1913), the American College of Physicians (founded in 1915), and the American Board of Medical Specialties (founded in 1933). While these organizations were concerned with the overall education and practice of physicians, the formation in 1951 of the organization that came to be known as The Joint Commission brought about a hospital partnership with medical associations to conduct regular peer review of physicians and other providers, not only to qualify for accreditation but also to address the linkage between provider ability and patient outcomes.

With the advent of Medicare (in 1965) and Medicaid (in 1966) as funders of medical care, the federal government entered the area of credentialing and privileging through the establishment of the Conditions of Participation (42 C.F.R. § 482.22), which mandated, among other things, the creation of organized medical staffs charged with the responsibility of patient outcomes within the hospital as well as in other practice venues. Since the federal government funds upward of 60 percent of all US healthcare expenditures through these programs, their mandates become standards for nearly all US healthcare providers to follow. Additional federal legislation included the Health Care Quality Improvement Act (HCQIA) of 1986, which established, among other things, the National Practitioner Data Bank requiring the submission of adverse actions related to licensure, hospital privileges, and professional societies; professional liability settlements or payouts of at least $10,000; loss of participation in federal programs such as Medicare or Medicaid; criminal convictions; and any drug license revocations or limitations. As a result of these mandates and regulations, the federal government has become a driving force in the standardization of medical staff credentialing and privileging. Additionally, the HCQIA established the immunity of medical staff members engaged in peer review and credentialing matters, protecting them from lawsuits (i.e., legal actions) by physicians who are adversely affected by credentialing/privileging efforts as long as the peer reviewers acted in good faith. This immunity provides more openness among peer reviewers, fosters an environment that is confidential and away from public view, and affords legal protection for healthcare peer evaluation. However, key to this immunity is a process that is driven by facts and not by bad-faith efforts that mask ulterior motives of anticompetitive or personal agendas.

Federal legislation such as the Health Insurance Portability and Accountability Act (HIPAA) and the Health Information Technology for Economic and Clinical Health (HITECH) Act has influenced credentialing/privileging efforts by forcing healthcare providers to add another layer to the process to ensure that patient information is only used as necessary and by users with a legitimate and direct need.

Perhaps the most significant development in the area of credentialing and privileging is the impact of court decisions finding meritorious actions of negligent credentialing and privileging. The first case to strike down the concept of the charitable immunity doctrine, or immunity granted to charitable organizations such as hospitals, was *Darling v. Charleston Community Memorial Hospital* (1965), in which the court found the hospital negligent in allowing a physician to practice at the hospital. This finding established the hospital's duty to allow staff medical privileges only to physicians who had been fully credentialed, recommended by the medical staff, and ultimately approved by the hospital's governing body. Subsequent hospital credentialing negligence cases have caused courts in more than 30 states to adopt the view that hospitals can be held accountable for negligent credentialing and negligent privileging of medical staff members, as well as other independent providers. Clearly, all healthcare managers must recognize the importance of due diligence in the process of determining the quality of their facility's medical staff.

Exhibit 4.1 provides a list of significant legal cases affecting issues of credentialing and privileging. This exhibit presents a chronological progression of the concept of negligent credentialing and shows how subsequent cases have shaped the process of physician credentialing and privileging. Beginning in 1965 with the *Darling v. Charleston Community Memorial Hospital* case, the hospital industry was placed on notice that credentialing and privileging could no longer be left exclusively to the medical staff and that issues of established practice problems and hospital privilege revocations should be factored into the decision-making process. The *Johnson v. Misericordia Community Hospital* (1980) case reinforced the hospital's duty to verify practice outcomes at other facilities. The next wave of judgments focused on issues of antitrust and disruptive behaviors that either affected patient care or had the potential to adversely affect patient care (*Hyde v. Jefferson Parish Hospital District No. 2* [1981], *Patrick v. Burget* [1988], *Mahmoodian v. United Hospital Center, Inc.* [1991]). Clearly, the courts found that nonclinical judgments and behaviors could lead to negative clinical outcomes. *Frigo v. Silver Cross Hospital* (2007) established that medical staff must adhere to their bylaws and

Case	Legal Issues Established
Darling v. Charleston Community Memorial Hospital 33 Ill. 2d 326, 211 N.E. 253 (1965)	This seminal case established that a hospital could be held liable for the actions of a physician on its staff and struck down the defense of charitable immunity.
Johnson v. Misericordia Community Hospital 97 Wis. 2d 521, 297 N.W.2d 501 (1980)	This case established that a hospital has a duty to check and verify information regarding a physician's prior and current malpractice claims and privileges at other facilities.
Hyde v. Jefferson Parish Hospital District No. 2 513 F. Supp. 532 (E.D. La. 1981)	The use of exclusive contracts for certain hospital-based medical services (anesthesiology, radiology, pathology) is not anticompetitive and does not violate the Sherman Antitrust Act.
Patrick v. Burget 486 U.S. 94 (1988)	Peer review of physicians must be conducted without an anticompetitive bias, and the process must not be "shabby, unprincipled, and unprofessional"; this case was the impetus for the Healthcare Quality Improvement Act (HCQIA) of 1986.
Mahmoodian v. United Hospital Center, Inc. 404 S.E.2d 750 (W. Va. 1991)	Otherwise competent physicians can be removed from the medical staff for disruptive behavior, as long as the disruption may lead to adverse patient care outcomes.
Frigo v. Silver Cross Hospital 377 Ill. App. 3d 43, 876 N.E.2d 697 (1st Dist. 2007)	The hospital granted advanced surgical privileges to a podiatrist who was not residency trained for such procedures as required in the hospital's medical staff bylaws, and the hospital did not provide any grandfathering provisions within its medical staff bylaws.
Larson v. Wasemiller 738 N.W.2d 300 (Minn. 2007)	The court found that negligent credentialing is "more directly related" to negligent selection of an independent contractor.
Poliner v. Texas Health Systems 537 F.3d 368 (5th Cir. 2008)	Under the HCQIA, peer reviewers must 1. Have a reasonable belief that action is in furtherance of quality healthcare, 2. Use reasonable efforts to obtain facts of the matter, 3. Offer adequate notice and hearing to the affected physician, and 4. Conclude with reasonable belief that the action is warranted by the facts known. This case reinforced the immunity provided to peer reviewers under the HCQIA.

EXHIBIT 4.1
Significant Cases Related to Credentialing/ Privileging

that practitioner privileges must be extended on the basis of demonstrated training and/or abilities. Further issues of credentialing revolved around the Healthcare Quality Improvement Act of 1986. *Poliner v. Texas Health Systems* (2008) determined that the actions of a medical peer review committee afforded immunity to peer reviewers who acted within the scope of the act, which states that members must (1) have a reasonable belief that action is in furtherance of quality healthcare, (2) use reasonable efforts to obtain facts of the matter, (3) offer adequate notice and hearing to the affected physician, and (4) conclude with reasonable belief that the action is warranted by the facts known. Exhibit 4.1 depicts the progression in the credentialing/privileging process and assists the reader in understanding how the system is framed.

Elements of the Credentialing/Privileging Process

As the most widely known and accepted accrediting body among healthcare facilities, The Joint Commission has promulgated over the years a prescriptive set of credentialing/privileging standards designed to "determine the competency of practitioners to provide high quality, safe patient care" (Joint Commission 2014, MS-22). These elements of the credentialing/privileging process "involves a series of activities designed to collect, verify, and evaluate data relevant to a practitioner's professional performance" (Joint Commission 2014, MS-22). Further, "these activities serve as the foundation for objective, evidence-based decisions regarding appointment to membership on the medical staff, and recommendations to grant or deny initial and renewed privileges" (Joint Commission 2014, MS-22).

The following are subsumed under The Joint Commission's Elements of Performance regarding credentials and privileges for physician members of an organization's staff:

- *Licensure.* This requirement entails that each applicant must have a current license from the jurisdiction of the facility's location. Primary source verification is required, or the institution must establish directly from the information source (state board of medical licensure) that the individual is currently licensed and must determine if any sanctions or actions have been taken against the individual's medical license.
- *Medical education.* The applicant must have successfully completed a course of study at a World Health Organization–approved medical school. Primary source verification is required.
- *Residency and specialty training.* This requirement establishes the applicant's exposure to and successful completion of an approved medical residency program. This program becomes the basis of core training, or what the specific residency program includes within

the prevailing standard of care according to which this specialty of medicine trains its residents, and serves to indicate what each resident has been exposed to and is competent to handle in practice. Further, in many residency programs, residents are required to keep a list of the procedures they have been exposed to and the level of care they assumed. For example, the progression of residents' participation goes from assisting to performing. Primary source verification is required.

- *Experience and quality outcomes.* This area concerns the practitioner's ongoing quality outcomes within the facility. These outcomes include mortality, morbidity, utilization, pathological reports, and any peer review issues. Also, this area includes any litigation pending or results of concluded suits.

- *Health status.* In this area, the facility is concerned with any impairments that must be considered when determining credentials and privileges. Routine physical health examinations may be required for physicians. Additionally, for practitioners with a history of impairment, the organization should have a mechanism to perform ongoing laboratory/toxicology testing to ensure compliance with any regulatory-based monitoring programs.

- *Regulatory and certification association sources.* This area concerns data provided by external associations concerned with regulation and certification of practitioners. Primary source verification is required.

  - *National Practitioner Data Bank.* As previously discussed, this entity provides any submissions of adverse action concerning medical licensure, hospital privileges and membership in professional societies, professional liability settlements/payouts of at least $10,000, loss of participation in federal programs such as Medicare or Medicaid, criminal convictions, or drug dispensing limitations.

  - *Office of Inspector General.* This entity provides information regarding a practitioner's removal from participation in Medicare and Medicaid funding amid issues of fraudulent billing activities.

  - *State medical licensure board.* The state board of medical licensure provides information on actions or investigations into a practitioner's license concerning practice limitations, suspension, or revocation.

  - *Professional certification societies.* Board certification societies may take actions that suspend or revoke a practitioner's board certification status.

Exhibit 4.2 provides a sample of the elements contained in a uniform credentialing application that has been adopted by Texas, Oklahoma, North Carolina, Maryland, Colorado, Georgia, and Minnesota. Other states and many major metropolitan areas have adopted similar standardized credentialing forms.

EXHIBIT 4.2
Elements
Contained in
Standardized
Credentialing
Applications

1. Demographic and personal information—typically includes US citizenship or visa status and military service, all with dates
2. Professional education—medical school dates of attendance, location, and contact information
3. Postgraduate education
   a. Internship dates, completion status, contact information of program director
   b. Residency dates, completion status, contact information of program director
   c. Fellowship dates, completion status, contact information of program director
   d. Other postgraduate education dates, completion status, contact information of program director
4. Licensure
   a. Type of licensure, date of issue, current status, expiration date
   b. Drug Enforcement Agency (DEA) number
   c. National Provider Identifier
   d. Medicare or Medicaid participant numbers
5. Board certification
   a. Status
   b. Initial certification dates, expiration dates
6. Work/employment history
   a. Current and previous professional practice locations with dates of service
   b. Gaps in employment, with explanations
7. Hospital affiliations
   a. Current and previous locations with dates of service
   b. Any restrictions on practice at all locations
8. Professional liability/claims history
   a. Current insurance provider with dates of issue
   b. Previous carriers with dates of issue and cancellation, and reasons for cancellation
   c. Current and previous claims with explanations for each
9. Disclosures
   a. Licensure: Have you ever been reprimanded; had your license denied, suspended, revoked, or restricted; or voluntarily surrendered your license?
   b. Hospital privileges: Has your medical staff membership ever been denied, suspended, revoked, restricted, denied renewal, voluntarily surrendered, or subject to probation?
   c. Education, training, board certification: Have you ever been placed on probation, disciplined, formally reprimanded, suspended, or

(continued)

EXHIBIT 4.2
Elements
Contained in
Standardized
Credentialing
Applications
*(continued from
previous page)*

asked to resign; been placed under investigation; voluntarily with-drawn from or prematurely terminated participation in any educa-tional or certification program; had a board certification revoked; or chosen not to recertify or to voluntarily surrender a certification?

d. DEA, Medicare, Medicaid, National Practitioner Data Bank, or other regulatory body: Have you ever been disciplined, excluded, debarred, suspended, sanctioned, censured, disqualified, or otherwise restricted from participation?

e. Malpractice claims history/criminal actions: Please state any actions within the last five years (or whatever length of time the facility chooses), and provide an explanation.

f. Health status: Provide any limitations to your ability to perform your job, including any use of chemical substances or illegal use of drugs/intoxicants. Do you pose a risk to your patients? Do you need any reasonable accommodations to perform your job?

Concerns and Issues of Credentialing and Privileging

With the advent of new and emerging medical procedures and devices, the credentialing committee is faced with the need to determine if a physician has the requisite skills to perform any new requested procedures. These new pro-cedures, or devices, obviously postdate the individual's training and experience. Therefore, the credentialing committee is faced with determining what new levels of expertise or experience are required for the use of the procedure or device to be added to the list of privileges assigned to the physician. With many new and emerging procedures or devices, manufacturers are quick to provide exposure to their products in the form of short continuing education events. However, the real issue of privileging is to make the determination that the physician has the proficiency and skills necessary to perform these procedures. This process entails much more than simply accepting the manufacturer's cer-tificate of training and must instead focus on what the literature has established concerning these new procedures or devices and what nationally recognized certifying boards or associations have addressed privileging issues. For an exam-ple, the field of bariatric surgery has been a newcomer to the field of general surgery. Only since the late 1990s has bariatric surgery training been included within the training curriculum of a general surgery residency. The privileging dilemma comes with trying to extend bariatric surgical privileges to physi-cians who did not have bariatric surgery included within their general surgery residency. In this example, these privileging issues have been addressed by the American Society for Metabolic and Bariatric Surgery (ASMBS). This entity developed guidelines (ASBS Bariatric Training Committee 2006) that hospitals may employ within the privileging process; for example, if the surgeon requests open bariatric surgery privileges, the surgeon must have operative experience of 15 open bariatric procedures during the general surgery residency or postresidency training supervised by an experienced bariatric surgeon (one who has experience with at least 200 bariatric procedures). These guidelines are only a brief example, and any real privileging must follow prescriptive guidelines that the relevant organization has promulgated concerning the specific area.

The issue of ongoing physician monitoring and quality assessment affects every medical provider within the organized medical staff, including both physicians and nonphysicians. The Joint Commission has developed the Ongoing Professional Practice Evaluation (OPPE) and Focused Professional Practice Evaluation (FPPE) mechanisms to address the routine oversight function (Joint Commission 2014). OPPE

has been designed to provide the facility with criteria that monitors and evaluates:
- review of operative and other clinical procedure(s) performed and their outcomes
- pattern of blood and pharmaceutical usage
- requests for tests and procedures
- length of stay patterns
- morbidity and mortality data
- practitioner's use of consultants
- other relevant criteria as determined by the organized medical staff

This information used in OPPE may be acquired through the following sources:
- periodic chart review
- direct observation
- monitoring of diagnostic and treatment techniques
- discussion with other individuals involved in the care of each patient including consulting physicians, assistants at surgery, and nursing and administrative personnel (Joint Commission 2014, MS-37–MS-38)

OPPE requires each facility to develop an institution-specific process that continually monitors and evaluates each physician's pattern of practice from an outcomes perspective. This outcomes perspective is intended to provide an objective system of evaluation that is quantifiable and not subject to broad interpretations. The key to this process is the determination of any trends or patterns of practice that suggest that the practitioner may need to be placed under FPPE, which can be viewed as a progressive step in the evaluation process. FPPE is

the process whereby the organization evaluates the privilege-specific competence of the practitioner who does not have documented evidence of completely performing the requested privilege at the organization. . . . This process may also be used when a question arises regarding a currently privileged practitioner's ability to provide safe, high quality care. Focused professional practice evaluation is a time-limited period during which the organization evaluates and determines the practitioner's professional performance. (Joint Commission 2014, MS-35–MS-36)

Under FPPE

the organized medical staff does the following:

- evaluates practitioners without current performance documentation at the organization
- evaluates practitioners in response to concerns regarding the provision of safe, high quality patient care
- develops criteria for extending the evaluation period
- communicates to the appropriate parties the evaluation results and recommendations based on results
- implements changes to improve performance (Joint Commission 2014, MS-38–MS-39)

FPPE serves a dual function in addressing both requests for new procedures and evaluation of practitioners who have exhibited alarming trends or patterns of practice. With practitioners requesting privileges to use new procedures or devices, the organization sets the bar to ensure that the practitioner has the requisite skills and ability to uphold the institution's mandate to provide safe, high-quality patient care. Privilege-specific credentialing is obviously limited to the requests in question and focuses on the evaluation of the practitioner's ability to use the newly requested procedure or device. On the other hand, the evaluation of a practitioner's overall ability or the totality of a practice will be more detailed and have a global perspective.

As an example, Ehrenfeld and colleagues (2012, 77) have demonstrated that the use of automatically captured electronic anesthesia objective data such as blood pressure monitoring, end tidal CO_2 monitoring, and timely documentation of compliance statements is helpful in OPPE and has provided a "key element of a comprehensive clinical performance evaluation that measures both technical and generalizable clinical skill sets." The use of such data does not completely accomplish OPPE objectives; rather, it serves as a preliminary starting point that is continuously monitored and becomes a benchmark or baseline for future quality practice improvements.

Likewise, Freed and colleagues (2006, 910) found that board certification, or efforts to become or remain board certified, among pediatricians was linked to "the premise [that] the development of recertification is the need to assure the public of the continued competence of physicians over the course of their professional careers." In this instance, board certification has become an organization-specific element in the OPPE process and serves to demonstrate the organization's commitment to safe, high-quality healthcare for its public.

Typical Credentialing/Privileging Encounter

The process begins with an initial appointment application from a physician. This process occurs the first time that a practitioner requests privileges from a hospital; all subsequent periods would constitute reappointment. While the ultimate goal is the same, the initial appointment involves a more detailed look at the education and training information, whereas in the case of reappointments this information would have already been determined. To begin the initial appointment, the application must be complete and is not reviewable until its completeness is established. The process would begin with current licensure within the state of the facility—exceptions would be in federal facilities such as the Veterans Affairs Medical Center, which only requires a license from any state. Contacting the appropriate state medical board would begin the process and would disclose any medical board actions. In the absence of such negative information, the application would progress to the issue of education and training. Each school or hospital involved in the educational process would be contacted. Information obtained from each facility would entail graduation from an approved medical school and successful completion of internship and residency training programs or reasons for noncompletion. While successful residency training is not an absolute requirement for all hospitals, most hospital medical staffs require completion of a residency program as a basic prerequisite for appointment. Additionally, the length of time the applicant took to complete the training is commonly reviewed. While a longer time to residency completion is not a negative predictor in and of itself, a longer period may signal other issues that need to be addressed. Likewise, changes in residency location also need to be discussed. Coupled with the residency program is the issue of specialty board certification. Again, board certification is not a requirement for every physician but may be a sign of competency. Therefore, board certification and testing results need to be addressed. From this point, the process would follow the questions displayed in Exhibit 4.2. Particular attention is focused on the "Disclosures" section of Exhibit 4.2. From the questions in this section, the facility would learn of issues that need to be more fully addressed and evaluated.

Typically, once the facility has gathered this information, the completed application and these findings are forwarded to the chairperson of the medical or surgical department in which the physician would be placed (e.g., pediatrics, general surgery, OB/GYN). After a review by the prospective department chairperson, the application, additional information, and a recommendation from the department chairperson would be forwarded to the medical staff credentialing committee for further evaluation and recommendation. Ultimately, the recommendation for either acceptance or rejection is sent to the facility's governing board for final approval. The ultimate decision rests with the governing body. According to prevailing medical staff bylaws, rules, and regulations, each applicant is afforded due process, or the right to contest the hospital's decision. While this process is fairly standardized, different facilities may have different levels of review and different evaluators. Of course, state laws may also apply in the process of credentialing and privileging and will govern each facility's process.

Future Trends in Credentialing and Privileging

Because the process of credentialing continues to evolve, issues of continuous outcome monitoring and new and emerging technology will continue to be at the forefront. Both OPPE and FPPE will continue to be tweaked to address whatever outcomes are germane at the time in question. And, with the dynamics of new technology, the credentialing process will be faced with new procedures; therefore, new privileges will have to be considered.

Additionally, the need to revamp the composition and focus of the credentialing committee's membership must also be considered. Historically, physician members of the credentialing committee were selected for limited terms (usually coinciding with the two-year credentialing period) and were not given the opportunity to gain additional experience or knowledge of the credentialing process. This situation, coupled with the reluctance to cast shadows on fellow medical staff colleagues stemming from a lack of credentialing knowledge, further resulted in credentialing and privileging decisions that failed to meet the goals of the process. Future changes in the composition and skills of the credentialing committee will include longer tenures for physician members, focused training in credentialing processes and outcomes evaluations, the appointment of nonphysician members to represent the governing body and executive administration with more potential for influence, the use of outside medical experts when the credentialing committee lacks the skill set to properly evaluate new and emerging technology, and a more proactive approach to the credentialing/privileging process (Hyde 2003). Clearly, the new credentialing committee will approach the tasks of credentialing and privileging in a systematic sense and will continually adapt to reflect the standards of care as they evolve.

Summary

From a healthcare management student's perspective, the process of credentialing and privileging may at first seem daunting and foreign, but this process ultimately determines the organization's quality of care, which ultimately determines the organization's viability. Therefore, prospective healthcare managers must gain at least a basic understanding of and appreciation for this process, and at the same time develop an understanding of the connections between patient outcomes and physician practice. As previously noted, the increasing number of state courts that have adopted negligent credentialing as a cause of action should send a clear and unequivocal message that hospitals must take the process of credentialing and privileging seriously, and credentialing/privileging committees must make an organizational investment of time and focus to fulfill their executive duties of being fiduciary stewards of the organization.

Discussion Questions

1. How does the use of telemedicine for interpretation of X-rays (by providers outside the organization and maybe out of the country) affect credentialing/ privileging decisions?

2. If a hospital learns that another facility has sanctioned one of its privileged physicians, how should the hospital react to such a situation?

3. Under the American with Disabilities Act, what type of accommodations can the hospital make? When may the accommodations have an adverse impact on patient outcomes?

4. Conduct an Internet search and find a state medical practice act. Under the terms of the act, what areas of practice are granted to the physician? Consider these parameters and discuss what areas

of credentialing are needed to fulfill these legal stipulations.

5. As the ultimate authority in credentialing/privileging decisions, what must the hospital's governing body do to satisfy its legal mandate?

6. Does physician ownership of a hospital, or any other medical facility, have any impact on credentialing/privileging decisions?

7. What sources should healthcare managers consider in obtaining outside medical/ peer evaluation when their medical staff do not have the requisite skills to make credentialing/privileging decisions?

8. Should the hospital and its medical staff consider some sort of practice reevaluation of elderly and aging physicians?

Experiential Exercise

In considering *Poliner v. Texas Health Systems*, 537 F.3d 368 (5th Cir. 2008), perform the following steps:

1. Do an Internet search to find the case and the final appellate court decision that reversed the initial jury finding awarding more than $300 million to Dr. Poliner for the hospital's breach of the HCQIA.

2. Identify the plaintiff's contention of sham peer review, and discuss how instrumental that cause was in the jury deliberations.

3. Prepare a brief summary of the chronology of the case events, and indicate how you see this ultimate finding influencing the willingness and diligence of future medical participants in the peer review/credentialing process.

References

ASBS Bariatric Training Committee. 2006. "American Society for Bariatric Surgery's Guidelines for Granting Privileges in Bariatric Surgery." *Surgery for Obesity and Related Diseases* 2 (1): 65–67. Accessed December 16, 2014. http://asmbs.org/wp/uploads/2005/10/GrantingPrivileges-Jan2006.pdf.

Ehrenfeld, J. M., J. P. Henneman, R. A. Peterfreund, T. D. Sheehan, F. Xue, S. Spring, and W. S. Sandberg. 2012. "Ongoing Professional Performance Evaluation (OPPE) Using Automatically Captured Electronic Anesthesia Data." *The Joint Commission Journal on Quality and Patient Safety* 38 (2): 73–80.

Freed, G. L., R. L. Uren, E. F. Hudson, I. Lakhani, J. R. C. Wheeler, and J. A. Stockman. 2006. "Policies and Practices Related to the Role of Board Certification and Recertification of Pediatricians in Hospital Privileging." *Journal of the American Medical Association* 295 (8): 905–12.

Hyde, J. 2003. "Physician Credentialing: Developing a Proactive Credentialing Process." *Journal of Legal Nurse Consulting* 14 (1): 3–8.

Joint Commission. 2014. *Hospital Accreditation Standards.* Oakbrook Terrace, IL: The Joint Commission.

Rolph, J. E., J. L. Adams, and K. A. McGuigan. 2007. "Identifying Malpractice-Prone Physicians." *Journal of Empirical Legal Studies* 4 (1): 125–53.

Williams, S. C., S. P. Schmaltz, D. J. Morton, R. G. Koss, and J. M. Loeb. 2005. "Quality of Care in US Hospitals as Reflected by Standardized Measures." *New England Journal of Medicine* 353 (3): 255–64.

5

WORKFORCE DIVERSITY

Rupert M. Evans Sr.

Learning Objectives

After completing this chapter, the reader should be able to

- accommodate cultural diversity of patients;
- strategize handling conflicts in a culturally diverse workplace;
- understand different kinds of diversity;
- understand how the proactive use of diversity principles can transform the organization's culture;
- understand the business case for diversity and inclusion in healthcare organizations;
- work toward creating an inclusive organizational culture;
- understand how to define the roles that healthcare providers, management, and governance play in building a business imperative for diversity within the organization; and
- discuss how healthcare leaders can develop a diversity program in their organizations.

Introduction

Demographic trends in the United States will result in an older and more racially and ethnically diverse population by 2060 (US Census Bureau 2012). The result of this significant demographic shift is that as the United States becomes more ethnically and racially diverse, healthcare systems and providers that can reflect and respond to an increasingly heterogeneous patient base are needed. Knowing how to serve people with different values, health beliefs, and alternative perspectives about health and wellness is a business imperative in the most diverse regions of the United States.

Diversity and inclusion continue to be issues on the mind of many healthcare leaders. In February 2012 the American College of Healthcare Executives, American Hospital Association (AHA), Association of American Medical Colleges, Catholic Health Association of the United States, and

National Association of Public Hospitals and Health Systems announced a call to action for the elimination of healthcare disparities. Their goals are to increase the collection of race, ethnicity, and language preference data; increase cultural competency training for clinicians and support staff; and increase diversity in governance and management. The coalition stated: "Addressing disparities is no longer just about morality, ethics and social justice: It is essential for performance excellence and improved community health" (Institute for Diversity in Health Management and Health Research & Educational Trust 2012).

When you hear the term *diversity*, what comes to mind? To some, the word means the differences between human beings related to race or ethnicity. To others, it means the uniqueness of each individual. A few people still may argue that it is just a code word for affirmative action.

Healthcare organizations across the United States are beginning to move toward embracing and fostering workforce diversity. This cultural change means adopting new values that are inclusive and appropriately managing a diverse workforce. In the future, diversity will drive the business practices of hospitals and other healthcare organizations, and this dynamic will require strong leadership. This chapter provides a definition of diversity and a framework for understanding the different ways people view the term. In addition, it highlights several studies and legal issues pertaining to this topic and enumerates methods for building a case for and establishing a diversity program.

Definition of Diversity and Inclusion

The Society for Human Resource Management defines diversity as "the collective mixture of differences and similarities that includes[,] for example, individual and organizational characteristics, values, beliefs, experiences, backgrounds, preferences, and behaviors." The organization goes on to define inclusion as "the achievement of a work environment in which all individuals are treated fairly and respectfully, have equal access to opportunities and resources, and can contribute fully to the organization's success" (Society for Human Resource Management 2008, 1, 2). These are formal definitions, but the reality is that people define diversity in many ways, depending on the way they live in and view society.

In his book *The 10 Lenses: Your Guide to Living and Working in a Multicultural World*, Mark Williams (2001) discusses the framework that explains the way people see the world:

1. The *assimilationist* wants to conform and fit in with the group to which he or she belongs.

2. The *colorblind* ignores race, color, ethnicity, and other cultural factors.

3. The *cultural centrist* seeks to improve the welfare of his or her cultural group by accentuating its history and identity.

4. The *elitist* believes in the superiority of the upper class and embraces the importance of family roots, wealth, and social status.

5. The *integrationist* supports breaking down all barriers between racial groups by merging people of different cultures together in communities and in the workplace.

6. The *meritocratist* lives by the adage "cream rises to the top"—the belief that hard work, personal merit, and winning a competition determine one's success.

7. The *multiculturist* celebrates the diversity of cultures, seeking to retain the native customs, languages, and ideas of people from other countries.

8. The *seclusionist* protects himself or herself from racial, cultural, and/or ethnic groups in fear that they may diminish the character and quality of his or her group's experiences within society.

9. The *transcendent* focuses on the human spirit and people's universal connection and shared humanity.

10. The *victim/caretaker* views liberation from societal barriers as a crucial goal and sees oppression as not only historical but also contemporary.

This framework can help explain why so many interpretations of the same idea exist. For the purposes of this chapter, diversity is described in the context of three key dimensions: (1) human diversity, (2) cultural diversity, and (3) systems diversity. Each dimension needs to be understood and managed in the healthcare workplace.

Human diversity includes the attributes that make a human being who he or she is, such as race, ethnicity, age, gender, family status (single, married, divorced, widowed, with or without children), sexual orientation, physical abilities, and so on. These traits are what frequently come to mind first when individuals consider the differences in people. Human diversity is a core dimension because it defines who we are as individuals. This dimension is with us throughout every stage of our lives, guiding how we define ourselves and how we are perceived by others. A workplace definition of diversity includes human diversity as a minimum.

Cultural diversity encompasses a person's beliefs, values, family structure practice (nuclear or extended family, independent living), and mind-set as a result of his or her cultural, community, and environmental experiences. This dimension includes language, social class, learning style, ethics or moral compass, religion, lifestyle, work style, global perspectives, and military views. Cultural diversity is a secondary dimension, but it can have a powerful impact on how a person behaves in the workplace. Cultural norms vary from one culture to another and influence how individuals interact with their work environments. For example, some religious groups are forbidden from working on the Sabbath, and this exemption has an impact on work scheduling and even hiring decisions.

Systems diversity relates to the differences among organizations in work structure and pursuits. This dimension includes teamwork reengineering, strategic alliances, employee empowerment, quality focus, educational development, corporate acquisitions, and innovation. Systems diversity deals with systems thinking and the ability to recognize how functions in the work environment are connected with diversity. In a multicultural, diverse, and inclusive workplace, organizational systems are integrated to enhance innovation, encourage teamwork, and improve productivity.

All of these dimensions are important and are present in the healthcare workplace, and all leaders should recognize them. The challenge is in seeing not only our differences but also our similarities as individuals, as professionals, and as members of a group. Leaders must develop effective strategies to manage the differences (and highlight similarities), and the use of these strategies will lead to building effective teams and a higher-performing organization (Guillory 2003).

Managing diversity is not an easy task, as a number of barriers often get in the way of achieving a harmonious working environment. Some of these barriers, which revolve around the diversity dimensions mentioned earlier, can be a great source of tension and conflict. For instance, a person's culture can be a barrier to a work team when other members of the group are not respectful or understanding of the person's values, beliefs, or even clothing, all of which may reflect that person's cultural background. Examples of a cultural difference may be the person's hairstyle or affinity for wearing religious artifacts. The education, race/ethnicity, work style, empowerment, and relationship/task orientation of an individual can also become barriers if they are not properly understood and managed.

Prejudice in the Workplace

Prejudice is a set of views held by individuals about members of other groups. Prejudice is prejudgment; hence, it is not based on facts or experience. It affects the way people react toward and think of other people, and it can be as innocent as children choosing not to play with children they deem different from themselves or as harmful as adults not associating with certain people because English is not their native language.

Formally, prejudice can be defined as a set of institutionalized assumptions, attitudes, and practices that has an invisible-hand effect in systematically advantaging members of more powerful groups over members of less dominant groups. This type of prejudice occurs in many healthcare institutions. Some examples include culturally biased assessment and selection criteria, cultural norms that condone or permit racial or sexual harassment, lower performance expectations for certain groups, and a collective misconception about a specific group that relegates the group's members to unfair positions. An example of the latter is stereotyping.

Stereotypes are generalizations about individuals based on their identity, group membership, or affiliations (Dreachslin, Weech-Maldonado, and Dansky 2004). A common stereotype in the healthcare management field is the assumption that black executives are not as qualified as their white counterparts. Thus, African-American executives are tested more often to prove their competence, while their white contemporaries are assumed to be capable from the start. (This fact is substantiated in the race/ethnic surveys discussed later in the chapter.)

The concept of "comfort and risk" relates to a human being's natural need to feel comfortable and to avoid risk. People tend to prefer to work with others from similar racial or ethnic backgrounds because doing so provides them with a certain amount of comfort and shields them from a certain amount of risk. Although subordinate–superior relationships that involve people from different backgrounds work sufficiently to allow people to get the job done, they often fail to lead to the close bonds that form between a mentor and a protégé.

Given the systemic existence of prejudice and the way it influences people's mind-set and behavior in the workplace, the fair and accurate assessment of minority employees (caregivers, support staff, and managers alike) remains an organizational dilemma rather than an established practice. For instance, the literature provides evidence that managers systematically give higher performance ratings to subordinates who belong to the same racial group as they do, while high performers from minority groups remain comparatively invisible in the managerial/leadership selection process (Thomas and Gabarro 1999).

The Business Case for Diversity

In 1900, one in eight Americans was nonwhite; in 2012, blacks represented one in five Americans and Hispanics represented one in six. By 2060 those ratios will be closer to one in four and one in three, respectively (US Census Bureau 2012). This trend means that the healthcare industry needs physicians, nurses, and other providers, but it also needs caregivers who reflect the diversity of the population because everyone, at one point or another, becomes a patient. The same is true for healthcare managers and executives.

Therefore, healthcare organizations must ensure that their caregivers and leaders represent the backgrounds of the communities they serve. In addition, healthcare executives must look for new insights, examples, and best practices to help navigate their organizations through a diversity journey. A key challenge in this journey is establishing a business case for having a diverse workforce. Another factor of the business case for diversity is understanding the key elements. They include the following:

- *Representation*—reflecting employees, patients, and communities
- *Inclusiveness*—in welcoming, listening, mentoring, training, and benefits
- *Cultural competency*—being respectful and responsive to cultural backgrounds and their impact on health outcomes
- *Broader definitions of diversity*—encompassing thought, education, skills and gender

The business case for diversity is unique for each organization. The circumstances, environment, and community demographics of one organization cannot be generalized to another institution. However, some elements that are common in all organizations can be the basis of a diversity program: the healthcare marketplace, employee skills and talent, and organizational effectiveness. These elements will drive the institution's investment in and commitment to diversity. An organization can achieve and sustain growth and profitability by doing the following:

- Expand market share by adding or enhancing services that target diverse populations.
- Link the marketplace with the workplace through recruiting, developing, and retaining employees with diverse racial/ethnic backgrounds.
- Create and implement workplace policies and management practices that maximize the talent and productivity of employees with diverse backgrounds.

The facts are that all members of minority groups buy and consume healthcare services, many of them are educated and trained to either provide healthcare services or manage operations, and many of them currently work within the field and understand its complexities. Hospitals and other healthcare organizations cannot afford to miss such opportunities. They can seek, cultivate, and retain minority talent to help them compete in today's diverse healthcare environment. Failure to take advantage of these opportunities will mean the difference between being a provider and employer of choice and losing ground to competitors (Dreachslin, Gilbert, and Malone 2012).

Governance Impact

The AHA developed an initiative called the Hospital Trustee Professionalism Program, led by the Institute for Diversity in Health Management and the Center for Healthcare Governance and assisted by many state hospital associations (Institute for Diversity in Health Management 2013). Several hundred candidates have participated in this orientation focused on hospital boards and their practices. The program has demonstrated no dearth of highly qualified leaders from minority communities, and a national registry of candidates is available (Center for Healthcare Governance 2014).

The challenge now is to improve placements on hospital boards to provide broader evidence of what many trustees already have experienced: Candidates drawn from minority communities can be the most effective trustees. In addition to the nation's shifting demographics, the wider health insurance coverage initiated in 2014 under the Affordable Care Act likely will increase diversity in patient populations, given the disproportionate share of minorities among the uninsured. For hospital trustees, reviewing the status of membership diversity on boards will be very important; resources such as the AHA's Minority Trustee Candidate Registry (Center for Healthcare Governance 2014) can be used to begin recruitment efforts. Doing this work will lead to one of the most important improvements trustees can make in building the strength of US hospitals and healthcare systems in the future: establishing boards and leadership that truly reflect the cultures of our communities.

Members of the board of trustees are the ultimate links to the communities served by a healthcare organization. They know the makeup of the population the organization serves and seeks to target, and they have insights into their communities' healthcare needs. Because board members are part of the community, they have an interest in making sure that the organization they represent is not only providing inclusive services but is also being a fair and equitable employer and neighbor. With this perspective in mind, governance should support a business strategy that promotes community goodwill, encourages growth, considers present social and demographic transformations and hence future needs, and emphasizes culturally competent and sensitive healthcare. Most importantly, members of the board should also reflect the multicultural mix of the surrounding communities.

Considering all of the challenges faced by any healthcare board, why should it be concerned with diversity? One of the many reasons is to protect the organization's bottom line. The financial impact of problems stemming from racial discrimination and discriminatory practices can be substantial. Cases of large organizations committing or turning their backs on such practices provide evidence of the extent of cost consequences. For example, in December 2012, a mill in South Dallas, Texas, agreed to pay $500,000 to 14 black employees to settle an Equal Employment Opportunity Commission (EEOC) race discrimination suit alleging violent, racist graffiti and racial slurs by coworkers and the display of nooses at an employee workstation. The employees alleged that the supervisors allowed the behavior to continue. The EEOC's response required the company to enact a graffiti abatement policy and undergo annual reviews of its compliance for two years (*EEOC v. Rock-Tenn Services Co.*; EEOC 2014). Similarly, in a lawsuit against Banner Health resolved in 2012, the EEOC alleged that the nonprofit healthcare system failed to accommodate an intellectually disabled individual who had worked for it since 1984 as a kitchen worker and dietary aide. During the course of his employment, the individual's requests for reasonable accommodation were ignored. In 2002, a settlement agreement in response to a charge of discrimination filed with the EEOC required the employer to notify the individual's brother, who had power of attorney, prior to taking any negative employment actions. However, when the individual requested an accommodation in 2005, Banner refused and instead fired the individual without notifying his brother. The settlement required Banner to pay $255,000 into a trust for the individual and provide injunctive relief, including training and postings (EEOC 2012). Another reason that a healthcare board should support diversity initiatives is to encourage and strengthen employee commitment to the organization. Simply, a diverse workforce is an asset. It differentiates an organization in the marketplace, giving it an edge against its competitors in terms of inclusiveness, cultural sensitivity and competency, and even progressive practice.

Board commitment to the principles of diversity may lead to shifts in the corporate culture as well, allowing all stakeholders to contribute to the overall success of the organization and its mission. Trustees should hold organizational leaders and managers accountable for setting and following high diversity standards. This practice will lead to an improved organization and to healthy communities.

Legal Issues

The debate continues over whether having a diversity program is the right thing to do or whether it enhances shareholder/stakeholder value. The answer is both—not only is it the right thing to do, but it also adds value to the organization. Educated, skilled, and experienced professionals and workers who are considered to be in the minority (including but not limited to women, racial and ethnic minorities, and people with physical challenges) bring strategic and unique perspectives into their roles, generate productive dialogue, and challenge the status quo. All of these are essential to the practices, products and services, and operations of a healthcare organization. If these reasons are not enough to maintain a diverse workforce, laws also prohibit employment discrimination.

The Civil Rights Act of 1964 was signed into law on July 2, 1964. This legislation was intended to ensure that the financial resources of the federal government would no longer subsidize racial discrimination (Wright 2013). This law bans discrimination in any activities, such as training, employment, or construction, that are funded by federal monies. Discrimination is also prohibited in entities that contract with organizations that receive federal funds. Every recipient of federal funds is required to provide written assurances that nondiscrimination is practiced throughout the institution. The Sullivan Commission Report, which was released in 2004, stated, "The civil rights movement of the 1960s eventually ended the more visible racial and ethnic barriers, but it did not eliminate entrenched patterns of inequality in health care, which remain the unfinished business of the civil rights movement" (Sullivan Commission 2004, 4). An important precedent of the Civil Rights Act was the decision of the US Court of Appeals for the Fourth Circuit on the case of *Simkins v. Moses H. Cone Memorial Hospital* (1963). The decision, which set a precedent against racial discrimination in organizations that received public funds, struck down the separate-but-equal provisions of the Hill-Burton Act and gave the federal government the legal standing that was the premise of Title VI of the Civil Rights Act of 1964 (Richardson and Luker 2014).

The Civil Rights Act also protects individuals whose native language is not English. The US Department of Justice issued its "Guidance to Federal Financial Assistance Recipients Regarding Title VI Prohibition Against National Origin Discrimination Affecting Limited English Proficient Persons" in 2002 (67 C.F.R. 117, 41455–72). This guidance, intended for recipients of federal funds, prohibits discrimination against people who have limited English-language proficiency. It requires federally funded entities to ensure that people whose primary language is not English can access and understand services, programs, and activities provided by these organizations. This mandate has had a serious impact on the way healthcare organizations, especially those in areas with large numbers of individuals who speak English as a second language (ESL), frame their service offerings. The National Council on Interpreting in Health Care (2008) has put together *The Terminology of Health Care Interpreting*, a glossary of terms intended to help healthcare leaders in developing programs for ESL patients; visit www.ncihc.org for more information.

See Chapter 2 for a comprehensive discussion of the Civil Rights Act and other laws that protect groups who are considered in the minority.

Diversity in Healthcare Leadership: Two Major Studies

Despite the demographic changes in the US population and hence in the healthcare field, few minorities are present in the executive suite. Two major studies have been undertaken to understand the factors behind minorities' difficult climb on the healthcare management ladder. As the findings of these studies indicate, although improvements are continually being made in terms of how workforce and leadership diversity is viewed and valued in healthcare organizations, much work remains to be done.

Study 1: Diversity and Disparities: A Benchmark Study of U.S. Hospitals

In 2011, the Institute for Diversity in Health Management, an affiliate of the AHA, commissioned the Health Research & Educational Trust of the AHA to conduct a national survey of hospitals to determine the actions that hospitals are taking to reduce healthcare disparities and promote diversity in leadership and governance (Institute for Diversity in Health Management and Health Research & Educational Trust 2012).

The survey results offer a snapshot of some common strategies used to improve the quality of care that hospitals provide to all patients, regardless of race or ethnicity. The survey results highlight that, while more work needs to be done, advancements are being made in key areas that can promote equitable care, such as collecting demographic data, providing cultural competency training, and increasing diversity in leadership and governance.

The survey included data collected through a national survey of hospitals mailed to the CEOs of 5,756 institutions, which represented all US registered hospitals at the time of the survey. The response rate was 16 percent (924 hospitals), with the sample generally being representative of all hospitals. The complete study can be found at www.hpoe.org/diversity-disparities.

Some core findings of this study indicate that cultural competency training is occurring: 81 percent of hospitals educate all clinical staff during orientation about how to address the unique cultural and linguistic factors affecting the care of diverse patients and communities, and 61 percent of hospitals require all employees to attend diversity training. In the area of leadership and governance, although minorities represent a reported 29 percent of patients nationally, they account for only 14 percent of hospital board members, an average of 14 percent of executive leadership positions, and 15 percent of first-level and midlevel management positions.

Study 2: Building the Business Case—Healthcare Diversity Leadership: A National Survey Report

In 2011, Witt/Kieffer, an executive search firm, completed a national survey that offered a progressive benchmark to build on its seminal survey conducted during 2006 and its original diversity survey conducted during 1998 (Witt/Kieffer 2006). Witt/Kieffer partnered with the Institute for Diversity in Health Management, Asian Health Care Leaders Association, National Association of Health Services Executives, and National Forum for Latino Healthcare Executives to conduct the 2011 survey, which attracted a diverse respondent pool: 55 percent African American, 13 percent Asian, 10 percent Hispanic, and 18 percent Caucasian. The 2011 sample was much more varied than the 2006 survey, in which 71 percent of the respondents were Caucasian. The 2011 survey also attracted more female respondents than the 2006 study (41 percent vs. 28 percent). More than half (54 percent) of the 464 respondents in 2011 were CEOs, C-suite executives, and vice presidents. The remaining 46 percent consisted of medical chiefs, administrators, directors, and other leaders. The study included an online survey conducted during July 2011 and 51 supplementary telephone interviews with survey respondents (Witt/Kieffer 2011).

The survey report identified the following main findings of the 2011 study:

- Respondents see diverse leadership as a valuable business builder, associating it with improved patient satisfaction, successful decision-making, reaching strategic goals, improved clinical outcomes, and a stronger bottom line.

- Respondents perceive more positive diversity activities within their own organizations when it comes to closing the minority leadership gap and giving equal consideration to minorities for leadership positions.

- While the pool of diverse candidates for healthcare leadership has grown over the last five years, respondents do not perceive the same growth within their own organizations.

- Minority representation is still weak, with only one-quarter reporting that minority executives are well-represented in their organizations' management teams and about the same percentage agreeing that the diversity of their management teams reflects patient demographics.

- The top five solutions for diversity success are being sensitive to cultural differences in the workplace, establishing strategic goals and standards that emphasize cultural diversity, seeking regular employee input about the organization's diversity initiatives, promoting minorities from within and mentoring people of color.

- Perceived barriers vary based on race/ethnicity. Minority respondents zero in on a lack of commitment from top management as the #1 barrier to success. Caucasian respondents focus on a lack of diverse candidates, access to them and a lack of candidates to promote from within.

- Respondents are in total agreement about best practices that will lead to the advancement of minority executives: mentoring programs, programs to expose young people to healthcare careers, sensitizing management, developing cultural sensitivity initiatives and communicating diversity initiatives to employees. (Witt/Kieffer 2011, 2)

Diversity Management

According to the Dotson and Nuru-Jeter (2012), finding strategies that lead to the development of high-quality healthcare in increasingly diverse patient populations has become a major challenge. To address the challenges of health and healthcare disparities, three effective strategies will lead organizations to become culturally competent. The first is to provide empirical evidence of a connection between diversity and performance. Second, link the organization's investment in diversity to strategic goals, financial incentives, and organizational success metrics. Finally, ensure that the leadership of the organization is responsible for cultural competence as a performance measure (Dotson and Nuru-Jeter 2012).

A study of the banking industry demonstrated an empirical link between diversity and performance; data showed that racial diversity was positively associated with performance of firms pursuing growth strategies and negatively associated with performance in firms going through downsizing (Dotson and Nuru-Jeter 2012). The study illustrated that racial diversity interacted with business strategies in determining productivity, return on equity, and market share. Through analysis of such studies, healthcare managers can develop their business cases using empirical data from other industries.

The Impact of Diversity on Care Delivery

As quoted in the *Praeger Handbook of Black American Health*, the first director of the center that became the National Institute on Minority Health and Health Disparities stated that "while the diversity of the American population is one of the nation's greatest assets, one of its greatest challenges is reducing the profound disparity in health status of America's racial and ethnic minorities" (Livingston 2004, 761). The Institute of Medicine's landmark report *Unequal Treatment: Confronting Racial and Ethnic Disparities in Health Care* (Smedley, Stith, and Nelson 2003) revealed the presence of significant disparities in the way white and minority patients receive healthcare services, especially in treatment for heart disease, cancer, and HIV. Addressing such disparities in care, including the disproportionate recruitment and selection of a minority workforce, and ensuring cultural competence of caregivers are interconnected. To minimize care disparities, institutions and providers have to develop cultural competence. To develop cultural competence, a diverse group of providers, support staff, and managers needs to be in place and diversity training and policies for all employees and caregivers have to be established. Simply, the lack of a culturally competent healthcare workforce is a possible contributor to the disparities in care.

Having examined how a diverse physician community also benefits healthcare, researchers Cohen, Gabriel, and Terrell (2002) posited at least four practical reasons for attaining greater diversity: (1) It advances cultural competency, (2) it increases access to high-quality care, (3) it strengthens the medical research agenda, and (4) it ensures optimal management. These findings are relevant and applicable to healthcare management and leadership as well. As stated by Cohen, Gabriel, and Terrell (2002, 90), "the first and perhaps most compelling reason for increasing the proportion of medical students and other prospective health care professionals who are drawn from underrepresented minority groups [is] preparing a culturally competent health care workforce."

Cultural competence may be defined as a set of complementary behaviors, practices, attitudes, and policies that enables a system, an agency, or individuals to effectively work and serve pluralistic, multiethnic, and linguistically diverse communities. The demographic makeup of this country will continue to change, and culturally competent and sensitive care is and will be expected from current and future healthcare professionals. To effectively provide such care, leaders, clinical staff, and all the employees in between must have a firm understanding of how and why belief systems, personal biases, ethnic origins, family structures, and other culturally determined factors influence the manner in which patients experience illness, adhere to medical advice, and respond to treatment. Such factors ultimately affect the outcomes of care. Physicians and other healthcare professionals who are not mindful of the potential impact of language barriers, religious taboos, unconventional views of illness and disease, or alternative remedies not only are unlikely to satisfy their patients but, more important, are also unlikely to provide their patients with optimally effective care (Cohen, Gabriel, and Terrell 2002).

A study finds that although African-American physicians make up only 4 percent of the total physician workforce in the United States, they care for more than 20 percent of African-American patients in the United States (Saha et al. 2000). The study suggests that African Americans prefer to get care from black physicians, and a contributing factor may be that many African-American physicians locate their practices in predominantly black communities and are therefore more geographically accessible to African-American healthcare consumers. If the hypothesis that minority consumers prefer care from physicians of their own race simply because of geographic accessibility is true, then organizational policies aimed at better serving the needs of minority communities need not consider physician race and ethnicity in the equation. If, however, minority patients have

EXHIBIT 5.1
Factors That
Influence
Disparities in
Healthcare

Patient-Related Factors	Health-System-Related Factors
Socioeconomic Low income and education **Health education** Lack of knowledge of health symptoms, conditions, and possible treatments **Health behavior** Patient willingness and ability to seek care, adhere to treatment protocols, and trust and work with healthcare providers	**Cultural competence** Insufficient knowledge of and sensitivity to cultural differences **Language** Inability to communicate sufficiently with patients and families whose native language is not English **Discrimination** Healthcare system and provider bias and stereotyping **Workforce diversity** Poor racial and ethnic match between healthcare professionals and the patients they serve **Payment** Insufficient reimbursement for treating Medicare, Medicaid, and uninsured patients

Source: Smedley, Stith, and Nelson (2003).

this preference because of a shared language or culture, for example, then increasing the supply of underrepresented minority physicians is justifiable and necessary.

An understanding of the factors that influence the disparities in health-care is essential in developing effective strategies to minimize the problem. Exhibit 5.1 presents two sets of factors: patient-related factors and health system–related factors. Patient-related factors are cultural characteristics of patients that prevent them from getting fair and adequate treatment in an organization that is not culturally competent or sensitive. Health-system-related factors are organizational dynamics (e.g., employee attributes and biases) that influence the methods used to treat patients.

Components of an Effective Diversity Program

Healthcare leaders can establish a diversity program that will lead to a more diverse and inclusive organization (see Exhibit 5.2). Actions that leaders can take toward this goal include, but are not limited to, the following:

- Ensure that senior management and the governing board are committed to the development and implementation of a diversity program.
- Broaden the definition of diversity to include factors beyond race and ethnicity.
- Recognize the business case for bringing in diversity at the leadership level.
- Tie diversity goals to business objectives.
- Hold recruiting events that target racial and ethnic groups, women, people with disabilities, older but capable workers, and others who are considered minorities.
- Encourage senior executives to mentor minorities.
- Develop employee programs that emphasize and celebrate diversity and inclusivity.

The business imperatives and organizational necessities for aggressively creating a diversity program include, but are not limited to, the following:

- *Reflection of the service population.* The healthcare organization's caregivers and support staff should mirror the diversity of the population that the institution serves. Toward this end, the organization should attract and take advantage of the talents, skills, and growth potential of minority professionals within the community.
- *Workforce utilization.* Minority employees have a lot to contribute to the organization. Leaders should recognize this fact and should

---

EXHIBIT 5.2
How to Create an Inclusive Culture

1. Study the culture, climate (i.e., what employees are thinking, feeling, or hearing about diversity issues), and demographics of the organization.
2. Select the diversity issues that allow the greatest breakthrough.
3. Create a diversity strategic plan.
4. Secure leadership's financial support for the plan.
5. Establish leadership and management accountabilities for the plan.
6. Implement the plan.
7. Provide continual training related to the new skills and competencies necessary to successfully achieve the plan goals.
8. Conduct a follow-up survey one or one-and-one-half years after implementing the plan.

be open to, sensitive to, knowledgeable about, and understanding of the cultures, mind-set, and practices of the organization's diverse workforce. Doing so will not only enhance staff productivity and overall performance but also boost staff morale.

- *Work–life quality and balance.* Leaders should recognize that work and personal activities are interrelated, not separate preoccupations. Both are performed on the basis of necessity, practicality, efficiency, and spontaneity.

- *Recruitment and retention.* Attracting and retaining a diverse workforce have a lot to do with the state of the workplace. Leaders should create an environment in which minorities feel included, professionally developed, and safe.

- *Bridging of generations.* Generational differences in expectations, education, and values exist between younger and older staff. Such gaps should be acknowledged, and attention should be paid to the physical, mental, and emotional well-being of all caregivers and staff at all ages regardless of backgrounds.

- *Cultural competence.* This competence is an in-depth understanding of and sensitivity to the values and viewpoints of minority staff, patients, and other customers. Leaders should master the skills necessary to work with and serve these groups and should provide training in this matter to all employees to ensure provision of culturally competent care.

- *Organization-wide respect.* Leaders should create an environment in which the differences in title, role, position, and department are valued and respected but not held too lofty above everything else. Each employee, regardless of his or her level within the organization, should be viewed as integral to the overall success of the team.

Summary

Health disparities that arise from a lack of access to care and contribute to poor health outcomes continue to disproportionately affect a growing segment of the population. While reports show some progress in reducing disparities, much work remains to be done. Healthcare organizations in the United States are beginning to make a commitment to embracing and fostering workforce diversity. This cultural change means adopting new values in terms of being inclusive and attracting a diverse workforce. The business case for diversity is unique for each organization because the circumstances, environment, and community demographics of one organization vary from those of another. However, certain elements (such as the marketplace and organizational effectiveness) that are common in all organizations can be the basis of a diversity program.

One of the many reasons that senior management and the governing board should pay attention to diversity issues is to protect the organization's bottom line. The financial costs of problems that stem from racial discrimination and discriminatory practices can be substantial. Studies have found disparities in two areas: (1) Minority healthcare administrators ascend in rank more slowly within their organizations than do their white counterparts, and (2) patients who belong to minority groups receive different medical treatments than patients who are white. Such disparities may be bridged with the development of a diversity program.

Discussion Questions

1. While this chapter discussed the many benefits of diversity, an alternative view suggests that no empirical evidence exists to show that a diverse workforce has a positive effect on organizational performance, employee commitment, and employee satisfaction. In fact, anecdotal evidence indicates that diversity can negatively affect business performance because of the possibility for internal conflict, dissension, and turnover. What is your reaction to this perspective in light of the content of this chapter? Do these arguments have merit? Why or why not?

2. Respond to this statement: Diverse leadership is a competitive advantage. What is the most compelling business argument for or against diverse leadership teams?

3. What are the legal, moral, and ethical consequences that prohibit hospitals from turning away patients on the basis of race? Why are no such consequences faced by patients who demand doctors, nurses, or workers of a specific race to administer their healthcare?

4. Can hospitals that adhere to gender- or race-based patient demands face discrimination lawsuits from their employees?

5. When an employer denies an employee (or a group of employees) his or her full employment opportunity based on the racial bias of customers, is the employer violating the employee's civil rights?

6. Does workforce diversity enhance organizational performance? Explain your answer.

7. Can an internal diversity program support an organization's overall mission and vision? How?

Experiential Exercise

Conley is the CEO of a major academic medical center in the midwestern United States. He is a middle-aged white male who has more than 20 years of management experience. Conley is not only the CEO but is also the chief diversity officer for his organization.

One afternoon while sitting at his desk, one of Conley's vice presidents notices an attractive young African-American woman walking by with a shiny diamond stud in her lip. His gut reaction was "No way." He stands up and heads for his door to tell the woman that the lip stud had to go. Just at that moment, Conley, the CEO, happens by. He points to the woman and says, "That young woman does a great job. I did not realize she was in your department. We need to make sure we keep her." In this moment, the vice president came face to face with the differences between personal preference and job performance. As the leader of an organization gains in diversity effectiveness, the organization as a whole gains, as do the employees of the medical center, at least those who are paying attention.

Later that afternoon, Conley met with the executive team at a strategic planning session. At the end of the session, he offered some closing comments. He said, "I have been thinking of requirements. The world is changing, our industry is changing, our community is changing, and I am not certain what requirements we need for our team of the future."

Written Assignment

Analyze this scenario using the following process:

1. Identify the key facts.
2. Identify the issues and the core problem(s).
3. Suggest and evaluate alternative solutions, using your learning from this chapter and the most current literature.
4. If you were Conley, what would you do to change the culture of your organization?
5. Recommend a course of action and specify the reason for choosing that direction.

In-Class Discussion

Discuss the following questions in groups:

1. What are some of the hidden biases or personal filters we each possess?
2. How do stereotypes filter a person's perceptions of others?
3. How can an individual begin a discussion about diversity and inclusion without intense emotions or misperceptions?

References

Center for Healthcare Governance. 2014. "Trustee Candidate Recruitment." Accessed December 16. www.americangovernance.com/trustee/index.shtml.

Cohen, J., B. Gabriel, and C. Terrell. 2002. "The Case for Diversity in the Healthcare Workforce." *Health Affairs* 21 (5): 90–102.

Dotson, E., and A. Nuru-Jeter. 2012. "Setting the Stage for a Business Case for Leadership Diversity in Healthcare: History, Research, and Leverage." *Journal of Healthcare Management* 57 (1): 38–42.

Dreachslin, J. L., J. M. Gilbert, and B. Malone. 2012. *Diversity and Cultural Competence in Health Care: A Systems Approach.* San Francisco: Jossey-Bass.

Dreachslin, J. L., R. Weech-Maldonado, and K. H. Dansky. 2004. "Racial and Ethnic Diversity and Organizational Behavior: A Focused Research Agenda for Health Services Management." *Social Science & Medicine* 59 (5): 961–71.

Equal Employment Opportunity Commission (EEOC). 2014. "Significant EEOC Race/Color Cases." Accessed November 23. www.eeoc.gov/eeoc/initiatives/e-race/caselist.cfm.

———. 2012. "Selected List of Pending and Resolved Cases Under the Americans with Disabilities Act (ADA)." Published November 8. www1.eeoc.gov/eeoc/litigation/selected/ada_11-12.cfm?renderforprint=1.

Guillory, W. 2003. "The Business of Diversity: The Case for Action." *Health & Social Work* 28 (1): 3–7.

Institute for Diversity in Health Management. 2013. "Trustee Education Program & Minority Trustee Candidate Registry." Updated August 2. www.diversityconnection.org/diversityconnection/education/About%20Trustee%20Prof%20Prog.jsp?fll=S5.

Institute for Diversity in Health Management and Health Research & Educational Trust. 2012. *Diversity and Disparities: A Benchmark Study of U.S. Hospitals.* Published June. www.hpoe.org/diversity-disparities.

Livingston, I. L. (ed.). 2004. *Policies and Issues Behind Disparities in Health.* Vol. 2 of *Praeger Handbook of Black American Health*, second edition. Westport, CT: Praeger.

National Council on Interpreting in Health Care. 2008. *The Terminology of Health Care Interpreting: A Glossary of Terms.* Revised August. www.ncihc.org/assets/documents/NCIHC%20Terms%20Final080408.pdf.

Richardson, C. M., and R. E. Luker. 2014. *Historical Dictionary of the Civil Rights Movement*, second edition. Lanham, MD: Rowman & Littlefield.

Saha, S., S. Taggart, M. Komaromy, and A. Bindman. 2000. "Do Patients Choose Physicians of Their Own Race?" *Health Affairs* 19 (4): 76–83.

Smedley, B. D., A. Y. Stith, and A. R. Nelson (eds.). 2003. *Unequal Treatment: Confronting Racial and Ethnic Disparities in Health Care.* Institute of Medicine report. Washington, DC: National Academies Press.

Society for Human Resource Management. 2008. "SHRM's Diversity & Inclusion Initiative." Accessed December 16, 2014. www.shrm.org/Communities/VolunteerResources/Documents/Diversity_CLA_Definitions_of_Diversity_Inclusion.ppt.

Sullivan Commission. 2004. *Missing Persons: Minorities in the Health Professions.* Report of the Sullivan Commission on Diversity in the Healthcare Workforce.

Embargoed September 20. http://depts.washington.edu/ccph/pdf_files/Sullivan_Report_ES.pdf.

Thomas, D., and J. J. Gabarro. 1999. *Breaking Through: The Making of Minority Executives in Corporate America*. Boston: Harvard Business School Press.

US Census Bureau. 2012. "U.S. Census Bureau Projections Show a Slower Growing, Older, More Diverse Nation a Half Century from Now." Published December 12. www.census.gov/newsroom/releases/archives/population/cb12-243.html.

Williams, M. 2001. *The 10 Lenses: Your Guide to Living and Working in a Multicultural World*. Sterling, VA: Capital Books.

Witt/Kieffer. 2011. *Building the Business Case: Healthcare Diversity Leadership: A National Survey Report*. Oak Brook, IL: Witt/Kieffer.

———. 2006. *Advancing Diversity Leadership in Health Care: A National Survey of Healthcare Executives*. Oak Brook, IL: Witt/Kieffer.

Wright, G. 2013. *Sharing the Prize: The Economics of the Civil Rights Revolution in the American South*. Cambridge, MA: Belknap Press of Harvard University Press.

JOB ANALYSIS AND JOB DESIGN

Myron D. Fottler

Learning Objectives

After completing this chapter, the reader should be able to

- distinguish between job analyses, job descriptions, and job specifications;
- describe the methods by which job analyses are typically accomplished;
- discuss the relationship of job requirements (as developed through job analyses, job descriptions, and job specifications) to other human resources management functions;
- enumerate the steps involved in a typical job analysis as well as the methods of job analysis;
- address the relationship between job analyses and strategic human resources management; and
- understand the changing nature of jobs and how jobs are being redesigned to enhance productivity.

Introduction

The interaction between an organization and its environment has important implications for the organization's internal organization and structure. For example, the environment affects how the institution organizes its human resources to achieve specific objectives and to perform different functions necessary in carrying out the organization's mission and goals. The organization formally groups the activities to be performed by its human resources into basic units referred to as jobs.

A *job* consists of a group of activities and duties that entail natural units of work that are similar and related. Each job should be clear and distinct from other jobs to minimize misunderstandings and conflict among employees and to enable employees to recognize what is expected of them. Some jobs are performed by several employees, each of whom occupies a separate position.

A *position* consists of certain duties and responsibilities that are performed by only one employee. For example, in a hospital, 40 registered nurses fill 40 positions, but all of them perform only one job—that of a registered nurse. Jobs that have similar duties and responsibilities may be grouped into a job family for purposes of recruitment, training, compensation, or advancement opportunities. For example, the nursing job family may be performed by registered nurses, the nursing supervisor, and the director of nursing services.

Healthcare organizations are continually restructuring and reengineering in an attempt to become more cost effective and customer focused. They have moved toward a smaller scale, less hierarchy, fewer layers, and more decentralized work units. As these changes occur, managers want their employees to operate more independently and flexibly to meet customer demands. To meet these demands, employees who are closest to the information and who are directly involved in the service delivery must make decisions. The objective is to develop jobs and basic work units that are adaptable and can thrive in a world of high-velocity change.

This chapter defines *job analysis, job description*, and *job specification*; indicates the processes that may be used to conduct job analyses; and identifies the relevance of and relationship between the results of job analysis (i.e., job descriptions and job specifications) and other human resources (HR) management functions. In addition, it emphasizes that these job processes provide the organization with a foundation for making objective and legally defensible decisions in managing human resources. The chapter discusses how healthcare jobs have been redesigned to contribute to organizational objectives while simultaneously satisfying the needs of the employees, and it reviews several innovative job design and employee-contribution techniques to enhance job satisfaction and organizational performance.

Definitions

Job analyses are sometimes called the cornerstone of strategic HR management because the information they collect serves so many HR functions. *Job analysis* is the process of obtaining information about a job by determining the job's duties, tasks, and/or activities. The procedure involves a systematic investigation in which predetermined steps are followed (Morgeson and Dierdorff 2011; Singh 2008). When the analysis is completed, a written report is created that summarizes the information obtained from studying 20 or 30 individual job tasks or activities. HR managers use these data to develop job descriptions and job specifications.

A *job description* is a written explanation of a job and the types of duties the job involves. Because no standard format for job descriptions exists, these documents tend to vary in appearance and content from one organization to another. However, most job descriptions contain the job title, a job identification section, and a job duties section. They may also include a job specification section, but sometimes this is presented as a separate document. A specific job description is a detailed summary of a job's tasks, duties, and responsibilities, emphasizing efficiency, control, and detailed work planning. This type of description fits best with a bureaucratic organizational structure, where well-defined boundaries separate functions and different levels of management.

A general job description, which is fairly new on the HR scene, emphasizes innovation, flexibility, and loose work planning. This type of job description fits best with an organization with a flat structure, where few boundaries exist between functions and levels of management (Pennell 2010). Only the most generic duties, responsibilities, and skills for a position are documented in a general job description.

Both general and specific job descriptions typically include approval signatures of the appropriate managers and a legal disclaimer. The disclaimer allows the employer to change the employee's job duties and/or request that the employee perform duties not listed. In other words, such job descriptions are not viewed as a contract between the employer and the employee (Pennell 2010). Each job description typically identifies the job's three to five most important responsibilities, and each responsibility begins with an action verb such as *diagnoses*, *treats*, or *plans*. All job descriptions should be updated periodically to retain their relevance (Mathis, Jackson, and Valentine 2014).

A *job specification* describes the personal qualifications an individual must possess to perform the duties and responsibilities contained in a job description, including necessary knowledge, skills, and abilities (also called KSAs). Typically, the job specification describes the skills required to perform the job and the physical demands the job places on the employee performing it. It usually includes education and experience, specialized knowledge or training, licenses, personal abilities and traits, and mental and physical requirements to do the job. It does not necessarily include the current employee's qualifications (Van Iddekinge, Raymark, and Eidson 2011). The physical demands of a job refer to the physical work environment, workplace hazards, and the amount of walking, standing, reaching, and lifting required by the job. The supplement at the end of this chapter provides an example of a combined job description/job specification document for the position of staff nurse in a hospital's labor and delivery department.

The Job Analysis Process

Exhibit 6.1 indicates how a job analysis is performed, including the functions for which it is used. Job analysis involves a systematic, step-by-step investigation. The end product of the analysis is a document that summarizes information about the job tasks or activities examined. This information is then used by HR managers in developing job descriptions and job specifications, which in turn are used to guide performance and to enhance different HR functions, such as developing performance appraisal criteria or the

EXHIBIT 6.1
The Process of
Job Analysis

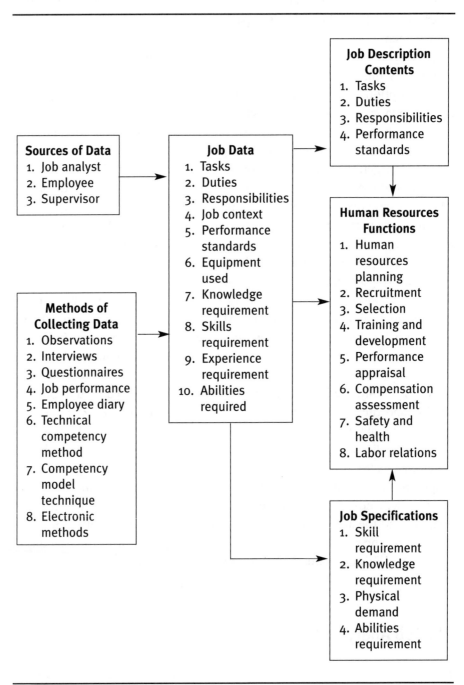

content of training classes (Morgeson and Dierdorff 2011). The ultimate purpose of a job analysis is to improve organizational performance and productivity. Studies have found a positive relationship between the quality of the job analysis process and improved employee and organizational performance (Safdar, Waheed, and Rafiq 2010).

Steps

The steps of a job analysis are as follows:

1. *Determine the purpose of the job analysis.* As a result of rapid growth or downsizing, jobs may have changed in their content. Such changes may cause employee salaries to be inequitable. The purpose of conducting the analysis should be explicit and tied to the organization's overall business strategy to increase the probability of a successful job analysis program.

2. *Identify the jobs to be analyzed.* All jobs are analyzed if no previous formal job analysis has been performed. If the organization has undergone changes that have affected only certain jobs or if new jobs have been added, then only those jobs are analyzed.

3. *Explain the process to employees, and determine their levels of involvement.* Employees should be informed of who will conduct the analysis, why the analysis is needed, whom to contact to answer questions and concerns, when the analysis will take place, and what roles they are expected to play in the process. In addition to receiving good communication, employees may elect a committee to serve as a verification check and to reduce anxiety. Such a committee can also help answer employee questions and concerns.

4. *Collect the job analysis information.* Managers must decide which method or combination of methods will be used and how the information will be collected. Alternatives are discussed in the next section of this chapter.

5. *Organize the job analysis information into a form that will be useful to managers and employees.* This form consists of job descriptions and job specifications. The job descriptions can vary from very broad to very specific and precise; the level of detail depends on the needs of the organization. The job specifications must be linked directly to the job description—that is, they must be relevant to the job.

6. *Review and update the job analysis information frequently.* Particularly in a dynamic environment such as healthcare, jobs seldom go unchanged for long periods of time. Even if no major changes have occurred within the organization, a complete review of all jobs should be performed every three years. More frequent reviews are necessary

when major organizational changes occur. Job information should be collected from a representative sample of job holders and checked for accuracy by their managers (Connell and Culbertson 2010).

Data Sources and Data Collection Methods

Conducting job analyses is usually the primary responsibility of the HR department or the individuals charged with this function. Although job analysts are typically responsible for the job analysis program, they usually enlist the cooperation of the employees and supervisors in the departments in which jobs are being analyzed. These supervisors and employees are the sources of much of the job information generated through the process.

Typically, the organizational chart is reviewed to identify the jobs to be included in the analysis. Often, restructuring, downsizing, a merger, or rapid growth initiates the job analysis. A job may be selected because its content has undergone undocumented changes. As new job demands arise and the nature of the work changes, compensation for the job also may have to change. The employee or the manager may request a job analysis to determine the appropriate compensation. The manager may also be interested in documenting change for recruitment, selection, training, and performance appraisal purposes.

Job information is collected in several ways, depending on the purpose identified by the organization. Managers should consider a number of methods to collect information because any one method is unlikely to provide all of the data needed for a job analysis. Among the most popular methods of data collection are observing tasks and behaviors of jobholders, interviewing individuals or groups, using structured questionnaires and checklists, performing the job, reviewing employee work diaries, asking job experts through the technical conference method, using a competency model, and using electronic or Web-based job analysis methods. Each method is described as follows:

- *Observations* require job analysts to observe jobholders performing their work. The observations may be continuous or consist of intermittent work sampling—that is, observing only a sampling of tasks performed. For many jobs, observation may be of limited usefulness because the job does not consist of physically active tasks. For example, watching an accountant review an income statement may not provide valuable information. Even with more active jobs, observation does not always reveal vital information such as the importance or difficulty of the task. Given the limitations of observation, incorporating additional methods for obtaining job analysis information is helpful.

- *Interviews* with employees who are knowledgeable about a particular job (i.e., the employee holding the job, supervisors, or former jobholders) can provide information on the specific work activities of the job. Usually a structured interview form is used to record information. The questions correspond to the data needed to prepare a job description and job specification. Employees may be suspicious of the interviewer's motives, especially if the interviewer asks ambiguous questions. Because interviewing can be a time consuming and costly method of data collection, managers and job analysts may prefer to use the interview as a means to get answers to specific questions generated from observations and questionnaires.

- The use of *structured questionnaires* and *checklists* is a quick and inexpensive way to collect information about a job. If possible, have several knowledgeable employees complete the questionnaire for verification. Such survey data often can be quantified and processed by computer. Follow-up observations and interviews are often necessary if a questionnaire or checklist is chosen as the primary means of collecting information. The questionnaire must be extremely detailed and comprehensive so that valuable data are not missed. Compared to other methods, questionnaires are cheaper and easier to administer but are more time consuming and expensive to develop. Management must decide whether the benefits of a simplified method of data collection outweigh the costs of its construction.

  Strategically, managers favor methods of data collection that do not require a lot of work and up-front costs if the content of the job changes frequently. One option may be to adopt an existing structured questionnaire. Among the more widely used structured questionnaires are the Position Analysis Questionnaire, the Management Position Description Questionnaire, and the Functional Job Analysis. Regardless of whether the questionnaire is developed in-house or purchased from a commercial source, rapport between analyst and respondent is not possible unless the analyst is available to explain items and to clarify mis- understandings. Without this rapport, such an impersonal approach may have adverse effects on the respondent's cooperation and motivation.

- The job analyst can *perform the job* in question. This approach allows exposure to the actual job tasks as well as the job's physical, environmental, and social demands. This method is appropriate for jobs that can be learned in a relatively short period. However, it is inappropriate for jobs that require extensive training and/or are hazardous to perform.

- The *diary method* requires jobholders to record their daily activities. Diaries are filled out at specific times during the workday for two to four weeks. This method is the most time consuming of all job analysis approaches, which adds to its cost.

- The *technical competency method* relies on supervisors who have an extensive knowledge of the job (frequently called "subject matter experts"). Job attributes are obtained from these experts. Although a good data-gathering method, it overlooks incumbent workers' perceptions of what their jobs actually entail (Mathis, Jackson, and Valentine 2014).

- The *competency model technique* is a popular form of job analysis today. A competency is an underlying characteristic of a person that results in effective and/or superior performance on the job by individuals or teams. It is also a cluster of related knowledge, skills, and attitudes that affects one's job performance. Competencies are focused on strategic goals and organizational outcome measures.

  Technical competencies refer to specific knowledge and skills relevant for a particular job. Behavioral competencies refer to *how* skills are used most effectively. Examples include communication effectiveness, adaptability, innovation, team orientation, and customer focus. The competency approach attempts to identify the competencies that have a positive impact on employee performance in a particular job (Sanchez and Levine 2009; Soderquist 2010).

  Most healthcare organizations have developed some form of competency-based job analysis. Future job analysis may integrate traditional task-based methods as well as competency-based job analysis models. One factor driving such an outcome is that many healthcare organizations are now attempting to identify strategic competencies in addition to job tasks and duties (Kucharova, Zavadska, and Sirotiakova 2010). Both approaches are needed because task-based analysis is likely to remain widely used because it is most defensible legally (McDaniel, Kepes, and Banks 2011).

- Employers are increasingly relying on *electronic or Web-based* job analysis methods. The manager or job analyst uses the Web to review information on the particular job and then sends this information electronically to job incumbents in remote locations. Responses are then discussed in video conferences. Face-to-face meetings are held to finalize the knowledge, skills, abilities, and competencies to be incorporated into the job description (Stone et al. 2013).

  - Many employers use Internet sources such as www.jobdescription.com to facilitate writing job descriptions.

- The Occupational Information Network (O*NET) of the US Department of Labor is an Internet database that includes about 20,000 occupations from the earlier printed *Dictionary of Occupational Titles* as well as an update of more than 3,500 additional occupations. The job descriptions in the database provide employee attributes and job characteristics, such as skills, abilities, knowledge, tasks, work activities, and experience-level requirements. The database is continually updated and is useful for a variety of HR activities, including job analysis, employee selection, career counseling, and employee training.

  O*NET's six-domain content model provides a framework for describing jobs in greater detail. Exhibit 6.2 shows the O*NET content model, which uses both job-oriented and worker-oriented descriptors. The model allows occupational information to be applied across jobs, sectors, or industries and within occupations. O*NET is free to use and provides comprehensive information on a wide variety of occupations (Morgeson and Dierdorff 2011). The website (see www.onetcenter.org) also offers downloadable detailed job analysis questionnaires that can be used for many purposes.

A combination of data collection methods is often appropriate. The job analyst should employ as many techniques as needed to develop valid and accurate job descriptions and job specifications.

Relation to Other Human Resources Functions

Job analysis provides the basis for tying all the HR functional areas together and for developing a sound HR program. Not surprisingly, job requirements as documented in job descriptions and job specifications influence many of the HR functions that are performed as part of managing employees. Consequently, job analysis has grown in importance as the workforce and jobs have changed over time (Morgeson and Dierdorff 2011). When job requirements are modified, corresponding changes must be made in other HR activities. Job analysis is the foundation for forecasting future needs for human resources as well as for planning such activities as recruitment, selection, performance appraisal, compensation, training, transfer, or promotion. Job analysis information is often incorporated into HR information systems.

Before attempting to attract capable employees, recruiters must know the job specifications for the positions that need to be filled, including the knowledge, skills, and abilities required for successful job performance. The information in the job specifications is used in job-opening notices and as a basis for attracting qualified applicants while discouraging unqualified

EXHIBIT 6.2
The Content
Model of O*NET

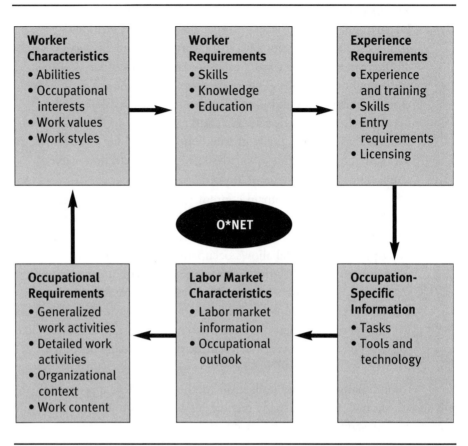

Source: O*NET Resource Center (2014).

candidates. Failure to update job specifications can result in a flood of applicants who are unqualified to perform one or more functions of the job.

Until 1971, job specifications used in employee selection decisions often were unrelated to the duties to be performed under the job description. In the case of *Griggs v. Duke Power Company*, 401 U.S. 424 (1971), the US Supreme Court ruled that employment practices must be job related. When discrimination charges arise, employers have the burden of proving that job requirements are job related or constitute a business necessity. Today, employers must be able to show that the job specifications used in selecting employees for a job are specifically associated with that job's duties.

Any discrepancies between the knowledge, skills, and abilities demonstrated by the jobholders and the requirements contained in the job description and specification provide clues for training needs. Career development is concerned with preparing employees for advancement to jobs at which their capabilities can be used to the fullest extent possible. The formal qualifications set forth in the job specifications for higher-level jobs serve to indicate how much more training and development are needed for employees to advance.

The requirements contained in the job description are the criteria for evaluating the performance of the jobholder. The appraisal may reveal, however, that certain performance criteria established for a particular job are not completely valid. These criteria must be specific and job related. If the criteria used to evaluate employee performance are overly broad, vague, and not job related, employers may be charged with unfair discrimination.

The relative worth of a job is one of the most important factors in determining the compensation for performing a job. This worth is based on what the job demands of an employee in terms of skill, effort, and responsibility as well as the conditions and hazards under which the work is performed. Information derived from a job analysis is also valuable in identifying safety and health considerations. If a job is hazardous (e.g., poses the possibility of contracting AIDS), the job description and specification should reflect this condition. Employers need to provide specific information about such hazards to enable jobholders to perform their jobs safely.

Job analysis information is also important to the employee-relations and labor-relations functions. When employees are considered for promotion, transfer, or demotion, the job description provides a standard for comparison of talent. Information obtained through job analysis can often lead to more objective HR decisions. Job analysis can be used in employee selection to determine whether an applicant for a specific job should be required to take a particular kind of test. The performance standards used to judge employee performance for promotion, rewards, discipline, and loyalty should be job related and based on the job description. Job analysis information can also be used to compare the relative worth of each job's contribution to the organization's overall performance. Finally, job analysis can be used to determine training needs by comparing current employee skills to skills identified in the job analysis. Training programs can then be put in place to reduce employees' skill gaps.

Legal Aspects

Although HR managers consider job descriptions a valuable tool for performing HR functions, they encounter the following problems when using these documents:

- Job descriptions are often poorly written and offer little guidance to the jobholder.
- They are generally not updated as job duties or specifications change.
- They may violate the law by containing specifications that are not related to job performance.

- The job duties included are often written in vague, rather than specific, terms.
- They can limit the scope of activities of the jobholder in a rapidly changing environment.

A major goal of job analysis is to help the organization establish the job-relatedness of its selection and performance requirements. Job analysis helps employees to meet their legal duties under equal employment opportunity law. Section 14.C.2 of the "Uniform Guidelines for Employee Selection Procedures" states, "There shall be a job analysis which includes an analysis of the important work behaviors required for successful performance. . . . Any job analysis should focus on work behavior(s) and the tasks associated with them" (Equal Employment Opportunity Commission [EEOC] 1978). Today's legal environment has created a need for higher levels of specificity in job analysis and job descriptions.

Federal guidelines require that the specific performance requirements of a job be based on valid job-related criteria (EEOC 1978). Employment decisions that involve either job applicants or employees and that are based on vague and non-job-related criteria are increasingly being challenged, and the challenges have mostly been successful. Managers of small healthcare organizations, where employees may perform many different job tasks, must be particularly concerned about writing specific job descriptions.

When writing job descriptions, employers must use statements that are terse, direct, and worded simply, excluding unnecessary phrases and terms. Typically, the sentences that describe job duties begin with verbs (see the end-of-chapter supplement). The term "may" is used for duties performed by only some workers on the job.

Excellent job descriptions are of value to both the employee and the employer. For the employee, job descriptions help them learn their job duties and remind them of the results they are expected to achieve. For the employer, job descriptions can minimize the misunderstandings that occur between supervisors and subordinates regarding job requirements. Good job descriptions also establish management's right to take corrective action in the event that the duties specified in the document are not performed at all or are performed at an inadequate or inappropriate level.

Job analysis is surrounded by several legal constraints largely because it serves as a basis for selection decisions, compensation, performance appraisals, and training. These constraints have been articulated in the "Uniform Guidelines for Employee Selection Procedures" and in several court decisions. Again, as the guidelines state, "Any job analysis should focus on work behavior(s) and the tasks associated with them." To determine this, organizations should assess the job skills, knowledge, and abilities needed to perform the jobs. After these items are known, selection procedures can be developed (EEOC 2002).

Organizations' failures to perform job analyses have resulted in successful challenges to the validity of the organizations' selection decisions; see *Albermarle Paper Company v. Moody*, 422 U.S. 405 (1975). Numerous court decisions regarding promotion and job analysis also exist. In *Rowe v. General Motors Corporation*, 457 F. 2d 348 (1972), the court ruled that a company should have written objective standards for promotion to prevent discriminatory practices. In *U.S. v. City of Chicago*, 573 F.2d 416 (7th Cir.) (1978), the court ruled that the standards should describe the job for which the person is being considered for promotion. In both cases, these objective standards can be determined through job analysis.

Before the enactment of the "Uniform Guidelines for Employee Selection Procedures" and the associated court decisions, labor contracts required consistent and equitable treatment of unionized employees. The information provided by job analysis is helpful to both management and unions in contract negotiations and in avoiding or resolving grievances, jurisdictional disputes, and other conflicts. For these reasons, unionized employers have found preparing written job descriptions and job specifications to be advantageous.

The passage of the Americans with Disabilities Act (ADA) also had a major impact on job analysis. Managers must now adhere to the legal mandates of the ADA when preparing job descriptions and job specifications. The ADA requires that job duties and abilities be essential functions for successful job performance. If the job requires the jobholder to perform certain essential physical and mental tasks, these requirements should be stated in the job description. Section 1630.2(n) of the ADA provides three guidelines for rendering a job function essential (EEOC 2002):

1. The reason the position exists is to perform a function.
2. A limited number of employees are available among whom performance of the function may be distributed.
3. The function may be highly specialized, requiring needed expertise or abilities to complete the job.

Managers who write job descriptions in terms of essential functions reduce the risk of discriminating on the basis of disability. Once the essential functions of a job are defined, the organization is legally required to make a reasonable accommodation to the disability of the individual.

The job analysis process is the basic method used to identify essential job functions. An *essential job function* is one that is fundamental to successful performance of the job, while a *marginal job function* is incidental to the main function of the job (i.e., a matter of convenience and not a necessity). Qualified individuals with disabilities are persons who have a disability but meet the skill, education, and experience of the job requirements and can perform the essential functions with or without reasonable accommodation.

Reasonable accommodation means that the employer may be required to alter the environment of a particular job to enable a person with a disability to perform all essential functions. However, employers cannot be required to make an accommodation that imposes undue hardship.

Other legislation also requires a thorough job analysis:

- The Fair Labor Standards Act categorizes employees as exempt and nonexempt on the basis of the job analysis.
- The Equal Pay Act requires equal pay for equal work. When pay differentials exist, job descriptions can be used to show whether jobs are substantially different in terms of skill, effort, responsibility, and working conditions.
- The Civil Rights Act often requires the use of job specifications to defend against charges of discrimination in initial selection, promotion, and other HR decisions.
- The Occupational Safety and Health Act requires that job applicants be shown in advance job descriptions that specify the elements of the job that may endanger employee health or be considered distasteful.

The Changing Environment

Traditional job analysis is a static view of a job as it currently exists. This approach is not aligned with current organizational trends emphasizing flexibility and innovativeness in all industries (Singh 2008). The traditional approach to job analysis assumes a static job environment, where jobs remain relatively stable apart from the incumbents who hold these jobs. It assumes that jobs can be meaningfully defined in terms of tasks, duties, processes, and behaviors necessary for job success. Unfortunately, these assumptions discount technological advances that are often so accelerated that jobs that are defined today may be obsolete tomorrow.

In a dynamic environment where job demands change rapidly, job analysis data can quickly become outdated and inaccurate. Obsolete job analysis information can hinder an organization's ability to adapt to change. Several approaches to job analysis may respond to the need for continuous change.

First, adopt a future-oriented approach to job analysis. This strategic analysis of jobs requires managers to have a clear view of how duties and tasks can be restructured to meet organizational requirements in the future. To perform this approach, researchers in one study asked experts on a particular job to identify aspects of the job, the organization, and the environment that might change in the next few years and how those changes might affect the nature of the job. The collected data were then used to describe the tasks, knowledge, skills, and abilities needed for the job in the future.

By including future-oriented information in job descriptions, health-care organizations can focus employee attention on new strategic directions. For example, one organization decided to change its strategic focus to increasing its "customer-consciousness" orientation (George 1990). Job descriptions were then amended to include tasks, knowledge, skills, and abilities related to customer contact and responsibilities. These new job descriptions focused more on what the organization wanted to be doing in the future.

Second, adopt a competency-based approach to job analysis that places emphasis on characteristics of successful performers rather than on standard job duties and tasks (Van Wart 2000). Healthcare organizations operating in fast-moving environments tend to rely on job profiles that look at both job duties and competencies or capabilities that the incumbent jobholder needs in order to adapt to new job changes. How the work is done is just as important as what work is done (Klas et al. 2010). These competencies will align with the organizational strategic plan and culture and often include interpersonal communication skills, the ability to work as part of a team, decision-making capabilities, conflict resolution know-how, adaptability, and self-motivation (Van Wart 2000).

The goal is to identify key competencies crucial to the organization's future success through focus groups, surveys, and interviews. This technique enhances a culture of continuous improvement in which organizational improvement is a constant aim. Both approaches to change-oriented job analysis have potential impracticalities, including dependence on the ability of managers to accurately predict future job needs, the uncertainty that the analysis will comply with EEOC guidelines, and the ambiguity in job descriptions resulting from their creation on the basis of estimates.

What distinguishes competency modeling from traditional job analysis? Is it the emphasis on the individual characteristic or specific performance (Sanchez and Levine 2009)? The objective of competency modeling is to outline and describe the competencies of successful employees for a series of related jobs. Competency models are particularly useful for developing career paths and relevant training experiences. Competency models list the knowledge, skills, and behaviors that employees must exhibit to get their multiple jobs done. Examples are skills (analyze financial statements), behaviors (diagnose based on symptoms), knowledge (clinical understanding), and experience (education and work experience). The goal is to summarize the competencies required for exceptional performance.

The International Council of Nurses has identified the following competencies for the nurse specialist: accountability, legal practice, ethical practice, health promotion, assessment, therapeutic communication, delegation and supervision, and quality improvement (Affra 2009). Such competency models have been shown in other industries to provide guidance for employee recruitment, selection, training, and performance appraisal (Campion et al. 2011).

Third, conduct a generic job analysis. The traditional job analysis approach serves to constrain desired change and flexibility by compartmentalizing and specifically defining presumably static job characteristics. It impedes shifting decision making downward in the organization, cross-training employees, and getting employees involved in quality improvement efforts. Reducing the number of job titles and developing more generic job descriptions can provide needed flexibility to manage unanticipated change.

The last item on a typical job description is often "any other duty that may be assigned." This statement is increasingly becoming *the* job description. This enlarged, flexible, complex job changes the way nearly every HR function is performed. For example, in recruitment and selection, individuals who possess only the technical skills required to perform the job are not viewed as ideal candidates anymore. HR managers are also looking for broader capabilities such as competencies, intelligence, adaptability, and an ability and willingness to work in teams.

The rapid pace of change in healthcare makes the need for accurate job analysis even more important. Historically, job analysis was conducted and then set aside for a reasonable time. Today, however, job requirements are in such a constant state of flux that job descriptions and specifications must be constantly reviewed to keep them relevant. By one estimate, people may have to change their entire skill sets three or four times during their careers (Snyder 1996). If this projection is right, the need for accurate and timely job analysis is becoming even more important. Organizations that do not revise or review job descriptions and specifications may recruit new employees who do not possess the needed skills or may not provide necessary training to update employee skills.

Managerial Implications

Several challenges may limit the impact and effectiveness of job analysis in healthcare organizations. Top management support of job analysis may be lukewarm or nonexistent, and updating of job descriptions and job specifications may not occur. The reason for these challenges may be a lack of understanding of and appreciation for the job analysis process and its significance in supporting the effective implementation of all HR functions. As a result, job analysis is not performed and job descriptions and specifications are not modified as jobs evolve over time. The organization, in turn, operates with outdated information, which adversely affects employee and organizational outcomes.

These situations may create the following challenges (followed by possible strategies to mitigate them):

- *Only single methods of job analysis may be used.* A combination of methods might provide better and more reliable data. In addition, input from job incumbents, supervisors, and experts may provide more usable and valuable data for job descriptions and job specifications.
- *The jobholder and supervisor may be excluded from the job analysis process.* Because of their extensive knowledge of the relative importance of job functions, both jobholders and supervisors should be involved in the process.
- *Sometimes the employee is involved in the process but is not allowed sufficient time to complete the job analysis with any level of quality.* This limitation often results in a poorly written, insignificant, vague, and nonspecific job description or specification that is of little value to the organization and may create legal liability. Obviously, employees should be allowed sufficient time during work hours to complete their input into the job analysis process.
- *Because neither managers nor employees are trained or motivated to generate quality data, their data may be distorted.* This problem could be overcome by training employees and managers, making employees aware of the importance of the process, and providing desirable rewards for good data.
- *Sometimes job descriptions imply that the job incumbent will perform only the job duties outlined in the description.* This implication could foster an "it's not my job" philosophy. Consequently, the last item of the job description should be phrased as "any other duty that may be assigned." Healthcare executives can no longer select individuals who possess only the narrow skills required to perform a job. They must go deeper and seek other competencies, such as ability to adjust and willingness to work in teams. Such qualities should be incorporated into job specifications.
- *Many job analyses do not go beyond the initial phase of reporting what the jobholder currently does.* The job should also be critiqued to determine whether it is being done correctly and whether other job functions may enhance the jobholder's contributions to achieving the organization's strategic objectives.

Finally, speed is of the essence. Job requirements are changing so rapidly that they must be constantly reviewed to keep them relevant. Yet the time that can be devoted to job analysis has diminished. "Job analysis at the speed of reality" has been developed as a shorter version of the interview method. Through this process, a validated job analysis can be completed in two to three hours (Hartley 2004).

Job Design

Job design is an outgrowth of job analysis and focuses on structuring and/or restructuring jobs to help improve organizational effectiveness, efficiency, and employee job satisfaction. It refers to organizing tasks, duties, responsibilities, and other job elements into a productive unit of work (Mathis, Jackson, and Valentine 2014). The process involves changing, eliminating, modifying, and enriching duties and tasks to capture the talents of employees so that they can contribute to the fullest and develop professionally. Job design should simultaneously facilitate the achievement of organizational objectives and recognize the capabilities and needs of those who perform the job (Foss et al. 2009).

Job design encompasses the manner in which a given job is defined and how it will be conducted. This process involves such decisions as how the job will be handled by an individual or by a team of employees and such determinations as how the job will fit into the overall organization. Organizing tasks, duties, and responsibilities into a unit of work to achieve a certain objective requires a conscious effort. Well-designed jobs in healthcare can provide several benefits to both the organization and the employee, including enhanced job performance, improved job satisfaction, reduced absenteeism and turnover, and enhanced employee physical and mental health (Ilies, Dimotakis, and De Pater 2010; Rao 2010).

Each job design process must acknowledge any unique skills possessed by a number of employees of a given profession and must incorporate appropriate professional guidelines or task limitations. In healthcare, most professionals are constrained by limitations on the functions and tasks they may legally perform and the level of supervision required. For example, many technical functions require performance either by a physician or by another professional under the direct supervision of a physician. Such legal constraints obviously reduce but do not obviate the flexibility of healthcare executives in designing jobs. Executives must make sure job expectations are clear, responsibilities and accountability are clarified, and integration with other jobs is appropriate (Holman, Frenkel, and Sørensen 2009).

Specialization in Healthcare

As a result of technological change, increased specialization, and the emergence of the hospital as the central focus of the healthcare system, approximately 700 different job categories exist in the healthcare industry. The most rapid growth in the supply of the healthcare workforce has occurred in new categories: More than two-thirds of all healthcare employees work in nontraditional allied health or support service positions (US Census Bureau 2012). The roles and job functions are controlled by state legislatures in the United States and evolve and change over time. A prime example is the evolving roles of primary care physicians, specialist physicians, physician assistants, and nurse practitioners (Beck 2014).

Specialization has inherent limitations and has been taken to extremes in healthcare. Because of the inherent disadvantages of specialization, new approaches to organizing work and job design are needed. The foremost criticism is that specialized workers may become bored and dissatisfied because their jobs may not offer enough challenge or stimulation. Boredom and monotony set in and absenteeism rises, introducing the possibility that the quality of work will suffer.

Not all employees have similar preferences regarding the degree of specialization in their jobs. Having a good fit between employees and the job requirements of their current positions is important (Avey, Luthans, and Youssef 2010). If not, either the person should be replaced or the job should be redesigned. As a result, different people will benefit from different kinds of work, and employee selection needs to focus on finding applicants with the proper fit (Boon et al. 2011).

To counter the problems of specialization and to enhance productivity and employee job satisfaction, healthcare executives have implemented a number of job design and job redesign options to achieve a better balance between organizational demands for efficiency and productivity and individual needs for creativity and autonomy. Four alternative redesign approaches are (1) job redesign (e.g., enlargement, enrichment, rotation), (2) employee empowerment, (3) workgroup redesign (e.g., employee involvement groups, employee teams), and (4) work schedule redesign. Each of these approaches is explored below.

Job Enlargement/Job Enrichment

Job enlargement involves changes in the scope of a job to provide greater variety to the employee. It is a *horizontal expansion* of duties with the same level of autonomy and responsibility. Alternatively, job enrichment adds additional autonomy and responsibility and is a *vertical expansion* of duties. One specific profession that was developed in response to the need for job enlargement or job enrichment is the *multiskilled health practitioner* (MSHP). These combined functions can be found in a broad spectrum of healthcare-related jobs and range in complexity from the nonprofessional to the professional level. The functions (skills) added to the worker's original job may be of a higher, lower, or parallel level.

Most theories of job enrichment stress that unless jobs are both horizontally and vertically enriched, little positive impact is made on motivation, productivity, and job satisfaction. Examples of job enrichment include giving an employee a complete job rather than just a piece, allowing more flexibility in how a job is performed, increasing an employee's accountability for results, and providing feedback directly to the employee.

Because the MSHP concept may involve horizontal, vertical, or both types of enrichment, whether it should be expected to enhance organizational outcomes is unclear. Research on the concept reveals that the outcomes have been positive in terms of enhanced productivity, job satisfaction, and patient satisfaction (Fottler 1996). However, those positive outcomes depend on many contingencies, such as whether the "right" employees are chosen for the program (i.e., those with higher needs for personal growth), implementation processes, available training opportunities, legal constraints, and continuing top-management commitment.

A related job design approach is "job crafting," which is a naturally occurring phenomenon whereby employees modify or enhance their original job task to better fit their existing or evolving skills, knowledge, ability, strengths, and motives (Tasler 2010). Employees who engage in job crafting tend to reshape their jobs with or without permission of their managers. The result is often higher levels of employee engagement and improved levels of organizational performance.

When healthcare organizations are restructured, such changes almost always create changes in employees' jobs. Most competitive challenges that result in restructuring require a committed and engaged workforce able to innovate and make decisions. Consequently, most jobs today in healthcare and beyond are being enriched, not simply enlarged or reduced in scope (Becker and Huselid 2010). A job enrichment process that has provisions for contact with patients and other clients is likely to enhance employee job satisfaction because employees learn directly how the customer experiences the service and how it affects him or her (Grant 2007).

Employee Empowerment

Job enlargement or job enrichment approaches, such as the development of the MSHP role, are programs by which managers and supervisors formally change the jobs of employees. A less structured approach is to allow employees to initiate their own job changes through the concept of empowerment. The process of empowerment entails providing employees with the skills and authority to make decisions that would traditionally be made by managers (Gomez-Mejia, Balkin, and Cardy 2012). The goal is to create enthusiastic and committed staff who perform their functions ably and enjoyably, having internal control over their activities. To support empowerment, organizations must share with the workforce information, knowledge, power to act, and rewards. Empowerment encourages employees to become innovators and managers of their own work and gives them more control and autonomous decision-making capabilities (Snell and Bohlander 2013).

Empowerment can involve employee control over the job content (functions and responsibilities), the job context (the environmental conditions under which the job is performed), or both (Ford and Fottler 1995). Most healthcare organizations are not ready for both and are advised to implement empowerment on an incremental basis. For empowerment to thrive and grow, organizations must encourage participation, innovation, access to information, accountability, and a culture that is open and receptive to change (Garcia 1997). Examples of organizations that have successfully implemented employee empowerment include Cigna, AT&T, MetLife, Costco, and Disney. Key management approaches relevant to employee empowerment include employee participation in decision making, receptivity to innovation, access to relevant information, and management and employee accountability for results (Snell and Bohlander 2013).

Work Group Design and Redesign

Work groups depend on a supervisor, while a team depends on its own members to provide leadership and direction. Groups or teams vary significantly in size from as few as two to as many as 80 members for virtual groups who collaborate over the Internet. Most teams should have fewer than five or six members for optimal purposes (Thompson 2011).

Several types of teams may periodically function beyond the scope of a staff member's normal job. Exhibit 6.3 outlines the six forms of work groups or teams currently being used in healthcare. Teams are groups of employees who assume a greater role in the service process. They provide a forum for employees to contribute to identifying and solving organizational problems. With work teams, managers accept the notion that the group is the logical work unit to resolve organizational problems and concerns.

Regardless of which team structure is employed, several team characteristics have been identified in successful teams. These characteristics include commitment to shared goals, motivated and energetic team members, consensus decision making, open and honest communication, shared leadership, a climate of trust and collaboration, valuing of diversity, and acceptance of conflict and its positive resolution. A good team also requires that team goals and scope of authority be defined by management, that employee selection partially consider the potential team member's interpersonal skills, and that extensive training for team members be provided (Wharton School 2009). Virtual teams, in particular, must guard against miscommunication, unresolved problems, and lower productivity (O'Leary and Mortenson 2010). The manager must also adapt to the role of leader (rather than supervisor) and not be threatened by the growing power of the team.

EXHIBIT 6.3
Types of
Employee
Teams in
Healthcare

Type	Description
Cross-functional team	A group staffed by a mix of specialists (nurses, physicians, and managers) and formed to accomplish a specific objective. Usually, membership on this team is assigned rather than voluntary.
Project team	A group formed specifically to design a new service. Members are assigned by management on the basis of their ability to contribute to team success. The group normally disperses after task completion.
Self-directed team (or autonomous work group)	A group of highly trained individuals who are accountable for a whole work process that provides a service or product to an internal or external customer. Members use consensus decision making to perform job duties, solve problems, or deal with internal or external customers.
Task force team	A group formed by management to resolve a major problem. This team is responsible for developing a long-term plan for problem resolution that may include implementing the proposed solution.
Process improvement team (or employee involvement group)	A group made up of experienced employees from different departments or functions and charged with improving quality, decreasing waste, or enhancing productivity in processes that affect all departments. Members are normally appointed by management.
Virtual team	A group with any of the above purposes that uses advanced computer and telecommunication technology to link geographically dispersed team members. Virtual teams are similar to project teams in that they do not require full-time commitment. Without some face-to-face communication, some teams may experience miscommunication, low productivity, and/or unresolved problems.

Sources: Beck (2014); Becker and Huselid (2010); Campion et al. (2011); Connell and Culbertson (2010); Dennis, Meola, and Hall (2012); Foss et al. (2009); Grant (2007); Kucharova, Zavadska, and Sirotiakova (2010); McDaniel, Kepes, and Banks (2011); Miguel and Miklos (2011); Pennell (2010); Petrecca (2013); Raiborn and Butler (2009); Safdar, Waheed, and Rafiq (2010); Singh (2008); Snell and Bohlander (2013); Stanley (2010); Stone et al. (2013); Tasler (2010); Thompson (2011); Van Hootegem et al. (2005); and Wildman et al. (2011).

Because many teams fail to operate at full potential, organizations must be aware of several obstacles to the effective functions of teams, including overly high expectations, inappropriate compensation, lack of training, and lack of power. For example, new team members must be retrained to work outside their primary functional area, and compensation systems must be constructed to reward individuals for team achievements. New career paths to general management and/or higher clinical positions must be created from the team's experience.

Finally, the roles of supervisors and managers change as they become team leaders and facilitators. Rather than giving orders, they assist the team, mediate and resolve conflict, and interact with teams and managers (Humphrey, Morgeson, and Mannor 2009). Management may need further training or incentives to work with teams. Comprehensive management training may also be needed to enhance skills in team leadership, goal setting, conducting of meetings, team decision making, conflict resolution, effective communication, and diversity awareness.

Work Schedule Redesign

Organizations are using many work schedule innovations based on industry demands, workforce needs, and other factors (Golden 2009). These innovations include the compressed workweek, flextime, job sharing, telecommuting, and contingent workers. In US industries as a whole, employers' most common options are flextime and telecommuting, while the compressed workweek, contingent workers, and job sharing are less common (Society for Human Resource Management 2010). A 2007 study by the American Business Collaboration showed that 64 percent of employers used some type of work schedule redesign. Similar to the Society for Human Resource Management 2010 study, it found the prevalence of each type as follows: flextime (33 percent), telecommuting (14 percent), compressed workweek (16 percent), contingent workers (9 percent), and job sharing (1 percent).

The goal of work schedule redesign is to give employees greater control over their time. Adjustments in work schedules alter the normal workweek of five eight-hour days in which everyone begins and ends their workday at the same time. Such adjustments are made to improve organizational productivity and morale by giving employees increased control over their work schedules.

By allowing employees greater flexibility in work scheduling, employers can reduce some of the most common causes of tardiness and absenteeism—that is, the time pressures of life. Employees can adjust their work schedules to accommodate their lifestyles, reduce pressure to meet a rigid schedule, and gain greater satisfaction. Employers can enhance their attractiveness when recruiting and retaining personnel while improving their customer service (poor service is a direct result of low levels of employee satisfaction). Productivity and quality may also be enhanced (Coombs 2011; Torpey 2007).

According to 68 percent of HR professionals surveyed, the quality of the employee's personal and family life is improved by flexibility at work (*HR Magazine* 2010). Such flexibility has also been found to improve recruitment and retention of high-quality employees (Brisco 2011), employee productivity, job satisfaction, and attendance (Brisco 2011; McMillan 2011).

Under the *compressed workweek* scheme, the number of days in the workweek is shortened by lengthening the number of hours worked per day. The four-day 40-hour week (4/40) is the most common form of compressed workweek, and the three-day 39-hour week (3/39) schedule is less common. Many workers in hospitals work three 12-hour shifts and then take off four days (Bloomberg BNA 2008).

The compressed schedule accommodates the leisure-time activities and personal appointments of employees. Potential barriers to this schedule design are the stringent rules under the Fair Labor Standards Act that require the payment of overtime to nonsupervisory employees who work more than 40 hours a week. Long workdays may also increase the amount of exhaustion and stress for employees and managers. A 2006 Society for Human Resource Management survey reported that 35 percent of the employer respondents offered some type of compressed workweek (Thompson 2006).

Flextime, or the use of flexible working hours, allows employees to choose daily starting and quitting times, provided that they work a certain number of hours per day or week. Flextime may be formal or informal, and may cover all employees or just a subset. Typically, employers designate a core period during the morning and afternoon when all employees on a given shift are required to be on the job. Most organizations have less than 10 percent of their employees on a flexible work arrangement, but these arrangements are very popular with employees who use them. They work best when the work is conducive to different schedules, the terms of the arrangement are clear, and sound performance management principles are followed (Golden 2009; Mayo et al. 2009; Stanley 2010).

In healthcare, flextime is most common in clerical or management functions, such as claims processing, health insurance, and human resources. Flextime is not appropriate for patient care positions because these functions must be staffed at all times, while communication and coordination are a continuing challenge in other positions.

The 2006 Society for Human Resource Management survey found that 57 percent of the employer respondents used some form of formal flextime (Thompson 2006). This percentage dropped slightly to 53 percent in 2011 (Coombs 2011). Flextime offers several advantages for both employers and employees. By allowing employees greater flexibility in work scheduling, employers may reduce absenteeism and tardiness (Zeidner 2008). Adjusting work schedules to accommodate particular lifestyles may also enhance employee job satisfaction, reduce employee commuting times, and improve customer service by extending operating hours. Finally, research demonstrates that flextime has a positive impact on the quantity, quality, and reliability of employee work (Baltes et al. 1999; Snell and Bohlander 2013).

Job sharing is an arrangement whereby two part-time employees share a job that otherwise would be held by a full-time employee. Job sharers sometimes work three days a week to create an overlap day for face-to-face conferencing. A survey of 1,020 employers by Hewitt Associates in 2005 showed that slightly more than 25 percent of the respondents offered some type of job sharing (Bach 2006). However, a Society for Human Resource Management survey in 2010 found that only 15 percent offered it, the lowest level in 13 years (Shellenbarger 2010). A major impediment is the reluctance of managers to hire and supervise managerial and professional employees on a part-time basis.

Job sharing can be scheduled to conform to peaks in the daily or weekly workload. However, more time may be needed to orient, train, and develop two employees who share one role. Job sharing partners need to operate as a team and communicate the details of their daily activities during handoffs in order to maintain their quantity, quality, and productivity of output (Miller 2007). Job sharing is best suited for employees who wish to work part time and can be helpful for older workers who wish to phase into retirement. Job sharing can reduce absenteeism because it allows employees to have time to accommodate their personal needs even when employed. It also aids in retention of valuable employees. Among notable healthcare organizations that have developed a job sharing program for physicians is HMO Kaiser Permanente in northern California.

Job sharing may pose problems for employers. Among the possible concerns are the time required to orient and train a second employee and prorating of employee benefits between the two job sharers. The key to making this approach work is good communication between partners through phone calls, e-mails, voice mails, or written updates. Job sharing is also helped if the two partners have worked in the organization together before they decide to share a job.

One of the most significant work schedule innovations is *telecommuting* or *telework*, which is the system of performing work at home or away from the office with the use of computers, networks, telephones, and fax machines. Telecommuting is more appropriate for companies or positions that are not engaged in direct patient care. A 2006 Society for Human Resource Management survey revealed that 58 percent of the employer respondents offered some type of telecommuting (Oettinger 2011). A 2013 sample of US employers found that 58 percent offer the option of telecommuting and another 4 percent plan to do so within 12 months (Statista

2014). Twenty-one percent offer full-time employees the option of telecommuting, and 24 percent of their employees report that they work at least some hours per week at home (Noonan and Glass 2012).

Evidence indicates that, when given a choice, employees prefer a mix of working part of the time from home and part of the time at the employer's premises (Garchiek 2006). Some jobs exhibit higher rates of telecommuting. For example, almost 45 percent of medical transcriptionists work from home (Bloomberg BNA 2012a). More than 13 million Americans work from home at least one day a week, with Fridays and Mondays the most common work-at-home days (Bloomberg BNA 2012b).

The two most important advantages of telecommuting are flexibility for employees and improved ability of organizations to attract workers who may not otherwise be available (Offstein 2010). Telecommuting also decreases overhead costs by eliminating or minimizing the need for office space. Drawbacks of telecommuting include the potential loss of employee creativity because of lower levels of face-to-face interaction, the difficulty of developing appropriate performance standards and evaluation systems, and the challenge of formulating an appropriate technology system for telecommuting. Telecommuting may also negatively affect employee–supervisor relationships. In addition, if some employees are denied the opportunity to work from home, they may pursue legal action or become dissatisfied.

Exhibit 6.4 summarizes the potential advantages and disadvantages of telecommuting for both employers and employees. Major advantages for both include lower overhead costs, improved employee productivity, enhanced employee recruitment and retention, and higher employee morale. Potential downsides include possible technology problems, employee career challenges, and lack of clarity regarding expectations in performance.

Since managers have less direct supervision of teleworkers, carefully worded policies need to be developed and implemented to avoid future problems. These policies include selection of employees, clarification of appropriate job tasks, time expectations, performance evaluation, addressing technology issues, communications, handling of expenses, expected outcomes, and other factors (Hutton and Norman 2010; Shadovitz 2011).

The technological flexibility exemplified by telecommuting also affects a much wider group of employees who are "always on call." For these employees, the line between work and personal life is not always clear. Such employees may find it difficult to find time to synthesize, reflect, and make good decisions (much less schedule personal time) in the 24/7 world that exists today. A personal strategy of "focus, filter, and forget" may help some adapt to this reality (Dean and Webb 2011). Otherwise, an inability to control technology may negatively affect their health and well-being (Petrecca 2013). A flexible workplace provides an opportunity for employees to lead

EXHIBIT 6.4
Potential
Advantages and
Disadvantages of
Telecommuting
for Employers
and Employees

Potential Advantages

- Cost reductions to lower overhead costs (employer)
- Improved productivity of employees (employer)
- Enhanced employee recruitment and retention (employer)
- Enhanced employee morale (both)
- Lower employee commuting costs (employee)
- Enhanced customer service (both)

Potential Disadvantages

- Possible need for supervisor retraining to manage teleworkers (employer)
- Career challenges of teleworkers (employee)
- Excessive teleworker hours—the "always working" syndrome (employee)
- Loss of employee creativity due to lack of face-to-face contact (both)
- Impersonal relationships between employer and employee (both)
- Lack of clarity for performance standards and employee evaluation standards (both)
- Potential technology problems (both)

Sources: Golden (2009); Hutton and Norman (2010); Mathis, Jackson, and Valentine (2014); Meinert (2011); Noonan and Glass (2012); Oettinger (2011); Raiborn and Butler (2009); and Shadovitz (2011).

fulfilling personal lives with better work–life balance so that they can reduce work-related stress (Westcott 2008). However, this opportunity will be wasted if managers insist on their subordinates being available 24/7.

Another work schedule innovation is the use of *contingent workers*. A contingent worker is not a permanent full-time employee but rather a temporary or part-time worker who is employed for a specific period or a specific type of work. The US Department of Labor separates contingent workers into two groups: (1) independent contractors and on-call workers, who are called to work only when needed, and (2) temporary or short-term workers. A number of contingent workers have contracts with employers that establish their pay, hours, job requirements, limitations, and time periods.

The reasons to use contingent workers include seasonal fluctuations in customer demand, project-based work, acquisition of skill sets not available among current employees, hiring freezes, rapid growth, and inadequate supply of certain occupations (e.g., registered nurses). Contingent workers may pose managerial challenges, such as unclear management reporting relationships, lack of accountability for performance, high relative compensation, low reten-tion rates, variable attitudes and work quality, and inadequate orientation and training. Contingent workers (like others) must have a good fit with their work situation (Boon et al. 2011). While some employees may view contin-gent work as desirable, others may view it as short-term and undesirable.

Contingent workers include temporary employees, part-time employ-ees, outsourced subcontractors, contract workers, and student interns. Con-tingent workers made up 26 percent of the total labor force in 2010 and included 27 million part-time employees, 10 million contract employees, and 1.2 million temporary employees (Gomez-Mejia, Balkin, and Cardy 2012).

Employers who seek temporary employees typically use private or tem-porary employment agencies, which charge fees enabling them to tailor their services to the specific needs of their employer clients. The largest healthcare staffing company in the United States is Maxim Staffing Solutions. Specifi-cally tailored to staffing of healthcare and medical professionals, Maxim has staffed more than 60,000 external employees throughout the nation and internally has about 2,500 personnel working in the field, nearly 800 staff coordinators and more than 900 corporate employees (Maxim Staffing Solu-tions 2014). Other healthcare staffing companies include Healthcare Staff-ing Incorporated, headquartered in Georgia, which has staffed more than 1,600 medical personnel across the nation (Healthcare Staffing Inc. 2013), and HealthCare Support Staffing, which ranked among the fastest growing private US companies in the *Inc.* 500 list in 2007 (Healthcare Support Staff-ing 2014).

Temporary employees, or temps, are typically used for short-term assignments or to meet temporary employer needs. Many are now being employed to fill positions once staffed by permanent employees. Temps give organizations flexibility because they can be hired and laid off as needed. The healthcare insurance costs may also be lower because they do not receive benefits and do not file healthcare insurance claims. Some temps are retirees, and others are those who do not wish to work full-time. Many who do wish to work full-time are often subsequently hired full-time by their employers. The process of working as a temp allows the employer and the employee to try one another out before a permanent commitment is made.

The federal government has expressed some legal concerns as to who is categorized as temporary. To prevent abuses, Congress, the US Depart-ment of Labor, and courts have established criteria that must be followed when hiring temps (Gray 2009). In addition, some employers have concerns that temps may have less of an incentive to be loyal and provide excellent customer service to clients than do permanent employees. Costs may also be a concern because private and temporary employment agencies charge fees to employers, employees, or both. For example, an employer commonly has to pay a fee of 25 to 30 percent of the individual's annual salary if the employer client hires an agency employee. Consequently, some employers are scaling back on the use of temps and hiring full-time employees to address temporary spikes in demand (Frauenheim 2011).

In sum, the healthcare industry can and does use all of the work schedule redesign approaches discussed here for positions that do not involve clinical care of patients. Positions that involve direct patient care must be staffed 24 hours a day, seven days a week. A compressed workweek and job sharing are the most appropriate work schedule adjustments for employees in such positions.

Summary

Job analysis is the collection of information relevant to the preparation of job descriptions and job specifications. An overall written summary of the task requirements for a particular job is called a *job description*, and an overall written summary of the personal requirements an individual must possess to successfully perform the job is called a *job specification*. Job analysis information developed in the form of job descriptions and job specifications provides the basic foundation for all HR management functions.

Some combination of available job analysis methods (observation, interviews, questionnaires, job performance, diary, technical competency, competency model, and electronic or Web-based methods) should be used because all have advantages and disadvantages. Key considerations regarding the choice of methods should be the fit between the method and the purpose, cost, practicality, and an overall judgment on the appropriateness of the method for the situation in question. The primary purpose of conducting a job analysis should be described clearly to ensure that all relevant information is collected. In addition, time and cost constraints should be specified before one or more of the available data-collection methods are chosen.

Healthcare executives should follow these steps when conducting a job analysis: (1) determine purpose, (2) identify jobs to be analyzed, (3) explain the process to employees, (4) collect job analysis information, (5) organize the information into job descriptions and job specifications, and (6) review and update the documents frequently. Job descriptions and job specifications, as derived from job analyses, must be prepared, and their processes must be valid, accurate, and job related. Otherwise, the healthcare organization may face legal repercussions, particularly in the areas of employee selection, promotions, and compensation.

The "Uniform Guidelines for Employee Selection Procedures" and associated court cases provide standards to help executives avoid charges of discrimination when developing documents from job analysis data. In today's rapidly changing healthcare environment, healthcare executives should consider the use of future-oriented job analyses when change is likely and generic job analyses when change is less likely. Both of these concepts may have legal or practical limitations that must be considered before the concepts are fully adopted.

New approaches to job design are required as healthcare organizations strive to overcome the effects of excessive specialization. Among the most significant of these approaches are the use of multiskilled health practitioners, employee empowerment, team concepts, and work schedule redesign.

Discussion Questions

1. Why should healthcare executives conduct a job analysis? What purpose does it serve?

2. What are job descriptions and job specifications? What is their relationship to job analysis? What will happen if a healthcare organization decides not to use any job descriptions at all?

3. Consider the position of the registered nurse in a large hospital. Which of the eight methods of job analysis will you use to collect data on this position, and why?

4. Describe the steps involved in the job analysis process.

5. How can the existence of a high-quality job analysis make a particular HR function, such as employee selection, less legally vulnerable?

6. Are healthcare jobs static, or do they change over time? What may cause a job to change over time? What implications does this change have for job analysis?

7. Describe and discuss future-oriented job analysis and generic job analysis. How may each be used to help healthcare executives cope with a rapidly changing and competitive environment? What are some potential pitfalls of each approach?

8. What are the advantages and disadvantages of using multiskilled health practitioners?

9. What types of work teams are most appropriate for achieving which objectives in the healthcare industry? Cite at least one successful team effort in healthcare.

10. Select one healthcare position with which you are familiar. What work schedule innovations make the most sense for this position? Why?

Experiential Exercises

Exercise 1 Imagine that you must form a team with four fellow students to make a 30-minute class presentation on the future of job analysis in the healthcare industry. All the work on this challenging project must be done by the entire team; however, your group cannot have any face-to-face meetings. Your virtual team must come up with ways to deal with the following issues:

1. How will you organize the virtual team? Would you select a team leader? If so, on what criteria would you base the selection?

2. On what criteria would you base the selection of team members?

3. Without face-to-face encounters, how will you ensure that every member of the team does his or her assigned tasks so that a high-quality presentation is produced?

Exercise 2 Form a team of four or five fellow students. As a group, select one healthcare job (e.g., registered nurse, physical therapist, receptionist) with which all of the team members have some familiarity. Basing your analysis solely on the group members' understanding of the selected job, outline the methods for conducting an analysis of the job. Draft a job description and a job specification that you believe represent the job. What future changes to the job do you think may affect your job description and job specification?

Exercise 3 You are a student in a master's in health administration program and have recently started your internship in a large, urban health system. Your preceptor has asked you to write a job description for your position, which is titled Student Intern in Health Services Administration. Review the job analysis data sources and data collection methods in this chapter. During your review, indicate the process and methods you will use to gather data. After completing those processes, write a model job description and job specification for your position.

References

Affra, F. 2009. *ICN Framework of Competencies for the Nurse Specialist.* Geneva, Switzerland: International Council of Nurses.

American Business Collaboration. 2007. *The New Career Paradigm: Flexibility Briefing.* Accessed December 22, 2014. www.shrm.org/Publications/HRNews/Documents/ABC_NCP_Flexibility_Briefing.pdf.

Avey, J. B., F. Luthans, and C. M. Youssef. 2010. "The Additive Value of Positive Psychological Capital in Predicting Work Attitudes and Behaviors." *Journal of Management* 36 (2): 430–52.

Bach, P. 2006. "Job Sharing Can Make for a Balanced Life." *Knight Ridder Tribune Business News*, January 31, A1.

Baltes, B. B., T. E. Briggs, J. W. Huff, J. A. Wright, and G. A. Neuman. 1999. "Flexible and Compressed Workweek Schedules: A Meta-Analysis of Their Effects on Work-Related Criteria." *Journal of Applied Psychology* 84 (4): 496–513.

Beck, M. 2014. "Battles Erupt over Filling Doctors' Shoes." *Wall Street Journal*, February 9.

Becker, B., and M. Huselid. 2010. "SHRM and Job Design: Narrowing the Divide." *Journal of Organizational Behavior* 31 (1): 379–88.

Bloomberg BNA. 2012a. "Telework Among Full-Time Employees Almost Doubled, Study Says." *Bulletin to Management*, June 12, 187.

———. 2012b. "13.4 Million Work from Home in 2010." *Bulletin to Management*, October 16, 330.

———. 2008. "Compressed Workweeks Gain Popularity, But Concerns Remain About Effectiveness." *Bulletin to Management*, September 16, 297.

Boon, C., D. N. Den Hartog, P. Boselie, and J. Paauwe. 2011. "The Relationship Between Perceptions of HR Practices and Employee Outcomes: Examining the Role of Person–Organisation and Person–Job Fit." *International Journal of Human Resource Management* 22 (1): 138–62.

Brisco, F. 2011. "Membership Has Its Privileges? Subcontracting in Access to Jobs That Accommodate Work–Life Needs." *Industrial and Labor Relations Review* 64 (2): 258–82.

Campion, M. A., A. A. Fink, B. J. Ruggeberg, L. Carr, G. M. Phillips, and R. B. Odman. 2011. "Doing Competencies Well: Best Practices in Competency Modeling." *Personnel Psychology* 64 (1): 225–62.

Connell, A. R., and J. S. Culbertson. 2010. "Eye of the Beholder: Does What Is Important About a Job Depend on Who Is Asked?" *Academy of Management Perspectives* 24 (2): 83–85.

Coombs, J. 2011. "Flexibility Still Meeting Resistance." *HR Magazine* 56 (7): 72.

Dean, D., and C. Webb. 2011. "Recovering from Information Overload." *McKinsey Quarterly*, January, 1–8.

Dennis, D., D. Meola, and M. J. Hall. 2012. "Effective Leadership in a Virtual Workforce." *Training and Development* 67 (2): 47–49.

Equal Employment Opportunity Commission (EEOC). 2002. *A Technical Assistance Manual on the Employment Provisions (Title 1) of the Americans with Disabilities Act: Addendum*. Washington, DC: EEOC.

———. 1978. "Uniform Guidelines for Employee Selection Procedures." *Federal Register* 43 (166): 38290–315.

Ford, R. L., and M. D. Fottler. 1995. "Empowerment: A Matter of Degree." *Academy of Management Executive* 4 (31): 21–29.

Foss, N. J., D. B. Minbaeva, T. Pedersen, and M. Reinholt. 2009. "Encouraging Knowledge Sharing Among Employees: How Job Design Matters." *Human Resource Management* 48 (6): 871–93.

Fottler, M. D. 1996. "The Role and Impact of Multiskilled Health Practitioners in the Health Services Industry." *Hospital & Health Services Administration* 41 (1): 55–75.

Frauenheim, E. 2011. "Companies Focus Their Attention on Flexibility." *Workforce Management* 90 (2): 3–4.

Garchiek, K. 2006. "Workers Pick Office over Telecommuting." *HR Magazine* 51 (9): 28–29.

Garcia, J. 1997. "How's Your Organizational Commitment?" *HR Focus* 74 (1): 22–34.

George, W. 1990. "Internal Marketing and Organizational Behavior: A Partnership in Developing Customer-Conscious Employees at Every Level." *Journal of Business Research* 20 (1): 63–70.

Golden, L. 2009. "Flexible Daily Work Schedules in US Jobs: Formal Introductions?" *Industrial Relations* 48 (1): 27–54.

Gomez-Mejia, L. R., D. B. Balkin, and R. L. Cardy. 2012. *Managing Human Resources*, seventh edition. Upper Saddle River, NJ: Pearson Education.

Grant, A. M. 2007. "Relational Job Design and the Motivation to Make a Prosocial Difference." *Academy of Management Review* 32 (2): 393–417.

Gray, K. G. 2009. "Dividing Lines." *Human Resource Executive Online*. Published September 8. www.hreonline.com/HRE/view/story.jhtml?id=251108192.

Hartley, D. E. 2004. "Job Analysis at the Speed of Reality." *Training and Development* 58 (9): 20–22.

Healthcare Staffing, Inc. 2013. "History and Introduction." Accessed December 23, 2014. www.healthcare-staffing.com/hcs-employers/history-and-introduction.

Healthcare Support Staffing. 2014. "History & Mission." Accessed December 23. www.healthcaresupport.com/about-hss/history-mission.

Holman, D., S. Frenkel, and O. Sørensen. 2009. "Work Design Variation and Outcomes in Call Centers." *Industrial and Labor Relations Review* 62 (4): 510–32.

Humphrey, S. E., F. P. Morgeson, and M. J. Mannor. 2009. "Developing a Theory of the Strategic Core of Teams: A Role Composition Model of Team Performance." *Journal of Applied Psychology* 94 (1): 48–61.

Hutton, J. E., and C. S. Norman. 2010. "The Impact of Alternative Telework Arrangements on Organizational Commitment." *Journal of Information Systems* 24 (1): 67–90.

Ilies, R., N. Dimotakis, and I. E. De Pater. 2010. "Psychological and Physiological Reactions to High Workloads: Implications for Well-Being." *Personnel Psychology* 63 (2): 407–36.

Klas, E. S., A. Papalexandris, G. Ioannou, and G. Prastacos. 2010. "From Task-Based to Competency-Based: A Typology and Process Supporting a Critical HRM Transition." *Personnel Review* 39 (3): 325–46.

Kucharova, V., Z. Zavadska, and M. Sirotiakova. 2010. "Comparison of Job Analysis: Traditional and Process Approach." *Human Resource Management & Ergonomics* 4 (1): 1–16.

Mathis, R. L., J. H. Jackson, and S. R. Valentine. 2014. *Human Resource Management*, fourteenth edition. Independence, KY: Cengage Learning.

Maxim Staffing Solutions. 2014. "About Us: FAQs." Accessed December 23. www.maximstaffing.com/aboutus/faq/employees.aspx.

Mayo, M., J. C. Pastor, L. Gomez-Mejia, and C. Cruz. 2009. "Why Some Firms Adopt Telecommuting While Others Do Not: A Contingency Perspective." *Human Resource Management* 48 (6): 917–39.

McDaniel, M. A., S. Kepes, and C. G. Banks. 2011. "The Uniform Guidelines Are a Detriment to the Field of Personnel Selection." *Industrial and Organizational Psychology* 4 (4): 494–514.

McMillan, H. S. 2011. "Constructs of the Work–Life Interface." *Human Resource Development Review* 10 (1): 6–25.

Meinert, D. 2011. "Make Telecommuting Pay Off." *HR Magazine* 56 (6): 33–37.

Miguel, R., and S. Miklos. 2011. "Individual Executive Assessment: Sufficient Science, Standards, and Principles." *Industrial and Organizational Psychology* 4 (3): 330–33.

Miller, S. 2010. "Flexible Hours in the Ranks." *HR Trend Book*, January, 16–17.

———. 2007. "Study Attempts to Dispel Five Myths of Job Sharing." Society for Human Resource Management. Published May 9. www.shrm.org/publications/hrnews/pages/xms_021497.aspx.

Morgeson, F. P., and E. C. Dierdorff. 2011. "Work Analysis from Technique to Theory." In *APA Handbook of Industrial and Organizational Psychology*. Vol. 2, *Selecting and Developing Members for the Organization*, edited by S. Zedeck, 3–41. Washington, DC: American Psychological Association.

Noonan, M. C., and J. L. Glass. 2012. "The Hard Truth About Telecommuting." *Monthly Labor Review*. Published June. www.bls.gov/opub/mlr/2012/06/art3full.pdf.

Oettinger, G. S. 2011. "The Incidence and Wage Consequences of Home-Based Work in the United States, 1980–2000." *Journal of Human Resources* 46 (2): 237–60.

Offstein, E. H. 2010. "Make Telework Work." *Strategic HR Review* 9 (2): 32–37.

O'Leary, M. B., and M. Mortensen. 2010. "Go (Con)Figure: Sub-groups, Imbalance, and Isolates in Geographically Dispersed Teams." *Organization Sciences* 21 (1): 115–31.

O*NET Resource Center. 2014. "The O*NET Content Model." Accessed October 15. www.onetcenter.org/content.html.

Pennell, K. 2010. "The Role of Flexible Job Descriptions in Succession Management." *Library Management* 31 (4/5): 279–90.

Petrecca, L. 2013. "Always Working." *USA Today,* March 7, 1A–2A.

Raiborn, C., and J. B. Butler. 2009. "A New Look at Telecommuting and Teleworking." *Journal of Corporate Accounting & Finance* 20 (5): 31–39.

Rao, H. 2010. "What 17th Century Pirates Can Teach Us About Job Design." *Harvard Business Review,* October, 44.

Safdar, R., A. Waheed, and K. H. Rafiq. 2010. "Impact of Job Analysis on Job Performance: Analysis of a Hypothesized Model." *Journal of Diversity Management* 5 (2): 17–36.

Sanchez, J. I., and E. L. Levine. 2009. "What Is (or Should Be) the Difference Between Competency Modeling and Traditional Job Analysis?" *Human Resource Management Review* 19 (2): 53–63.

Shadovitz, D. 2011. "Telework Hits a Roadblock." *Human Resource Executive Online.* Published July 14. www.hreonline.com/HRE/view/story. jhtml?id=533340007.

Shellenbarger, S. 2010. "Job Sharing: Appealing But Little Used." *Wall Street Journal.* Published August 2. http://blogs.wsj.com/juggle/2010/08/02/job-sharing-appealing-but-little-used/.

Singh, P. 2008. "Job Analysis for a Changing Workplace." *Human Resource Management Review* 18 (2): 87–99.

Snell, S., and G. Bohlander. 2013. *Managing Human Resources.* Mason, OH: South-Western Cengage Learning.

Snyder, D. 1996. "The Revolution in the Workplace: What's Happening to Our Jobs?" *Futurist* 30 (2): 8.

Society for Human Resource Management. 2010. *2010 Benefits Survey.* Alexandria, VA: SHRM/Colonial Life.

Soderquist, K. E. 2010. "From Task Based to Competency Based." *Personnel Review* 39 (3): 325–46.

Stanley, R. 2010. "Effective Ways to Manage Teleworkers." *Workspan,* January, 83.

Statista. 2014. "Share of Employers Offering/Planning to Offer Telecommuting Options to Employees in the United States as of 2013." www.statista.com/statistics/256020/us-employers-offering-telecommuting-benefits/.

Stone, D. L., K. M. Lukaszewski, E. F. Stone-Romero, and T. L. Johnson. 2013. "Factors Affecting the Effectiveness and Acceptance of Electronic Selection Systems." *Human Resource Management Review* 23 (1): 50–70.

Tasler, N. 2010. "Help Your Best People Do a Better Job." *Business Week.* Published March 26. www.businessweek.com/managing/content/mar2010/ca20100325_310839.htm.

Thompson, L. L. 2011. *Making the Team: A Guide for Managers,* fourth edition. Upper Saddle River, NJ: Pearson Prentice Hall.

Thompson, S. 2006. "Working Mothers Flex Their Scheduling Muscle." *Advertising Age,* November, 72–80.

Torpey, E. 2007. "Flexible Work: Adjusting the When and Where of Your Job." *Occupational Outlook Quarterly,* June, 14–27.

US Census Bureau. 2012. *Statistical Abstract of the United States.* Washington, DC: Government Printing Office.

Van Hootegem, G., J. Benders, A. Delarue, and S. Procter. 2005. "Teamworking: Looking Back and Looking Forward." *International Journal of Human Resource Management* 16 (2): 167–73.

Van Iddekinge, C. H., P. H. Raymark, and C. E. Eidson Jr. 2011. "An Examination of the Validity and Incremental Value of Needed-at-Entry Ratings for a Customer Service Job." *Applied Psychology* 60 (1): 24–45.

Van Wart, M. 2000. "The Return to Simpler Strategies in Job Analysis." *Review of Public Personnel Administration* 20 (3): 5–23.

Westcott, S. 2008. "Beyond Flextime: Trashing the Workweek." *Inc.,* August, 30–31.

Wharton School. 2009. "Teamwork: The Dark Side." University of Pennsylvania. Published June 19. http://knowledge.wharton.upenn.edu/article/teamwork-the-dark-side/.

Wildman, J. L., A. L. Thayer, M. A. Rosen, E. Salas, J. E. Mathieu, and S. R. Rayne. 2011. "Task Types and Team-Level Attributes: Synthesis of Team Classification Literature." *Human Resource Development Review* 11 (1): 97–129.

Zeidner, R. 2008. "Bending with the Times." *HR Magazine* 53 (7): 10.

JOB TITLE   Staff Nurse

DEPARTMENT   Nursing–Labor and Delivery

FLSA STATUS   Nonexempt

JOB SUMMARY

Assesses, prescribes, delegates, coordinates, and evaluates the nursing care provided. Ensures provisions of quality care for selected groups of patients through utilization of nursing process, established standards of care, and policies and procedures.

SUPERVISION

A. SUPERVISED BY: Unit Manager, indirectly by Charge Nurse

B. SUPERVISES: No one

C. LEADS/GUIDES: Unit Associates/Ancillary Associates in the delivery of direct patient care

JOB SPECIFICATIONS

A. EDUCATION
   — Required: Graduate of an accredited school of professional nursing
   — Desired: Continuing nursing education

B. EXPERIENCE
   — Required: None
   — Desired: Previous clinical experience
   — LICENSES, CERTIFICATIONS, AND/OR REGISTRATIONS: Current RN state license; BCLS and certifications specific to areas of clinical specialty preferred.

C. EQUIPMENT/TOOLS/WORK AIDS: PCA infusers, infusion pumps and other medical equipment, computer terminal and printer, facsimile machine, photocopier, and patient charts.

D. SPECIALIZED KNOWLEDGE AND SKILLS: Ability to work with female patients of childbearing age and newborn patients in all specialty and subspecialty categories, both urgent and nonurgent in nature.

E. PERSONAL TRAITS, QUALITIES, AND APTITUDES: Must be able to (1) perform a variety of duties, often changing from one task to another of a different nature without loss of efficiency or composure; (2) accept responsibility for the direction, control, and planning of an activity; (3) make evaluations and decisions based on measurable or verifiable criteria; (4) work independently; (5) recognize the rights and responsibilities of patient confidentiality; (6) convey empathy and compassion to those experiencing pain or grief; (7) relate to others in a manner that creates a sense of teamwork and cooperation; and (8) communicate effectively with people from every socioeconomic background.

(continued)

F. <u>WORKING CONDITIONS:</u> Inside environment, protected from the weather but not necessarily temperature changes. Subject to exposure to infection, contagious disease, combative patients, and potentially hazardous materials and equipment. Variable noise levels. Also subject to rapid pace, multiple stimuli, unpredictable environment, and critical situations.

G. <u>PHYSICIAL DEMANDS/TRAITS:</u> Must be able to: (1) perceive the nature of sounds by the ear; (2) express or exchange ideas by means of the spoken word; (3) perceive characteristics of objects through the eyes; (4) extend arms and hands in any direction; (5) seize, hold, grasp, turn, or otherwise work with hands; (6) pick, pinch, or otherwise work with the fingers; (7) perceive such attributes of objects or materials as size, shape, temperature, or texture; and (8) stoop, kneel, crouch, and crawl. Must be able to lift 50 pounds maximum with frequent lifting, carrying, pushing, and pulling of objects weighing up to 25 pounds. Continuous walking and standing. Must be able to identify, match, and distinguish colors. Rare lifting of greater than 100 pounds.

7

RECRUITMENT, SELECTION, AND RETENTION

Bruce J. Fried and Michael Gates

Learning Objectives

After completing this chapter, the reader should be able to

- understand the major steps and decisions involved in designing and implementing a recruitment effort,
- discuss the factors considered by potential employees in deciding whether to accept a job offer,
- design a recruitment and selection effort for a particular job,
- address the advantages and disadvantages of internal and external recruitment and other sources of job applicants,
- explain the concepts of person–job and person–organization fit,
- identify alternative selection tools and how they can be used in the selection process, and
- discuss the challenges inherent in designing a retention strategy.

Introduction

In this chapter, attention turns to the processes of recruitment, selection, and retention. These three topics are explored together because they are integrally related not only to each other but also to other human resources management (HRM) functions. A successful recruitment effort generates sufficient applicants so that the employer can be selective in the process of identifying the most suitable applicant. The stringency of criteria used for selecting job applicants depends, to a large degree, on the success of the recruitment effort. An organization can be more selective when a relatively large supply of qualified applicants is available. Retention, in turn, is at least partially related to the selection process. The likelihood of retaining an employee is generally higher when the employee, the job, and the organization are well matched. Of course, some factors that affect retention are largely out of the control of the organization. In general, however, employees are more likely to stay with an organization if they achieve success in their job.

Successful recruitment and retention also depend on other key HRM functions. Before a recruitment plan for a position is developed, an accurate, current, and comprehensive job description, as well as explicit identification of job requirements and the desired qualifications of successful applicants, is absolutely essential. A rigorous review of the job is a necessary step in the recruitment and selection process. Without a clear understanding of the job, the selection process can become chaotic, and may cause conflict and misunderstanding among stakeholders and decision makers.

In developing selection criteria, managers may find themselves in the position of focusing exclusively on the technical and regulatory (e.g., credentials, licenses) aspects of the job. The desired knowledge and skills and possession of the necessary credentials are certainly essential for the successful applicant. However, the key to a successful employee may lie beyond technical competencies. Depending on the job, such factors as motivation, commitment, career goals, adaptability, and ability to work on a team may be critical to success. While these less tangible qualities are more difficult to assess than technical readiness for the job and credentials, methods for assessing many of them are available. These methods are addressed later in this chapter. As with all HRM functions, recruitment and selection processes must be carried out within the legal and regulatory environment. For example, federal and state laws related to employment discrimination must be taken into account in the design and implementation of employee selection processes.

With the exception of positions that are temporary or otherwise time-limited, organizations place a high value on employee retention. Turnover is costly, and not simply in financial terms. Turnover can affect the quality and continuity of care, job satisfaction and morale, and teamwork. While a position is unfilled, organizations may face the extra cost of hiring temporary employees, which in some cases (including some nursing positions) is more costly than hiring a full-time permanent employee. New employees are likely to be less productive, and training is therefore another cost associated with turnover. Many factors affect employee retention, including the effectiveness of orientation and onboarding procedures, as well as factors outside of the control of the organization. Recruitment and selection play an important role in retention. Consequently, an important measure of the effectiveness of recruitment and selection is the extent to which the organization is able to attract committed and high-performing employees who remain with the organization over a specified period.

These three functions are highly interdependent, but they are addressed separately and sequentially in this chapter. The concepts related to these functions include the following:

- Recruitment steps
- Sources of job applicants
- Organizational fit, and its importance in the selection process
- Reliability and validity of selection decisions
- Selection instruments
- Types of selection interviews and ways to improve their effectiveness
- Factors and strategies related to employee retention and turnover

Recruitment

Human resources (HR) executives consistently report that their single greatest workforce challenge is to create or maintain their organizations' capacity to attract talented employees to their organization. The goal of recruitment is to generate a pool of qualified job applicants. Specifically, recruitment refers to the range of processes an organization uses to attract qualified individuals on a timely basis and in sufficient numbers and to encourage them to apply for jobs in the organization. When recruitment strategies are considered, attention often focuses on a set of key questions:

- Should the organization recruit and promote from within, or should it focus on recruiting external applicants?
- Should the organization consider alternative approaches to filling jobs with full-time employees, such as outsourcing, flexible staffing, and hiring contingent workers?
- Should the organization find applicants who have precisely the right technical qualifications or applicants who best fit the culture of the organization but may require additional training to improve their technical skills?

The success of recruitment depends on many factors, including the attractiveness of the organization, the community in which the organization is located, the work climate and culture of the organization, managerial and supervisory attitudes and behavior, workload, and other job-related considerations. Before exploring these aspects, this chapter first addresses recruitment from the perspective of applicants and potential employees. What factors influence an individual's decision to apply for and accept employment with a particular organization? If applicants and employees are considered as customers, then an understanding of their needs and expectations is central to the development and implementation of effective recruitment strategies.

Factors That Influence Job Choice

What do potential employees look for in a job? Once an individual is offered a position, how does that person make the decision to accept or reject the offer? People consider a number of factors related to the attractiveness of the position and the organization, as well as factors specific to the individual. Applicants consider their own competitiveness in the job market and whether alternative positions that provide better opportunities are available. They are also sensitive to the attitudes and behaviors of the recruiter, or whoever is their first contact with the organization. First impressions are very potent because the issue of "fitting in" with the organization is often decided at this stage, and early negative first impressions may be difficult to reverse. Questions foremost in the applicant's mind are "Is this the kind of place I can see myself spending 40 or more hours a week?" and "Will I fit in?" Applicants may also be concerned with opportunities for career mobility and promotion.

Considerable research has been conducted on the factors associated with attracting applicants to organizations. Job choice has both cognitive and emotional elements. On the cognitive side, applicants evaluate compensation, opportunities for growth, and other tangible factors. On the emotional side, a consistent finding is that applicant attraction to an organization is maximized when an applicant is familiar with the organization and sees the organization as having a positive reputation and possessing values and attributes consistent with the values of the job seeker. The implications of these findings are clear. First, more information is better: The more applicants know about the organization, the more likely they are to seek employment, assuming that they perceive a fit between their values and those of the organization. Second, organizations must be cognizant of their own image and reputation in the labor market. Related to this factor is the importance of organizations' assessment of their own promotional strategies to ensure that the image they seek to present is in fact having a positive impact. Where the organization's public image is inconsistent with the organization's ideal view of itself, strategies must be developed to better understand public perceptions and, ultimately, to design messaging to improve the image.

The factors that predict actual job choice decisions are difficult to establish because of the multiple dynamics and elements involved in a particular job choice decision. The relative importance of factors varies, depending on the individual, the organization, the job, and environmental factors such as the level of unemployment. Understanding the factors that affect job choice is central to developing effective recruitment strategies. A helpful way to think about the reasons for a job choice is to consider the characteristics of the organization and job; individual needs, preferences, and values; and the fit between the organization and the individual, as well as the fit between the individual and the specific job.

Individual characteristics are personal considerations that influence a person's job decision. The factors considered by a family physician to accept employment with a rural health center may be quite different from the factors that drive a nurse's decision to accept employment with an urban teaching hospital. An almost infinite number of individual factors potentially affect job choice, but for any individual at a particular point in time, a few selected factors may play a decisive role. One's life or career stage, for example, may affect the salience of these decision factors.

Organizational characteristics, on the other hand, are factors associated with the organization as a whole, as well as specific job-related factors, notably total compensation, advancement opportunities, job security, and geographic location. Each of these factors is explained below.

Total compensation, which includes wages and benefits, is most often thought of as the key element affecting an individual's decision to accept a position with an organization. For some positions in healthcare, additional compensation may be offered by providing a hiring bonus, incorporating additional pay into base pay, providing relocation assistance, slotting a job into a higher pay grade than would normally be warranted, and more frequently reviewing an individual's salary once the person starts working with the organization. These methods are sometimes referred to as "hot skill" premiums and are associated with jobs requiring scarce and in-demand skills (Berthiaume and Culpepper 2008).

The relative importance of compensation to potential employees is varied and complex. Under some circumstances, employees may leave an organization for another only to obtain an incremental increase in compensation. In other instances, employees may choose to stay with an organization even when a substantially more generous offer is made by another organization. In sum, compensation is a part—but certainly not the entirety—of one's decision to accept a job offer.

The amount of challenge and responsibility inherent in a particular job is frequently cited as an important job choice factor, and this element is likely even more salient in healthcare organizations, where professionals seek out positions that maximize use of their professional knowledge, training, and skills. Similarly, many applicants place value on jobs with substantial advancement and professional development opportunities. While the availability of such opportunities is relevant for all applicants, these opportunities are likely to be a particularly important determinant for professionally trained individuals (Lu et al. 2012) as well as individuals aspiring to management roles.

A study of public health nurses' job satisfaction funded by the Robert Wood Johnson Foundation revealed interesting findings about the relationship between compensation, job satisfaction, and promotional opportunities.

The survey found that 85 percent were happy with their career choice, and 90 percent felt they were making a contribution to their communities. Regarding compensation, 40 percent reported that they were being compensated fairly, and 30 percent felt their salaries were inadequate. Most striking, however, was the finding that 56 percent felt they would not be able to receive a promotion, and 64 percent said they hoped to obtain additional training to advance their career. Fewer than half (49 percent) reported that their health department recognizes employee accomplishments through promotions or other methods. These findings were reinforced by a parallel survey of key informants within local and state health departments: About 70 percent of local health departments and 63 percent of state health departments reported that promotion opportunities were often unavailable to registered nurses (University of Michigan Center of Excellence in Public Health Workforce Studies 2013).

Traditionally, advancement opportunities for clinically or technically trained individuals have been relatively scarce in healthcare because the sole avenue to advancement was often through promotion to supervisory or management responsibilities. For many clinicians, taking on supervisory responsibilities may lead to a feeling of loss of their professional identity. In healthcare (and other industries as well), dual career ladders have been established to enable highly talented clinicians to move up while not forcing them to abandon their clinical interests and expertise. A dual career ladder is a method by which employees can move up in the organization without requiring them to assume managerial responsibilities (Society for Human Resource Management 2012b). Dual career ladders have been used frequently in healthcare as well as in other industries with technically trained professionals. Dual career development plans allow upward mobility for employees without requiring that they be placed into supervisory or managerial positions. This type of program has typically served as a way to advance employees who may have particular technical skills and/or education but who are not interested or inclined to pursue a management or supervisory track. The Cleveland Clinic (2014a), for example, has a career ladder "designed to promote and recognize excellence in practice, foster professional growth, and retain compassionate caregivers in direct care settings."

Job security is clearly an important determinant of job choice. The current healthcare and general business environment is characterized by an unprecedented number of mergers, acquisitions, and reorganizations, which lead to frequent downsizing and worker displacement. This phenomenon was once limited largely to blue-collar workers, but professionals and employees in middle and senior management roles are equally at risk. An illustrative manifestation of the importance of job security is evident in union organizing and collective bargaining. Traditionally, compensation and benefits were the most highly valued issues in labor negotiations. However, job security has become a matter of great importance in employees' decision to unionize (Carlson 2014), and it remains a key factor in contract negotiations (Algier 2013). In fact, it is not unusual for unionized employees to make wage concessions in return for higher levels of job security (Alonzo 2014).

Job applicants may also consider geographic location, along with other lifestyle concerns, particularly for individuals in dual-income families, where the employment of a spouse can be a significant determinant of job acceptance. In healthcare, location is a particularly serious issue because healthcare organizations are often, by necessity, located in less-than-desirable locales that may not be attractive to applicants.

As employees consider their preferences, employers go through a similar process of trying to make their organizations attractive to prospective employees. As discussed later in this chapter, determining if the applicant will fit into the organizational culture is a challenge for both the organization and the job applicant. Applicants are more likely to accept positions in organizations that share their values, beliefs, and work style. Implicitly or explicitly, organizations engage in a signaling process, in which they communicate their values to the public. This process of communicating values can and should occur early in the process of employee selection, and certainly at the time of a job interview. At this time, the hiring manager can emphasize what is important to the organization, convey how it goes about its work, and provide the applicant an opportunity to withdraw if the applicant does not find the corporate culture appealing (Lukens 2014). Signals are also included in the recruitment messages that the organization sends to potential job applicants. Typically, recruitment messages convey information about the organization's mission and values, as well as the nature of the work environment. In the case of nurse recruitment, Magnet hospital designations by the American Nurses Credentialing Center receive prominence in recruitment materials. Consider this extract from the nurse recruitment message for the Cleveland Clinic, which highlights the organization's clinical leadership, support for nurses, and personal and professional development activities for nurses:

> As a large research and teaching hospital, we offer nurses opportunities to work on the cutting edge of nursing care, using state-of-the-art technology and new treatment options, and having at hand a broad spectrum of support to affect nursing practice and improve patient care. Cleveland Clinic strives to provide unique benefits and opportunities for our nurses both in and out of the workplace. (Cleveland Clinic 2014b)

Similarly, the Mayo Clinic's recruitment message includes statements about its commitment to patient-centered care and high level of professionalism:

> Working at Mayo Clinic is making a difference. It's providing the highest quality patient care by placing the needs of patients first. At Mayo Clinic, you'll discover a culture of teamwork, professionalism and mutual respect—and most importantly, a life-changing career. (Mayo Clinic 2014a)

The Mayo Clinic also highlights its status, earned continuously for 14 consecutive years, of being listed among *Fortune* magazine's 100 Best Companies to Work For. In its statement, the chief executive officer provides an empowering message to its current employees, assigning credit to its employees for the "Best Company" designation:

> We congratulate our employees for earning Mayo Clinic this distinction. . . . Their bright minds and passionate service give Mayo Clinic its world reputation as a place of hope and solutions for patients. We have 60,000 individuals who link arms with one another to support our patients and their families. (Mayo Clinic 2014b)

In its effort to attract new nurse graduates, Kaiser Permanente promotes its New Grad Program, which is designed to "ease the transition of a new graduate RN into professional practice" through skills development (Kaiser Permanente 2014). Similarly, Johns Hopkins Medicine appeals to job applicants by describing the diversity of its workforce and work settings:

> Our patients come from all over the country. And so do our staff. They come to be part of the most professional, diverse and reputable health care teams. They come to work beside the unequaled talent of Johns Hopkins physicians, nurses and staff. And they come for the benefits and unlimited opportunities for personal and professional growth. From community settings to an academic medical center, and from the city to the suburbs, Johns Hopkins Medicine is defined by our family of diverse work environments. (Johns Hopkins Medicine 2014)

Healthcare organizations vary in their ability to attract and retain a talented workforce, and rural hospitals face particularly challenging obstacles (Brimmer 2012), requiring targeted recruitment efforts (Punke 2013). To attract physicians, rural hospitals may have to offer very attractive compensation and benefits packages, and may rely on such programs as the National Health Service Corps to meet physician staffing needs. In other instances, hospitals increase their use of midlevel providers, such as nurse practitioners and physician assistants. Other approaches to physician recruitment include loan repayment programs, which usually include an obligation to work in an underserved rural community for a specified period, and physician shares, which may involve joint contracts with physicians between hospitals (Kutscher 2013).

Exhibit 7.1 illustrates how different job applicants may assess the relative importance of job features. Although the depiction in the exhibit oversimplifies the job choice process, it shows how individuals value different aspects of the job depending on personal preferences and life circumstances. The first column briefly describes each applicant. The second column states each applicant's minimum standards for job acceptance along four dimensions: pay, benefits, advancement opportunities, and travel requirements. These four dimensions are sometimes categorized as noncompensatory standards—that is, no other element of the job can compensate if these standards are not met, or, more simply, these elements are "deal killers." Thus, Person 3, who does not like to travel, will be unlikely to accept a job that requires substantial travel, regardless of anything else; similarly, for Person 2, health insurance coverage is an absolute requirement for job acceptance.

The lower half of the exhibit shows summaries of three potential jobs. Assessing how each of these three hypothetical job applicants would evaluate each job should not be difficult. Person 1, for example, would be unlikely to be interested in the research assistant position, largely because it seems to lack promotional opportunities.

The Recruitment Process

The foundation of a recruitment process is the organization's HR plan. An *HR plan* includes specific information about the organization's strategies, the types of individuals required by the organization, recruitment and hiring approaches, and a clear statement of how HR practices support organizational goals. Those involved in recruitment and selection must, of course, have a thorough understanding of the position that needs to be filled, including job requirements and its relationship with other positions within and, at times, external to the organization. The recruitment process should begin with a job analysis, which addresses questions of job tasks, knowledge, skills, and abilities, and development of specific qualifications required of applicants (see Chapter 6 for discussion of job design).

The early stages of the recruitment process involve an examination of the external environment, particularly the supply of potential job applicants and the relative competitiveness of the position. This analysis should also examine compensation and benefits given to individuals who hold similar jobs in the organization as well as in competing organizations. With any position, organizations are concerned with being externally competitive, that is, being able to compete successfully for job applicants, while also ensuring that salaries are internally equitable. Another helpful approach is to evaluate external recruitment sources, such as colleges, competing organizations, and professional associations, to determine which of them proved to be successful recruitment sources in the past. Other aspects to consider in this assessment

EXHIBIT 7.1
Preferences Among Three Hypothetical Job Applicants

Job Applicant	Minimum Standards for Job Acceptance	Three Potential Jobs
Person 1: 23 years old, single	**Pay:** At least $50,000 **Benefits:** Health insurance: Essential Dental insurance: Important Paid vacation: Essential Disability and life insurance: Of minor importance 401(k)/Roth 401(k): Somewhat important Personal and sick time: Important **Advancement opportunities:** Very important **Travel restrictions:** None	**Insurance company provider relations coordinator** **Pay:** $50,000 **Benefits:** Health insurance, dental insurance, paid vacation, disability and life insurance, 401(k)/Roth 401(k), personal and sick time **Advancement opportunities:** Recruitment done internally and externally **Travel requirements:** Average 25 percent travel
Person 2: Sole wage earner, married with plans to raise a family	**Pay:** At least $50,000 **Benefits:** Health insurance: Family coverage essential Dental insurance: Important Paid vacation: Essential Disability and life insurance: Highly important 401(k)/Roth 401(k): Somewhat important Personal and sick time: Important **Advancement opportunities:** Very important **Travel restrictions:** Minor restrictions	**Healthcare consultant** **Pay:** $60,000 **Benefits:** Health insurance, dental insurance, paid vacation, disability and life insurance, personal and sick time **Advancement opportunities:** Strong history of promotions within one year **Travel requirements:** Average 50 percent travel
Person 3: Spouse of high-wage earner; family of five	**Pay:** At least $45,000 **Benefits:** Health insurance: Not important Dental insurance: Not important Paid vacation: Not essential Disability and life insurance: Somewhat important 401(k)/Roth 401(k): Important Personal and sick time: Very important **Advancement opportunities:** Relatively unimportant **Travel restrictions:** Cannot travel more than one week per year	**Research assistant in academic medical center** **Pay:** $42,000 **Benefits:** Health insurance, paid vacation, 401(k)/Roth 401(k), personal and sick time **Advancement opportunities:** Generally hires externally for higher-level positions **Travel requirements:** Little or none

are the logistics and timing of a recruitment effort; for some positions, seasonal factors play a role in the recruitment process, such as graduation dates from nursing school.

The process should then review past recruitment efforts for the position and similar ones: Will this job require an international, national, or regional search, or will the local labor market suffice? Optimally, a *human resources information system* (HRIS) will provide useful information during the recruitment process. While the sophistication of an organization's HRIS varies, many such systems include some or all of the information described in Exhibit 7.2. A *skills inventory* database maintains information on every employee's skills, educational background, training acquired, seminars attended, work history, and other job-development data. This inventory optimally should also include data on applicants who were not hired. A well-managed database broadens the pool of possible applicants from which to draw.

An initial question in the recruitment process is applicant sourcing, or specifying where qualified job applicants are located. As the Internet and social media have emerged, recruitment has undergone massive changes. Recruitment has transitioned from the traditional print classified advertisements to the Internet and, most recently, to mobile devices. In addition to individual companies' use of the Internet for recruitment, the use of job search websites continues to grow. Exhibit 7.3 reports the most popular job search engines. Some websites are general in scope, while others market to a particular industry or job category. Idealist, for example, specializes in nonprofit, volunteer, and internship opportunities. Functionality also varies

HRIS Data	Uses in Recruitment
Skills and knowledge inventory	Identifies potential internal job candidates
Previous applicants	Identifies potential external job candidates
Recruitment source information • Yield ratios • Cost • Cost per applicant • Cost per hire	Helps in the analysis of cost effectiveness of recruitment sources
Applicant tracking	Provides a method to automate many labor-intensive aspects of recruitment
Employee performance and retention information	Provides information on the success of recruitment sources used in the past

EXHIBIT 7.2
Human Resources Information System Recruitment Data

EXHIBIT 7.3
Most Common
Job Search
Engines

Website	URL
Indeed	www.indeed.com
CareerBuilder	www.careerbuilder.com
Monster	www.monster.com
Craigslist	www.craigslist.org
LinkedIn	www.linkedin.com
Simply Hired	www.simplyhired.com
Glassdoor	www.glassdoor.com
Mediabistro	www.mediabistro.com
Dice	www.dice.com
Internships.com	www.internships.com
TweetMyJobs	www.tweetmyjobs.com
Idealist	www.idealist.org

Source: Adapted from Griffith and Bergen (2014).

among websites and may include resume storage, RSS feeds, and employee-generated content on companies. TweetMyJobs communicates the best job matches to users through social media such as Twitter. Many search engines specialize in healthcare jobs, such as JobsInHealthcare.com and HealthECareers.

The use of technology has extended to the use of mobile devices for recruitment. Mobile devices enable job seekers to conveniently apply for employment from any location, often speeding up the recruitment process. Because this transition requires optimizing websites for mobile devices, organizations have been somewhat slow to adapt to the use of mobile devices as a recruitment tool; however, this transition in recruitment is unmistakable. A survey conducted by TheLadders, a job search site, found that "57 percent of customers wouldn't recommend businesses with poorly designed mobile sites and 40 percent have gone to a competitor's site after a bad mobile experience with a company's site" (Onley 2014). Numerous publications provide guidance to job seekers on the use of social media (see, e.g., Hellmann 2014 and Waldman 2013). Interestingly, one proponent of using social media for job searches recommends that a job hunt should consist of 80 percent personal networking, 10 percent talking to headhunters, and only 10 percent using online search engines (Griffith and Bergen 2014).

Just as new technologies are used by job seekers, online technologies are used by employers to evaluate job applicants. This use of technology may take the form of resume scanning and online employment assessments by employers (Frauenheim 2011). These assessments may be company-specific or use externally developed tools. Virtual assessments have been developed by such companies as Starbucks, Sherwin Williams, and several banking institutions. Through an online simulation, Virtual Job Tryout evaluates applicants' cultural and team fit, and may also be used to assess job-specific skills. This simulation also provides applicants with a realistic preview of a job so that the prospective employee can assess fit with the organization (Zielinski 2011). New technologies not only identify potential job applicants but also provide information on their suitability for the job (Richtel 2013).

A fundamental question in recruitment is whether to recruit internally through promotions or transfers, or to seek candidates from outside the organization. Organizations may have preferences for internal or external hiring but tend to use a combination of strategies depending on the specific circumstances. Each strategy has merit and potential risks.

Exhibit 7.4 summarizes the advantages and disadvantages of internal and external recruitment. On the positive side of internal recruitment, candidates are generally already known to the organization—the organization is familiar with their past performance and future potential and is aware of their expectations. Internal candidates also tend to be well acquainted with specific organizational processes and procedures and may not require as much socialization and start-up time. Internal recruitment may also be used as a motivator, morale builder, and retention strategy because of the opportunities provided for upward mobility in the organization.

Recruiting from within may encourage highly valued and productive employees to stay with the organization. A study of employees in the banking industry systematically examined the performance of internal versus external hires. The study found that internally promoted workers exhibited significantly higher levels of performance for the first two years than those hired from outside the organization. Internal recruits also had lower rates of voluntary and involuntary turnover. Interestingly, external hires were found to be paid about 18 percent more than internal recruits, and workers who were promoted and transferred simultaneously exhibited lower levels of performance than those promoted from within (Bidwell 2011).

On the negative side of internal recruitment, however, is the possible manifestation of the Peter Principle, a common phenomenon in which successful employees continue to be promoted until they reach one position above their level of competence (Peter and Hull 1969). With the Peter Principle, employees may be promoted regardless of their aptitude for the new

Advantages	Disadvantages
Recruiting Internal Candidates	
• May improve employee morale and encourage valued employees to stay with the organization • Permits greater assessment of applicant abilities; candidate is a known entity • May be faster, and may involve lower cost for certain jobs • Good motivator for employee performance • Applicants have a good understanding of the organization • May reinforce employees' sense of job security	• Possible morale problems among those not selected • May lead to inbreeding • May lead to conflict among internal job applicants • May require strong training and management development activities • May manifest the Peter Principle • May cause ripple effect in vacancies, which need to be filled
Recruiting External Candidates	
• Brings new ideas into the organization • May be less expensive than training internal candidates • Ensures candidates do not have preexisting dysfunctional relationships with others and are not embroiled in organizational politics	• May identify candidate who has technical skills but does not fit the culture of the organization • May cause morale problems for internal candidates who were not selected • May require longer adjustment and socialization • Uncertainty about candidate skills and abilities, and difficulty obtaining reliable information about applicant

position. This phenomenon is noteworthy in healthcare, where individuals with strong clinical skills may be promoted into supervisory and management roles without the requisite skills and training for those responsibilities. For example, a world-renowned clinician and researcher may be promoted to vice president of medical affairs even though that person is not the best candidate. Effective organizations seek to prevent this phenomenon by ensuring the accuracy of job descriptions and by requiring internal (and external) candidates to meet the specified job qualifications. If an individual who does not possess all the job qualifications is hired, a manager has to be cognizant of the person's need to be trained in the areas requiring remediation. Companies such as Microsoft and GlaxoSmith Kline avoided the Peter Principle in their selection of CEOs through intensive scrutiny and testing of eventually successful internal hires (Carey and Useem 2014). Internal recruitment may also have the disadvantage of causing disarray in the organization. At times, promotion creates a ripple effect—one individual moves into a different position, leaving a vacancy; this vacancy, in turn, is filled by someone else who causes another vacancy, and so forth.

External recruitment refers to using applicant sources outside the organization, often through the Internet and social media, but also including job fairs and educational institutions, such as high schools, vocational schools, community colleges, and universities. For some jobs (and in some labor markets), nontraditional candidates including prisoners, senior citizens, and workers from abroad may be employed (Waldo 2012). An advantage of external recruitment is that candidates may bring in new ideas. In addition, the organization may be able to more specifically target candidates with the skills needed rather than settle for an internal candidate who may be acquainted with the organization but may lack specific skills and knowledge. External candidates also tend to be unencumbered by political problems and conflict and therefore may be easier to bring into a difficult political environment than an internal applicant. This advantage is often a rationale for selecting a CEO from outside.

Many applicants are not easy to characterize as coming from either an internal or an external source. For example, hiring candidates who have worked for the organization in a contingent or part-time capacity, including contract employees, is not uncommon. This practice is increasingly common in nursing, where traveling or agency nurses may apply or be recruited for a full-time position. As a general rule, it is advantageous to obtain as many qualified job applicants as possible. From the organization's perspective, having a large number of applicants permits choice and sometimes may even stimulate a rethinking of the content of the job. For example, an applicant may be found to have additional skill sets that are not necessarily relevant to the job as currently designed but are useful nonetheless. Successful organizations are flexible enough to take advantage of these opportunities. Designing recruitment efforts in such a way that they yield applicants who have at least the minimum qualifications is advisable. Processing a large number of unqualified applicants can be expensive as well as a waste of time for both the organization and applicants. As noted earlier, many organizations have automated the screening process through resume-scanning programs.

Employee referral is an excellent source because the current employee knows the organization and the applicant and can thus act as the initial screen. A person identified and hired through this mechanism may therefore bring advantages common to both internal and external recruitment. Yield ratios tend to be higher with employee-referred applicants than others. They have also been found to yield employees who stay longer with the organization and exhibit higher levels of loyalty and job satisfaction than do employees recruited through other mechanisms (Schwartz 2013). Evidence also indicates that employees who make referrals are more productive than other employees and are less likely to quit after making a referral (Burks et al. 2013). Interestingly, other evidence suggests that employees recruited through employee referral may have a mistaken perception of the organization, and join the organization with erroneous expectations (Hsieh and Chen 2011). Some employee referral programs give monetary rewards to employees whose referrals were successful—that is, if the new hire remains with the organization for a defined period. Keeping the information of employee-referred applicants who were not hired is advisable because such referrals may be mined for open positions in the future.

Former employees may be a fruitful source of applicants. Employees who have left under good conditions—that is, as a result of other employment opportunities, organizational downsizing and restructuring, relocation, or other personal factors—sometimes may seek or be available for reemployment with the organization. Their capabilities and potential are already usually well known to the organization. Returning employees may also send an implicit message to current employees that the work environment is sufficiently positive to attract them back to the organization.

Depending on the position involved, employment agencies and executive search firms (both state sponsored and private) may be useful as applicant search and screening vehicles. Agencies may specialize in different types of searches and typically work either on a commission or on a flat-fee basis.

Content of the Recruiting Message

An important objective of recruitment is to maximize the possibility that the right candidate will accept the organization's job offer. What are the appropriate messages to include in recruitment? Four types of information should be communicated to applicants:

1. *Applicant qualifications:* education, experience, credentials, and any other preferences that the employer has within legal constraints
2. *Job basics:* title, responsibilities, compensation, benefits, location, and other pertinent working conditions (e.g., night work, travel, promotion potential)
3. *Application process:* deadline, resume, cover letter, transcripts, references, and contact person and address for the application packet

4. *Organization and department basics:* name and type of organization, department, and other information about the work environment

Recruitment Messages and Realistic Job Previews

The *recruitment message* is considered to be an important aspect of both recruiting applicants and filling job openings. Researchers have found that applicants frequently lack information about a position they are considering, and this lack of information makes them less likely to accept a position (Barber and Roehling 1993). Allen, Mahto, and Otondo (2007) found that providing additional information about a job was linked to position attractiveness and that more information increased the credibility of the information. Of particular interest is the view, supported by research, that providing realistic information about a job results in applicants' obtaining clearer and more realistic information about the job (Breaugh 2010).

Considerable research is available on the effectiveness of the *realistic job preview.* The goal of a realistic job preview is to present practical information about job requirements, organizational expectations, and the work environment. The preview should include negative and positive aspects of the job and the organization, and it may be presented to new hires before they start work. The use of realistic job previews is related to higher performance and lower attrition from the recruitment process, lower initial expectations, lower voluntary turnover, lower turnover overall, and higher ratings of role clarity and organizational honesty (Breaugh 2013; Earnest, Allen, and Landis 2011; Phillips 1998). A realistic job preview can be presented in a number of ways: verbally, in writing, or through the media. Certainly the most straightforward approach is for the prospective or new employee to hold frank discussions with coworkers and supervisors. In addition, the new employee may observe the work setting and perhaps shadow an employee who is doing a similar job.

Regardless of the approach used, preventing surprises and providing the employee with an honest assessment of the job and the work environment are key.

Evaluating the Recruitment Function

Assessing the effectiveness of recruitment efforts is critical. Such an evaluation process depends on the existence of reliable and comprehensive data on applicants, a well-functioning HRIS, the quality of applicants, the applicants' disposition, and recruitment costs. Numerous metrics may be used to evaluate the effectiveness and efficiency of recruitment and selection processes, as well as the usefulness of specific recruitment strategies and sources. Exhibit 7.5 illustrates the variety of measures that may be used to evaluate the recruitment process. Again, a good HRIS and cost-accounting system can help the organization establish the costs associated with recruitment and selection.

EXHIBIT 7.5
Measures of
Recruitment
Effectiveness
and Efficiency

Type of Cost	Expenses
Cost per hire	• Advertising, agency fees, employee referral bonuses, recruitment fairs and travel, and sign-on bonuses • Staff time: salary; benefits; and overhead costs for employees to review applications, set up interviews, conduct interviews, check references, and make and confirm an offer • Processing costs: opening a new file, medical examination, drug screening, and credential checking • Travel and lodging for applicants, relocation costs • Orientation and training
Application rate	• Ratio-referral factor: number of candidates to number of openings • Applicants per posting • Qualified applicants per posting • Number of internal candidates per posting; number of qualified internal candidates per posting • Number of external candidates per posting; number of qualified external candidates per posting • Yield ratio: the number of applicants at one stage of the recruitment process compared with the number of applicants at the subsequent stage
Diversity	• Diversity hire ratio: percentage of employees hired who self-identify as coming from a diversity group (overall and per job posting) • Female hire ratio: percentage of externally hired employees who are female
Hiring	• Time between job requisition and first interview • External hire rate: people hired externally as a percentage of head count • Internal hire rate: people hired internally as a percentage of head count • Time to hire: time between job requisition and offer • Time to start: the number of calendar days from the date of a requisition to the start date of the newly hired employee (may be calculated for internal and external hires) • Offer acceptance rate: number of offers accepted as a percentage of all new hire offers extended (may also be calculated separately for internal and external hires, and by recruitment source) • Time between job offer and offer acceptance

(continued)

Recruitment source effectiveness	• Offers by recruitment source • Hires by recruitment source • Employee performance (using performance evaluation information and promotion rates) • Employee retention by recruitment source
Recruiter effectiveness	• Response time, time to fill, cost per hire, acceptance rate, employee performance, and retention
Miscellaneous	• Materials and other special or unplanned expenses, new employee orientation, reference checking, and drug screening • Sign-on bonus percentage: number of new hires receiving a sign-on bonus as a percentage of new hires

EXHIBIT 7.5
Measures of Recruitment Effectiveness and Efficiency *(continued from previous page)*

Source: Adapted from Fitz-enz and Davison (2002); Society for Human Resource Management (2014).

Common measures of the success of a recruitment function include the following:

- *Quantity of applicants.* The proper use of recruitment methods and sources will yield a substantial number of candidates (depending on the market supply) who meet at least the minimum job requirements. Having a sufficiently large pool of applicants allows the organization a better chance of identifying the most qualified candidates. However, attracting many applicants is also associated with increased recruitment costs. Therefore, the minimum job requirements need to be established to maintain a balance among the number of candidates, the quality of applicants, and the cost.

- *Quality of applicants.* A well-designed recruitment effort will bring in employees who have the appropriate education, qualifications, skills, and attitudes.

- *Overall recruitment cost and cost per applicant.* A recruitment effort's costs are often unacceptable to the organization. The overall cost per applicant and the cost of the recruiting methods and sources should be examined. This analysis provides the opportunity to determine the cost effectiveness of alternative recruitment methods. The financial impact of using part-time or temporary help while looking for the right applicant should also be considered because these costs can be substantial.

- *Diversity of applicants.* Assuming that one goal of the recruitment program is to identify and hire qualified candidates who represent the diversity of the service population or to address diversity goals, the organization can consider its recruitment goal met if it can show that candidates from diverse cultural and demographic backgrounds have been considered or are holding positions for which they are qualified.

- *Recruitment time or time-to-fill.* The more time spent on proper recruitment, the greater the chance that the ideal candidate will emerge. However, a lengthy recruitment process also results in greater costs, disruption of service or work, and potential dissatisfaction of current employees who end up filling in for the missing jobholder.

International Recruitment

A topic of great interest is that of recruiting health professionals from other countries to address health workforce shortages in the United States. In an increasingly interconnected world, the movement of people and information across international borders has become a phenomenon that is often taken for granted. As skilled healthcare providers, physicians and nurses have had opportunities to seek employment internationally for several decades, and foreign-trained professionals are important parts of the healthcare systems in many countries. In the United States alone, about 26 percent of practicing physicians are graduates of non-US medical schools (American Medical Association 2013) and about 4 percent of nurses were educated overseas (Aiken et al. 2004; Cooper and Aiken 2006). This percentage is substantially higher in such states as California and New York, where about 20 percent or more of employed nurses are foreign educated. Since 2008, the economic recession has led to a decline in foreign-educated nurses (Pittman et al. 2014).

The implications of *international migration* of physicians and nurses are complex and have become a source of increasing debate. While physicians and nurses who migrate to other countries can benefit from better working conditions or salaries in their destinations, their movement can exacerbate inequalities in the worldwide distribution of healthcare workers. These developing countries not only lose their investments in education and training, income tax revenue, and potential for national growth, but they also see adverse health effects on their populations. In nations where healthcare workforce shortages are already severe, the need to replace healthcare professionals who have left for other countries only further depletes the health system's resources—funds that normally go toward health system strengthening. In addition, the lack of highly skilled care providers prevents these countries from meeting their own needs for healthcare innovation and problem solving. These factors exacerbate the existing inequalities in healthcare between high- and low-income countries.

Recruitment of workers from abroad has important ethical implications, which have been addressed by international organizations and specific countries.

The World Health Organization (WHO 2010) established the Global Code of Practice, which is largely voluntary. Other countries, such as the United Kingdom, have established similar policies that are also mostly voluntary in nature (NHS Employers 2014). Interestingly, a study of 42 key informants in Australia, Canada, the United Kingdom, and the United States reported that 93 percent of respondents indicated that no specific changes were made in their work as a result of the WHO Global Code of Practice, and 60 percent indicated that their colleagues were unaware of the code (Edge and Hoffman 2013).

The movement of international medical and nursing graduates into the US healthcare system raises several important issues for managers and leaders. In particular, managers must be aware of issues of ethical recruitment, regulation (visas), credentialing, and adaptation for foreign-trained physicians and nurses. Careful consideration of all of these areas is necessary to facilitate the successful recruitment and incorporation of foreign-trained healthcare professionals into the US healthcare system and to minimize the migration's negative effects on sending countries.

Selection

Employee selection is the process of collecting and evaluating applicant information that will help the employer to extend a job offer. To a great extent, the selection process is a matter of predicting which person, among a pool of potential hires, is likely to achieve success in the job. Of course, the definition of success is not always straightforward. Job performance may be defined in terms of technical proficiency, but the goals of a selection process may also include longevity in the position as well as fit with the culture and goals of the organization. Thus, evaluating the effectiveness of a selection process may include not only the time taken to fill the position but also the hired individual's performance and length of service, among other factors.

Selection must be distinguished from simple hiring (Gatewood, Feild, and Barrick 2011). In selection, an applicant's knowledge, skills, and abilities are carefully analyzed, as well as attitudes and other relevant factors. Ideally, the applicant who scores highest on the specified selection criteria is then extended an employment offer. Not infrequently, however, offers are made with little or no systematic collection and analysis of job-related information. A common example is the hiring of an individual based on political considerations or based on the applicant's relationship with the owners of or the managers in the organization. In such instances, these non-job-related factors may take precedence over objective measures of job suitability. In circumstances where a position has to be filled in a short time, or when a labor shortage exists in a particular area, an organization may simply hire whoever is available, assuming the individual possesses the minimum level of qualifications. This occurrence is frequent in the staffing of health centers in remote or otherwise undesirable locations. Applicant availability, rather than the comparative competence of the applicant, is the key criterion for selection in such situations.

The Question of Fit

Traditional selection processes are based on ensuring person–job fit. As noted earlier in this book, an accurate job description, based on sound job analysis, provides the foundation for selecting a candidate who has the required qualifications for the job. In practice, managers tend to be concerned mostly with applicant competencies, assessing whether the person has the knowledge, skills, and abilities to perform the job. Of increasing importance is the idea of *person–organization fit*—the extent to which an applicant will fit in with the values and culture of the organization. Person–organization *value congruence* is perhaps the overriding principle of person–organization fit (Hoffman et al. 2011).

Weyland (2011) notes that organizational fit involves more than simply the values of the organization. It actually includes how work is done in the organization, how people are treated, what behaviors are rewarded, and whether the culture is characterized by competition or cooperation. Research suggests that applicants conduct their own assessments of person-organization fit, and these perceptions are likely to change throughout the recruitment process and affect job choice decisions (Swider, Zimmerman, and Barrick 2014). This finding dramatically changes the dynamic of hiring, from a selection method that is based on concrete and observable indicators of *person–job fit* to a selection approach that seeks to assess person–organization fit. However, selection methods to assess fit are far from perfect and are largely untested. Arthur and colleagues (2006) state that if person–organization fit is used as a selection criterion, then measures must be held to the same psychometric and legal standards that apply to more traditional selection tests.

While the idea of person–organization fit is appealing, among the questions asked by researchers and managers is whether it is actually associated with job performance. That is, while applicants and employers intuitively seek to incorporate person–job fit into selection decisions as a means of reinforcing job satisfaction and organizational culture, does fit predict job performance? The evidence shows mixed results. Hoffman and Woehr (2006) found that person–organization fit is weakly to moderately related to job performance, organizational citizenship behavior, and turnover. In their meta-analysis of studies in this area, Kristof-Brown, Zimmerman, and Johnson (2005) revealed that person–organization fit is strongly associated with job satisfaction and organizational commitment and is moderately correlated with intention to quit, satisfaction, and trust. However, the same study found a low correlation between fit and overall job performance. This evidence should not discourage efforts to achieve person–organization fit, but institutions need to have realistic expectations for higher levels of performance as a result of fit.

What does this line of inquiry imply for healthcare organizations? First, in some cases, considering fit, either person–job or person–organization, is not possible. For example, in positions that are difficult to fill, whoever meets the minimum qualifications may need to be hired. Known to some sardonically as the "warm body" approach, this situation was defined by Rosse and Levin (2003, 9) as when a manager hires "anyone with a warm body and the ability to pass a drug test." Whether this type of hiring is effective in the long run is debatable, and certainly hiring without concern for fit has been shown to lead to poor long-term outcomes. Second, in situations in which fit can be taken into consideration, the importance of job fit versus organizational fit depends on the nature of the job and work environment. No fixed rule can be used for deciding on the appropriate balance between the two types of fit, but this balance should be discussed explicitly among hiring decision makers. Both person–job and person–organization fit have great importance in hiring a nurse on a psychiatric unit. However, person–organization fit may be less important in hiring a medical data-entry clerk, although an argument could be made for the importance of person–organization fit.

Among the most well-known approaches to measuring fit is the Organizational Culture Profile (OCP) (O'Reilly, Chatman, and Caldwell 1991). However, the main difficulty with the OCP is that it is labor intensive and is thus susceptible to respondent fatigue. Therefore, if person–organization fit is used as a selection criterion, an easy-to-administer, valid measure of person–organization fit needs to be established for use in parallel with measures that assess technical job competency and person–job fit. The use of fit as a selection criterion has potential legal implications and concerns for diversity. If we exclude people who are not "like us," does this action reflect a closed culture in which hiring managers are interested only in people from a very narrow segment of society?

Perhaps the flip side of hiring for fit is the practice of "ritual hiring," in which organizations or individuals apply well-worn but possibly obsolete hiring practices without assessing whether these procedures predict performance or perhaps even favor lower-performing applicants (Rosse and Levin 2003, 9). Organizations and jobs change, and so do job requirements. Thus, selection methods need to be current and consistent with the demands of the job. Managers must question "tried and true" selection methods to determine if they are in fact useful and helpful, and these methods deserve serious discussion by those involved in and affected by hiring decisions.

Through such processes as targeted selection and behavioral interviews, successful selection based on person–organization fit can be made. For example, Women & Infants Hospital of Rhode Island made an explicit effort to select employees on the basis of their fit with the culture, believing that a "person must be qualified to do the job, but they also require the right personality" (Greengard 2003, 56). After starting a hiring program using behavior-based interviews and in-depth analysis of candidates, the hospital saw patient satisfaction rise from the 71st percentile to the 89th percentile nationally, while turnover was reduced by 8.5 percent. Labor disputes also decreased, while productivity increased (Greengard 2003). The choice between seeking internal or external candidates is not often clear, and simultaneous pursuit of both internal and external candidates is not unusual. At the University of North Carolina (UNC) at Chapel Hill, UNC Hospitals use the Targeted Selection (Development Dimensions International 2014) approach, in which all employees are assessed on core values and attitudes specific to the organization.

Job Requirements and Selection Tools

The primary goal of selection is to identify among a group of applicants the person to whom a job offer should be made. On what basis should such a decision be made? A variety of selection tools can be used to evaluate each applicant's knowledge, skills, and abilities. Selection tools refer to any procedures or systems used to obtain job-related information about job applicants. Selection tools include the job application form, standardized tests, personal interviews, simulations, references, and any other mechanism that yields valid information about job applicants (see Exhibit 7.6). However, having a clear understanding of job requirements should precede the choice of selection tools. While this statement may seem obvious, not uncommonly a selection process moves forward without adequate information about job requirements and necessary competencies.

Selection tools should evaluate the full range of job requirements, including the more intangible requirements of the job, such as interpersonal skills, attitude, judgment, values, fit, ability to work in teams, and management abilities. Without an in-depth understanding of the job, the organization runs the risk of hiring someone who is a poor fit for the job, the organization, or both. As the organization moves into the hiring process, conducting a job analysis is therefore advisable. In particular, the job needs to be analyzed with respect to its current and future content and requirements. Jobs change, and using the content of the job from three years ago can easily overlook some of the most critical aspects of the job. The analysis may include seeking out the views of individuals who currently hold the position or who are in a similar position and obtaining the perspectives of supervisors and coworkers.

Selection Tool	Purpose
Cognitive tests	Evaluate reasoning, memory, perceptual speed and accuracy, and skills in arithmetic and reading comprehension, as well as knowledge of a particular function or job
Physical ability tests	Measure the physical ability to perform a particular task or the strength of specific muscle groups, as well as strength and stamina in general
Sample job tasks, such as performance tests, simulations, work samples, and realistic job previews	Assess performance and aptitude on particular tasks
Medical inquiries and physical examinations, including psychological tests	Assess physical or mental health
Personality tests and integrity tests	Assess the degree to which a person has certain traits or dispositions, such as honesty, dependability, cooperativeness, or safety, or aim to predict the likelihood that a person will engage in undesirable conduct, such as theft, absenteeism, and conflict
Criminal background checks	Provide information on arrest and conviction history
Credit checks	Provide information on credit and financial history
Performance appraisals	Reflect a supervisor's assessment of an individual's performance
English proficiency tests	Determine English fluency

EXHIBIT 7.6
Common
Selection Tools

Source: Adapted from Equal Employment Opportunity Commission (2010).

A more formalized *critical incident analysis* may also be used for discovering the hidden or less formal aspects of a job. A critical incident analysis is designed to generate a list of good and poor examples of job performance by current or potential jobholders. Once these examples of behaviors are collected, they are grouped into job dimensions. Evaluative measures are then developed for each of these job dimensions. The critical incident approach involves the following steps:

1. *Identify job experts, and select methods for collecting critical incidents.*
   Incidents can be obtained from the jobholder, coworkers, subordinates,

customers, and supervisors. Collection of critical incidents can be done in a group setting, with individual interviews, or through administration of a questionnaire. Note that different job experts may have varied views of the same job and thus may identify dissimilar critical incidents; this range of perspectives is, in fact, the strength of this method.

2. *Generate critical incidents.* Job experts should be asked to reflect on the job and identify examples of good and poor performance. Note that critical incidents may also be used as a form of performance appraisal, whereby the supervisor maintains a list of employee incidents illustrative of excellent and less than optimal behavior. According to Bowns and Bernardin (1988), each critical incident should be structured such that

   - it is specific and pertains to a specific behavior;
   - it focuses on observable behaviors that have been, or can be, exhibited on the job;
   - it briefly describes the context in which the behavior occurred; and
   - it indicates the positive or negative consequences of the behavior.

3. *Define job dimensions.* Job dimensions are defined by analyzing the critical incidents and extracting common themes. This information may then be used to inform the selection process.

Exhibit 7.7 provides examples of critical incidents associated with four different jobs, including the job dimensions related to each incident. This exercise yields a thorough understanding of the job's technical requirements, the job's formal qualifications, and the informal but critical aspects of successful job performance. Not only does a critical incident analysis provide a solid foundation for selection, but it also provides protection against charges of unfair hiring practices as it specifically identifies how key job requirements are related to job performance.

Reliability and Validity of Selection Tools

Not all selection tools are equal in their ability to predict job performance. Ideally, applicants who score better on selection instruments should consistently exhibit higher levels of job performance than individuals who score at lower levels. Therefore, to be useful, selection tools must ultimately be both reliable and valid.

From a measurement perspective, reliability is defined as the repeatability or consistency of a selection tool. Under this definition, a selection tool is deemed reliable if it provides the same result over and over again, assuming that the trait the selection tool is attempting to measure does not change. In other words, a reliable selection tool is one that yields the same

EXHIBIT 7.7
Critical Incident Approach to Identifying Job Requirements

Job	Critical Incident	Job Dimensions
Staff physician, rural hospital	• In an administrative staff meeting to review plans for the coming year, this individual exhibited strongly condescending and rude behaviors toward other team members. • The physician effectively communicated with a non-English-speaking immigrant family with no interpreter available.	• Ability to work in teams • Respect for other professionals • Communication skills • Resourcefulness
Nurse, emergency department	• After a school bus accident, the emergency department was overwhelmed with children and frightened parents. This nurse effectively and appropriately managed communication with parents and successfully obtained further assistance from elsewhere in the hospital. • When an upset spouse of a family member with a nonurgent condition became angry and potentially violent, the nurse effectively defused the individual's anger while maintaining normal triage procedures in the emergency department.	• Creativity and resourcefulness • Leadership • Community relations • Negotiation skills • Conflict resolution • Crisis management
Medical director, local public health department	• The local media reported an outbreak of salmonella that resulted in the hospitalization of one child with this serious condition. The outbreak was traced to a fast-food restaurant that was inspected by health department personnel less than one week before the incident. The health department was blamed for not preventing the outbreak. This medical director conducted a thorough internal investigation and found that this outbreak was an isolated incident caused by mishandling of food on a single occasion. She communicated effectively at a press conference, defending the health department and assuring the public of the safety of local eating establishments.	• Ability to work effectively under crisis conditions • Strong interpersonal skills • Effective crisis manager • Strong communication and media skills • Strong sense of public accountability
Medical director, community hospital	• At an open community meeting, the medical director succeeded in defusing anger among community members resulting from the closing of a hospital service line. • On numerous occasions, the medical director successfully engaged other professionals in quality improvement activities.	• Conflict management • Community relations • Leadership • Multidisciplinary orientation • Understanding of quality improvement philosophy

findings regardless of who administers the tool or in what context (e.g., time of day, version of the tool) the tool is used. In general, physical and observable traits and skills (such as height and weight, the ability to lift a given weight, and the ability to compute manually) are more reliably measured than are psychological or behavioral traits (such as competitiveness, intelligence, and tolerance). Exhibit 7.8 provides an overview of the relative reliability of the measurement of different human attributes.

In contrast, validity refers to the relationship between a selection instrument and job criteria. In essence, validity addresses the question of whether a selection instrument measures something that is related to job performance. That is, validation of a selection test addresses the question of whether individuals who receive high scores on a selection test will perform well on the job (Farr and Tippins 2010). *Content validity* is the extent to which a selection tool representatively samples the content of the job for which the measure will be used. According to this strategy, a selection tool that includes a sufficient amount of actual job-related content is

EXHIBIT 7.8
Relative Reliability of Measurement of Human Attributes

Level of Reliability	Human Attributes
High	*Personal* Height Weight Vision Hearing
Medium	*Attitudes and Skills* Dexterity Mathematical skills Verbal ability Intelligence Clerical skills Mechanical skills
Medium to low	*Interests* Economic Scientific Mechanical Cultural
Low	*Personality* Sociability Dominance Cooperativeness Tolerance

Sources: Adapted from Albright, Glennon, and Smith (1963); Gatewood, Feild, and Barrick (2011).

considered valid. Expert judgment, rather than statistical analysis, is typically used to assess content validity. One may look at content validity in designing a knowledge-based selection tool for laboratory technicians. A test that requires applicants to describe procedures associated with the most common laboratory tests is likely to be judged to have content validity.

More specifically, *construct validity* refers to the degree to which a selection tool actually measures the construct it intends to measure; this concept ultimately determines the conclusions that can be legitimately drawn from the tool's use. For example, most organizations are concerned with the integrity of their employees, defined as employees' honesty, dependability, trustworthiness, and reliability. If an organization administers an integrity test to job applicants, how certain can the organization be that the test actually measures the construct of integrity? A criticism of this type of test is that applicants may fake their responses, that is, respond in a way that creates the desired impression. Construct validity is commonly equated with criterion-related validity. *Criterion-related validity* is the extent to which a selection tool is associated with or predicts actual job performance. Criterion-related validity can be demonstrated through two strategies. The first of these strategies, *concurrent validity*, involves administering a selection tool to a group of current employees. These employees' scores are then correlated with actual job performance. For the selection tool to demonstrate concurrent validity, a strong correlation must exist between the score on the selection tool and the actual job performance.

An alternative and more complex approach to assessing a selection tool's criterion-related validity is by assessing a tool's *predictive validity*. Here, the selection tool is administered to a group of job applicants but is not used as a means of selection. Because the selection tool has not yet been validated, actual selection decisions are made on the basis of other measures and criteria. Over time, data are obtained on the actual job performance of those selected for the job. The two sets of scores—those from the selection tool being validated and scores derived from employee's actual performance measures—are correlated and examined for possible relationships. A strong correlation between performance on the selection tool and future job performance would provide evidence that the selection tool is valid.

Unfortunately, many organizations employ a range of selection tools but pay little or no attention to issues of reliability and validity. In the following section, the reliability and validity of some common selection tools are examined and suggestions are offered on how they can be improved.

Reference Checks

Organizations typically perform background checks on prospective employees, which may include verifying educational credentials, assessing legal status to work in the United States, checking credit references, reviewing criminal records, and performing online searches. Employers face many restrictions on background checks, many on a state level. For example, several states restrict the use of credit histories in hiring decisions, while other states prohibit private employers from asking applicants about their criminal records on written applications (Roberts 2011).

To avoid negligent hiring, checking references from former employers is a potentially useful tool. However, many organizations refuse to provide information about former employees for fear of defamation lawsuits. A study conducted by the Society for Human Resource Management found that while 98 percent of respondents indicated that their organizations verify dates of employment for current or former employees, 68 percent would not discuss work performance, 82 percent would not discuss character or personality issues, and 8 percent would not disclose a disciplinary action (Meinert 2011). This finding certainly limits the usefulness of reference checks beyond verifying past employment. The Equal Employment Opportunity Commission (2014) has established guidelines for employer background checks that address a variety of issues, including the need to obtain an applicant's written permission to conduct a background check and the importance of applying the same standards to all applicants.

Adding to the difficulty in using information from references is the lack of data on the reliability of using reference checks to gauge performance in previous jobs. In studies that have been conducted, researchers have sought to determine the level of agreement (interrater reliability) between different individuals who provide a reference for the same applicant. Reliability estimates are typically poor, at a level of 0.40 or less. This finding may be explained by a number of factors, including the reluctance of many referees to provide negative feedback and the real possibility that different raters may be evaluating different aspects of job performance. Studies of the validity of reference checks have found that this tool has moderate predictive validity (Hunter and Hunter 1984; Meinert 2011). Several explanations have been suggested for the poor predictive power of reference checks:

- Many measures used in reference checks have low reliability; where reliability is low, validity must be low as well.
- Individuals who provide references frequently only use a restricted range of scores—typically in the high range—in evaluating job applicants. If virtually all reference checks are positive, they are still unlikely predictors of performance success for all individuals.
- In many instances, job applicants preselect the individuals who will provide the reference, and applicants are highly likely to select only those who will provide a positive reference.

How can the validity of reference checks be improved? Research in this area offers the following conclusions (Gatewood, Feild, and Barrick 2011):

- The most recent employer tends to provide the most accurate evaluation of an individual's work.
- The reference giver has had adequate time to observe the applicant, and the applicant is the same gender, ethnicity, and nationality as the reference giver.
- The old and new jobs are similar in content.

Exhibit 7.9 provides some basic guidelines for the appropriate use of references.

Job Interviews

The job interview is used for virtually all positions largely because those involved in hiring simply wish to find out more than can be obtained from the application, references, and other documentation. The result of the interview is often given the greatest weight in hiring decisions. Job interviews, however, typically have low reliability and validity, are often unfair to applicants,

---

EXHIBIT 7.9
Guidelines for the Appropriate Use of Reference Checks

1. Ask for and obtain only job-related information.
2. As the conversation proceeds, describe the job under consideration and the relationship the reference had with the applicant.
3. Do not ask for information in an application or personal interview that may be deemed illegal.
4. Applicants should provide written permission to contact references.
5. Individuals who check references should be trained in interviewing techniques, including methods of probing and accurately recording reference information.
6. Reference information should be recorded in writing immediately after the interview.
7. Use the reference-checking process to confirm information provided by the application and to identify gaps in the employment record.
8. Be aware of the possibility that the individual who provides a reference could be trying to damage a prospective employee by giving a negative reference.
9. Use the references provided by the applicant as a source of additional references or information.
10. While asking about an applicant's attendance record is permissible, avoid questions dealing with the employee's medical or disability status, use of sick leave or medical leave, or workers' compensation issues. Similarly, avoid questions related to the individual's home life and family.

and may be at least partially illegal. They are frequently not reliable because questions vary from interviewer to interviewer, and two applicants vying for the same position are sometimes asked different questions altogether. Similarly, the manner in which answers to interview questions are interpreted and scored by interviewers may vary substantially as well. Strong evidence also suggests that some people are capable of, and often engage in, "faking" of answers such that they appear more appealing to the organization, and that individuals with particular personality profiles are more likely to engage in this behavior (O'Neill et al. 2013). While differentiating between honest and faking interviewees can be difficult, the less transparent the interview format, that is, the less apparent the socially desired response, the better the chance of identifying the right person for the job.

The predictive validity of the job interview—that is, does a positive interview actually forecast job success?—has also been questioned. Job interviews present several problems. First, the questions are usually not provided to applicants in advance and may bear little relationship with the candidate's performance in the future. This format may be seen as unfair because candidates are not given the opportunity to prepare answers that would showcase their knowledge, skills, and abilities. On the other hand, not providing questions in advance may reduce the opportunity for applicants to game the system by preparing socially desirable responses. Second, interview questions are often not standardized, causing applicants to be treated inequitably because each interviewer poses different questions and each applicant is asked a different set of questions. This lack of standardization prevents the interviewer and the organization from obtaining the information necessary to make informed decisions. Third, untrained interviewers have a tendency to pose legally dubious questions that violate the law or compromise ethical principles, such as inquiries about plans for starting a family or for maternity leaves.

Notwithstanding these problems, the job interview can be an effective and efficient method of acquiring job-competency information and assessing the applicant's suitability for a position and fit within the organization. Furthermore, it can be used as a valuable recruitment tool because it allows the interviewer to highlight the positive features of the organization, the department, and the job.

Those involved in selection can choose between unstructured and structured interview techniques. *Unstructured interviews* present few constraints in how interviewers go about gathering information and evaluating applicants. As a result, unstructured interviews may be very subjective and thus tend to be less reliable than structured interviews. However, because of the free rein frequently given to interviewers, unstructured interviews may be more effective than the structured type in screening unsuitable candidates.

In a *structured interview*, the questions are clearly job related and based on the result of a thorough job analysis. A discussion before the interview among the selection team members is advantageous because it provides the team an opportunity to decide on what responses would be considered high and poor quality. This decision, in turn, allows the team to score applicant responses. Situational, experience-based, job-knowledge, and worker-requirement questions are most commonly posed during a structured interview.

Situational questions relate to how an applicant may handle a hypothetical work scenario, while experience-based questions ask how the candidate previously handled an issue that is similar to an issue that may be encountered on the new job. Following is an example of a scenario and related situational and experience-based questions. The constructs being assessed in this case are the ability to handle a stressful situation, competency in dealing with the public, and professionalism.

> *Scenario:* Seven pediatricians work in a busy medical practice, and Monday morning is the busiest time of the week at the clinic. The waiting room is overcrowded, and two of the pediatricians are unexpectedly called away from the office—one for a personal situation and the other to attend to a patient in the hospital. Children and their parents now have to wait up to two hours to see the remaining doctors, and their level of anger and frustration increases as they wait. They are taking out their anger on you.
>
> *Situational questions:* How would you handle this situation? What and how would you communicate with the remaining physicians about this situation?
>
> *Experience-based questions:* Think about a situation in your last job in which you were faced with angry and upset patients or customers. What was the situation? What did you do? What was the outcome?

Situational questions should be designed in a way that allows alternative, not just expected, responses to be evaluated or scored. If a panel—two or more people—conducts the interview, each panelist should be able to confirm answers and their meaning with each other.

Job-knowledge questions assess whether the applicant has the knowledge to do the job. These questions and follow-up probes are predetermined and are based on the job description. Similarly, worker-requirement questions seek to determine if the candidate is able and willing to work under the conditions of the job. For example, applicants for a consulting position may be asked if they are able and willing to travel for a designated portion of their work.

Whatever form is used, job interviews must be conducted with the following guidelines in mind:

1. Prepare yourself. For an unstructured interview, learn the job requirements. For a structured interview, become familiar with the questions to be asked. Review information about the job applicant.

2. Create a respectful physical environment for the interview.

3. Describe the job, and invite questions about the job.

4. Put the applicant at ease, and convey an interest in the person. A purposely stressful interview is not desirable, as other reliable and more ethical methods can be used to assess an applicant's ability to handle stress. Furthermore, a purposively stressful interview may reflect poorly on the organization.

5. Do not come to premature conclusions (positive or negative) about the applicant. This guideline is particularly important for unstructured interviews.

6. Listen carefully, and ask for clarity if the applicant's responses are vague.

7. Observe and take notes on relevant aspects of the applicant's dress, mannerisms, and affect.

8. Provide an opportunity for the applicant to ask questions.

9. Do not talk excessively. Remember that the interview is an opportunity to hear from the applicant.

10. Do not ask questions that are unethical or that put the organization in a legally vulnerable position (see Exhibit 7.10).

11. Explain the selection process that comes after the interview.

12. Evaluate the applicant as soon as possible after the interview. This evaluation includes engaging with other interviewers who may be interviewing the same applicant.

EXHIBIT 7.10 Inappropriate and Appropriate Job Interview Questions	**Personal and Marital Status**
Inappropriate:	• How tall are you? • How much do you weigh? (acceptable if these are safety requirements) • What is your maiden name? • Are you married? • Is this your maiden or married name? • With whom do you live? • Do you smoke?
Appropriate:	• After hiring, inquire about marital status for tax and insurance forms purposes. • Are you able to lift 50 pounds and carry it 20 yards? (acceptable if this is part of the job)

(continued)

Parental Status and Family Responsibilities

Inappropriate:
- How many kids do you have?
- Do you plan to have children?
- What are your child care arrangements?
- Are you pregnant?

Appropriate:
- Would you be willing to relocate if necessary?
- Travel is an important part of this job. Would you be willing to travel as needed by the job?
- This job requires overtime occasionally. Would you be able and willing to work overtime as necessary?
- After hiring, inquire about dependent information for tax and insurance forms purposes.

Age

Inappropriate:
- How old are you?
- What year were you born?
- When did you graduate from high school and college?

Appropriate:
- Before hiring, asking if the applicant is above the legal minimum age for the hours or working conditions is appropriate, as this is in compliance with state or federal labor laws. After hiring, verifying legal minimum age with a birth certificate or other ID and asking for age on insurance forms are permissible.

National Origin

Inappropriate:
- Where were you born?
- Where are your parents from?
- What is your heritage?
- What is your native tongue?
- What languages do you read, speak, or write fluently? (acceptable if this is relevant to the job)

Appropriate:
- Are you authorized to work in the United States?
- May we verify that you are a legal US resident, or may we have a copy of your work visa status?

Race or Skin Color

Inappropriate:
- What is your racial background?
- Are you a member of a minority group?

Appropriate:
- This organization is an equal opportunity employer. Race is required information only for affirmative-action programs.

EXHIBIT 7.10
Inappropriate and Appropriate Job Interview Questions
(continued from previous page)

(continued)

EXHIBIT 7.10
Inappropriate
and Appropriate
Job Interview
Questions
*(continued from
previous page)*

Religion or Creed

Inappropriate:
- What religion do you follow?
- Which religious holidays will you be taking off from work?
- Do you attend church regularly?

Appropriate:
- May we contact religious or other organizations related to your beliefs to provide us with references, per your list of employers and references?

Criminal Record

Inappropriate:
- Have you ever been arrested?
- Have you ever spent a night in jail?

Appropriate:
- Questions about convictions by civil or military courts are appropriate if accompanied by a disclaimer that the answers will not necessarily cause loss of job opportunity. Generally, employers can ask only about convictions and not arrests (except for jobs in law-enforcement and security-clearance agencies) when the answers are relevant to the job performance.

Disability

Inappropriate:
- Do you have any disabilities?
- What is your medical history?
- How does your condition affect your abilities?
- Please fill out this medical history document.
- Have you had recent illnesses or hospitalizations?
- When was your last physical exam?
- Are you HIV-positive?

Appropriate:
- Can you perform specific physical tasks (lifting heavy objects, bending, kneeling) that are required for the job?
- After hiring, asking about the person's medical history on insurance forms is appropriate.
- Are you able to perform the essential functions of this job with or without reasonable accommodations?

Affiliations

Inappropriate:
- To what clubs or associations do you belong?

Appropriate:
- Do you belong to any professional or trade groups or other organizations that you consider relevant to your ability to perform this job?

Note: Questions listed here are not necessarily illegal. For example, it is not illegal to ask an applicant's date of birth, but it is illegal to deny employment to an applicant solely because he or she is 40 years of age or older. In this case, the question is not illegal, but a discriminatory motive for asking is illegal. Unknown or ambiguous motive is what makes any question with discriminatory implications inappropriate. If an individual is denied employment, having asked this and similar questions can lead to the applicant claiming that the selection decision was made on the basis of age, gender, or other characteristic for which it is illegal to discriminate.

Applications and Resumes

Application forms and resumes usually contain useful information about job applicants. The major drawback of these tools is that they may misrepresent qualifications. Several methods can be used to improve the usefulness of application forms. First, create an addendum to the application that asks applicants to provide information that is specific to the open position. This way, particular knowledge, skills, and abilities can be targeted for different jobs. Second, include a statement on the application form that allows the applicant to indicate that all the information he or she reported is accurate; the applicant should then be required to sign or initial this statement. Third, ensure that illegal inquiries about personal information (e.g., marital status, height, weight) are excluded from the form.

Ability and Aptitude Tests

Ability and aptitude tests (including personality, honesty, integrity, cognitive reasoning, and fine motor coordination tests) are available, and many of them demonstrate reliability and validity. A number of firms specialize in developing and assessing tests; see, for example, Walden Personnel Testing and Consulting at www.waldentesting.com. Debate is brewing about the issue of situational validity—the notion that the nature of job performance differs across work settings and that the validity of tests may vary according to the setting. In general, studies tend to conclude that results of a test on basic abilities are generalizable across work settings, assuming that the test itself is valid and reliable. The key is to ensure that such tests are actually representative of the work involved in a particular job.

Assessment Centers

The use of assessment centers is a highly sophisticated and multidimensional method of evaluating applicants. The term *assessment centers* may refer to the physical locations where testing is done, but it may also refer to a series of assessment procedures that are administered, professionally scored, and reported to hiring personnel. Traditionally, assessment centers have been used to test an applicant's managerial skills, but they are also employed for a variety of hiring situations. Typical assessment formats include paper-and-pencil tests, leaderless group discussions, role-playing intelligence tests, personality tests, interest measures, work-task simulations, in-basket exercises, interviews, and situational exercises. Evidence indicates that positive statistical relationships exist between assessment center scores and job performance (Jackson, Stillman, and Englert 2010; Lehman et al. 2011).

Turnover and Retention

Among the most important healthcare workforce challenges is staff shortage, and associated with this issue are employee turnover and retention. Larger environmental and systemic pressures contribute to the chronic shortages in healthcare. Although turnover is not appreciably increasing in healthcare, rates are higher in this industry than in others. A number of factors affect the high demand for healthcare workers, including population growth, the aging of the population, the expansion of health insurance coverage to tens of millions of previously uninsured individuals via the enactment of healthcare reform, declining labor productivity in the healthcare sector, and advances in technology (Carnevale et al. 2012).

An example of the high demand for healthcare workers can be seen in the projected growth of the nursing workforce. According to the Bureau of Labor Statistics (2013), the number of employed registered nurses will grow from 2.71 million nurses in 2012 to an expected 3.24 million nurses in 2022, an increase of more than 19 percent. These projections also explain the need for an additional 525,800 nurses to replace nurses leaving the workforce, bringing the total number of job openings for nurses due to growth and replacement to more than 1.05 million by 2022. Even though the stability and supply of the nursing workforce is heavily influenced by the aging of registered nurses, the surge of younger nurses entering the profession, and the uncertainty of the lingering effect of the expansion of the nursing work-force that took place during the 18-month recession that began in December 2007, the growth in demand for nurses will continue to outpace the supply (Auerbach, Buerhaus, and Staiger 2011; Auerbach et al. 2013). Although estimates of the future nurse shortage vary, one analysis estimates a shortfall of about 260,000 nurses by the year 2025 (American Association of Colleges of Nursing 2014).

These broad societal factors are largely out of the control of healthcare organizations, and they substantially influence the worker vacancy rates in hospitals. These vacancy rates, in turn, highlight the need for organizations to do a better job at recruiting, selecting, and retaining staff. This section explains the concern with turnover, enumerates the costs associated with turnover, discusses the factors that contribute to turnover, and explores the methods proven to improve retention. Although the nursing shortage is used as a basis to explore the issues of turnover and retention, shortages are also present in other healthcare professions, such as among radiologic technicians, primary care physicians, and pharmacists. The lessons in the discussion of the nursing shortage are applicable to other professions as well.

A distinction has to be made between the separate, although related, concepts of turnover and retention. Many organizations view retention as the inverse of turnover, and as a result, they miss critical trends that are happening within their systems. A *turnover rate* is a simple ratio that provides only a summary of the gross movement in and out of the organization during a specific time frame (usually one year), or the number of times on average

that employees must be replaced during a year. A *retention rate*, on the other hand, is the percentage of employees who are employed at the beginning of a period and who remain with the organization at the end of the period (Society for Human Resource Management 2012a). The key distinction is that retention views an individual or a group as an entity; therefore, retention allows for a more thorough examination of how the loss of one individual or cohort influences retention strategies and productivity.

For example, an organization that experiences a slight decline in turnover (say, from 20 percent to 18 percent) over a five-year period may think that it is doing well in addressing its retention problem. However, during that same five-year time span, the retention rate of individuals who have 5 to 15 years of service declined (say, from 70 percent to 35 percent). These rates indicate that the organization has difficulty with retaining experienced employees and needs to explore and implement new retention strategies. Overall, organizations need to thoroughly examine both turnover and retention rates to successfully deal with the challenge of staff shortages.

Studies on Nursing Turnover

The demand for healthcare workers has increased, but the quality of their work life has decreased. The average annual turnover rate for hospital workers is about 14.7 percent, with substantially higher percentages for particular professional groups. At any one time, the national nurse vacancy rate ranges from 5 percent to 23 percent, with about 27 percent of US hospitals experiencing a vacancy rate of 17 percent or more. About 43 percent of hospitals report having difficulties filling vacancies (Nursing Solutions Inc. 2014). Generally, registered nurse turnover in hospitals ranges between 4.3 percent and 31 percent, with a national average of 15.1 percent (Nursing Solutions Inc. 2014). Nursing homes face an even bleaker situation, with 90 percent of nursing homes lacking sufficient nursing staff to provide even basic care (American Health Care Association 2014). A 2012 study found that the turnover rate in nursing homes for direct care staff (registered nurses, licensed practical nurses, and certified nursing assistants) was a staggering 50 percent (American Health Care Association 2014).

Nurse dissatisfaction has been cited as a key reason for turnover and even departure from the profession. In a study of nurse satisfaction and burnout, 24 percent of hospital nurses providing direct patient care and 27 percent of nursing home nurses reported dissatisfaction in their current job, while 34 percent of hospital nurses and 37 percent of nursing home nurses reported feeling burned out in their current job (McHugh et al. 2011). These findings are consistent with an earlier worldwide study of nurses, which found that the United States had the highest rate of nurse job dissatisfaction at 41 percent, which is four times higher than the dissatisfaction

score of the professional workforce in general (Aiken et al. 2001; Albaugh 2003). Twibell and colleagues (2012) summarize the main causes of nurse turnover as heavy workloads, disillusionment about scheduling, lack of autonomy, lack of intrinsic and extrinsic workplace rewards, insufficient time with patients, and dissatisfying relationships with peers, managers, and colleagues. A Jackson Healthcare (2012) report identifies the top five drivers of nurse dissatisfaction: (1) poor, unsupportive, unresponsive management; (2) work overload; (3) low compensation; (4) inadequate staffing; and (5) lack of respect and appreciation from management.

The impact of turnover and other nurse staffing concerns on healthcare quality have been documented in a number of studies. Stevens and colleagues (2011) found that insufficient nurse staffing was related to higher patient mortality rates, and that when a nurse's workload increases because of high turnover, the risk of mortality increases. Similarly, in a study focused on the impact of mandatory nursing ratios in California hospitals, Aiken and colleagues (2010) found that hospital nurse staffing ratios mandated in California were associated with lower mortality and nurse outcomes predictive of better nurse retention. In a study examining the impact of nurse factors and patient satisfaction, McHugh and colleagues (2011) found that patient satisfaction levels are lower in hospitals with more nurses who are dissatisfied or burned out. These studies present the connection among nurse dissatisfaction, turnover, and quality of care.

In addition to the effect on quality, shortages and turnover also have significant financial implications. The costs associated with employee termination, recruitment, selection, hiring, and training represent a substantial non-value-adding element in the organizational budget. A 2004 study of turnover estimated the costs associated with turnover in an academic medical center (Waldman and Arora 2004). Depending on assumptions made in the analysis, the total cost of turnover reduced the annual operating budget of the medical center between $7 million and $19 million, or between 3.4 percent and 5.8 percent. This research indicates that, at this medical center, more than one-fourth of the total turnover costs were attributable to nurse turnover. Several studies have focused specifically on the cost of nursing turnover. While nurse turnover is difficult to measure, both the Advisory Board Company (1999) and Jones (2005, 2008) have attempted to capture not only the direct costs of nurse turnover but the hidden costs of reduced productivity (e.g., predeparture, vacancy, new employee onboarding) as well. The estimated cost of a single nurse leaving is $42,000 (Advisory Board Company 1999) and $64,000 (Jones 2008), and these estimates support the claim that nursing turnover has significant financial implications for all healthcare organizations. The following example reiterates this point: Assuming a turnover rate of 13 percent and the cost of nurse turnover ranging

between $42,000 and $64,000 per nurse, a hospital that employs 600 nurses would face yearly estimated nursing staff replacement costs of between $3.25 million and $5 million per year.

Turnover can be viewed as costly in terms of patient care, financial stability, and staff morale. Nurse turnover affects communication among nurses and between nurses and other healthcare professionals, the quality of care, and care continuity. The work of teams is disturbed as well, as team composition and skills change when a member comes or goes, and members who are left behind often feel low morale and a sense of rejection.

Retention Strategies

Many of the factors associated with effective recruitment are also applicable to retention because a person's reasons for accepting an employment offer are basically the same as the reasons for staying with that employer. Therefore, retention strategies are a necessary follow-up to recruitment. With the opportunities available to nurses in other organizations and professions, viewing retention as an essential HRM function, like compensation and training, is critical.

One study examined the strategies used by nurse managers who have succeeded in achieving low turnover rates; high satisfaction among patients, employees, and providers; good patient outcomes; and positive working relationships (Manion 2004). The study found that these nurse managers were able to develop a "culture of retention." Through their daily work, these managers created an environment where people want to stay because they enjoy their work and where staff contribute to this sense of attachment. These managers emphasized caring sincerely for the welfare of their staff, forging authentic connections with each staff member, and focusing on results and problem solving.

In today's healthcare environment, much of the turnover that occurs is beyond the control of a single organization. Employee commitment to employers has virtually evaporated. Except in rare instances, the market profoundly affects the movement of employees. Organizations can still control turnover, but their influence is becoming limited. Retention strategies have simply not achieved the type of consistent success once anticipated. Furthermore, each organization needs to develop its own retention strategies and tailor them to the particular circumstances of the institution (Hirschkorn et al. 2010).

Several generic retention strategies have been shown to work. First, offer competitive compensation. Compensation comes in many forms, including signing bonuses, premium and differential pay, forgivable loans, bonuses, and extensive benefits. Second, structure jobs so that they are more appealing and satisfying. This structure can be achieved by carefully assigning

and grouping tasks, providing employees with sufficient autonomy, allowing flexible work hours and scheduling, enhancing the collegiality of the work environment, and instituting work policies that are respectful of individual needs. In the nursing environment, job design encompasses elements such as nurse–patient staffing ratios and mandatory overtime. Third, put in place a superb management and supervisory team. The idea that people quit their supervisors, not their jobs, is true in nursing, as nurses sometimes leave because of poor working relationships with their managers or other health-care professionals. Fourth, make opportunities for career growth available. Providing career ladders is becoming increasingly difficult as organizations become flatter and widen their spans of control. Alternatives to promotions need to be developed and implemented.

The American Nurses Credentialing Center established the Magnet Recognition Program to acknowledge and reward healthcare organizations that exhibit and provide excellent nursing care. Designated Magnet hospitals are characterized by fewer hierarchical structures, decentralized decision making, flexibility in scheduling, positive nurse–physician relationships, and nursing leadership that supports and invests in nurses' career development (American Nurses Credentialing Center 2014). Magnet hospitals have been found to have better patient outcomes and higher levels of patient satisfaction (Aiken et al. 2008; McHugh et al. 2013). Compared to other hospitals, Magnet institutions have lower turnover and higher job satisfaction among nurses (Huerta 2003; Upenieks 2002). These findings suggest that becoming a Magnet healthcare organization has the potential to increase nurse satisfaction and improve retention (Drenkard 2010).

Many guides to effective nurse retention have been published, and their recommendations generally pertain to the topics discussed earlier. These topics include issues related to ensuring value congruence, improving job satisfaction, reducing stress, improving intrinsic and extrinsic rewards, focusing on improvements in hiring or onboarding processes, increasing professional autonomy, and reducing patient-nurse ratios (Dotson et al. 2014). Note that not all strategies aimed at improving nurse satisfaction also improve retention. In an early review of nurse recruitment and retention strategies, the Health Care Advisory Board (2001) distinguished between strategies that boost morale and those that enhance retention. While this review has not been replicated since its publication, the distinction it makes is important. The Health Care Advisory Board summarized the findings into four types:

1. *Strategies that neither increase morale nor improve retention.* Examples are providing individualized benefits, concierge services, and employee lounge areas.

2. *Strategies that increase morale but do not improve retention.* Examples include forming morale committees, offering on-site childcare, creating recognition programs, and providing educational benefits.

3. *Strategies that do not increase morale but improve retention.* Examples are improving screening of applicants, monitoring turnover in key areas, and tracking turnover of key employees.

4. *Strategies that increase morale and improve retention.* Examples include establishing staffing ratios, providing career ladders, implementing buddy programs, and allowing flexible scheduling.

The Health Care Advisory Board's review yielded five effective retention strategies: (1) selecting the right employees; (2) improving orientation and onboarding processes by creating a buddy program and other opportunities that help new employees establish professional and personal relationships with colleagues; (3) monitoring turnover to identify specific root causes, including identifying managers whose departments have high turnover rates; (4) developing and implementing ways to retain valued employees; and (5) although marginal in its effectiveness, systematically attempting to reverse turnover decisions.

Every organization faces different challenges in its efforts to retain valued employees. The success of a retention program depends on the ability of the organization to correctly determine the causes of turnover and to enact strategies that appropriately target these causes. Also, the organization must recognize the advantages and usefulness of alternative retention strategies.

Summary

Recruiting, selecting, and retaining employees continue to be important HRM functions, especially in a competitive, pressurized environment like healthcare. Healthcare organizations and their HR departments face enormous challenges. From a recruitment and selection standpoint, they need to seek employees who (1) have specialized skills but are flexible to fill in for other positions, (2) bring in expertise and are able to work in groups whose members are not experts, (3) are strongly motivated yet are comfortable with relatively flat organizational structures in which traditional upward mobility may be difficult, and (4) represent diversity yet also fit into the organizational culture. From a retention standpoint, they need to identify factors related to retention and develop innovative strategies to improve retention. By doing so, healthcare organizations will be better able to meet challenges in the coming decades.

Discussion Questions

1. Given two equally qualified job applicants—one from inside and one from outside the organization—how would you go about deciding which one to hire?

2. For various reasons, some healthcare organizations are unable to pay market rates for certain positions. What advice would you give such an organization about possible recruitment and retention strategies?

3. The use of work references is increasingly viewed as unreliable. How can employers legally and ethically obtain information about an applicant's past performance? What measures can be taken to verify information contained in a job application or resume?

4. What are the advantages and disadvantages of recruiting through the Internet? What advice do you give to a hospital that is considering using the Internet for recruitment?

Experiential Exercises

Case **Sexual Orientation Discrimination**

Note: This case was written by Brian Cooper.
Kathleen, director of physical therapy at Wabash Community Health Center, smiled as she reflected on her meeting with Jerry, the chief medical officer (CMO) of the health center. Jerry had just made the decision to unfreeze a vacant position in Kathleen's department, a position that had been vacant for more than a year. Since one of the physical therapists (PTs) retired one year ago, the remaining four PTs in the department had begun to feel burned out. Only one PT could take vacation or be off work at a time so that the health center would have enough PTs to staff its physical therapy clinic. Until now, the vacant position had been frozen by the CMO because of the health center's recent financial troubles and declining volumes. Even if the position had been available, finding a PT to fill it would

have been difficult because the health center was located in a rural county in Mississippi.

Kathleen was interested in finding a new hire, not only to fill a much-needed position in the department, but also to introduce some diversity into the team. The current PTs were all white women, the youngest aged 42 years. Kathleen was concerned that in the future she would struggle to keep the clinic staffed because the current PTs would continue to retire with a shortage of replacements to fill the void.

Kathleen was therefore very pleased when she received the application of Keith, an African-American man who had just graduated from the University of Alabama at Birmingham. She received the application one week after HR posted the position, and thus far Keith was the only applicant. Kathleen was unsure whether she should interview Keith immediately or wait for more applications to emerge. *I should probably reel in the first catch I get*, she thought. *After all, a bird in the hand is worth two in the bush.*

While looking over Keith's application materials, Kathleen noticed that he did not have any physical therapy experience on his resume, but he had only graduated from the program a month ago. Kathleen wondered why Keith chose to move to Wabash County after living in a large city like Birmingham, where he might find higher-paying work, but she surmised that he might have been from the area originally and that he probably moved back to be around family.

Kathleen decided to bring Keith in for an interview. When Keith walked into her office on Monday morning, he seemed very polite and professional. He appeared to be in his midtwenties and to be in good health, capable of doing the necessary work of a PT. Before proceeding with the official interview questions, Kathleen wanted to make some brief conversation, during which she curiously inquired about what brought Keith to Wabash County. Expecting to hear something about family, she was surprised when she heard him explain, "My partner lives here, and I moved to Wabash to be close to them." Kathleen did not notice a ring on Keith's finger and was surprised that when Keith referred to his partner in the previous statement, he used the pronoun "them." Kathleen thought nothing of it at the time, and she began asking the professional questions. Keith did very well when answering the questions concerning clinical physical therapy practices, and he even showed promise as a leader when answering questions about his methods of interpersonal conflict resolution and personal initiative.

When the interview was complete, Kathleen thanked Keith for coming in. She sat at her desk for a moment, reviewing her notes from the interview. She was certain that Keith would be a great fit for the team and that Keith had terrific competency concerning the duties of the job.

While Kathleen was reflecting on this, one of the PTs whom she supervised rushed into her office and closed the door behind her without saying a word. Kathleen's head shot up from her paperwork and she stared, bewildered, at the very concerned face of Linda. The PT clinical supervisor, Linda managed the other three PTs on staff, creating work schedules and serving as support if needed.

"That young man that was just in here, who just walked out, that's one of the men who just moved into my neighborhood!" Linda exclaimed, taking a seat while slowly regaining composure. She cleared her throat and explained, "One of my neighbors, Becky, told me that two men just moved into our neighborhood, you know, together. They're living an 'alternative lifestyle.'" She demonstrated the quotes with her fingers in the air as she said the last two words.

Kathleen was taken aback by this remark, almost in shock that her PT clinical supervisor, who was usually very professional and appreciative of diversity, was choosing to point out this fact to her. After coming back from two seconds of speechlessness, Kathleen asked, "Well, if in fact what you have just said is true, is that an issue for you?"

"Yes," Linda stated, almost with a pedagogical tone. "I can accept a lot of things about people. But I will not accept someone who lives that kind of lifestyle. It's just not morally right."

Kathleen was once again taken aback, but she tried to calm Linda down and to perform damage control in the situation. "Linda," she softly said, "I advise you to think about what you're saying. We don't know that this information is true about Keith. Even if it *is* true, this is not a factor that I would consider when assessing an applicant. I realize that his choices may violate your personal beliefs, but you and I both know that we need to work with people who have different beliefs from our own."

"You're going to hire him, aren't you? I can see it already. Why, the job has only been posted for one week and you're just going to hire the first guy that comes in?" Linda held up her index finger as she ordered, "Do not hire him. I do not want him on my staff."

Kathleen leaned forward in her chair and answered, "Keith is an excellent applicant and he *will* be considered for this position. If you have a behavioral or experiential issue to point out about him I'm happy to hear about it, but I will not entertain the issue of sexual orientation among our criteria for hiring someone."

Linda became very angry and rose from her chair. "If you think I'm going to have a homosexual on my staff, you're dead wrong." She pointed at the door and continued, "If you hire him, I'm going to walk right out that door and you will have to find another supervisor." With a huff, she marched out of the room.

Kathleen sat at her desk, unsure of how to react to this situation. *Was Linda simply blowing off steam, or was she making a real threat to leave if Keith was hired? Linda did have a tendency to get emotional, especially when changes occurred around the health center. Perhaps she would get over this in a day or two.* Kathleen decided to leave

the matter alone for now and to have a talk with Linda the next day.

At 8:05 the next morning, Kathleen got a phone call from the personal assistant of Jerry, the CMO of the health center, asking for Kathleen to be present in the second-floor conference room at 8:30 a.m. When Kathleen walked into the room, Linda and Jerry were already sitting at the conference table. Jerry motioned for Kathleen to take a seat, and began speaking.

"I understand that you and Linda had a disagreement yesterday concerning an applicant that is under consideration for employment. I understand and appreciate diversity as much as you do, Kathleen, but Linda has raised some important concerns about this applicant. The residents of this county do not appreciate the lifestyle that this applicant is alleged to have, and the practice of physical therapy involves a great deal of touching and general interaction with patients. I am concerned that his sexual orientation will lead to problems in our delivery of care. You know how quickly news travels in this community, and patients will not want to receive services from a homosexual physical therapist. If he is hired here, I am concerned that patients will either mistreat him or that they will take their business elsewhere. The health center is already hurting due to lack of volume, and I am afraid that the decision to hire this applicant would ultimately result in a collapse of your department. I, therefore, ask that you do not hire him. If you're concerned about staffing, keep in mind that the job has only posted for one week. If we have made it this long without a fifth PT, we can make it until the right applicant comes along. Do you understand?"

Discussion Questions

1. What would you do in Kathleen's situation?
2. Identify the facts of the case. Try to distinguish the facts of the case from what has been alleged or perceived.

3. Is it feasible for Kathleen to not hire Keith without liability?
4. Do you think Linda has any hidden motives to prevent Keith from being hired?
5. How often do you think this type of discrimination occurs in healthcare?

Project Chronic and worsening healthcare workforce shortages are likely in the foreseeable future. The objective of this project is to learn about how hospitals and other healthcare organizations are coping with healthcare workforce shortages. Specifically, how do organizations perceive the causes of turnover, and what strategies have they found successful in improving both their recruitment and retention?

1. Identify one professional group (e.g., nurses, laboratory technicians, radiologic technicians, information technology personnel) that is known to be experiencing recruitment and retention problems.
2. Choose two healthcare organizations that employ this professional group.
3. Locate the individual or individuals most directly accountable for recruiting and retaining professionals in this group. This person may be a staff member in the HR department, a nurse recruiter, or another employee.
4. Find the approximate number of professionals in this group needed by the organization.
5. Obtain the following information on this group:

   a. Current vacancy rate
   b. Turnover and retention rates for the last five years

6. Discuss with the appropriate individuals their perception of the causes of recruitment challenges and of turnover and the reasons people choose to stay with their organizations. If possible, interview front-line staff in this professional group to obtain their perceptions on these issues.
7. If possible, explore the costs associated with recruitment, retention, and turnover at the facilities you have selected. Do the organizations keep track of these costs? If not, why? If so, do they use this information to make decisions concerning future recruitment and retention efforts?
8. In your discussions, explore the strategies both organizations have used to increase the success rate of their recruitment and retention efforts. Do the organizations know which strategies have been successful and unsuccessful? If so, which strategies have proven successful? Which strategies have not been effective? What strategies may be effective but are difficult to implement?

References

Advisory Board Company. 1999. "A Misplaced Focus: Reexamining the Recruiting/ Retention Trade-off." *Nursing Watch* 11: 1–14.

Aiken, L. H., J. Buchan, B. Sochalski, B. Nichols, and M. Powell. 2004. "Trends in International Nurse Migration." *Health Affairs* 23 (3): 69–77.

Aiken, L. H., S. P. Clarke, D. M. Sloane, E. T. Lake, and T. Chenney. 2008. "Effects of Hospital Care Environment on Patient Mortality and Nurse Outcomes." *Journal of Nursing Administration* 38 (5): 223–29.

Aiken, L. H., S. P. Clarke, D. M. Sloane, J. A. Sochalski, R. Busse, H. Clarke, P. Giovannetti, J. Hunt, A. M. Rafferty, and J. Shamian. 2001. "Nurses' Reports on Hospital Care in Five Countries." *Health Affairs* 20 (3) 43–53.

Aiken, L. H., D. M. Sloane, J. P. Cimiotti, S. P. Clarke, L. Flynn, J. A. Seago, J. Spetz, and H. L. Smith. 2010. "Implications of the California Nurse Staffing Mandate for Other States." *Health Services Research* 45 (4): 904–21.

Albaugh, J. 2003. "Keeping Nurses in Nursing: The Profession's Challenge for Today." *Urologic Nursing* 23 (3): 193–99.

Albright, L. E., J. R. Glennon, and W. J. Smith. 1963. *The Use of Psychological Tests in Industry*. Cleveland, OH: Howard Allen.

Algier, A. J. 2013. "L+M Offers Bonuses, Urges Vote on Contract." *The Westerly Sun*. Published December 12. www.thewesterlysun.com/news/westerly/3132613-129/lm-offers-bonuses-urges-vote-on-contract.html.

Allen, D. G., T. V. Mahto, and R. F. Otondo. 2007. "Web-Based Recruitment: Effects of Information, Organizational Brand, and Attitudes Toward a Web Site on Applicant Attraction." *Journal of Applied Psychology* 92 (6): 1696–1708.

Alonzo, A. 2014. "YRC Union Workers Approve New Labor Pact." *Kansas City Business Journal*. Published January 26. www.bizjournals.com/kansascity/news/2014/01/26/yrc-union-workers-approve-new-labor-pact.html?page=all.

American Association of Colleges of Nursing. 2014. "Nursing Shortage Fact Sheet." Updated April 24. www.aacn.nche.edu/media-relations/fact-sheets/nursing-shortage.

American Health Care Association. 2014. "American Health Care Association 2012 Staffing Report." Accessed December 31. www.ahcancal.org/research_data/staffing/Documents/2012_Staffing_Report.pdf.

American Medical Association. 2013. *International Medical Graduates in American Medicine: Contemporary Challenges and Opportunities*. AMA-IMG Section Governing Council position paper. Published January. http://nycsprep.com/pdf/international-medical-graduates.pdf.

American Nurses Credentialing Center. 2014. "Forces of Magnetism." Accessed December 31. www.nursecredentialing.org/ForcesofMagnetism.aspx.

Arthur, W., S. T. Bell, A. J. Villado, and D. Doverspike. 2006. "The Use of Person–Organization Fit in Employment Decision Making: An Assessment of Its Criterion-Related Validity." *Journal of Applied Psychology* 91 (4): 786–801.

Auerbach, D. I., P. I. Buerhaus, and D. O. Staiger. 2011. "Registered Nurse Supply Grows Faster Than Projected amid Surge in New Entrants Ages 23–26." *Health Affairs* 30 (12): 2286–92.

Auerbach, D. I., D. O. Staiger, U. Muench, and P. I. Buerhaus. 2013. "The Nursing Workforce in an Era of Health Care Reform." *New England Journal of Medicine* 368 (16): 1470–72.

Barber, A. E., and M. V. Roehling. 1993. "Job Postings and the Decision to Interview: A Verbal Protocol Analysis." *Journal of Applied Psychology* 78 (5): 845–56.

Berthiaume, J., and L. Culpepper. 2008. "'Hot Skills': Most Popular Compensation Strategies for Technical Expertise." Society for Human Resource Management. Accessed December 30, 2014. www.shrm.org/hrdisciplines/compensation/articles/pages/popularcompensationstrategies.aspx.

Bidwell, M. 2011. "Paying More to Get Less: The Effects of External Hiring Versus Internal Mobility." *Administrative Science Quarterly* 56 (3): 369–407.

Bowns, D. A., and H. J. Bernardin. 1988. "Critical Incident Technique." In *The Job Analysis Handbook for Business, Industry, and Government*, edited by S. Gael, 1120–37. New York: Wiley.

Breaugh, J. A. 2013. "Employee Recruitment." *Annual Review of Psychology* 64: 389–416.

———. 2010. "Realistic Job Previews." In *Handbook of Improving Performance in the Workplace*, edited by R. Watkins and D. Leigh, 203–18. San Francisco: Pfeiffer.

Brimmer, K. 2012. "Rural Hospitals Struggle with Physician Recruitment, but Can Focus on Improved Quality Scores." *Healthcare Finance News*. Published August 8. www.healthcarefinancenews.com/news/rural-hospitals-struggle-physician-recruitment-can-focus-improved-quality-scores.

Bureau of Labor Statistics. 2013. "Employment Projections: 2012–2022." Published December 19. www.bls.gov/news.release/pdf/ecopro.pdf.

Burks, S., B. Cowgill, M. Hoffman, and M. Housman. 2013. "The Facts About Referrals: Toward an Understanding of Employee Referral Networks." Social Science Research Network paper. Published December 11. http://ssrn.com/abstract=2253738.

Carey, D., and M. Useem. 2014. "How Microsoft Avoided the Peter Principle with Nadella." *Harvard Business Review*. Published February 6. www.hbr.org/2014/02/how-microsoft-avoided-the-peter-principle-with-nadella/.

Carlson, J. 2014. "Reform, New Labor Issues Likely to Keep Unions Busy in 2014." *Modern Healthcare*. Published January 15. www.modernhealthcare.com/article/20140115/NEWS/301159931.

Carnevale, A. P., N. Smith, A. Gulish, and B. H. Beach. 2012. *Healthcare*. Washington, DC: Georgetown University Public Policy Institute.

Cleveland Clinic. 2014a. "Career Development." Accessed December 31. http://my.clevelandclinic.org/nursing-institute/career-growth-development/career-development.aspx.

———. 2014b. "Employment." Accessed December 31. http://my.clevelandclinic.org/nursing-institute/career-growth-development/employment.aspx.

Cooper, R. A., and L. H. Aiken. 2006. "Health Services Delivery: Reframing Policies for Global Migration of Nurses and Physicians—a US Perspective." *Policy, Politics, and Nursing Practice* 7 (3, suppl.): 66S–70S.

Development Dimensions International. 2014. "Targeted Selection." Accessed December 31. www.ddiworld.com/products/targeted-selection.

Dotson, M. J., D. S. Dave, J. A. Cazier, and T. J. Spaulding. 2014. "An Empirical Analysis of Nurse Retention: What Keeps RNs in Nursing?" *The Journal of Nursing Administration* 44 (2): 111–16.

Drenkard, K. 2010. "Going for the Gold: The Value of Attaining Magnet Recognition." *American Nurse Today* 5 (3): 50–52. Accessed December 31, 2014. www.americannursetoday.com/going-for-the-gold-the-value-of-attaining-magnet-recognition/.

Earnest, D. R., D. G. Allen, and R. S. Landis. 2011. "Mechanisms Linking Realistic Job Previews with Turnover: A Meta-analytic Path Analysis." *Personnel Psychology* 64 (4): 865–97.

Edge, J. S., and S. J. Hoffman. 2013. "Empirical Impact Evaluation of the WHO Global Code of Practice on the International Recruitment of Health Personnel in Australia, Canada, UK and USA." *Globalization and Health* 9:60. Accessed January 2, 2015. www.globalizationandhealth.com/content/pdf/1744-8603-9-60.pdf.

Equal Employment Opportunity Commission. 2014. "Background Checks: What Employers Need to Know." Accessed April 17. www.eeoc.gov/eeoc/publications/background_checks_employers.cfm.

———. 2010. "Employment Tests and Selection Procedures." Modified September 23. www.eeoc.gov/policy/docs/factemployment_procedures.html.

Farr, J. L., and N. Tippins. 2010. *Handbook of Employee Selection*. New York: Routledge.

Fitz-enz, J., and B. Davison. 2002. *How to Measure Human Resources Management*. New York: McGraw-Hill.

Frauenheim, E. 2011. "More Companies Go with Online Tests to Fill in the Blanks." *Workforce Management* 90 (5): 12–13.

Gatewood, R. D., H. S. Feild, and M. Barrick. 2011. *Human Resource Selection*, seventh edition. Mason, OH: Southwestern Cengage Learning.

Greengard, S. 2003. "Gimme Attitude." *Workforce Management* 81 (7): 56–60.

Griffith, E., and J. Bergen. 2014. "The Best Job Search Websites and Apps." *PC Magazine*. Published May 22. www.pcmag.com/slideshow/story/294523/the-best-job-search-websites-apps.

Health Care Advisory Board. 2001. *Competing for Talent: Recovering America's Hospital Workforce*. Washington, DC: Advisory Board Company.

Hellmann, R. 2014. *Your Social Media Job Search: Use LinkedIn, Twitter, and Other Tools to Get the Job You Want!* New York: Robert Hellmann LLC.

Hirschkorn, C. A., T. B. West, K. S. Hill, B. L. Cleary, and P. O. Hewlett. 2010. "Experienced Nurse Retention Strategies: What Can Be Learned from Top-Performing Organizations." *Journal of Nursing Administration* 40 (11): 463–67.

Hoffman, B. J., B. H. Bynum, R. F. Piccolo, and A. W. Sutton. 2011. "Person–Organization Value Congruence: How Transformational Leaders Influence Work Group Effectiveness." *Academy of Management Journal* 54 (4): 779–96.

Hoffman, B. J., and D. J. Woehr. 2006. "A Quantitative Review of the Relationship Between Person–Organization Fit and Behavioral Outcomes." *Journal of Vocational Behavior* 68 (3): 389–99.

Hsieh, A. T., and Y. Y. Chen. 2011. "The Influence of Employee Referrals on P–O Fit." *Public Personnel Management* 40 (4): 327–39.

Huerta, S. 2003. "Recruitment and Retention: The Magnet Perspective." *Journal of Illinois Nursing* 100 (4): 4–6.

Hunter, J., and R. Hunter. 1984. "The Validity and Utility of Alternative Predictors of Job Performance." *Psychological Bulletin* 96 (1): 72–98.

Jackson, D., J. A. Stillman, and P. Englert. 2010. "Task-Based Assessment Centers: Empirical Support for a Systems Model." *International Journal of Selection and Assessment* 18 (2): 141–54.

Jackson Healthcare. 2012. *Vital Signs 2012: A National Nursing Attitudes & Outlook Report*. Accessed January 2, 2015. www.jacksonhealthcare.com/media/164537/nursestrendsreport_ebook0113_lr.pdf.

Johns Hopkins Medicine. 2014. "Employment Opportunities." Accessed October 22. www.hopkinsmedicine.org/employment/index.html.

Jones, C. B. 2008. "Revisiting Nurse Turnover Costs: Adjusting for Inflation." *Journal of Nursing Administration* 38 (1): 11–18.

———. 2005. "The Costs of Nursing Turnover, Part 2: Application of the Nursing Turnover Cost Calculation Methodology." *Journal of Nursing Administration* 35 (1): 41–49.

Kaiser Permanente. 2014. "New Grad Program." Accessed October 22. http://nursingpathways.kp.org/scal/learning/newgrad/.

Kristof-Brown, A. L., R. D. Zimmerman, and E. C. Johnson. 2005. "Consequences of Individuals' Fit at Work: A Meta-analysis of Person–Job, Person–Organization, Person–Group, and Person–Supervisor Fit." *Personnel Psychology* 58 (2): 281–342.

Kutscher, B. 2013. "The Rural Route: Hospitals in Underserved Areas Taking Different Roads to Recruit, Retain Physicians." *Modern Healthcare* 43 (18): 30–31.

Lehman, M. S., J. R. Hudson Jr., G. W. Appley, E. J. Sheehan Jr., and D. P. Slevin. 2011. "Modified Assessment Center Approach Facilitates Organizational Change." *Journal of Management Development* 30 (9): 893–913.

Lu, H., K. L. Barriball, X. Zhang, and A. E. While. 2012. "Job Satisfaction Among Hospital Nurses Revisited: A Systematic Review." *International Journal of Nursing Studies* 49 (8): 1017–38.

Lukens, M. 2014. "Getting Engagement from the Get-Go." *HR Magazine* 59 (2): 54–55.

Manion, J. 2004. "Nurture a Culture of Retention." *Nursing Management* 35 (4): 28–39.

Mayo Clinic. 2014a. "Jobs at Mayo Clinic." Accessed January 2, 2015. www.mayoclinic.org/jobs.

———. 2014b. "Mayo Clinic: One of FORTUNE Magazine's 100 Best Companies to Work For." Accessed January 2, 2015. www.mayoclinic.org/jobs/fortune-100-best-companies-to-work-for.

McHugh, M. D., L. A. Kelly, H. L. Smith, E. S. Wu, J. M. Vanak, and L. H. Aiken. 2013. "Lower Mortality in Magnet Hospitals." *Medical Care* 51 (5): 382–88.

McHugh, M. D., A. Kutney-Lee, J. P. Cimiotti, D. M. Sloane, and L. H. Aiken. 2011. "Nurses' Widespread Job Dissatisfaction, Burnout, and Frustration with Health Benefits Signal Problems for Patient Care." *Health Affairs* 30 (2): 202–10.

Meinert, D. 2011. "Seeing Behind the Mask." *HR Magazine* 56 (2): 30–37.

NHS Employers. 2014. "Code of Practice for International Recruitment." Published March 18. www.nhsemployers.org/your-workforce/recruit/employer-led-recruitment/international-recruitment/uk-code-of-practice-for-international-recruitment.

Nursing Solutions Inc. 2014. *2014 National Healthcare RN Retention Report.* Published February 19. www.nsinursingsolutions.com/Files/assets/library/workforce/StaffingStrategiesSurvey2014.pdf.

O'Neill, T. A., N. M. Lee, J. Radan, S. J. Law, and R. J. Lewis. 2013. "The Impact of 'Non-targeted Traits' on Personality Test Faking, Hiring, and Workplace Deviance." *Personality and Individual Differences* 55 (2): 162–68.

Onley, D. S. 2014. "Mobile Recruiting on the Rise." Society for Human Resource Management. Published March 18. www.shrm.org/hrdisciplines/technology/articles/pages/mobile-recruiting-rising.aspx.

O'Reilly, C. A., J. Chatman, and D. F. Caldwell. 1991. "People and Organizational Culture: A Profile Comparison Approach to Assessing Person–Organization Fit." *Academy of Management Journal* 34 (3): 487–516.

Peter, L. J., and R. Hull. 1969. *The Peter Principle.* New York: William Morrow.

Phillips, J. M. 1998. "Effects of Realistic Job Previews on Multiple Organizational Outcomes." *Academy of Management Journal* 41 (6): 673–90.

Pittman, P., C. Davis, F. Shaffer, C. N. Herrera, and C. Bennett. 2014. "Perceptions of Employment-Based Discrimination Among Newly Arrived Foreign-Educated Nurses." *American Journal of Nursing* 114 (1): 26–35.

Punke, H. 2013. "6 Tips for Recruiting Physicians to Rural Hospitals." *Becker's Hospital Review.* Published August 16. www.beckershospitalreview.com/hospital-physician-relationships/6-tips-for-recruiting-physicians-to-rural-hospitals.html.

Richtel, M. 2013. "How Big Data Is Playing Recruiter for Specialized Workers." *New York Times.* Published April 27. www.nytimes.com/2013/04/28/technology/how-big-data-is-playing-recruiter-for-specialized-workers.html.

Roberts, B. 2011. "Close-up on Screening." *HR Magazine* 56 (2): 22.

Rosse, J. G., and R. A. Levin. 2003. *The Jossey-Bass Academic Administrator's Guide to Hiring.* San Francisco: Jossey-Bass.

Schwartz, N. D. 2013. "In Hiring, a Friend in Need Is a Prospect, Indeed." *New York Times.* Published January 27. www.nytimes.com/2013/01/28/business/employers-increasingly-rely-on-internal-referrals-in-hiring.html.

Society for Human Resource Management. 2014. "Metrics Calculators." Accessed January 2, 2015. www.shrm.org/templatestools/samples/metrics/Pages/default.aspx.

———. 2012a. "Retention: How Do I Calculate Retention? Is Retention Related to Turnover?" Accessed January 2, 2015. www.shrm.org/templatestools/hrqa/pages/calculatingretentionandturnover.aspx.

———. 2012b. "What Is a 'Dual Career Ladder'?" Accessed January 2, 2015. www.shrm.org/TemplatesTools/hrqa/Pages/termdualcareer.aspx.

Stevens, S. R., C. L. Leibson, P. Buerhaus, M. Harris, J. Needleman, and V. S. Pankratz. 2011. "Nurse Staffing and Inpatient Hospital Mortality." *New England Journal of Medicine* 364 (11): 1037–45.

Swider, B. W., R. D. Zimmerman, and M. R. Barrick. 2014. "Searching for the Right Fit: Development of Applicant Person–Organization Fit Perceptions During the Recruitment Process." *Journal of Applied Psychology.* doi:10.1037/a0038357.

Twibell, R., J. St. Pierre, D. Johnson, D. Barton, C. Davis, M. Kidd, and G. Rook. 2012. "Tripping over the Welcome Mat: Why New Nurses Don't Stay and What the Evidence Says We Can Do About It." *American Nurse Today* 7 (6). Published June. www.americannursetoday.com/tripping-over-the-welcome-mat-why-new-nurses-dont-stay-and-what-the-evidence-says-we-can-do-about-it/.

University of Michigan Center of Excellence in Public Health Workforce Studies. 2013. *Enumeration and Characterization of the Public Health Nurse Workforce: Findings of the 2012 Public Health Nurse Workforce Surveys.* Published June. www.sph.umich.edu/cephw/docs/Nurse%20Workforce-RWJ%20Report.pdf.

Upenieks, V. 2002. "Assessing Differences in Job Satisfaction of Nurses in Magnet and Nonmagnet Hospitals." *Journal of Nursing Administration* 32 (11): 564–76.

Waldman, J. 2013. *The Social Media Job Search Workbook: Your Step-by-Step Guide to Finding Work in the Age of Social Media.* Tigard, OR: Career Enlightenment Press.

Waldman, J. D., and S. Arora. 2004. "Measuring Retention Rather Than Turnover: A Different and Complementary HR Calculus." *Human Resource Planning* 27 (3): 6–9.

Waldo, M. 2012. "Second Chances: Employing Convicted Felons." *HR Magazine* 57 (3): 36–40.

Weyland, A. 2011. "How to Recruit People Who Fit." *Training Journal*, July, 41–45.

World Health Organization. 2010. *The WHO Global Code of Practice on the International Recruitment of Health Personnel.* Published May. www.who.int/hrh/migration/code/code_en.pdf?ua=1.

Zielinski, D. 2011. "Effective Assessments." *HR Magazine* 56 (1): 61–64.

PERFORMANCE MANAGEMENT

Bruce J. Fried

After completing this chapter, the reader should be able to

- define performance management, and describe the key components of a performance management system;
- discuss the reasons that organizations engage in performance management;
- identify the characteristics of good rating criteria for performance appraisal;
- enumerate sources of information about job performance, and discuss the strengths and shortcomings of each;
- describe the types of performance information that may be used and the rationale for each type of information;
- distinguish between rating errors and political factors as sources of distortion in performance appraisal; and
- conduct a performance appraisal interview with an employee, taking into consideration the techniques that make such an interview successful.

Introduction

The goal of human resources management (HRM) systems is to foster high levels of performance and commitment from individuals and teams. This chapter discusses performance management, which comprises all of the organization's activities related to individual performance, including measurement using performance information. Performance management coordinates the efforts of human resources (HR) systems that affect performance. Performance management also specifically involves collecting performance information and using that information to conduct formal and informal improvement efforts. While performance management can be considered a tool for evaluating and improving individual performance, a performance management system can also be used to assess the success of other HR functions. A well-functioning performance management system can provide insight into the effectiveness of an organization's selection processes, can help determine whether training programs are effective, and can indicate whether compensation and reward systems are successful in meeting performance goals. Exhibit 8.1 provides examples of how performance management is related to other HR functions.

In this chapter, the term *performance management* refers to a set of tools and practices used for setting performance goals with employees, measuring individual performance, designing strategies with employees to make and sustain improvement, monitoring employee progress toward achieving goals, and providing ongoing feedback and coaching by supervisors and perhaps peers and subordinates. While the phrase *performance appraisal* is often used, that term tends to limit the process to measurement, which is a necessary but insufficient part of performance management. As discussed in this chapter, performance management encompasses more than collecting performance information; it is a data-informed system for improving performance. In this chapter, the term *performance appraisal* is sometimes used to refer to aspects of the process that deal with obtaining performance information.

Issues of employee performance and productivity are at the forefront in healthcare organizations. The Joint Commission and the Baldrige Performance Excellence Program both include specific references to performance management. The Joint Commission requires accredited healthcare organizations to assess, track, and improve the competence of all employees. Its standards include such phrasing as the following (Joint Commission 2014):

- "The organization evaluates staff based on performance expectations that reflect their job descriptions" (HRM.01.07.01).
- "The organization evaluates staff performance in accordance with law and regulation and organization policy, but at least once every three years. This evaluation is documented" (HRM.01.07.01).
- "If the organization has conducted any performance improvement activities that relate to staff providing direct care, treatment, or services, and performance findings from these activities are available, the organization uses those findings when evaluating staff performance" (HRM.01.07.01).
- "The organization confirms each staff member's adherence to organization policies, procedures, rules, and regulations" (HRM.01.07.01).
- "Staff participate in education and training to maintain or increase their competency. Staff participation is documented" (HRM.01.05.01).

HRM Function	Effects of Performance Management	Effects on Performance Management
Job analysis and job design	Performance information may suggest how jobs should be redesigned	Accurate information about jobs is central to developing criteria for performance appraisal
HR and succession planning	Performance information provides a performance profile of the workforce and helps identify individuals who may be promoted into higher-level positions; employee performance information can identify vital skill gaps in the organization	Current and future workforce needs may be used to identify critical employee performance dimensions that may be integrated into performance appraisal tools
Recruitment and selection	Performance information provides managers with information about the effectiveness of alternative sources of recruitment and the effectiveness of their selection criteria and procedures; may provide information helpful in predicting the performance of job applicants	The organization's ability to recruit and select employees may affect the criteria and standards developed for performance appraisal
Training and development	Performance management systems provide information on employees' training and development needs; information on employee performance after training can be used to assess the effectiveness of training	Performance appraisal tools may be designed to assess the impact of training programs
Compensation	Compensation systems may be designed such that performance appraisal information has an impact on employee compensation	A fair and equitable compensation system may lead to higher levels of employee performance

EXHIBIT 8.1
Relationship of Performance Management to Other Human Resources Management Functions

In addition, the requirements of the prestigious Baldrige Performance Excellence Program (2013) for healthcare organizations make numerous mentions of performance management, employee engagement, training, and employee development, asking the organization to analyze the following:

- "How the ability to identify and meet workforce capability and capacity needs correlates with retention, motivation, and productivity" (p. 9).

- ". . . your workforce capability and capacity needs, how you meet those needs to accomplish your organization's work, and how you ensure a supportive work climate. The aim is to build an effective environment for accomplishing your work and supporting your workforce" (p. 10).
- ". . . services, facilities, activities, and other opportunities [such as] personal and career counseling; career development and employability services; recreational or cultural activities; formal and informal recognition; non-work-related education; child and elder care; special leave for family responsibilities and community service; flexible work hours and benefits packages; outplacement services; and retiree benefits, including extended health care and ongoing access to services" (p. 11).
- ". . . engagement is characterized by performing meaningful work; having clear organizational direction and performance accountability; and having a safe, trusting, effective, and cooperative work environment. In many organizations, employees and volunteers are drawn to and derive meaning from their work because it is aligned with their personal values. In health care organizations, workforce engagement also depends on building and sustaining relationships between administrative/operational leaders and independent practitioners" (p. 11).
- "Learning and development opportunities might occur inside or outside your organization and could involve on-the-job, classroom, e-learning, or distance learning, as well as developmental assignments, coaching, or mentoring" (p. 12).
- "Individual learning and development needs. To help people realize their full potential, many organizations prepare an individual development plan with each person that addresses his or her career and learning objectives" (p. 12).

Performance management makes sense. The adage "you can't manage what you can't measure" is applicable to performance management. However, performance management has a well-deserved reputation for being very poorly implemented. It is perhaps the most misunderstood and misused HR function. Measuring and improving employee performance is also among the most highly examined aspects of management, both in scholarly works and in the popular press. Perhaps because it has met with so much disappointment and failure, it is also one of the areas of management most prone to passing fads, which have been widely adopted in popular management literature and by countless consulting firms that seek to identify and promote quick fixes to improve employee productivity.

This chapter describes the essential components of performance management and presents the countless pitfalls that may be faced in designing and implementing performance management systems. To the extent possible, the discussion avoids the jargon and fashions that come and go and maintains a focus on the processes found to have the highest likelihood of leading to improved and sustained employee performance. Specifically, the chapter explores the following:

- Why organizations develop and implement performance management systems
- Types and sources of information about employee performance
- Performance criteria, criterion deficiency, criterion contamination, reliability, and validity
- Multisource or 360-degree performance management approaches
- Advantages and disadvantages of common formats for collecting and summarizing performance information
- The annual or periodic performance review
- Common sources of errors and other problems in performance appraisal
- Guidelines for conducting effective performance management interviews

Every manager seeks to have employees who are highly motivated and productive. This goal is challenging for a number of reasons. First, employee motivation is in itself a complex phenomenon and is influenced by many things outside of the manager's control. Second, whether managerial interventions are effective in improving performance is unclear. For instance, compensation clearly has some motivational potential for most employees, but money is not an effective motivator in all circumstances. In healthcare organizations with very small margins, the availability of performance-based rewards tends to be very limited. Third, employee performance is often difficult to observe and measure in a reliable manner. This factor, of course, varies by job. For example, assessing the performance of an employee doing medical equipment sales is relatively easy, but evaluating the performance of a case manager for individuals with chronic mental illness is much more challenging. As with all HR functions, performance management activities are carried out within a legal context, and performance management procedures must abide by relevant employment laws.

Performance management has many negative connotations. Edward Deming, perhaps the greatest innovator in quality improvement, stated that performance appraisal systems "leave people bitter, crushed, bruised, battered, desolate, despondent, dejected, feeling inferior, some even depressed, unfit for weeks after receipt of rating, unable to comprehend why they are inferior," and are, in essence, a "deadly disease" (Deming 2000, 102). This view was reinforced by Culbert (2010) in the *Wall Street Journal*:

> This corporate sham is one of the most insidious, most damaging, and yet most ubiquitous of corporate activities. Everybody does it, and almost everyone who's evaluated hates it. It's a pretentious, bogus practice that produces absolutely nothing that any thinking executive should call a corporate plus.

Why has this process earned such an emotionally volatile reaction, not just from writers, but also from employees? Perhaps the most fundamental issue is that performance management is frequently viewed as a punitive process. Indeed, managers may implement performance management systems in such a manner, particularly if they themselves were treated in this way. The negative associations with performance management may also lead employees to believe that one of the benefits of moving up in the organization is that they will no longer be subject to this uncomfortable process. This view may also be based on the assumption that higher-level employees *do not need* supervision in the same manner as lower-level employees. This attitude may be based in perceptions of social class. That is, the perception may be that lower-level employees are motivated entirely by money and need to be coerced to work and carefully monitored. Higher-level—and higher-paid—employees are seen as having a different level of motivation and as being driven to work by the intrinsic value of the work. Such people are perceived as "above" performance appraisal and management processes.

Managers need to understand that even with the best of intentions, performance management processes—and annual reviews in particular—may be perceived as being harshly judgmental, condescending, or demeaning. This perception may not reflect the manager's intention, but employee perceptions are often based on how they have been evaluated and spoken to since childhood. Employees may also be skeptical about the fairness of the performance appraisal process and may therefore view the process in a perfunctory manner. Their beliefs about the fairness of the system may very well be based in reality. Understandably, then, employees may become highly defensive when the negative emotional history associated with performance management is enmeshed with perceived unfairness and the serious issues of employment security and compensation.

Given the unpleasant baggage that comes with performance management, one should not be surprised that performance management processes tend to be ignored or passively implemented by managers. Perhaps the most common introduction to a performance management interview is "Let's get this over with." Given the importance of employee performance, the fact that this process has been plagued by such perceptions is unfortunate.

Notwithstanding all of these issues, performance management is a vital process for all members of the organization, including—and perhaps especially—the CEO and senior managers. Indeed, evidence in the literature indicates that the higher the position, the less likely a performance appraisal is to be conducted. Appraisals of senior-level employees may be poorly and haphazardly done. However, much evidence also suggests that executive-level employees have a strong desire to obtain information about their performance (Longenecker and Gioia 1992).

The bottom line is that performance management is for everyone in the organization. Further, the process need not be demeaning to any employee, whether at a lower level or at an executive level. Because of the tendencies for even well-designed performance management systems to be poorly implemented, all organizations should critically examine their systems to determine their impact, costs, and benefits (Scullen 2011).

The Role of Performance Management

Performance management consists of an array of processes that collectively are goal oriented and directed toward maximizing the productivity of individuals, teams, and the organization. Ultimately, performance management helps to align the work of individuals and teams with the goals of the organization. Performance management is an ongoing process. One of the most common performance management mistakes is to focus exclusively on the annual review, which typically includes paperwork and an interview, both of which are often unpleasant for all parties. Without stretching the analogy, this approach is similar to the focus that most of us give to the annual physical, the one and only time in the year we think about our health. An annual performance review is not unimportant; it plays a role but is not the central feature of performance management systems.

Annual appraisals are necessary, but performance management is ideally carried out on a daily basis. An effective supervisor provides feedback continuously and addresses and manages performance problems when they occur. To extend the analogy further, if a child is experiencing an earache, a parent will likely not wait to address this problem until the child's next scheduled physical. Performance management is an ongoing function that includes the following managerial responsibilities and activities:

- Setting specific performance goals with the employee, and ensuring mutual understanding of these goals
- Developing performance criteria, and communicating these criteria to the employee

- Establishing development plans with the employee
- Monitoring and measuring employee progress toward performance goals
- Providing continual coaching, training, and education as necessary
- Evaluating performance and conducting periodic performance reviews, modifying the employee's development plan as needed

The annual or periodic performance review is only one part of the performance management process, but it is commonly used in organizations and thus requires attention. Essentially, the periodic performance review provides an opportunity for the supervisor and employee to reflect and plan. The review may include discussions about personnel decisions, such as promotion, compensation, disciplinary action, transfer, or recommendation for training. The review is not a time to deliver dramatically new information or surprises to employees. Supervisors should continually provide employees with feedback on their performance, and supervisors and employees should come into the annual review with a problem-solving mind-set aimed at developing improvement strategies. The performance review should be reserved for the following:

- Giving employees the opportunity to discuss performance and performance standards
- Addressing employee strengths and weaknesses
- Identifying and recommending strategies for improving employee performance
- Discussing personnel decisions, such as compensation, promotion, and termination
- Defining a variety of regulatory requirements that deal with employee performance, and discussing compliance methods

The periodic performance review has both administrative and developmental purposes. Administrative purposes commonly refer to using performance information to make decisions about promotion, termination, and compensation. To defend against charges of discrimination, organizations attempt to maintain accurate and current performance appraisal information on employees.

Modern approaches to performance management view the periodic review as not simply evaluating or appraising performance but helping to improve performance. As a developmental process, the periodic review uses performance information to improve performance; appraisal information identifies employee strengths and weaknesses, which then become the basis for developing improvement strategies. The review also provides an opportunity for employees to discuss concerns, and for the manager and employee to improve communication. Organizations can, of course, use appraisals for both administrative and developmental purposes. However, whether a manager or supervisor can actually conduct an honest developmental appraisal in concert with discussions that affect the employee's income, promotion potential, and other bread-and-butter issues is the subject of considerable debate. To expect an employee to focus on his or her development while also waiting for the all-important information about compensation is difficult and sometimes unrealistic. A common practice is to temporally separate the periodic performance review from the process of informing employees about compensation decisions, perhaps providing the latter information several weeks after the formal review.

Establishing Job Standards and Appraisal Criteria

As is the case with many other HR activities, an effective performance management system must begin with a clear job description, job standards, and appraisal criteria. Of particular importance is the need for managers and employees to agree on the content of the job description and to have a shared understanding of job expectations. Once agreement is reached, employees and managers together must identify job standards and the specific measurable criteria by which performance will be evaluated. These criteria need to be job related and relevant to the needs of the organization. Developing criteria is a challenging task and requires employee–manager collaboration. Criteria must be agreed on well in advance of a formal performance appraisal interview. Managers must avoid the situation where performance standards and appraisal criteria are set in isolation and without employee input. Employees should not feel they are being evaluated on standards and criteria that were not agreed on. Thus, the issue of evaluation criteria is critical. How should performance criteria be defined? What are the characteristics of useful criteria?

First, criteria should have strategic relevance to the organization as a whole. For example, if patient satisfaction is an important organizational concern, then including patient-relations criteria for employees who interact with customers makes sense. Criteria for individual performance appraisal are in many ways an extension of criteria used to evaluate organizational performance and in fact are consistent with a management-by-objectives approach, as discussed later in this chapter.

Second, criteria should be comprehensive and take into consideration the full range of an employee's major functions as defined in the job description. Criterion deficiency occurs when performance standards focus on a single criterion to the exclusion of other important, but perhaps less quantifiable, performance dimensions (Snell, Morris, and Bohlander 2015). For example, counting the number of visits made by a home care nurse may be relatively simple, but assessing the quality of care provided during those visits is certainly more difficult (but no less important). *Criterion contamination* occurs when factors out of the employee's control have a significant influence on his or her performance. This problem is commonly encountered in healthcare because of the complexity of patient care and the interdependence of the factors that affect quality and clinical outcomes. Clinicians, for example, may have little control over patient volume or the speed with which laboratory test results are reported. Therefore, to avoid criterion contamination, appraisal criteria should include only the items over which the employee has control.

Third, criteria should be reliable and valid. *Reliability* refers to the consistency with which a manager rates an employee in successive ratings (assuming consistent performance) or the consistency with which two or more managers rate performance when they have comparable information. Criteria can be made more reliable by selecting objective criteria and by training managers in applying the criteria. *Validity* is the extent to which appraisal criteria actually measure the performance dimension of interest. For example, in measuring a nurse's ability to carry out the nursing responsibilities during emergency medical procedures, is it sufficient to assess knowledge of these responsibilities rather than actual performance under real emergency conditions? Questions of validity are also difficult when attitudes deemed important for a particular job are measured.

Collecting Job Performance Data

In traditional performance appraisal processes, performance information is generated by the employee's supervisor. Typically, the supervisor observes the employee's performance using whatever format the organization has designed for performance appraisal (described later in this chapter) and records the appraisal information. Given the complexity of many jobs, however, having one individual accurately describe each employee's performance is often impossible. Alternative approaches to obtaining performance data have therefore been developed.

A *self-appraisal* is an evaluation done by the employee on himself or herself; it is generally done in conjunction with the manager's appraisal. This approach is very effective when a manager is seeking to obtain the involvement of the employee in the appraisal process, which is desirable under virtually all circumstances. Because of the obvious potential for bias on the part of the employee, self-appraisals are almost always done for developmental rather than administrative purposes.

Ideally, employee performance should be evaluated by the person or persons most knowledgeable about the employee's performance. Those persons providing performance information should have had the opportunity to observe the employee's performance. How can a manager's performance as a supervisor be evaluated? In all likelihood, the manager of that person is not in the best position to observe the employee's performance as a supervisor of other people. In this instance, having the employee's subordinates provide performance data on the employee's performance as a supervisor makes sense. *Subordinate appraisal* presents many benefits, among which are identifying managers' blind spots and improving managerial performance. From the subordinate's perspective, this type of appraisal has obvious risks, as not all managers may take kindly to critiques and opinions. The risk of retaliation may discourage subordinate appraisal. Thus, such appraisals should be done anonymously; where anonymity is not possible, the appraisal is unlikely to yield useful results and likely should not be done at all. To increase the likelihood of honest assessments, this type of performance evaluation is most useful for developmental rather than administrative purposes.

Team-based appraisal is beneficial in that it explicitly reinforces the importance of teamwork. Measuring team accomplishments sends a message that the organization places a high value on team performance. Organizations may link team performance with pay, and numerous models for distributing team rewards are available. For example, an organization may establish a team-based incentive system whereby team members share in the savings to the organization, usually through reduced labor costs. *Team-based compensation* may exacerbate anxieties and frustrations with the "free-rider" syndrome, where one or more team members benefit from team rewards without putting forth corresponding effort. Employees may also feel that they have little control over their compensation and that a single poor performer can jeopardize the rewards for the entire team (Merriman 2009). However, team-based compensation is not a necessary component of team-based appraisal. In using team-based appraisal, with or without compensation, team members must agree on behavior-based and outcome-based appraisal criteria. Team members may also be involved in assessing the performance of other team members. Again, this approach reinforces the value that the organization places on teamwork and team citizenship, and it has the potential for building team cohesion and enhancing communication. When using team-based appraisal, several questions need to be addressed, including the manner in which team members are involved in appraisals: Are all team members involved in appraising every other team member? Who should provide feedback to members? While this approach may help build teams, it also presents the risk of alienation and conflict if feedback is provided in a divisive manner. Therefore, whoever is selected to provide the feedback should be trained in interviewing and feedback techniques.

Among the most useful ways to collect job performance information is using multiple sources. *Multisource appraisal*—also known as 360-degree appraisal or multirater assessment—acknowledges that for many jobs, relying on one source of performance information is incomplete and inadequate. To obtain a comprehensive assessment of performance, perspectives must be obtained from those within and outside the organization, including the manager or supervisor, peers, subordinates, clients, and other internal and external customers. The advantages of multisource appraisal include the following:

- Emphasizes aspects of performance valued by the organization
- Recognizes explicitly the importance of customer focus
- Reinforces the value of teams and team development
- Contributes to employee involvement and development
- Reduces bias because it incorporates multiple perspectives

Typically, multisource appraisal is done for developmental purposes, but it must be designed and administered with great care. Following are some of the limitations and potential pitfalls of multisource appraisal:

- Employees must have a level of trust in the organization such that they feel safe providing feedback without fear of retribution or other negative consequences.
- Anonymity is critical, which may limit the use of multisource appraisal in a small organization or in a setting where a manager has a small span of control.
- Employees may use the process for purposes of retribution.
- Multiple sources of information may be difficult to integrate or combine.
- The method of feedback must be done by a trained individual in a manner that encourages insight and growth.

Regardless of the source of performance information, decisions need to be made about the content of the information to be obtained in performance appraisals. In general, four types of information may be obtained:

1. *Individual traits* refer to individual characteristics, such as aptitude, interpersonal abilities, and personality characteristics. One may think of traits as inborn characteristics in large part biologically created, or perhaps nurtured through many so years so that they have become relatively permanent individual characteristics.

2. *Behaviors* are more likely than traits to have developed through experience. Behaviors may refer to general characteristics such as the ability to work in teams, customer service skills, and leadership skills, as well as behaviors specific to a particular job.

3. *Results or outcomes* refer to the outputs of an individual: what is actually produced. Results are varied and may include financial goals, patient satisfaction, and clinical outcomes. As evaluation criteria, outcomes should, of course, be under the control of the individual.

4. *Competencies* represent a relatively new approach to evaluation, and may be thought of as the core capabilities required to successfully perform a job. Competencies differ from simply identifying knowledge, skills, and abilities in that they "shift the level of analysis from the job and its associated tasks, to the person and what he or she is capable of" (Soderquist et al. 2010, 327).

One can think of competencies as a combination of traits, behaviors, and outcomes: What attributes are necessary to perform a job successfully? In this sense, competency models provide an approach that is future oriented and may provide an organization with greater flexibility and improve its ability to innovate. Competencies and competency models may be developed along a number of dimensions. They may, for example, be generic or organization specific, and skill based or behavior based. While competencies are attributes critical to successful job performance, they are not strictly bound to the tasks required for a particular job. Whether traits, behaviors, outcomes, or competencies are used for evaluation, how is this information obtained? This section describes methods of collecting and organizing performance information. Each approach has its strengths and shortcomings, and each approach is useful for particular types of jobs and circumstances.

Graphic Rating Scale

Graphic rating scale refers to any rating scale that uses points along a continuum and that measures traits or behaviors. This method is the most common way to assess performance, largely because it is easy to construct and can be used for many different types of employees. In its simplest form, rating scales evaluate such employee traits as reliability, accuracy, interpersonal skills, and communication. As shown in Exhibit 8.2, such a scale aims to measure a series of dimensions through anchor points (e.g., 1 through 6) that indicate different levels of performance. As the example in the exhibit shows, both traits and behaviors of the employee are assessed. Note, however, that many of the items included in the exhibit, such as "flexible," are prone to subjective judgment, and among the main criticisms of graphic rating scales is that they are subjective and prone to bias.

EXHIBIT 8.2
Example of a
Graphic Rating
Scale

Please answer the following questions about this employee.						
Question	**Scale**					
1. Rate this person's pace of work.	1 slow	2	3	4	5	6 fast
2. Assess this person's level of effort.	1 below capacity	2	3	4	5	6 full capacity
3. What is the quality of this person's work?	1 poor	2	3	4	5	6 good
4. How flexible is this person?	1 rigid	2	3	4	5	6 flexible
5. How open is this person to new ideas?	1 closed	2	3	4	5	6 open
6. How much supervision does this person need?	1 a lot	2	3	4	5	6 a little
7. How readily does this person offer to help out by doing work outside his or her normal scope of work?	1 seldom	2	3	4	5	6 often
8. How well does this person get along with peers?	1 not well	2	3	4	5	6 very well

Another drawback of graphic rating scales is that the items may be quite general, often not representing specific job-related behaviors that indicate positive or negative performance. The scale frequently does not yield information on how any item can be changed because the questions and statements for the behaviors or traits being rated are general. Because of this subjectivity, raters may be uncomfortable using this method, particularly when ratings are linked with compensation. Graphic rating scales can be improved by the use of behaviorally anchored rating scales, where specific observable behaviors are associated with each point on a scale.

Perhaps the most important drawback of graphic rating scales is that they typically do not weight behaviors and traits according to their importance to a particular job. In Exhibit 8.2, for example, pace of work (item 1) may be extremely relevant to the job of some employees but may be relatively unimportant to others. Thus, certain criteria may be less relevant for particular jobs. Related to this drawback is the common practice of using a one-size-fits-all approach to criteria—sometimes a scale is borrowed from another organization, and at other times a scale is adapted for another position, all without giving consideration to how the scale applies to the particular job or organization.

Ranking

Ranking is a simple method of performance appraisal in which managers rank employees simply from best to worst on some overall measure of employee performance. Such a method is typically employed for administrative purposes, such as making personnel decisions (e.g., promotions, layoffs). The major advantages of the ranking method are that it forces supervisors to distinguish among employees and that it does not have many of the problems associated with other appraisal methods. Among the disadvantages of ranking are the following:

- Focuses on aggregate work effectiveness and may not take into account the complexity of work situations
- Becomes cumbersome with large numbers of employees, forcing appraisers to artificially distinguish among employees
- Simply lists employees in order of their performance but does not indicate the relative differences in employees' effectiveness
- Provides no guidance on specific deficiencies in employee performance and therefore is not useful in helping employees improve

One type of ranking, which may involve the use of different types of performance measures, is known as *forced ranking* or forced distribution. With forced ranking, employee evaluations are not based on each employee's own set of objectives but are based on a comparison to other employees. Among the drivers behind their use is to keep managers from being too lenient in their evaluation, and to improve the competitiveness of the organization by rewarding the highest-performing employees and encouraging others to leave. Managers are instructed to force evaluations of employee performance into a particular distribution, which is similar to grading students on a curve. For example, managers may be directed to distribute 15 percent of employees as high performers, 20 percent as moderately high, 30 percent as average, 20 percent as below average, and 15 percent as poor. Forced ranking has been rationalized in a number of ways, including (1) to ensure that lenient managers do not systematically inflate appraisals, (2) to push managers to distribute their rankings, and (3) to limit bonuses and other financial payouts. Although these objectives may be met by using forced ranking, they may corrupt one of the key purposes of performance appraisal, which is to obtain honest information that can be used for employee development and improvement.

The most controversial use of forced ranking is to force out poor performers, sometimes referred to as "rank or yank." This approach, also known as "stack ranking," was made famous by Jack Welch, former CEO of General Electric (Welch and Byrne 2003). This strategy was known as the 20-70-10 plan. Variants of this approach exist, but in essence it works this way: Managers are required to identify the top 20 percent, middle 70 percent, and lowest

10 percent of employees. The bottom 10 percent are told to improve or they will be terminated. The validity of this approach is hotly debated. One study of HR executives, half of whom worked in organizations that use forced ranking, reported that this approach resulted in lower productivity, inequity, and skepticism and has negatively affected employee engagement, morale, trust in management, and collaboration (Novations Group 2004; Pfeffer and Sutton 2006). In addition, lawsuits filed at companies such as Ford Motor Company and Goodyear have challenged the legality of forced ranking, claiming that the process discriminates against older workers. Interestingly, Ford abandoned forced distribution in 2001 and settled two class-action cases for about $10.5 million (Boehl 2008). Forced stack ranking has also been implicated as a key issue in some of Microsoft's competitive shortcomings, in commentary pointing to, among other things, the negative impact of forced ranking on teamwork:

> "The behavior this [stack ranking] engenders, people do everything they can to stay out of the bottom bucket," one Microsoft engineer said. "People responsible for features will openly sabotage other people's efforts. One of the most valuable things I learned was to give the appearance of being courteous while withholding just enough information from colleagues to ensure they didn't get ahead of me on the rankings." (Eichenwald 2012)

When forced ranking is used, the implicit assumption is that 10 percent of employees (or whatever percentage is selected) are poor employees and therefore perform at a level deemed worthy of dismissal. The usefulness of this approach in healthcare is particularly problematic because of critical staff shortages. That is, a hospital that is facing a nurse shortage would likely not consider a "rank or yank" strategy for its nursing staff.

Behavioral Anchored Rating Scale

A *behavioral anchored rating scale* (BARS) is a significant improvement over traditional graphic rating scales. This scheme provides specific behavioral descriptions (or anchors) for each numerical rating on a rating scale. Exhibit 8.3 is an example of a BARS that measures aspects of the performance of a clinical trials coordinator. Note that the scale assesses the four dimensions of leadership, communication, delivery of results, and teamwork. In some instances, the behavioral measures are relatively easy to observe (e.g., delivery of results), while in other instances, the measures may be a bit more subjective (e.g., teamwork). Using BARS, a manager is able to explain the reason behind the ratings, rather than vaguely state "unacceptable" or "average" on the performance criteria. With BARS, a manager can explicitly state his or her expectations for improved performance.

Task Dimension	Scale	Definition
Leadership	4	Identifies alternative methods that enhance productivity and quality and that eliminate unnecessary steps
	3	Takes the initiative to bring attention to productivity problems
	2	Has difficulty with change and with providing support for the required change
	1	Uses inappropriate interpersonal skills, and creates unproductive working relationships
Communication	4	Communicates openly, completely, and straightforwardly with management, peers, and coworkers
	3	Listens and seeks intent of communication
	2	Has difficulty with expressing decisions, plans, and actions
	1	Is unable to communicate accurately with team members
Delivery of results	4	Completes 90 percent to 100 percent of all projects within time frame and budget and according to standards
	3	Completes 75 percent to 90 percent of all projects within time frame and budget and according to standards
	2	Completes 50 percent to 75 percent of projects within time frame and budget; sometimes produces substandard work
	1	Completes less than 50 percent of projects within time frame and budget; frequently produces substandard work
Teamwork	4	Contributes positively to problem definition and takes responsibility for outcome
	3	Respects suggestions and viewpoints of others
	2	Has trouble with interactions with others and with understanding individual differences
	1	Does not contribute positively to team functioning

EXHIBIT 8.3

Behavioral Anchored Rating Scale for a Clinical Trials Coordinator

The advantages of BARS include the following:

- Reduces rating errors because job dimensions are clearly defined for the rater and are relevant to the job being performed
- Clearly defines the response categories available to the rater
- Is more reliable, valid, meaningful, and complete
- Has a higher degree of acceptance and commitment from employees and supervisors
- Minimizes employee defensiveness and conflict with the manager because employees are appraised on the basis of observable behavior
- Improves a manager's ability to identify areas for training and development

Developing a BARS for each job dimension for a particular job is not a trivial task. Among the disadvantages of a BARS is the amount of time, effort, and expense involved in its development. Use of this approach is most justifiable when a large number of jobholders are performing in the same position (e.g., nurses, transporters). BARS is most appropriate for jobs whose major components consist of physically observable behaviors.

A variation of BARS is the *behavioral observation scale* (BOS), a system that asks the rater to indicate the frequency with which the employee exhibits specified highly desirable behaviors. Desirable behaviors are identified through job analysis and discussions with managers and supervisors. Exhibit 8.4 is an example of a BOS for a patient relations representative. As seen in the exhibit, six desirable behaviors for this job are identified, and the rater indicates the frequency with which each behavior is observed in the patient relations representative. As with BARS, those who use BOS should have a clear understanding of the types of behaviors expected.

Critical Incident

The *critical incident* approach involves keeping a record of unusually favorable or unfavorable occurrences in an employee's work. This record is created and maintained by the employee's manager. A major strength of this method is that it provides a factual record of an employee's performance and can be very useful in subsequent discussions with the employee. The approach does require that the manager closely and continuously monitor employee performance, which is not always feasible, although linking a critical incident method with 360-degree feedback raises the possibility that incidents may be observed and recorded by a number of different individuals in the organization.

	Almost Never				Almost Always
1. Responds to patient or family concerns within 24 hours	1	2	3	4	5
2. Conducts investigations into complaints effectively	1	2	3	4	5
3. Communicates results of investigations to relevant parties	1	2	3	4	5
4. Follows up with patient or family after investigation	1	2	3	4	5
5. Identifies and analyzes both immediate and distant causes of patient complaints	1	2	3	4	5
6. Makes useful and practical recommendations for improvement based on results of investigation	1	2	3	4	5

EXHIBIT 8.4

Behavioral Observation Scale for a Patient Relations Representative

Documentation of critical incidents need not be very lengthy, but it should be tied to one or more important performance dimensions. This example of a critical incident for a mental health case manager demonstrates the importance of creativity and negotiation skills for case managers.

In speaking with her client—an individual with severe mental disorder—the case manager discovered that the client was about to be evicted from her apartment for nonpayment of rent. She was able to work with the client and the landlord to work out a payment plan and to negotiate successfully with the landlord to have much-needed repairs in the apartment done. She followed up with the client weekly regarding payment to the landlord and the home repairs, and positive outcomes have been achieved in both areas.

Results-Based Evaluation Systems

A results-based evaluation system evaluates individual performance by assessing how well employees achieved a set of results or outcomes. The most well-known and popular application of this approach is management by objectives (MBO). The basic premise of MBO is as follows: (1) The organization defines its strategic goals for the year; (2) these goals are then communicated throughout the organization; (3) on the basis of organizational goals, each employee in turn defines his or her goals for a specified period; and (4) managers provide continuous feedback on goal achievement. Achievement of these goals becomes the standard by which each employee's performance is assessed.

MBO has three key characteristics (Heery and Noon 2008):

1. Through collaboration of employees and managers, it establishes specific and objectively measurable goals for employees.
2. Goals are set at a level that is challenging but attainable.
3. Managers assess and provide feedback to employees on the extent to which objectives have been met by the employee, feeding this information into the performance management system.

MBO has been found to be most effective when specific, difficult goals are set, and where employees are actively engaged in the goal-setting process. Like most managerial practices, MBO is most effective when it is supported by and has the commitment of senior management. MBO requires managers to obtain substantial training in goal setting, giving feedback, and coaching. While goal setting is central to MBO, the process by which goals are set is of great importance as well (DeCenzo, Robbins, and Verhulst 2013).

Depending on the position of the jobholder, organizations may use a variety of results-oriented methods such as MBO. These approaches are most useful when the work yields objectively measurable outcomes. MBO is most commonly used for senior executives, for whom objectively measurable bottom-line concerns may be paramount; salespeople; and sports teams and individual athletes. The approach may be combined with other performance appraisal methods, particularly for jobs in which both the manner in which work is done and the outcomes are important and measurable.

The Cynicism About Performance Management

Many managers and employees are cynical about performance management. This cynicism grows out of a perception that aspects of performance management are distasteful and uncomfortable. Managers are often ill at ease about sitting down and discussing concerns with employees, and employees may resent the paternalism and condescension that often accompany such processes. This cynicism is clearly based in the reality that performance appraisals are traditionally punitive in nature and, particularly when tightly tied to employee compensation, have high emotional content.

Regardless of the type of data used in performance appraisal, what persists are "rating errors," as social psychologists call them. *Rating errors* are simply distortions in performance appraisal ratings—whether positive or negative—that reduce the accuracy of appraisals. The most common rating errors are as follows:

- *Distributional.* These errors come from the tendency of raters to use only a small part of the rating scale. They come in three forms:
  - *Lenient:* Some raters tend to be overly generous with giving positive ratings and thereby avoid conflict and confrontation.
  - *Strict:* Some raters tend to be overly critical of performance and therefore are deemed unfair when compared with other raters without such a tendency.
  - *Central:* Some raters tend to rate every employee as average and thereby avoid conflict and confrontation.
- *Halo effect.* These errors result from the propensity of some raters to rate employees high (or low) on all evaluation criteria, without distinguishing between different aspects of the employees' work. This effect leads to evaluations that may be overly critical or overly generous.
- *Personal bias.* These errors arise because of some raters' tendency to rate employees higher or lower than is deserved because of the rater's personal like or dislike of the employee. In particular, stereotyping based on cultural bias can certainly influence appraisal—and it is illegal (Pfeffer 2009). The key point is that we all have biases, but conducting an effective and fair performance evaluation requires that managers develop an awareness of and manage their biases (Krell 2011).
- *Familiarity or similarity bias.* These errors stem from the likelihood of some raters to judge those who are similar to them more highly than they would those who are not like them. Research shows that the strongest impact of similarity occurs when a manager and an employee share demographic characteristics, such as race and age group (Stepanovich 2013).
- *Contrast effect.* These errors are created when raters compare employees with each other rather than use objective standards for job performance.

The most important strategy for overcoming these rating errors is user training in different rating methods. Typically, training helps to increase managers' familiarity with rating scales and the specific level of performance associated with different points on these scales. The ultimate objective of such training is to increase each manager's consistency in using rating scales and to improve interrater reliability among managers. As a result, error rates are minimized. At a minimum, managers need to be aware of potential rating errors in performance appraisal. Strategies may be offered to help managers both identify their errors and develop strategies to avoid making errors. For example, managers may avoid distributional errors by improving their awareness of the appraisal tool and their understanding of the objective standards used to evaluate performance. Of course, the success of training efforts is contingent on the existence of valid and reliable assessment instruments and clear performance standards.

The reality in organizational life is that, even with well-developed assessment tools and presumably effective management training programs, the process of performance appraisal is often tarnished not because of subtle or unconscious distortions but because of political pressures. Organizations are political organizations, and as much as managers are encouraged to make rational decisions and conduct themselves in an objective manner, they are subject to acute political pressures, and these pressures may cause distortions in the performance appraisal process. Political pressures may cause a manager to inflate, deflate, or completely avoid doing a performance review. One common source of political pressure is the reality that a manager will have to continue working with a particular employee. A mediocre or poor review (although realistic), then, may be perceived as a blemish in the employee–manager relationship and may upset the workplace climate and productivity. In such instances, a manager may inflate an appraisal to avoid the potential personal and workplace negative effects.

A manager may also artificially inflate an appraisal to permit awarding the employee a merit increase or other financial reward. While this destroys the intent of both the performance management and the compensation system, when faced with bread-and-butter issues, managers may choose to err on the side of generosity toward the employee. Managers may also inflate an appraisal to prevent an employee from having a written record of poor performance, to avoid a confrontation with an employee, or to reward an employee's improved performance. Quoting a manager's observations about performance appraisal, Longenecker, Sims, and Gioia (1987, 185) noted:

> The mere fact that you have to write out your assessment and create a permanent record will cause people not to be as honest or as accurate as they should be. . . . We soften the language because our ratings go in the guy's file downstairs [the personnel department] and it will follow him around his whole career.

As emphasized in this chapter, performance should be assessed using objective criteria. While improved performance may be recognized and discussed during a performance review session with an employee, managers should stick with the criteria when assigning a rating to an employee's performance. Although somewhat rare, instances in which a manager inflates an appraisal to enable an employee to be promoted "up and out" of the organization can occur. This strategy obviously has highly questionable legal and ethical aspects. Finally, managers may sometimes give a break to an employee who is having personal problems.

Deflating an appraisal is also sometimes done to shock an employee into improving or to teach a rebellious employee a lesson. No evidence exists that such shock treatments are effective, but managers often use strategies with unproven effectiveness. Because careful documentation is usually required for employee termination, managers may also deflate an appraisal to speed up the termination process. Furthermore, providing an overly critical review could be viewed as a way of sending a message to an employee that he or she should think about leaving the organization. Exhibit 8.5 summarizes these and other political distortions to the appraisal process. Altering the appraisal process for political purposes is not condoned here, but tampering occurs, and recognizing the potential for this behavior is important. An enduring aspect of performance appraisal systems is that implementation is often fraught with problems; therefore, when designing performance management systems and training managers in their use, HR managers need to be cognizant of the many opportunities for abuse and misuse.

Conducting Effective Performance Management Interviews

As noted earlier, the ultimate objective of performance management is to improve employee performance. Because performance management has historically focused on the evaluation or measurement aspects, relatively little attention has been given to its improvement aspects.

Reasons to Inflate	Reasons to Deflate
• Maximize merit increases for an employee, particularly when the merit ceiling is considered low • Avoid hanging dirty laundry out in public if the appraisal information is viewed by outsiders • Avoid creating a written record of poor performance that would become a permanent part of the individual's personnel file • Avoid confrontation with an employee with whom the manager recently had difficulties • Give a break to a subordinate who had shown improvements • Promote an undesirable employee "up and out" of the organization	• Shock an employee back onto a higher performance track • Teach a rebellious employee a lesson • Send a message to an employee that he or she should think about leaving the organization • Build a strongly documented record of poor performance that may speed up the termination process

EXHIBIT 8.5
Reasons Managers Inflate or Deflate a Performance Appraisal

Source: Adapted from Longenecker, Sims, and Gioia (1987).

A key step in the improvement process is to provide performance information to the employee. Many managers are reluctant to provide feedback because of fear of confrontation and conflict. These concerns are real for both managers and employees, given many employees' negative experiences with performance management. In informal surveys that the authors of this chapter conduct with students, the great majority of students typically report that they either rarely have a performance evaluation or have had a poorly done evaluation. Finding a student who has had a well-implemented appraisal is relatively unusual. Therefore, remember that managers are not naturally skilled in providing feedback to employees. In fact, managers tend to be emotionally challenged by the process. Manager training is therefore critical to have a useful performance management system. Further, evaluating whether and how well managers are performing this essential management responsibility is important.

The following are techniques for a valuable performance evaluation:

- *Ensure that the criteria used to assess performance are job related and under the control of the job holder.* In addition, employees need to know the basis on which they will be evaluated *at the beginning of the appraisal period.* Managers and employees should agree on these criteria and expected standards of performance.
- *Provide feedback on an ongoing basis.* Checking on how an employee is performing should be a regular occurrence, not just done during the formal appraisal process. Giving continuous feedback is, after all, a key responsibility for managers. By providing ongoing feedback, surprises at the formal appraisal can be avoided.
- *Evaluate the frequency of a formal performance appraisal.* The frequency of formal appraisals varies depending on an employee's performance and longevity in the organization. For a high performer, an annual appraisal (as well as ongoing informal feedback) may be sufficient; such an assessment is usually done to reward good work, to reinforce existing levels of performance, and to discuss employee development and promotion possibilities. For an average performer, more frequent appraisals may be necessary to ensure that improvement goals are on track and will be achieved. For marginal or poor performers, formal appraisals may need to be held monthly (or perhaps more often) to provide an opportunity for closer coaching and, if necessary, disciplinary action.
- *Prepare for the performance appraisal.* At the appraisal session, the manager should have a set of clear goals for the appraisal, be equipped with data, have a strategy for presenting performance information, be able to anticipate employee reactions, and be prepared to engage the

employee in problem solving and planning. An appropriate physical location should be found, and relevant supporting information should be available as a reference.

- *Use multiple sources of information.* Consistent with multirater or 360-degree appraisal, obtaining performance information from several sources is useful. This information is particularly important in situations in which the manager is unable to adequately observe an employee's work, the job is highly complex, or the employee must interact with multiple individuals inside and outside the organization.

- *Encourage employee participation.* Employee self-appraisal is commonly used as part of the appraisal process. The employee may have greater insight into his or her own performance concerns, and these insights are often consistent with the manager's assessment. An atmosphere should be created in which the appraisal is structured to benefit the employee, rather than be punitive. This positive environment may be difficult to create given many employees' negative perceptions of the performance appraisal process. Employee participation is also vital because the employee must assume accountability for improvement, and the first step in being accountable is understanding what needs to be done and being involved in developing strategies toward that effort. Improvement should be viewed as a partnership between the manager and the employee.

- *Focus on future performance and problem solving.* Reviewing past performance during an appraisal is important, but the emphasis of such a review should be on setting goals for the future and on generating specific strategies for meeting those goals. In many cases, the employee will identify factors outside of his or her control that may contribute to lower-than-expected levels of performance. These factors are certainly appropriate to discuss during an appraisal session. Follow-up sessions should also be scheduled as appropriate.

- *Focus on employee behavior and results, not personal traits.* In almost all cases, the purpose of performance feedback is to help employees improve their work, not to change the person. The performance evaluation session is not the time to change an employee's values, personality, motivation, or fit with the organization. If these factors represent true problems, they should have been considered during the selection process. The manager should focus on behaviors and outcomes, not the value of the person. Doling out condescending criticisms and reciting a litany of employee problems are rarely useful and are more likely to generate defensiveness and resentment from the employee.

- *Reinforce positive performance.* Performance appraisal sessions have gained the reputation of being punitive and negative. One of the most effective ways for managers to ally themselves with employees is to ensure that the interview focuses on all aspects of performance, not just the negative. As in other areas of life, rewarding and reinforcing positive performance are essential aspects of productive human relationships.

- *Ensure that performance management is supported by senior managers.* The best way to destroy any effort at implementing a performance management system is for word to get out that senior management is either unsupportive of or ambivalent about the process. Senior management must assert and communicate that performance management is important to meeting organizational goals and that it must be done at all levels of the workforce. If this message is absent or weak, the performance management system will either fade away or become a meaningless bureaucratic exercise.

- *Plan follow-up activities and pay attention to expected outcomes and timetables.* Given the complex and hectic nature of organizations, losing focus on the important but not urgent aspects of work is easy. If plans are put into place, they should be accompanied by timetables, expectations, and concrete plans for follow-up. Without follow-up, the integrity of the performance management process is put into great jeopardy.

The Special Case of Bullies and Toxic Managers

In a typical executive management class, when students are asked who has worked with a bully or for a toxic manager, a sizeable number of students raise their hands. When those who did not raise their hands are asked if they have a close acquaintance who has had such an experience, nearly all of them raise their hands. Follow-up discussions usually reveal that the behaviors of bullies and toxic managers are rarely changed. The most common way people deal with these situations is to eventually leave the department or organization.

Bullies present a unique performance challenge. What are bullies and toxic managers and how did they get this way? Beginning with definitions, the Workplace Bullying Institute (WBI 2014a) defines bullying as

repeated, health-harming mistreatment of one or more persons (the targets) by one or more perpetrators. It is abusive conduct that is:
- Threatening, humiliating, or intimidating, or
- Work interference—sabotage—which prevents work from getting done, or
- Verbal abuse.

The WBI annual survey of workplace bullying (WBI 2014b) reports that 27 percent of Americans have suffered abusive conduct at work; another 21 percent have witnessed it; and 72 percent are aware that workplace bullying occurs. About 69 percent of bullies are men, and women are more likely than men to be the target of bullying. Interestingly, while 56 percent of bullying is top-down (supervisor bullying a direct report), one-third of bullying is done by coworkers, and 11 percent is "bottom-up" bullying (an employee bullying the supervisor). Perhaps most distressing are data on employer reactions to bullying. According to the WBI (2014b),

- 25 percent of employers *deny* that bullying takes place;
- 16 percent *discount* the impact of bullying;
- 15 percent *rationalize* the bullying behavior, usually as the way of doing business;
- 11 percent *defend* the behavior, particularly when the perpetrators are executives or managers; and
- 5 percent *encourage* the bully or the practice of bullying, often because it is viewed as necessary if an organization is to remain competitive.

On the positive side, 6 percent of employers condemn bullying, often through a zero-tolerance policy; 10 percent acknowledge that bullying takes place by showing concern for the victims; and 12 percent seek to eliminate bullying by creating and enforcing policies and procedures (WBI 2014b).

Bullying overall in society is a problem (for example, see www.stop bullying.gov, a US Department of Health and Human Services website devoted to bullying in schools). While not a scientific way to assess the prevalence of bullying, an Amazon.com search for "workplace bullying" turned up 1,896 books (a search for "bullying" turned up 13,481 publications). Guidebooks are available for employees, teachers, parents, counselors, and virtually anyone else affected by bullying. Most deal with how to stop or respond to bullies.

From the individual victim's perspective, bullying can result in emotional distress, post-traumatic stress disorder, physical health issues, feelings of helplessness, depression, family problems, and any number of other impacts cascading from the bullying behavior. Organizations feel the impact of bullying through absenteeism, turnover, loss of productivity, costs associated with legal fees and investigations, a climate that is steeped in fear, gaps in quality due to the climate of fear, and perhaps difficulty recruiting people to the organization.

Healthcare organizations face particular and more difficult bullying challenges. In fact, the prevalence of bullying in healthcare led The Joint Commission to issue a Sentinel Event Alert addressing what it called disruptive behaviors, stating that "intimidating and disruptive behaviors can foster medical errors . . . and [contribute] to preventable adverse outcomes" (Joint Commission 2008). Larson (2013) notes the pervasiveness of bullying among nurses, describing both vertical bullying (a manager bullying a subordinate nurse) and horizontal bullying (in which nurses bully their colleagues). In addition, the American Nurses Association published a booklet on the bullying epidemic, providing guidelines for developing a positive workplace culture and ensuring a safe workplace, and offering advice to nurses who are confronting bullying (American Nurses Association 2012).

Bullying is often exacerbated by rigid hierarchies and power differentials. Hierarchies are omnipresent in healthcare, and in particular, status differences are present between physicians and others. This power differential is very high between physicians and nurses, particularly newly graduated nurses. Studies conducted as part of the Robert Wood Johnson Foundation's RN Work Project found that early-career nurses experiencing moderate abuse were significantly younger than those experiencing no abuse, and expressed a lower intent to stay and lower organizational commitment. In addition, verbal abuse from physicians correlated with high levels of abuse from nurse colleagues (Brewer et al. 2013).

How prevalent is bullying in healthcare compared with other industries? In an unscientific study of people who self-reported being bullied, the breakdown by industry suggests that healthcare employees may be particularly at risk. The unscientific sample of 401 respondents fell into the following industries (Workplace Bullying Institute 2013):

- Healthcare (27 percent)
- Education (23 percent)
- Public services (e.g., law enforcement, postal service) (16 percent)
- Service industry (e.g., retail, hospitality, restaurant) (10 percent)
- Information technology (5 percent)
- Manufacturing (5 percent)
- Other (14 percent)

Some important characteristics of bullies make them particularly difficult to manage. First, they tend to be organizational survivors, and have had their behavior enabled or sanctioned, usually passively, through the years. Second, notwithstanding their destructive behavior, they add value to the organization and may be difficult to replace. Consider the secretary who has been in the family medicine department for 20 years and knows every nuance of how the department functions—and is likely to keep that information to herself. Among physicians, consider the orthopedic surgeon who generates millions of dollars annually for the hospital. A senior manager facing a complaint from a low-level employee may have two choices: help the victim by confronting (and perhaps angering) the surgeon, or ignore the complaint, ensuring the surgeon's continued contentment (and abusive behavior).

Bullies may come from all levels of the organization, and in most cases, the bully is the manager of the target. A recent poll of people who were targets of bullying found that 82 percent were bullied by their boss, 47 percent by coworkers and peers, and 16 percent by a subordinate (Workplace Bullying Institute 2012). The dynamics, however, vary among these three levels of bullies. Because of power differentials, bosses have the ability to affect their targets' lives, and it is easier for a boss to bully a subordinate than for a subordinate to bully the boss. One method a subordinate can use to bully a boss is by sabotaging the work of a higher-ranking target. This sabotage could potentially have a destructive impact on the boss's career. The most common form of bullying by peers is associated with the use of social exclusion and ostracism to harm targets (Workplace Bullying Institute 2012).

Perhaps the most difficult aspect of preventing and eliminating bullying behavior is changing the organizational culture, particularly when changing the culture may affect an organization negatively, at least in the short term. While an organization may not explicitly promote bullying, it may still provide fertile ground for its growth. For example, an organization that thrives on competition among its employees may tolerate behavior that hinges on bullying and may evolve into bullying. An organization with a highly competitive culture may also find that it is selecting employees who have a competitive mind-set, which may be dysfunctional. Distinguishing between an employee who brings a healthy competitive spirit and one whose competitive nature turns pathological may be difficult. Certainly, a zero-tolerance culture sends a message to employees about the seriousness of the issue. However, even if the organization states that it has a zero-tolerance culture, this statement provides no assurance that individual employees will feel safe lodging complaints against bullies. The fear of retribution (or, perhaps, earning a reputation as a complainer) may be sufficient to convince an employee that living with the situation is better than confronting the issue.

Dealing with bullying is a problem for both the individual victim and for the department or organization where the bullying occurs. From an individual's standpoint, one can approach the issue from a survival and coping perspective as well as from the viewpoint of eliminating the behavior or ridding the organization of the bully. Numerous recommendations for dealing with bullies have been proposed. The following recommendations are based on the assumption that the bully is of the "manageable" variety—that is, a boss who is subject to occasional flare-ups as opposed to a boss who may be subject to legal sanctions based on his behavior (Taylor 2009; Smith 2013):

- Intervene early as warning signs appear.
- Set limits and avoid personal martyrdom to accommodate the bully.
- Speak to coworkers to assess how widespread the bullying is and to get advice on coping strategies.
- Use positive reinforcement with the bully, rewarding positive and civilized behavior.
- Be a good role model by serving as an example of good behavior for the bully.
- Consult with the HR department.
- Where abusiveness is out of control, seek assistance from coworkers, other managers, or outside counsel.

Taylor (2009) notes that directly confronting the boss is rarely effective and is not advised.

On the organizational side, the following strategies may help to prevent or eliminate the bullying behavior:

- Conduct thorough background checks on job applicants, and be sure that treatment of others is part of the selection process.
- Include treatment of others in performance appraisal and reward systems; this process may include the use of multisource appraisals.
- Assess if the bullying behavior is a result of a treatable physical condition, such as drug dependence, anxiety, depression, or attention-deficit/hyperactivity disorder.
- Coach abusive employees.
- Be prepared to terminate employees whose bullying behavior is not changeable.

Some reason for hope exists in this area. Comparing bullying to sexual harassment is instructive. In the not-so-distant past, sexual harassment was widely (and passively) accepted and was usually not taken seriously. Only relatively recently has public attention focused on sexual harassment, partly as a result of several highly visible cases, and the fact that it is illegal under Title VII of the Civil Rights Act. Similar attention has begun to be given to bullying. Although bullying involves nothing that is explicitly illegal, its presence throughout society, and particularly among children, has propelled the issue into prominence. Several tragic stories about children dying as a result of bullying behavior have received great attention in the media (Bazelon 2013), and the nation may have reached a turning point in its tolerance of bullying. Whether the changing narrative around bullying maintains its momentum and results in measurable changes remains to be seen.

Summary

Historically, performance appraisal focused primarily on judging employee behavior. The process was often viewed as negative and punitive in nature and was generally avoided by both managers and employees. Although change has occurred only gradually, many organizations are taking a more enlightened and helpful approach, focusing on improvement, coaching, and aligning individual goals with those of the organization. Performance management implies an improvement-focused process in which efforts are made not only to assess performance but also to develop specific collaborative strategies to enhance performance. Recognizing that employee performance results from an employee's skills, motivation, and facilitative factors in the work environment, improvement strategies may include training, work process redesign, and other changes that are both internal and external to the employee.

An important aspect of performance management is the development of relevant appraisal criteria for the employee's position and the expectations of the organization. Appraisal data may be gathered through a variety of mechanisms, including self, subordinate, team members, and multisource or 360-degree feedback. Methods for organizing these data may involve a graphic rating scale, ranking, BARS, BOS, a critical incident record, and achievement of outcomes or objectives. The choice of approach depends on the job, the organizational goals, and, perhaps most important, the culture of the organization, particularly its readiness to confront performance issues honestly and openly.

Discussion Questions

1. What is the distinction between performance appraisal and performance management?

2. Why does The Joint Commission require hospitals and other healthcare organizations to have a performance management system?

3. What is the relationship between performance management and continuous quality improvement?

4. What are the advantages and disadvantages of including discussions of compensation in a performance management interview?

5. What is the difference between performance appraisal rating errors and political factors that influence the accuracy of performance appraisal information?

6. How does a manager decide how often to conduct formal performance management interviews?

7. Why is employee participation in the performance management process important? Under what circumstances is employee participation not necessarily important?

Experiential Exercises

Case 1   Summit River Nursing Home (SRNH) is a 60-bed nursing home that serves a suburban community in the Midwest. The facility provides a broad range of services to residents, including recreational activities, clinical laboratory services, dental services, dietary and housekeeping services, mental health and nursing services, occupational and physical therapies, pharmacy services, social services, and diagnostic X-ray services.

The facility has a good reputation in the community and is well staffed. Licensed practical nurses administer medications and perform certain treatment procedures. Each nursing home resident receives at least two hours of direct nursing care every day. Certified nursing assistants perform most of the direct patient care. A dietary service supervisor manages the daily operations of the food service department along with a registered dietitian. Activity coordinators provide nonmedical care designed to improve cognitive and physical capabilities. Two social workers on staff work with residents, families, and other organizations, and an important part of their role is to ease residents and their families' adjustment to the long-term-care environment. They also help to identify residents' specific medical and emotional needs and provide support and referral services. Environmental service workers maintain the facility with a goal of providing a clean and safe facility for the residents. Housekeeping staff also have considerable contact with residents on a day-to-day basis. SRNH has contractual relationships with a dental practice, physical therapists, a pharmacist, a psychologist, and a multispecialty physician practice.

The management team at SRNH consists of an administrator, a finance director, an HR director, a director of nursing, and administrative support personnel. Recently, concerns about quality have emerged at the nursing home. Several instances of communication breakdown among staff have occurred, and several instances of medication error have also taken place. A resident satisfaction survey also revealed problems of which management had been unaware. Some of the problems concern contract staff who have not been included in the organization's performance management process.

Discussions with management and employees established that a team atmosphere among staff was lacking. Each member of the management team was asked to develop a strategy to improve the level of teamwork in the facility. The HR director agreed to take action in three areas:

1. Ensure that all job descriptions address teamwork and that these changes are discussed with employees.
2. Develop and implement a team-building training program for all employees, including contract staff.
3. Revise the performance management approach so that it focuses on teamwork as well as individual skills and accomplishments.

The first two strategies were relatively easy to complete. Job descriptions were revised, and supervisors met with employees to discuss these changes. With the assistance of an outside consultant, a training program was implemented to teach employees communication and conflict management skills. Several, but not all, contract employees attended the training program.

The third strategy raised some difficulties. The existing performance management system was traditional, using a 12-item graphic rating scale (some with behavioral descriptions) that measured aspects of work such as attitude, quality of performance, productivity, attention to detail, job knowledge, reliability, and availability. The form also provided room for comments by both supervisors and employees. This rating approach, however, was found to be incapable of addressing the team components of the jobs. An additional problem is that several staff members are on contract and are not fully integrated into the organization. Other employees are obtained for temporary employment through local staffing agencies. These staff members do not go through the organization's performance management process; only full-time permanent employees are integrated into the performance management process.

The HR director wants to modify the performance management process so that it includes methods to assess and improve team performance for both full-time permanent as well as contract employees.

You are a consultant to the HR director. Your job is to develop a method by which teamwork will be integrated into the performance management process.

Case Questions

1. How would you proceed with the task of modifying the performance management process to include a teamwork component?

2. How would one go about collecting information about an employee's performance as a team member?

3. Given that some members of the organization are not full-time permanent employees, how would you involve them?

4. How could the compensation system be used to reinforce positive team behaviors? What are the advantages and potential pitfalls of using teamwork as a factor in making compensation decisions?

Case 2

Note: This case was written by Lee Ellis, Dawn Morrow, and Adia Bradley.

Introduction

Kristen closes the reminder on her calendar. She has 15 more minutes until a 90-day performance review of Leslie, her newest direct report. Kristen has been director of marketing at Englewood Hospital for almost a year, and this is the first time she has supervised an employee who is not meeting expectations. She pushes the papers around her desk

as she thinks about how to handle the meeting. She remembers her first hospital position ten years ago, right after she graduated.

Background

Ten years ago, Kristen had just started her first job as a manager at Bayside Healthcare, the same system where only a year earlier she had completed her administrative fellowship under the chief operating officer (COO). As a fellow, she formed great working relationships with many of the hospital's administrators, including her new boss, Jessie, director of public affairs. During her fellowship, Kristen worked on several projects for Jessie and thought of her as a mentor. After several months under her, however, Kristen realized that Jessie was not as easy to work for as she had expected. During the hiring process, Kristen was told that she would contribute to several public relations projects for Bayside Healthcare's outpatient clinics and that she would be directly responsible for two large, revenue-generating projects in the emergency department each year. This type of work was what she had always wanted to do, and she was excited to get started on these projects right away. However, after her first month on the job, Kristen had not been informed of what the first project in the emergency department would be, nor had Jessie posted the required formal work plan on the hospital's online project-management system.

Several months later, Corey, a former manager in Bayside Healthcare's physician practice, was hired as Kristen's counterpart. Corey's job description was the same, with responsibility for two large, revenue-generating projects per year based in the outpatient clinics. He was excited to start his new position, but he was also experiencing a tense working relationship with Jessie. In his first week on the job, Jessie sat down with her two new managers to discuss her expectations. She said she would be sending them work daily and expected the work to be completed quickly. She would closely monitor their performance until they were able to win her trust. She wanted them to type minutes for any meetings they attended without her. They both asked when they would get the details of their first major projects, the primary focus of their position, but Jessie brushed them off, promising that she would inform them later.

Two weeks passed, and Kristen and Corey grew more frustrated with their jobs. Their work plans were still not entered in the project management system, and they were only working on small projects assigned daily by Jessie. Moreover, their offices had not been completed, forcing both of them to move from desk to desk wherever space was available. They finally decided to set up a meeting with Jessie to discuss their frustrations. They developed an agenda for the meeting that included a discussion of the work they completed; proposals for their first projects; and a list of things they required to effectively perform their jobs, including a consistent work space. They framed the meeting as a time to develop a structured work plan, as they were unsure of their current role expectations. Unfortunately, the meeting did not go as smoothly as planned. Jessie felt attacked and was defensive. Although they talked through their agenda items, they did not reach solutions on any issue. Everyone left the meeting feeling uneasy and suspicious.

The next day, Jessie scolded Corey for the previous day's events, saying that he and Kristen needed to learn their place. He walked away flabbergasted and found Kristen to tell her about the encounter. She was still on a six-month probation period, during which she could be fired with few questions asked. He, however, had served the system for four years and could not be terminated as easily. Nonetheless, he called his former boss and explained his situation. The boss offered him an open position, and he turned in his resignation, only one month after he began.

Kristen was now left alone and had few options except to do as she was told to survive her probationary period. Jessie finally posted a work plan for her, but the plan and its expected results were vague. Jessie continued to assign daily tasks, but they all had unrealistic deadlines. Although

Kristen presented several proposals for her first project, Jessie continued to dismiss her.

More weeks passed and Kristen learned from a close colleague that Jessie had made a disparaging comment about her during a meeting attended by many service line managers. Apparently, Jessie said, "Well, that was a mistake," in reference to having hired Kristen. Also, the colleague reported that the grapevine was abuzz with talk that Jessie had been making derisive comments around the hospital about Kristen. Kristen was furious about this news and was worried about its impact on her reputation. Not knowing what to do, she decided to leverage the relationships she had developed during her time as the fellow to save her reputation. She set up meetings with several vice presidents and even her former boss, the COO, to discuss the situation. These meetings did not prove especially helpful, but she felt vindicated and avenged in some ways. Kristen grew increasingly bitter about Jessie's unrealistic demands, especially the requirement to provide minutes for any meeting that she attended alone. Jessie had access to Kristen's calendar and carefully monitored it, sending her reminders about when she should send the minutes. Kristen finally quit scheduling meetings on her electronic calendar, opting instead to stop by someone's office if she needed to meet or to call for an appointment and jot down a reminder on her paper calendar. If her boss wanted to play games, then she could play too.

Two weeks before her six-month review, Kristen received a meeting request from Jessie and Bruce, vice president of outpatient services. She expected that this meeting would not be good news, so she prepared a rebuttal the night before. As expected, Kristen was informed that her employment with the hospital was not working out and she could either be fired and given 30 days'

severance pay or resign, effective immediately. The reasons cited included (1) insubordination that negatively affected teamwork and customer service and (2) failure to provide quality and quantity of work expected. Kristen resigned and left immediately.

Current Situation

Kristen was devastated by that experience, but she moved on. Right after her termination, she went to work for a competing hospital, where she stayed for several years. Although the sting of that first job has faded, she can still remember it and does not want her new direct report, Leslie, to have the same experience. Kristen wishes now that she had given Leslie consistent feedback throughout the past six months instead of waiting until now, her formal review date.

Leslie is a recent graduate of a top-tier master of health administration (MHA) program. Six months ago, she accepted a position with Englewood Hospital, a private, secular, not-for-profit system that consists of a medical school, five hospitals, and a large ambulatory care facility. The system is consistently ranked among the top 25 hospitals in the United States, and it is world-renowned in oncology and cardiology. Before attending graduate school, Leslie was a healthcare consultant in a small firm, where she was responsible for strategic planning projects with hospital clients. At that firm, she was a consistently good performer and worked her way up from analyst to contract manager. After earning her MHA, she wanted to apply the skill sets she had obtained in a different healthcare setting, so she applied for a position as a marketing manager for Englewood Hospital's outpatient clinics.

In preparation for Leslie's performance evaluation, Kristen reviewed the job description she had given Leslie when she joined the team (see Exhibit 8.6).

EXHIBIT 8.6
Job Description

Job Overview
- Responsible for managing development of the strategic marketing plan for the orthopedic, cardiology, and endocrinology clinics.
- Required to perform market analyses and develop strategies to increase the number of patients who receive services at these three clinics.

Supervisor: Reports to director of marketing for Outpatient Services
Direct reports: Three research analysts

Essential Job Functions
- Identify and address critical issues within each clinic pertaining to the marketing of services/service line expansion, and recommend solutions; win "buy-in" from management/physicians for plans.
- Lead segmentation activities for each clinic.
- Analyze emerging market opportunities, and develop justification for service line development.
- Target patient populations based on competitive strengths.
- Assess feasibility of meeting targets' needs.
- Monitor competitive environment.

Manage Resources
- Implement expansion of clinical services, and coordinate launch activities.
- Lead cross-functional groups, including Patient Satisfaction, Quality Improvement, Operations, Marketing, Communications, Legal, and Finance/Accounting.
- Recommend and implement pricing strategies and cost-reduction measures to optimize profitability.
- Establish and achieve quarterly profitability goals.

Deliverables Include
- Monthly report of progress on annual goals and quarterly summary statistics on clinic performance
- Semiannual report of the activities of competitive activity relating to the three service lines
- Brief reports on clinic staff and departmental meetings
- Written performance reviews for direct reports
- Other reports as requested

Core Behaviors
- Leads strategically
- Builds alignment
- Communicates directly
- Drives performance
- Collaborates
- Energizes others
- Develops people

Leslie's Performance

On several occasions in the last six months, Kristen had been disappointed with Leslie's performance:

- The local newspaper reported that a local hospital was launching a new service line consisting of freestanding orthopedic clinics. However, Leslie had not mentioned this new development, even though it could have a direct impact on the outpatient clinics for which Leslie was responsible.
- One departmental director informed Kristen that the marketing department had no representation at 9 out of the last 12 Patient Satisfaction and General Clinic Operations meetings.
- Leslie submitted a preliminary draft of profitability goals, but Kristen noticed several errors in the assumptions used to develop the goals. Additionally, the goals seemed shortsighted and arbitrary.

Despite these issues, Leslie has received praise from her direct reports and colleagues, including the following comments:

- "Leslie is smart, and a great person to work with. She does not micromanage and is always available. She gives me constructive feedback and makes me feel that I am a valued team member. She is also a team player. I remember an instance during my first month working with her when one of the clinics asked me to do a data analysis that used software that I was unfamiliar with, and I had been working on it for hours and still couldn't figure it out. I finally went and talked to her about it, and she not only knew how to use it but also walked me through the process without ever making me feel stupid."
- "It was a pleasure having Leslie in our staff meeting today. She spoke clearly and perceptively about the issues facing our clinic. She knew the key issues we faced and the threats that we were seeing from our competitors. She advised us on clinic positioning for maximum growth and recommended several initiatives for both short-term and long-term growth, offering to develop and lead the implementation teams. We really feel like she helped us take a giant step forward."

Kristen believes that although Leslie has not performed up to expectations so far, she has a lot of potential. Kristen wants to retain and develop Leslie and give her some meaningful feedback.

Discussion Questions

1. Assume that the performance review is still a few days away. How should Kristen prepare for this meeting? Personally, how should she prepare to maximize the effectiveness of the review?
2. What additional information should Kristen have gathered before the meeting?
3. What could Kristen have done to prevent the current situation with Leslie?

4. If you were Kristen, how would you give feedback to Leslie? Outline an agenda for the performance review, and think about how you will discuss each agenda topic.

5. What reaction do you anticipate Leslie will have to Kristen's concerns about her performance, and how should Kristen respond to this reaction? Every story always has multiple sides, and this scenario is no exception. Kristen's perception of Leslie's performance may represent only a portion of a bigger story. How do you expect Leslie to talk about this situation?

6. How will Kristen determine if the performance review was successful? What outcomes should she expect?

References

American Nurses Association. 2012. *Bullying in the Workplace: Reversing a Culture.* Silver Spring, MD: American Nurses Association.

Baldrige Performance Excellence Program. 2013. *2013–2014 Baldrige Health Care Criteria for Performance Excellence: Category and Item Commentary.* Accessed January 2, 2015. www.nist.gov/baldrige/publications/hc_criteria.cfm.

Bazelon, E. 2013. "Defining Bullying Down." *New York Times.* Published March 11. www.nytimes.com/2013/03/12/opinion/defining-bullying-down.html?_r=0.

Boehl, S. 2008. "Keeping Forced Ranking Out of Court." *Training* 45 (5): 40–46.

Brewer, S. C., C. T. Kovner, R. F. Obeidat, and W. C. Budin. 2013. "Positive Work Environments of Early-Career Registered Nurses and the Correlation with Physician Verbal Abuse." *Nursing Outlook* 61 (6): 408–16.

Culbert, S. A. 2010. "Yes, Everyone Really Does Hate Performance Reviews." *Wall Street Journal.* Published April 11. www.wsj.com/articles/SB127093422486175363.

DeCenzo, D. A., S. P. Robbins, and S. L. Verhulst. 2013. *Fundamentals of Human Resource Management.* Hoboken, NJ: Wiley.

Deming, W. E. 2000. *Out of the Crisis.* Cambridge, MA: MIT Press.

Eichenwald, K. 2012. "Microsoft's Lost Decade." *Vanity Fair.* Published August. www.vanityfair.com/business/2012/08/microsoft-lost-mojo-steve-ballmer#.

Heery, E., and M. Noon. 2008. "Management by Objectives." In *A Dictionary of Human Resource Management*, second revised edition. Oxford, UK: Oxford University Press.

Joint Commission. 2014. "Prepublication Requirements: Revised Human Resources (HR) Chapter for Behavioral Health Care, Now Called Human Resources Management (HRM) Chapter." Issued June 20. www.jointcommission.org/assets/1/18/PrepublicationRpt_BHC_HRM_Run20140627.pdf.

———. 2008. "Behaviors That Undermine a Culture of Safety." *Sentinel Event Alert* 40. Published July 9. www.jointcommission.org/assets/1/18/SEA_40.PDF.

Krell, E. 2011. "An Impartial Review." *HR Magazine* 56 (10): 97–99.

Larson, J. 2013. "Bullying: A Persistent Problem in Nursing." RN.com. Accessed January 2, 2015. http://w3.rn.com/news/news_features_details.aspx?Id=41619.

Longenecker, C. O., and D. Gioia. 1992. "The Executive Appraisal Paradox." *Academy of Management Executive* 5 (2): 25–35.

Longenecker, C. O., H. P. Sims, and D. A. Gioia. 1987. "Behind the Mask: The Politics of Employee Appraisal." *Academy of Management Executive* 1 (3): 183–93.

Merriman, K. K. 2009. "On the Folly of Rewarding Team Performance While Hoping for Teamwork." *Compensation and Benefits Review* 41 (1): 61–66.

Novations Group. 2004. "Uncovering the Growing Disenchantment with Forced Management Performance Management Systems." White paper. Boston: Novations Group.

Pfeffer, J. 2009. "Low Grades for Performance Reviews." *Business Week*, August 8, 68.

Pfeffer, J., and R. I. Sutton. 2006. *Hard Facts, Dangerous Half-Truths, and Total Nonsense: Profiting from Evidence-Based Management.* Boston: Harvard Business School Press.

Scullen, S. E. 2011. "Why Do You Have a Performance Appraisal System?" *Drake Management Review* 1 (1): 8–11.

Smith, J. 2013. "How to Deal with a Bullying Boss." *Forbes.* Published September 20. www.forbes.com/sites/jacquelynsmith/2013/09/20/how-to-deal-with-a-bullying-boss/.

Snell, S., S. Morris, and G. Bohlander. 2015. *Managing Human Resources*, seventeenth edition. Boston: Cengage Learning.

Soderquist, K. E., A. Papalexandris, G. Ioannou, and G. Prastacos. 2010. "From Task-Based to Competency-Based: A Typology and Process Supporting a Critical HRM Transition." *Personnel Review* 39 (3): 325–46.

Stepanovich, P. L. 2013. "Pernicious Performance Appraisals: A Critical Exercise." *Journal of Behavioral and Applied Management* 14 (2): 107–39.

Taylor, L. 2009. *Tame Your Terrible Office Tyrant: How to Manage Childish Boss Behavior and Thrive in Your Job.* Hoboken, NJ: Wiley.

Welch, J., and J. A. Byrne. 2003. *Jack: Straight from the Gut.* New York: Warner Business Books.

Workplace Bullying Institute. 2014a. "The WBI Definition of Workplace Bullying." Accessed December 31. www.workplacebullying.org/individuals/problem/definition/.

———. 2014b. *2014 WBI U.S. Workplace Bullying Survey.* Accessed December 31. www.workplacebullying.org/multi/pdf/WBI-2014-US-Survey.pdf.

———. 2013. *2013 WBI Survey—Bullying by Industry.* Accessed December 31. www.workplacebullying.org/multi/pdf/WBI-2013-Industry.pdf.

———. 2012. *The WBI Website 2012-H Instant Poll: Workplace Bullying Perpetrators' Rank & Numbers.* Accessed January 18, 2015. www.workplacebullying.org/multi/pdf/WBI-2012-IP-H.pdf.

COMPENSATION PRACTICES, PLANNING, AND CHALLENGES

Bruce J. Fried and Howard L. Smith

Learning Objectives

After completing this chapter, the reader should be able to

- describe the purposes of compensation and compensation policy in healthcare organizations;
- distinguish between extrinsic rewards and intrinsic rewards and understand the value of each to employees;
- understand the concepts of balancing internal equity and external competitiveness in compensation;
- enumerate the objectives of job evaluation, and discuss the comparative merits of alternative approaches to job evaluation;
- articulate the challenges and problems faced in designing and implementing incentive programs; and
- see how different practice settings affect physician income and physician compensation strategies.

Introduction

People work for a variety of reasons, although they may not always be able to articulate them. Employee motivation has been studied for many years. Findings from research and practice suggest that several factors lead to job satisfaction and performance, including interest in work, competent supervision, and personal reward. Rewards include both intrinsic rewards, or the satisfaction and pride an individual takes in one's work, and extrinsic rewards, which are visible rewards such as pay, promotion, and benefits. Personal rewards may thus be both financial and nonfinancial in nature. Financial compensation itself can be broken down into direct financial compensation and indirect compensation, which includes health insurance, paid time off, and a variety of other benefits. Total compensation, which includes both direct and indirect forms, is normally addressed in discussions of compensation.

A healthcare organization's compensation system is one element of the overall motivational structure of the organization. An individual's motivation may be considered to be a combination of extrinsic factors, including such tangible rewards as compensation, and intrinsic factors, notably the satisfaction and self-fulfillment one feels as a result of the work. Although healthcare professionals are commonly thought of as driven by the satisfaction they get from their work, they are also influenced to work for and stay with the organization by the financial rewards they receive for their efforts. A good compensation system is particularly important in an industry such as healthcare in which professional shortages occur cyclically, leaving organizations to compete with other providers for the limited supply of applicants. Money does not explain all motivation, but it has a significant effect on the workplace. Employees draw conclusions about their own value to the organization on the basis of both the amount of compensation they receive for their work and how their pay compares to that of others. Compensation sends a powerful message to employees about what their organizations value. Employees focus on whether their compensation is comparable to the rates offered in the general market and the rates given to coworkers who perform the same job. A compensation system must be internally equitable; people should be rewarded according to a consistently applied methodology (discussed later in this chapter). However, a compensation system must also be externally competitive, that is, capable of successfully recruiting and retaining employees. Balancing these two goals is a constant challenge in all organizations.

Beyond issues of internal and external equity, an organization's compensation system must accomplish several objectives:

- It must fairly reward individuals for labor performed and expertise applied.
- It must align employee incentives with the goals of the organization.
- It should reduce or eliminate undesirable behavior—that is, practices that prevent the successful accomplishment of required tasks and achievement of objectives.
- It should have sentinel features to provide information about how job requirements and disciplines are changing and about the emergence of new jobs and disciplines. This requirement is particularly important in highly technical and dynamic industries, such as healthcare.
- It should be comparable to or even exceed the compensation systems of similar organizations in the market to give the organization a competitive advantage. This goal is especially critical in healthcare.

Healthcare organizations have unique characteristics and missions that set them apart from other organizations. Beyond achieving their own goals, healthcare organizations have a supplementary set of objectives related to improving population health and the processes used to deliver health services. Ideally, the design of compensation systems in healthcare encourages providers to engage in behaviors that improve health, such as fostering prevention and health promotion activities and complying with clinical guidelines. This goal is one of the bases for pay-for-performance plans in healthcare organizations. Compensation can also facilitate quality and process improvements, such as implementing electronic medical records and other innovations. Large healthcare organizations may also have a complex web of service lines, and each service line contributes in a different manner and to a different degree to organizational goals. This complexity raises a number of questions, not least of which is whether the organization should financially reward people differently if they work on particularly "valuable" service lines.

The healthcare sector presents other complexities and nuances that often are not encountered in other service or manufacturing sectors. First, a substantial number of healthcare employees are professionals with advanced education and training who must obtain and maintain licensure. Professional associations may exert an influence over expectations for compensation. Second, shortages of skilled professionals drive up salaries and wages, allowing healthcare professionals to enjoy both high mobility and lucrative compensation. In some instances, market forces drive up salaries and may create internal inequities and wage compression. Third, healthcare providers cannot always determine the price of services because of third-party payer reimbursement policies. Consequently, third-party payment confounds the need to meet rising wage and salary levels in the marketplace.

In sum, compensation is always at the forefront of human resources (HR) management in healthcare, requiring continuing vigilant attention. Healthcare managers can better respond to these challenges by understanding the basics of compensation planning and policymaking as well as the unique compensation needs of physicians and other healthcare providers.

This chapter reviews the strategic role of compensation, considers operational issues involved in determining individual compensation, discusses the need for healthcare organizations to establish a process for determining the monetary value of jobs, describes common forms of job evaluation, examines different types of incentive compensation, defines the challenges encountered in developing and implementing compensation plans, and analyzes compensation practices unique to physicians and other healthcare personnel.

The Strategic Role of Compensation Policy

An organization's compensation policy has an impact on multiple aspects of organizational performance and employee satisfaction and turnover. Employees cite a number of factors associated with their desire to stay with an organization, including specific job elements, such as responsibilities and challenge;

opportunities for professional growth; supervisors' behavior; the culture of the organization; and compensation. One's decision to stay with or leave an organization is complex and varies by the individual, and reliably predictive models remain elusive. A review of the literature on nurse turnover illustrates the complexity of the issue, and identifies compensation as one of several factors affecting turnover. Compensation remains important—including the competitiveness of compensation relative to other organizations—but is not the sole predictor of employee behavior. Figure 9.1 illustrates the major findings of this review.

In light of studies that confirm the importance but not the criticality of money in healthcare employees' decision to remain with their employers, organizations should develop a compensation policy that aims to enhance other employee motivators. In addition, this policy should align employees' efforts with the objectives, philosophies, and culture of the organization, highlighting and rewarding employees' contributions when organizational goals are achieved. A strategic compensation policy that balances individual needs with organizational interests typically includes the following goals:

- Rewards employee performance
- Achieves internal equity within the organization
- Maintains external competitiveness in relevant labor markets
- Aligns employee behavior and performance with organizational goals
- Attracts and retains high-performing employees
- Maintains the compensation budget within organizational financial constraints
- Complies with legal requirements

EXHIBIT 9.1
Research Findings: Retention of Experienced Nurses in Top-Performing Organizations

Nurse retention is a central issue in healthcare given the high cost of turnover, in terms of both cost and quality. Of particular importance is the retention of experienced nurses who possess substantial institutional knowledge and contribute positively to high-quality patient care. Today's hospital environment is characterized by higher patient acuity, fewer expert-level registered nurses (RNs) practicing at the bedside, and increased scrutiny of healthcare quality by regulators and payers. The situation is made more dire by the finding that about 55 percent of nurses plan to retire between 2011 and 2020.

A review article based on several studies conducted with the support of the Robert Wood Johnson Foundation (Hirschkorn et al. 2010) summarizes the key retention strategies of organizations that have had proven success with experienced nurse retention. These organizations include both healthcare and nonhealthcare organizations; however, the authors note the applicability of these successful strategies to healthcare organizations. Among

(continued)

the most important organizational practices are the following:

- Mentoring programs
- Alignment of compensation and benefits to support retention objectives
- Innovative phased-retirement programs
- Involvement of nurses in master planning and design
- Flexible benefits design tied to employees' life cycle
- Flexible work environments
- A business case for retention of experienced RNs

Noteworthy among these findings is the relatively small role played by compensation. This finding does not necessarily imply that compensation is not important; rather, it is consistent with the view of Herzberg that salary and what he termed "hygiene" factors were necessary to prevent dissatisfaction (Herzberg, Mausner, and Snyderman 1959). That is, adequate compensation is a necessary but insufficient tool to generate job satisfaction. Other factors considered to be motivational include intrinsic satisfiers, such as the sense of professional achievement and feeling of responsibility.

Focusing on the role of nursing leadership and nurse performance, Germain and Cummings (2010) identified several nonfinancial factors associated with nurse performance and found the following key predictors of nurse performance:

- Autonomy
  - "When nurse leaders express confidence in their subordinates' ability to perform at a high level, nurses feel empowered to perform" (Germain and Cummings 2010, 433).
  - "Empowered nurses are eager to implement evidence-based practices to ensure quality of care" (438).
- Work relationships
  - "Interpersonal relationships developed through good communication skills are related to effective nurse performance" (434).
  - "Nurses who felt that expectations were known and clear felt increased ability and confidence to perform their job well" (434).
- Access to resources
  - "Nurses who had increased access to information and resources had increased perceived work effectiveness" (435).
  - "When nurses have access to appropriate resources, such as necessary equipment, the availability of support services frees the nurse to plan, implement and evaluate care" (435).

These reviews and other studies demonstrate the importance of placing compensation in perspective: Fair and equitable compensation alone is not necessarily sufficient to generate satisfaction and retention. Particularly in a competitive labor market, multiple organizational factors may play a critical role in determining satisfaction and retention.

EXHIBIT 9.1
Research Findings: Retention of Experienced Nurses in Top-Performing Organizations *(continued from previous page)*

The strategic contribution of compensation is apparent in these goals. Compensation directly affects an organization's ability to achieve its fundamental mission and strategic objectives, to maintain fiscal integrity while delivering high-quality services, and to ensure customer satisfaction.

Compensation Decisions and Dilemmas

Strategic compensation goals may come into conflict in certain situations. For example, higher compensation offered to attract certain types of employees can disrupt internal equity. Recruiting physical therapists is a case in point. Physical therapists are in short supply in many parts of the United States (Zimbelman et al. 2010). As a result, some organizations may have to offer certain employees compensation packages that are inconsistent with existing pay rates in the organization. The discrepancy between an employee's worth (relative to other employees in the organization) and the amount that the employee is paid is often determined by the market. This conflict between the goals of internal equity and external competitiveness is one of the major challenges in establishing an enlightened compensation policy, a conflict that is particularly acute in healthcare because of periodic shortages of professionals. In certain communities where competition for employees is acute, organizations monitor compensation trends carefully (often on a weekly basis) for key professional groups.

Managers must make a number of other decisions when developing a compensation policy for their organization, which in turn may affect the goals and architecture of the organization's current compensation programs. First, a determination must be made on whether to pay above, below, or at prevailing rates; this decision may be made explicitly or implicitly. Typically, organizations earn a reputation for the level at which they pay employees. Second, the types of employee performance, practices, or contributions that are rewarded must be identified. This decision may seem trivial, but the factors chosen to be rewarded usually signal what the organization values. For example, annual raises that are not explicitly tied to performance tend to reward longevity and seniority in an organization, rather than performance. Rewarding longevity seems to contradict the general movement toward a value-based culture. On the other hand, retaining employees may be as important a goal as providing incentives for high performance. Retention bonuses in fact aim to encourage longevity in the organization.

The trend toward paying for performance is now well established in healthcare. The idea behind a pay-for-performance system is not only to compensate employees for their contributions but also to encourage good performance for the sake of maintaining and attracting high-level service

reimbursements for the organization. This system is being enacted in the hospital sector and is seriously discussed in seminars and formal education programs. One of the criticisms of organizational "reimbursement" for performance is that payers may be rewarding high levels of performance that are attributable more to environmental circumstances than to specific strategies undertaken by the organization to motivate high performance. Managers in poorly performing hospitals argue that punishing poorly performing organizations only reinforces historical inequities that may have caused differences in performance in the first place. The fact that organizational performance is affected by factors outside of the institution's control, such as being located in a community with high numbers of uninsured people, is well accepted. The dilemmas that plague organization-level pay for performance parallel those for incentive schemes for employees.

Among the first decisions necessary in designing a pay-for-performance system is establishing the performance criteria to be used in determining compensation. While criteria associated with productivity-oriented pay-for-performance policies are generally established internally, increasingly third-party payers are establishing pay-for-performance programs that tie financial incentives to meeting quality- or outcome-oriented goals using externally established criteria. These sometimes competing criteria can result in unanticipated consequences when certain aspects of performance are rewarded. For example, when excessive emphasis is placed on fiscal concerns, especially cost containment, an imbalance can result in other critical outcomes such as quality, access, and consumer satisfaction. Managers must therefore be especially vigilant about the causal relationship between compensation and outcomes. Careful attention is necessary when defining performance criteria, and caution is also critical when establishing prudent measures and data collection. Additionally, managers must extrapolate from intended policy to desired results and must anticipate dysfunctions associated with policy.

Other concerns are inherent when designing, improving, and implementing compensation programs:

- The worth of individual jobs must be determined.
- The value that an employee's education and experience contribute to the position must be assessed.
- Guidelines on keeping salaries and incentives confidential to the recipient and managers must be formulated and communicated to all concerned.

The point here is sobering: Developing and improving employee compensation policies and practices is a never-ending challenge. Changes in the marketplace, trends within the healthcare professions, redirection of organizational

goals and objectives, and other factors suggest that compensation policies and plans are seldom, if ever, stable, reinforcing the fact that compensation is a critical strategic issue in organizations.

Intrinsic Versus Extrinsic Rewards

Compensation should be considered in the context of the overall reward structure of an organization. Rewards can be intrinsic (internal) or extrinsic (external). *Intrinsic rewards* are largely intangible and may include recognition such as praise from a supervisor for completing an assignment or for meeting established performance objectives; it may also include feelings of accomplishment, recognition, or belonging to an organization. *Extrinsic rewards* are tangible (and viewing compensation from a "total compensation" perspective is important) and include direct monetary compensation (i.e., wages, salaries), benefits, payment for time not worked (e.g., vacation pay), and stock options. In today's environment, job applicants are extremely sensitive to the benefit structure offered, in particular health insurance. From the organization's perspective, the cost of indirect compensation is not trivial. In 2013, private industry employers spent an average of $29.63 per hour worked. Of this amount, 70.1 percent ($20.76) percent consisted of wages and salaries while the remaining 29.9 percent ($8.87) was for benefits (Bureau of Labor Statistics 2014).

Determining which type of reward drives each employee is difficult because in most instances employees are motivated by a combination of intrinsic and extrinsic rewards. In one early approach to defining reward systems and understanding motivation, Herzberg, Mausner, and Snyderman (1959) suggested that employees first must have their basic "hygiene" needs met. By "hygiene," they were referring to salary and decent working conditions. In their view, fulfillment of these needs does not produce employee motivation or job satisfaction but is a precondition that ushers in motivation. Thus, extrinsic "hygiene" rewards are necessary but insufficient elements for encouraging employees to contribute and subsequently feel a sense of accomplishment. The presence of extrinsic factors may prevent dissatisfaction but does not necessarily lead to satisfaction. This perspective is similar to Maslow's (1970) view that individuals must have their basic needs (biological and safety) met before they are able to achieve high esteem and fulfillment goals that are usually associated with high levels of engagement and performance. Managers, therefore, need to be cognizant of these two types of rewards and understand their functions and limitations.

The distinction between intrinsic and extrinsic rewards has substantial implications for managing healthcare professionals and support staff. Simply devising a well-orchestrated plan for compensation is not sufficient because pay in and of itself is only part of a complex equation that affects employee satisfaction. Managers must also attend to rewards that may not require

financial resources. Encouraging employees, establishing a collegial and safe practice environment, setting consistent performance objectives, and conducting periodic performance assessments are all strategies whose costs tend to be measured more in terms of time and commitment than in terms of direct financial expenditures. Assuming a prudent span of management, fiscally challenged healthcare providers can pursue these strategies in establishing a fertile reward environment. See Exhibit 9.2 for an example of balancing intrinsic and extrinsic rewards for academic physicians.

Low- or no-cost rewards are particularly of interest to nonprofit and financially stressed healthcare organizations with limited budgets. In these circumstances, managers should be especially mindful of the potential for

EXHIBIT 9.2
Balancing Intrinsic and Extrinsic Rewards in Academic Medical Settings

Academic physicians have traditionally been drawn to universities because of opportunities to combine education and research with clinical care. Fiscally strapped academic medical centers and schools of medicine have progressively asked faculty to provide more clinical service as a means to raise revenue. So-called revenue-based compensation (RBC) pays academic physicians according to the clinical revenue they generate, thereby raising faculty members' income as well as that of the medical center and rewarding physicians who generate high revenue.

Richard Gunderman (2004) of the School of Medicine at Indiana University argues that RBC is insidious as far as the intrinsic rewards of academic medicine are concerned. He underscores that RBC can distract faculty members and encourage them to focus on remuneration, eroding their commitment and loyalty to the academic mission. Specifically, potential erosion can occur under RBC in the following intrinsic rewards:

- Institutional prestige
- Intellectual discourse
- Opportunities for collaboration
- Quality of intellectual discourse
- Infrastructure

The end result is greater potential for faculty to migrate out of academic medicine.

The solution? Gunderman suggests that RBC plans should define revenue in measurable and objective terms, that expectations should be transparent, and that compensation plans should promote the mission of the medical school and the academic departments. As Natalia Fijalkowski and colleagues (2013) demonstrated in a study of ophthalmologists, otolaryngologists, neurosurgeons, and neurologists in the University of California healthcare system, incentives for high publication performance led to more academic productivity. This finding suggests that strategies addressing multidimensional objectives consistent with the complex missions of academic medicine will do more to ensure that compensation is balanced with intrinsic aspects of the academic role.

using intrinsic rewards to supplement limited extrinsic rewards. This delicate balancing point eventually may result in the perception among employees that their salaries are not comparable to the compensation given in competing organizations. How much imbalance staff members will tolerate is rarely certain. Fiscally challenged organizations need to pursue intrinsic rewards to the greatest extent possible to minimize turnover and its associated costs.

Internal Equity and External Competitiveness

As noted earlier, every organization must maintain a balance between internal equity and external competitiveness in its reward system. Equity theory (Adams 1963; Homans 1961) is a useful and well-tested framework for understanding the impact of perceived equity and inequity on individual motivation and performance. *Equity* is the perceived fairness of the relationship between what a person contributes to an organization (inputs) and what that person receives in return (outcomes). *Inputs* are such things as an individual's education, seniority, skills, effort, loyalty, and experience. *Outcomes* include pay, benefits, job satisfaction, opportunities for growth, and recognition.

According to equity theory, employees calculate the ratio, or balance, between their outcomes and inputs. They then compare their own ratio to the ratio of other people ("referent others") in their organization or another organization. Particularly where professionals are concerned, comparisons may be made to people who hold similar jobs in other organizations. For example, an operating room nurse in a hospital will likely compare his or her ratio with the ratio of other operating room nurses in the same hospital, with other nurses performing different tasks, with other types of staff members (to determine the comparability of their outcomes in relation to their inputs), and with nurses who perform similar work in other organizations. The result of this comparison is a belief by the employee that he or she is being treated either equitably or inequitably. Feelings of inequity create discomfort, and people naturally seek to restore a sense of equity or leave the organization (or field) for a more equitable situation.

Perceived inequity comes in two types. The more common phenomenon of *underpayment inequity* is a perception that occurs when an employee perceives that his or her ratio is smaller than the referent's. In such a situation, an employee is likely to attempt to restore a sense of equity either by decreasing inputs or by increasing outcomes received from work. With a perception of underpayment, employee motivation, morale, and performance are likely to decline (Bell 2011). *Overpayment inequity* is a person's belief that his or her ratio is greater than that of the referent. Depending on the person's predisposition, overpayment inequity may lead to feelings of guilt, which can result in efforts to restore equity such as putting in greater effort (Harris, Anseel, and Lievens 2008).

This comparing feature of equity theory is pervasive in all organizations. Consider, for example, the interest generated when the salaries of senior executives in *Fortune* 500 firms are publicized in the media. Of course, the comparative judgments made by employees may be highly subjective and based on limited or inaccurate information. Regardless of how subjective these assessments may be, managers must contend with these perceptions because motivation and performance are affected by perception, not reality. Managers must be attentive not only to *their own perception* of the fairness of the reward system but also to *employee perceptions* of the fairness or equity of rewards.

Healthcare managers face a substantial challenge in addressing pay equity. Salaries and wages in most healthcare professions are common knowledge because they are widely communicated for recruitment purposes. Consequently, some staff will allude to these differentials as a strategy to seek higher compensation. In addition to acknowledging these perceptions, managers can emphasize and develop the intrinsic rewards offered by their organization. This strategy may help to defuse that differential and encourage staff to focus on the bigger picture, an approach that is especially appropriate to the professions.

Equity issues are particularly troublesome because of shortages in certain healthcare professions. Newly graduated nurses, for example, may be hired at a salary level that approaches the compensation of seasoned and experienced nurses. While the experienced employee may have a cognitive understanding of the market-based reasons for this inequity, the impact of this inequity is likely to remain. Such an employee is faced with several choices: accept the situation, seek additional compensation, change jobs within the organization, take on additional responsibilities, or move to another organization to achieve the financial benefits of being newly hired. In some markets, job hopping is a tried-and-true method of increasing one's compensation.

As mentioned earlier, employees who perceive inequity may attempt to equalize the situation in two ways: (1) increase their outcomes or (2) decrease their inputs. Increasing their outcomes can be accomplished by working harder, and perhaps as a result, the employee will obtain additional compensation or a promotion (note that working harder may also increase the inputs side of the ratio); by organizing other employees, possibly in the form of unionization; and by engaging in illegal activities, such as theft or false reporting of hours worked. The second approach, decreasing inputs, can be accomplished through working fewer hours (e.g., coming in late, leaving early, being absent) and putting forth less effort. Employees may also attempt to restore a sense of equity by changing their perceptions of the inputs or outcomes of others. For example, an employee may convince herself that her referent employee has more experience and is therefore entitled to a higher level of rewards. Similarly, an employee may conclude that while his salary may be lower than that of a referent, working conditions are much better at his organization than at the other organization. In other instances, employees may simply change their frame of reference—that is, they may change the person with whom they compare themselves.

While organizations seek to ensure internal equity, they must also pursue external competitiveness to recruit staff. To be externally competitive, organizations must provide compensation that is perceived to be equitable to the salary given to employees who perform similar jobs in other organizations. If an organization is not externally competitive, it is likely to face problems of turnover and staff shortages, particularly in geographic areas where the supply of certain professionals is scarce. Healthcare employers have traditionally faced tight labor markets for physicians, nurses, and medical technicians, which lead to difficulty in attracting and retaining these and other clinical providers. This competition results in an ascending spiral of wages, salaries, benefits, and other forms of compensation that the market cannot afford and that inflates organizational cost structures and eats away at margins. In such a situation, emphasizing intrinsic rewards or intangible incentives can contribute to attracting and retaining high-quality staff.

When confronting a tight labor market, organizations should formulate specific strategies to position themselves in the labor market. As far as pay is concerned, these positioning strategies typically follow a quartile strategy. An employer that pays at the second quartile is paying the market rate, and implicitly believes that this strategy enables the organization to balance employer cost pressures while also attracting and retaining employees. On the other hand, a pay follower employs a first-quartile strategy, choosing to pay below-market compensation. Employers take this position for several reasons. First, shortage of funds or an inability to pay more may converge with the need to continue to meet strategic organizational objectives. Second, if a large number of applicants with lower skills are available in the labor market, this strategy can be used to attract sufficient workers at a lower cost. A major disadvantage of using a first-quartile strategy is high turnover, and, if the labor supply tightens, the organization may have difficulty attracting and retaining workers. Quality-of-care ramifications in nursing homes that operate in the lower quartile are illustrated in Exhibit 9.3.

A third-quartile strategy, in which employees are paid at above-market value, is more aggressive. This strategy may be used to ensure that a sufficient number of employees with the required capabilities are attracted and retained; it also allows an organization to be more selective. However, the expectation in most organizations is that employees who are paid above-market rates must be more productive and must deliver higher-quality services and products.

Mohr and colleagues (2004) studied nursing homes in the lowest tier — that is, facilities that house mainly (> 85 percent) Medicaid residents. They note that nursing homes with high proportions of Medicaid patients have correspondingly fewer resources to hire staff and that poor, frail, and minority residents in these facilities tend to receive substandard care. In particular, their analyses suggest that staffing intensity is statistically lower in Medicaid-dominated nursing homes. Fewer RNs are found on staff in lower-tier nursing homes, but not fewer licensed practical nurses. This finding led the authors to conclude that less-expensive and less-qualified staff are used as substitutes for higher-trained staff by fiscally constrained Medicaid facilities. Physician extenders and administrators are also less prevalent in lower-tier nursing homes.

Quality-of-care indicators suffer in lower-tier nursing homes, according to the study. Medicaid-dominated facilities report higher incidences of pressure ulcers, higher use of physical restraints, and higher use of antipsychotic medications. Clearly, poor quality of care is associated with restricted use of RNs as well as limited administrative resources and physician extenders. Mohr and colleagues (2004) acknowledge that lower staffing intensity is accompanied by fewer resources to hire and train clinical and administrative staff. In sum, economic constraints lead to higher turnover, lower retention, and ultimately lower quality of care.

EXHIBIT 9.3
Quality-of-Care Ramifications of a Low-Quartile Position

Determining the Monetary Value of Jobs

Job evaluation is a formal process for determining the monetary value of jobs. Development and maintenance of an intelligent wage-and-salary system begin with accurate job descriptions and job specifications for each position. This information is used to perform job evaluations and to conduct pay surveys. These activities ensure that a pay system is both internally equitable and externally competitive. Data gathered in the job evaluation process and pay surveys are used to design or improve pay structures.

In theory, job evaluation is used to obtain an objective assessment of a job's worth or contribution to the organization. This level of contribution is then translated into monetary terms. After this monetary value is determined, compensation levels are typically adjusted to better reflect market compensation levels (Martocchio 2011). However, in tight labor markets, the use of job evaluation information for setting compensation levels may be limited. In certain types of jobs, information from wage and salary surveys may be the dominant or sole method used to set compensation levels. Periodic job evaluations may be conducted, but over extended periods (often, several years), salary decisions may be made almost exclusively on market information. Smaller organizations are also likely to use market data for compensation decisions. This discussion of job evaluation, therefore, needs to be placed in the context of volatile and unpredictable labor markets.

In a job evaluation, a job is examined and ultimately priced according to each job's relative importance to an organization; the knowledge, skills, and abilities each job requires; and the difficulty of each job. The premise of a job evaluation is that jobs that require greater qualifications, involve more responsibility, and assign more complex duties should pay more than jobs with lower requirements or lesser tasks. Job evaluation is also a way of ensuring that employees perceive equity in the compensation system. To motivate staff, a fair pay value must be assigned to each job.

When conducting a job evaluation, benchmark jobs are identified. These benchmarks require similar knowledge, skills, and abilities and are performed by individuals who have been assigned relatively similar duties. Benchmark jobs are used to establish a basis on which other comparable jobs are evaluated.

Methods of Evaluating Job Value
Ranking

Perhaps the simplest job value assessment technique, the ranking method lists jobs in order of their inherent value to an organization. The entire job, rather than individual components of the job, is considered. Those who rank jobs use their judgment when ranking, and consequently this method is extremely susceptible to subjectivity. Managers may have difficulty explaining why one specific position is ranked higher than another. Additionally, this method is cumbersome to use in large organizations because of the sizeable number of jobs in such institutions.

Job Classification Systems

Job classification systems categorize jobs on the basis of predetermined requirements based on *compensable factors*. A compensable factor is a job element that is essential for effectively doing a job. These elements may include skill requirements, working conditions, educational requirements, responsibility, supervisory responsibilities, and decision-making autonomy. Compensable factors are established by the organization, as are the relative weights assigned to different factors. Jobs are then evaluated and rated according to the level of compensable factors in the job. In other words, the organization does not pay for the job, but pays for the compensable factors present in the job.

In a job classification system, jobs of similar value (as determined by an evaluation of compensable factors) are slotted into groups. Jobs within a group are paid at an established rate, with adjustments made for such factors as tenure in the organization. The job classification method is most common in the public sector. In the US government, jobs are classified according to the federal government's General Schedule (GS) of 15 grades (special provisions are made for jobs above a GS-15 rating). In the GS system, each job is classified into one of these grades on the basis of eight compensable factors: difficulty and variety of work, supervision received and exercised, judgment exercised, originality required, nature and purpose of interpersonal work relationships, responsibility, experience, and knowledge required. Each grade is associated with a salary range, which varies by geographic location.

Similar to ranking, job classification systems are subject to considerable subjectivity and are vulnerable to manipulation. Jobs can be misclassified, or perceived as misclassified, because of assumptions made by the job analyst. Job classification is problematic when applied to multisystem organizations because two jobs with the same title may entail very different responsibilities in different settings. For example, RNs in a skilled nursing facility perform roles that are substantially different from those performed by RNs in an outpatient surgery center.

Broadbanding

Job classification systems assign jobs to categories known as pay bands. The *broadbanding* approach to compensation is a response to the constraints imposed by rigid classification systems. For example, if someone's job is classified as a "band 3" in a job classification system, asking this person to take on responsibilities above his or her pay grade without adjusting the salary would be difficult. Traditional classification systems have narrow pay ranges for jobs classified in a particular band. In a job classification system with many pay bands, an employee's maximum compensation may be limited by this narrow salary range. If the employer wishes to provide additional compensation to an employee who assumes new responsibilities or learns new skills, traditional classification systems provide little flexibility in how this person is compensated; promotion to a new position and reclassifying the position are the main options. Broadbanding collapses multiple salary bands into fewer bands with larger salary ranges (Giancola 2009), such that jobs in these broader bands are more varied and exhibit wider pay ranges. This potentially provides greater flexibility for the organization and employee.

A broadband is a single, large salary range that spans pay opportunities formerly covered by several separate small salary ranges. Numerous jobs and salary levels can be included within a single broadband. A major advantage of broadbanding is that it provides more flexibility when managing an employee's compensation within a particular pay range. Levels of compensation can be changed without the necessity of changing job titles or reclassifying jobs. Individuals can be moved between jobs without concern for dramatic changes in salary. For example, an employee may be reluctant to move into another position because of the possibility of a salary decrease. With broadbanding, both jobs may be in the same salary range, allowing for stability in salary. Employees can also be more easily rewarded within a broad pay grade for taking on new responsibilities or obtaining new skills. In a work environment characterized by flatter organizations, promotional opportunities occur less frequently. For the employee, a broadbanding approach may be helpful in redefining career growth from a traditional approach based on promotions to one based on acquiring new knowledge and skills (O'Neil 2012).

Broadbanding may be especially appropriate because it is consistent with trends toward flatter, less hierarchical organizations and the use of cross-functional job positions. Cross-functional positions enable organizations to respond quickly to competitive pressures. With broadbanding, employees can more easily shift responsibilities as market and organizational requirements change. Broadbanding offers several potential advantages. First, it may enable organizations to base compensation decisions on the characteristics of people who perform jobs rather than on the characteristics of the job alone. Second, authority for compensation decisions is largely decentralized to operating managers. Therefore, managers can more easily gain approval for changes in compensation because broadbanding enables them to reward employees without going through the myriad justifications required in a traditional classification system. Additionally, the wider spread between pay grades gives managers more flexibility to recognize and reward different levels of individual contribution. Third, because broadbanding results in fewer pay groupings, job evaluation is potentially simpler because organizations no longer need complex job evaluation schemes. Managers can encourage employees to move into other job areas that may broaden their knowledge, skills, and abilities. Broadbanding also allows employees to evaluate their own skill acquisition and cross-training opportunities in terms of professional development and personal growth, rather than focus on pay grades.

Broadbanding, however, is not appropriate for every organization and organizational culture. The narrow range of the traditional pay system may serve as an automatic cost-control mechanism that keeps compensation expenses in check. With broadbanding, all employees may potentially float to the maximum pay level within their band, resulting in higher-than-market compensation for many or most employees. New employees who replace those with seniority may discover that they are paid at significantly lower levels, an artifact of time on the job of their more senior counterparts. However, such an explanation may provide little solace. Perceptions of inequity may become an irritant and may lower morale.

The most difficult aspect of implementing broadbanding is helping employees to think differently about how they are paid. Pay grades have long been used to determine status, titles, and eligibility for perquisites. Consequently, employees sometimes have difficulty relinquishing these preconceptions. Broadbanding also implies fewer upward promotion opportunities. With a smaller number of bands, employees recognize that promotions to a higher grade level will occur less frequently than before. Employees must assume significantly greater job responsibilities to warrant placement in a higher band.

Point System

The point system is a widely used job evaluation tool and is compatible with job pricing methodologies and competency-based pay (Kilgour 2008). As with job classification systems, a basic assumption behind this method is that organizations do not pay for jobs but for specific aspects of these jobs, known as *compensable factors*. Examples of compensable factors include knowledge and skill requirements, job experience, accountability, supervisory responsibilities, and working conditions. These compensable factors are determined through job analysis and are then assigned values or weights—points—based on the extent to which each factor is present. Compensation levels and pay ranges are then linked to these points, although actual compensation for a particular job may vary based on market and other factors.

The point method is popular because it is relatively simple; is based on job analysis; may be used for many jobs; and, once established, is relatively easy to update. However, this method does have several drawbacks, including the amount of time needed to develop the system and the tendency to reinforce traditional organizational structures and job rigidity. Furthermore, as discussed earlier, compensation levels for particular jobs may be based more on salary survey data than on the results of job evaluation. Often, significant differences exist between compensation levels derived from job evaluation and compensation levels according to market pay rates.

Following are the general steps in developing and implementing a point system:

1. Compensable factors must be acceptable to all parties.
2. Compensable factors must validly distinguish among jobs.
3. Compensable factors must be relevant to the jobs under analysis.
4. Jobs must vary on the compensable factors selected so that meaningful differences in jobs can be identified.
5. Compensable factors must be measurable.
6. Compensable factors must be independent of each other.
7. Job evaluation and market pay rates must be reconciled.

Implementing the point system requires a number of key steps, with some variation in how each step is carried out (see, for example, Dessler [2014, 2–15] for a 16-step methodology). An initial step in implementing a point system is the identification of compensable factors, and this important procedure is generally done by a committee. Weights are then assigned to each compensable factor on the basis of the value of the factor to the organization. Each factor is then assigned degrees, which define the extent to which a job contains a particular factor. Each degree is then assigned a point value. Exhibit 9.4 provides a simplified example of a point system. After the points are developed, jobs are evaluated according to the point system. Jobs may then be arrayed on a wage curve, which shows the relationship, based on current wages, between points and salaries. Some jobs will fall above and others below the wage curve, and decisions need to be made about how to reconcile jobs that are out of line. In some cases, a job needs to be above the wage curve because of market forces. In other instances, a job that appears below the wage curve may need to have its salary adjusted upward for equity purposes.

Factor Comparison

The factor comparison method is a combination of the ranking and point methods. It differs from point systems in that compensable factors for a job are evaluated against compensable factors in benchmark jobs in the organization. Benchmark jobs are important to employees and the organization, vary in their requirements, have relatively stable content, and are used in salary surveys for wage determination.

Benchmark jobs are typically evaluated against a set of compensable factors, such as skill, mental effort, physical effort, responsibilities, and working conditions. A pay rate is assigned to each compensable factor for each benchmark job. For example, the job of an emergency room (ER) nurse may be identified as a benchmark job. Analysis determines that of the $28 hourly

EXHIBIT 9.4
Hypothetical
Points
Allocated in a
Point System

Factors	First Degree	Second Degree	Third Degree	Fourth Degree	Fifth Degree
Educational requirements (500 maximum points)	100	250	350	450	500
Supervisory and delegation responsibilities (200 maximum points)	0	100	160	180	200
Working conditions (170 maximum points)	50	100	140	160	170
Customer interactions (130 maximum points)	15	80	120	125	130

wage paid to an ER nurse, $10 is paid for mental effort, $5 for responsibility, and so forth. Similarly, we may use a hospital medical technologist's job as a benchmark, and we may decide that of the $26 hourly wage paid to this individual, $7 is paid for mental effort, $5 for responsibility, and so forth. A factor comparison scale is developed to evaluate other jobs in the organization. Thus, to evaluate the job of an occupational therapist, the mental effort, skill, and other factors of that job are compared to that of the ER nurse and the medical technologist.

Key advantages of the factor comparison approach are that it can be tailored to one organization and it indicates which jobs are worth more and how much more, making factor values more easily converted into monetary wages. Disadvantages of this method include complexity, time required to establish comparable factors, and difficulty explaining the methodology to employees.

Market Pricing

The approaches to valuing jobs discussed in the previous section focus almost exclusively on ensuring equity within the workplace. However, healthcare organizations are also almost always heavily dependent on labor supply and market wages, as well as the role of unions. Thus, market information should always be included in compensation decisions. Ideally, the wages in an organization take into consideration the objective value of jobs as well as market considerations. Managers learn about market wages largely from salary surveys carried out by organizations, the government, associations, and external consulting firms. These surveys are helpful in ensuring that an organization's wages do not fall too low or too high relative to other organizations. The Bureau of Labor Statistics conducts annual surveys on area and industry wages as well as surveys of professional, administrative, technical, and clerical positions. Private consulting firms that conduct salary surveys include the Hay Group, Heidrick & Struggles, and Aon Hewitt. The Society for Human Resource Management and Financial Executives International also conduct wage surveys. In the healthcare sector, the American Hospital Association conducts a series of annual wage and salary surveys. The Internet may also be used to obtain market salary information; see, for example, salary.com, a website that provides market information for a variety of jobs across industries.

Limitations of market pricing of jobs include questionable methodologies that may be used to obtain salary information. Relying on the market to set compensation can also lead to wide variations and fluctuations in salary as shortages ebb and flow. Furthermore, using job titles to inform compensation rates may not take into consideration the wide differences in actual job responsibilities across organizations, which may result in misleading information about appropriate salary levels.

Variable Compensation and Performance-Based Pay

While the need for flexibility in compensation structures has been mentioned, the discussion thus far has addressed compensation in a relatively static manner. This section discusses variable pay, which is often linked to performance metrics. Performance-based pay is not new; the history of pay based on incentives is long. Straight piecework, where employees are paid based on each unit produced, is perhaps the most well-known type of plan. In fact, fee-for-service (FFS) medicine has many piecework features. Piecework also has many variations. For example, under a differential piecework system, employees who produce higher than the standard output receive a higher rate of pay for all of their work. Piecework is attractive because it is easy to implement, assuming that the units of output can be easily measured, when quality is less important than quantity, when the work is standardized, and when a constant flow of work can be maintained. Healthcare organizations frequently violate these assumptions; quality *is* critical, and the work is often unpredictable and therefore less standardized than work in other settings. Compensation systems based on individual productivity may create dysfunctional competition and inhibit cooperation among employees. Also, when employees are focused on volume, the competition generated by piecework may work against a culture that emphasizes cooperation and teamwork (Gómez-Mejía, Balkin, and Cardy 2012, 368–69). Furthermore, employees may be skeptical of piecework because they may perceive that management is arbitrarily raising production targets without a commensurate increase in compensation.

Commission-based pay is another traditional method of incentive compensation, and is most commonly used in sales. Such plans are usually combined with a salary plan. Commonly used systems also include lump-sum merit pay, where a bonus does not alter an individual's base pay. Merit-based pay has numerous problems, including the expectation that merit pay will always be awarded, and the pervasive problem of identifying valid measures of performance.

Company-wide compensation arrangements, whereby individuals receive rewards based on company-wide performance metrics, also have a substantial history. Profit-sharing plans distribute a predetermined percentage of an organization's profits to employees, while gain-sharing plans reward employees for improving productivity, reducing costs, or achieving other company objectives.

Team-Based Incentives

Healthcare providers increasingly structure service delivery around work teams, causing HR managers to consider compensation systems that reward team performance. Team-based rewards can be used to boost productivity and performance, improve quality and customer service, and increase retention. Unfortunately, the actual development of team-based compensation systems is often constrained by the need to reward individual performance. Among the challenges faced in team-based incentive compensation is whether to provide the same-size reward for each member or variable-size rewards for different members depending on such factors as contribution, seniority, and skill levels.

For example, a care delivery team made up of an obstetrician, a case manager, a social worker, and a nurse's aide may be rewarded for a productivity outcome of delivering more infants, experiencing minimal adverse cases, and receiving high patient satisfaction. What level of reward should be assigned to the team? What percentage of the respective base salaries of each team member will the reward constitute? Will inequities in rewards cause some team members to work less in achieving team objectives? These questions are representative of those that must be addressed before a team-based compensation system is implemented.

Healthcare organizations that are interested in rewarding team performance need to strike a balance between individual rewards and team rewards. Paying the same amount to everyone on the team regardless of a team member's competencies or contributions may create pay-equity problems. It also may be unpopular with high-achieving employees, who may feel that the team has free riders and that they are carrying the weight for the team. Team incentives are most commonly incorporated as variable pay—that is, a team-based incentive is added to base pay. While base pay is determined by job evaluation and market information, variable pay is added according to team performance.

Skills-Based or Competency-Based Pay

In skills-based compensation systems, employees are paid according to valued work-related skills and competencies that they develop while in the organization. An important rationale for using competency-based pay is that it addresses the issue of rapid changes in the content of jobs. Where jobs are dynamic, rewarding employees on the basis of blocks of relevant skills may be more useful than relying on a soon-to-be-obsolete job description. Competencies may be defined broadly and could include such areas as technical skills, leadership, and acquiring licensure or certification. Note that this approach is also consistent with broadbanding, where employees can earn increases in compensation by acquiring new packages of knowledge and skills. Typically, employees begin at a base pay level and are given the opportunity to increase their compensation by acquiring new skills, knowledge, or competencies, thereby making themselves more valuable to the organization (Martocchio 2011). The reward structure of this approach is based on the range, depth, and types of skills that individual employees possess. Compensation is increased after an employee demonstrates the ability to perform specific, desired skills. Competency-based pay differs from a point system in that point systems focus on the value of the job, while competency-based pay focuses on the value the employee adds in supporting the organization (DeCenzo, Robbins, and Verhulst 2013).

This compensation approach is based on the idea that employees with a broad range of skills allow the organization more flexibility in deploying its staff. Typically, an employee is hired and is provided training for that job. The employee may then join a work team and be given the opportunity to learn new skills through additional training and on-the-job experience. As the employee learns new jobs, his or her compensation is increased. This approach reinforces the concept of the autonomous work group, where members work interdependently.

Skills-based pay can follow a stair-step approach, in which a logical, well-defined progression is followed in skills development. Pay is increased as skills are mastered. A job-point accrual model is used when the organization has a variety of jobs for which an employee may be trained. Jobs are given a point rating that is based on the difficulty of mastering job skills, and compensation is increased in accordance with points earned. A cross-department model is one in which employees may be trained to work in jobs in other parts of the organization, and compensation increases as the employee masters these jobs (Gómez-Mejía, Balkin, and Cardy 2012, 336).

A challenge in skills-based pay is the need for appropriate training to facilitate skill acquisition, and, of course, the system needs to be adequately funded. A promising application of skills-based pay in healthcare is related to generational differences between baby boomers and generation Y employees. In comparison with earlier generations, generation Y employees tend to be less dedicated to the organization but more interested in personal professional development. Therefore, a skills-based compensation model, in which employees are rewarded for obtaining additional competencies, may be more motivating than a compensation model based only on rewarding one's current skills (Haeberle 2014).

Pay for Performance in Healthcare

Pay-for-performance systems are built on the principles that good work deserves to be rewarded and that pay based on good work produces improved performance. In a pay-for-performance system, managers evaluate the work of their employees according to preestablished goals, standards, or company values. On the basis of this judgment, employees are given variable or contingent financial rewards. Individual compensation is directly linked to personal performance and attainment of objectives consistent with the organization's mission. Alternatively, individual rewards may be linked to team, department, or organizational performance.

Reward systems in healthcare organizations are increasingly reflective of transformations in how health services as a whole are being financed. Methods of payment for healthcare services in the United States are undergoing great change, with a continuing transition from volume-based FFS payment to a system based on value and outcomes. Hospitals are under increasing pressure from payers to achieve outcome targets, and parallel developments have occurred in physician compensation, which has seen a transition from volume-based to process- and outcome-based compensation. Bonus-type compensation structures have also shifted to ones in which providers' revenues are earned. Known as value-based systems, these approaches put some financial risk on providers, and seek to reduce medical costs and improve patient outcomes. These value-based approaches have been adopted by Medicare as well as selected commercial payers (Madden 2013). Financial incentives are also embedded within the Affordable Care Act.

Healthcare organizations continue to move toward network models, exemplified by the concepts of medical homes, accountable care organizations, and physicians who are aligned with the goals and interests of the organization and network. Payers, including Medicare and commercial payers, are establishing accountable healthcare contracts with hospitals, and hospitals, in turn, are applying these same accountability concepts in their contracts with physicians. This accountability translates into compensation models that incorporate quality outcomes, patient satisfaction measures, and other metrics. Notwithstanding these trends, quality metrics remain a relatively small part of physician compensation. According to a 2012 estimate, primary care physicians derived only 3 percent of their total compensation from quality metrics (Beaulieu 2013). However, the trajectory is moving toward systems in which a larger proportion of physician payment is linked to performance metrics rather than to current FFS metrics (Herman 2014). For example, a physician search firm reported that in 2013, 39 percent of its search assignments that offered a production bonus also included payments based on quality metrics (Beaulieu 2013). A long list of quality metrics may be used in physician compensation, including participation in the incentive programs for meaningful use of health information technology, the use of e-prescribing, participation in the Physician Quality Reporting System, and measures of patient satisfaction. Several classic studies of physician compensation models are described in Exhibit 9.5.

As noted earlier, pay-for-performance systems in healthcare are moving toward a value or quality focus. Seeking to align physician or organization incentives with the delivery of high levels of care, *quality-focused pay for performance* has increased greatly since the late 1990s; however, it is still far less common than productivity-focused pay for performance (Beaulieu 2013). Pay-for-quality programs reward activities and practices that are likely to improve healthcare outcomes, including increasing the use of prevention

EXHIBIT 9.5
Financial
Incentives
for Physician
Productivity

While the area of physician compensation and productivity has been dynamic and controversial, several earlier studies shed light on physician interests and concerns related to compensation. The results of these studies remain relevant as we consider ways in which to reward physicians in a manner that aligns their interests with those of the organization while also abiding by their professional interests.

In 2002, Conrad and colleagues explored the relationship of financial incentives with physician productivity in 102 medical groups and 2,237 physicians in the Medical Group Management Association (MGMA). The sample is admittedly a small proportion of MGMA's membership of 5,725 practices at the time of the study (out of 19,478 medical groups in the United States); however, the advantage of this study group is the valuable information it supplied on resource-based relative value scale units established in 1997. Data were derived from MGMA's annual surveys—the Compensation and Production Survey and the Cost Survey.

The conceptual basis underlying this study relates back to a seminal analysis that Gaynor and Pauly (1990) completed on medical group partnerships. These researchers discovered that physician productivity is extremely sensitive to individual compensation. Tying compensation completely to productivity (i.e., productivity determines 100 percent of a physician's total salary) increased productivity by 28 percent. In practical terms, physicians respond favorably to incentive-based compensation.

Conrad and colleagues' findings reaffirm those of Gaynor and Pauly. Physicians in medical groups that base pay on individual performance are more productive than physicians not practicing in large groups. Moreover, the results suggest that bonuses heighten the productivity effect. The individual characteristics of the physicians also play a role in responses to incentives, according to further in-depth study. Physician experience is associated with modest increases in productivity. Gender appears to have some impact, although the statistical results in the Conrad study are affected by the fact that female physicians tended to work fewer hours per week than did their male counterparts.

With respect to productivity pay in large groups, Rosenthal and colleagues (2006) documented in a national study of health plans that 52.1 percent used pay for performance. However, HMOs (health maintenance organizations) that did not require patients to designate primary care providers (PCPs) were less likely to implement pay for performance. The Rosenthal study, like that of Conrad and colleagues, suggested that large group size is correlated with pay for performance because of the presence of administrative infrastructure to implement the system.

Turning to incentive effects on each group as the unit of analysis, the findings suggest an inverse relationship with group size—that is, as the size of groups becomes larger, the impact of incentives dissipates. The sense of participating in a cohesive, close-knit professional team seems to be adversely affected by a larger number of providers. In effect, physicians may

(continued)

be less motivated psychologically because they are only one provider among many in a large group practice, possibly leading them to remain at the average production capacity rather than strive to exceed this average. These findings are important because they indicate that large, vertically integrated delivery systems can be inimical to high productivity.

Conrad and colleagues' study has important practical implications for all healthcare providers. It infers that production of services is linked to the availability of incentives. As healthcare costs continue to escalate and healthcare organizations seek higher productivity from clinicians, the scope and depth of incentive compensation plans will likely continue to grow.

EXHIBIT 9.5
Financial
Incentives for
Physician
Productivity
*(continued from
previous page)*

screenings, ensuring up-to-date patient vaccinations, investing in information technology designed to reduce medical errors, and consistently adhering to evidence-based medical guidelines. By improving outcomes, quality-focused pay-for-performance programs hope to produce healthier and more satisfied patients and ultimately reduce costs.

Evidence that quality-focused pay-for-performance programs have been effective at giving physicians or organizations the incentive to improve quality levels is modest at best. Among the most notable successful examples is the large demonstration program by the Centers for Medicare & Medicaid Services (CMS), which showed moderate quality improvements (Lindenauer et al. 2007). Despite the limited evidence, pay-for-quality programs remain of great interest to both private and public third-party payers, both of which are expected to continue to experiment with the system to find the formula that will achieve desired outcomes. Notably, the Deficit Reduction Act of 2005 mandated that CMS implement value-based pricing in hospitals for Medicare patients by 2009. As Petersen and colleagues (2006) showed in a systematic analysis of 17 studies addressing the association of pay for performance and quality, and as Hartmann and colleagues (2012) showed in a study of healthcare-associated infections in Medicare and Medicaid patients, considerable work needs to be done to properly understand the possible unintended effects of incentive pay on quality care.

Several researchers and commentators have raised significant questions about the relationship between pay-for-performance and healthcare quality (Carroll 2014; Lee et al. 2012; Bardach et al. 2013; Werner et al. 2011). While some studies show modest improvements in quality, improvements are often short-lived and inconclusive. Changing physician behavior is a complex endeavor, and factors affecting patient outcomes, such as income, housing, and education, are frequently outside of the control of physicians. Furthermore, pay-for-performance systems risk being detrimental as physicians respond to financial rewards at the expense of intrinsic motivations (Carroll 2014) and may in fact have detrimental effects (Rangle 2010; Woolhandler and Ariely 2012). Like all people, physicians have complex motivations, and simply offering financial incentives for higher quality (or productivity) may not actually cause the intended outcome.

Furthermore, implementing quality-focused pay for performance is complicated and can be expensive. Clearly, for such a program to be effective, the magnitude of the incentives must exceed the costs incurred in meeting the program's targets. These costs can be considerable and may include designing new procedures, training employees on their implementation, and collecting data on process and outcome measures necessary to support the program's reporting requirements. The latter often involves substantial investment in information technology development and support. Additionally, the cost of unreimbursed time that physicians, nurses, and other staff must spend with patients to implement new procedures or to carry out necessary administrative tasks must be considered. For this reason, hospitals and large practice settings with extensive management and information technology support are generally in a better position than smaller physician practices without such resources to successfully implement this type of pay for performance. Another complicating factor is that most physician practices have contracts with multiple third-party payers, each of which places unique demands on the organization.

Notwithstanding questions about pay for performance, quality-focused pay for performance will continue to merit significant management attention for the foreseeable future. Exhibit 9.6 highlights the experiences that some practice executives have had in implementing pay-for-performance programs.

Criticisms of Pay for Performance

Some argue that pay-for-performance systems increase quality differentials, decrease the focus on customer needs, increase the loss of accurate information about defects and improvement opportunities, discourage achievement of stretch goals, reduce risk taking and innovation, and discourage cooperation (Milkovich, Newman, and Gerhart 2014). These disadvantages have been cited because pay-for-performance systems may make the supervisor the most important customer; under these circumstances, employees play to their supervisors rather than to external customers or patients. Also, paying a bonus for doing less—that is, providing only necessary evidence-based care—can be politically awkward even if doing less means a better outcome (Gosfield 2004).

The system may also deprive providers of essential information because managers learn less about defects and changes that need to be made. Under a pay-for-performance plan, employees may be reluctant to report problems because doing so may have a negative impact on their compensation. Pay-for-performance approaches may also encourage employees to set lower goal

Although no clear formula has yet emerged for giving healthcare providers an incentive to improve quality of care through pay-for-performance programs, an examination of the role that practice executives play in the implementation of these programs may be instructive. Practice executives are administrators responsible for negotiating quality targets and incentives with health plans. They are responsible for implementing pay-for-performance programs in their organizations. The implementation decisions they make can affect the success of these programs.

To this end, Bokhour and colleagues (2006) conducted a series of qualitative interviews with practice executives from 69 physician organizations in Massachusetts. These practice executives were responsible for implementing pay-for-performance programs that affected more than 5,000 primary care physicians. The findings of this qualitative study outline the careful and detailed consideration that must be given to program implementation:

- Practice executives indicated that physicians find quality-oriented incentives to be better aligned with their inherent desires to provide high-quality care than were productivity- or utilization-oriented incentives.
- Practice executives did not come to a general agreement that the incentives motivated individuals to achieve quality improvement goals.
- Several issues may explain the failure of pay-for-quality programs to achieve their goals:
  - Physicians said that some measures used were outside of their scope of control. For example, measures for achieving a certain level of preventive screenings relied on patient cooperation.
  - Physicians said that data recording and reporting for the programs were inaccurate or did not represent a true measure of quality. Additionally, these measures lagged behind current clinical or state-of-the-art practices, creating a conflict that reduced the power of the incentives.
- The method of distributing rewards affects the power of the incentives to motivate change. For example, distributing rewards equally to all physicians is much less motivating than distributing rewards based on each physician's achievement of goals. The latter method, however, was sometimes found to be unfair in cases where several physicians were involved in the treatment of a particular patient but only one of them got credit toward program measures.
- Some organizations recognize that delivery of quality care depends not only on physicians but also on the active participation of all members of the practice. These organizations choose to retain program rewards for reinvestment in infrastructure that facilitates delivery of quality care rather than for distribution to individuals. While reinvestment provides no direct incentives to the individual, this system is a move toward improving quality through system-level changes. Still, other organizations create a balance by using a hybrid approach to distributing rewards. That is, some of the reward is reinvested and some is given to individuals to motivate provider-level change.

EXHIBIT 9.6
Practice Executives' Experiences with Implementing Pay-for-Quality Performance Programs

aspirations. When goals are set in advance, employees may argue for less ambitious goals instead of stretch goals to ensure that they receive performance-related rewards. Finally, pay-for-performance systems may hamper change because innovation disrupts tried-and-tested ways of delivering services, thus lowering efficiency and affecting goal accomplishment. This effect is especially detrimental in healthcare because constant breakthroughs in performance require substantial changes in the way employees do their work (Berwick 1995; Pfeffer 1998). Pay-for-performance plans may discourage risk taking and reduce creativity because the fear of not getting the reward may make people less inclined to take risks or explore alternative approaches to work. Thus, the efficacy of incentive plans is a topic of considerable debate.

In addition, pay for performance may be viewed as inconsistent with the trend toward transparency. Pay-for-performance programs create an arrangement between payer and physician to accomplish a task, such as increasing the rate of generic prescriptions. However, this goal may be hidden from the consumer, who may have no idea that the physician is given an incentive to prescribe generics to meet some predetermined goal. Consumerism in healthcare depends on creating a transparent process—the consumer must have a full understanding of how and why the physician is acting in a certain way. As a result, pay for performance may actually slow the complete adoption of transparency in healthcare.

Those who support incentive plans point to the fact that most people are, in reality, motivated by money. In other words, most people would rather have more money than less money; therefore, money can be used to change employee behavior. Supporters of pay for performance assert that behaviors that are rewarded are repeated and behaviors that are not rewarded (or punished) are eliminated. Therefore, when rewarding behaviors, organizations must ensure that all relevant aspects of behavior are measured. Incomplete measurement may result in incomplete performance, with employees only doing tasks or engaging in behaviors that are rewarded. Rewards also provide an opportunity for management to communicate values to employees.

In sum, pay for performance in healthcare and the use of this strategy as a managerial policy for stimulating desired behaviors and outcomes have faced much criticism. Recognizing that the healthcare field will continue to evolve in incentive payment designs, Van Herck and colleagues (2011) outline a series of 23 necessary steps in implementing a pay-for-performance system using the Model for Implementing and Monitoring Incentives for Quality (MIMIQ). Their approach includes identifying priority quality dimensions and priority patient groups, identifying a suitable combination of structure, process, and outcome variables, and considering key points in developing the incentive structure. Pay for performance is not a panacea. However, if these 23 steps are properly orchestrated, healthcare executives, providers, and organizations may be able to position themselves to better achieve accessible, low-cost, high-quality care.

The Future of Variable Compensation Arrangements

In an effort to achieve greater levels of effectiveness and efficiency, new compensation arrangements will likely continue to emerge in healthcare. In particular, pay-for-performance programs will evolve as third-party payers develop a formula that provides an incentive to healthcare providers to deliver higher quality. Change can be good, but healthcare managers should proceed cautiously because compensation is a highly charged topic. Tampering with compensation arrangements can have disastrous effects, so consequences cannot be overlooked or underestimated. Nonetheless, the difficult constraints that bind healthcare providers call for taking bold action. Perhaps the most important element in ensuring success in this regard is to involve employees at all levels in the design and implementation of compensation plans. In this way, the plan is more effective and meets broader acceptance.

Special Considerations for Compensating Physicians

Before World War II, most physicians were general practitioners who delivered care in independent practices on a fee-for-service basis (Starr 1982, 198–235). Medicine was considered one of the more successful cottage industries. This practice changed radically after the war, with the emergence of medical subspecialties nurtured by battlefield needs, the rise of care within hospitals instead of at home, and the advent of employer-based medical insurance. Once consumers of care (patients) were no longer directly responsible for the cost of care they received, payers of the services (i.e., employers or government) and providers of care (i.e., physicians) were no longer obliged to justify costs to consumers. The checks and balances that typically exist in any economic interaction were lost. The result was a system that paid physicians whatever they requested, without the system attempting to validate the appropriateness of those services. This series of events led to the managed care movement (Burchell, Smith, and Piland 2002).

With the development of managed care, attention shifted to using payment mechanisms as a means to modify clinical behavior. Analysts have expressed widespread concern globally that the use of medical evidence in decision making is frequently lacking. For example, two patients with the same condition may receive vastly different therapies, or two patients with distinct diseases may be treated virtually the same. Allowing for the "art of medicine" does not explain the inconsistent use of clinical practice guidelines that have been shown to improve outcomes. Furthermore, variation in practice is widespread and is not linked to medical differences in populations. Two adjacent communities, with similar populations and demographics, may have dramatically different rates of surgery or use of certain modalities. Scientific justification for such discrepancies usually does not exist, suggesting that variations in care come from physician choice and habit, not medical data.

A key objective of health policy in the early 1990s was to leverage reimbursement mechanisms to address variation in treatment processes and outcomes. However, the track record for reducing practice discrepancies or improving practice behaviors since that time has been disappointing. Modifying physicians' forms of reimbursement has been a notable failure. Capitation is a system that pays a physician a certain amount for each patient assigned to his or her panel or list of patients. The fee is meant to cover professional services required to care for each patient. The challenge for the practitioner is to provide these services within the limits of capitated payment. As an incentive, any funds left over after delivering care revert to the physician as revenue. Capitation was initially seen as an incentive to physicians to perform the appropriate level of care without generating excess costs.

In contrast, FFS encourages the use of (and reimbursement for) excessive services and the tendency to neglect preventive measures. The argument was that compensating physicians a set amount per patient (a capitated payment) would encourage them to do as much as possible to keep patients healthy, thereby avoiding the need for expensive services. The Achilles' heel of capitation was that it put physicians at risk when they treated patients who had preexisting conditions or medical predispositions over which physicians had no control. Capitation also rendered physicians responsible for patients whom they had never seen before. While many physician groups initially were enthusiastic about accepting risk payment, mainly because of the increased payments it brought, they usually failed to understand the full implications of being responsible for a population versus caring for individual patients.

Bankruptcies of medical groups were not uncommon because of their inability to manage the very problems with physician behavior that capitation was supposed to solve. As a result, risk payment methods became increasingly unpopular as a payment option. Because of capitation's inability to change practice patterns (Grumbach et al. 1999; *Managed Care Outlook* 1999) and its adverse impact on both physician group viability and the willingness of groups to participate in such plans, other compensation approaches have surfaced.

An important element that affects the potential for compensation models to change behaviors is the continued growth in physician income. In the early 1990s, the general belief was that by putting the brakes on the rise in salaries, physicians could be brought in line with the directions that health plans and employers wanted them to go. This concept is frequently referred to as *aligning incentives*. However, numerous studies have demonstrated the ability of physicians to continue to increase their incomes in spite of cost-control measures; the target-income hypothesis addresses this effect (Folland, Goodman, and Stano 2012, 305–8).

The ability to increase volume even as the cost per unit decreases has largely protected most physicians from experiencing radical shifts in income. Furthermore, unlike other professions, in medicine an increased supply of physicians has actually led to higher levels of health spending. Unlike in other industries in which more suppliers typically result in lower overall costs and revenues, in healthcare, competition has had minimal impact on total costs.

Payment Mechanisms Associated with Practice Settings

Most variations in how doctors are paid come from the settings in which physicians practice or are employed. Each setting offers benefits and drawbacks to compensation, depending on the goals of the particular practice. To provide an understanding of how practice settings will continue to evolve in the future, a look at how they developed is instructive.

Office Practice

Three broad categories of office practice are solo practices, group practices, and independent practice associations (IPAs). One practitioner defines a solo practice, and a group practice is composed of two or more physicians who have established a legal entity to deliver care together. An IPA usually consists of a collection of practices, including both solo and group practitioners, that join forces in taking advantage of economies of scale for contracting, business services, or ancillary services (such as laboratory). The IPA may negotiate on behalf of its practitioner members, and typically it has signature authority to establish contracts and distribute reimbursements.

Office-based physician practice is the classic model in which two or more physicians work together in an office setting. The degree of affiliation between the physicians can range from tight to very loose. A closely knit group comprises physicians who have a common philosophy and approach and who may share both business and clinical functions. A loosely connected group is made up of physicians who share office services, such as clerical and billing, but who practice independently in all other regards, especially concerning fiscal matters.

For solo and group practice physicians, the dominant reimbursement mode is pure FFS and salary plus incentive. Over the preceding ten years, fee schedules used in determining payments have been significantly reduced by private payers and government payers. An unintended, but not unexpected, consequence has been an increase in utilization of services so that even as the price of each unit of service has declined, the number of units provided has increased. This increase in service has further resulted in higher incomes for physicians in many specialties even as fee schedules are driven lower. As fee schedules are lowered, or discounted, physicians have an incentive to increase volume to make up the difference in their income.

IPAs may seek risk contracts from a payer, particularly if the IPA is large and well integrated. This approach implies a shared philosophy of care among physicians, with a high degree of self-discipline. Such groups actively monitor utilization internally, usually comparing it to national standards and scientifically validated treatment guidelines. Physicians who deviate significantly from these norms are either reeducated by their peers or are asked to leave the group. Frequently, a sophisticated information-gathering system is in place within the group to facilitate monitoring of outcomes and utilization. Information allows a group to control costs and to maximize efficiency. This system creates a climate for accepting financial risk.

Few IPAs have the ability to accept significant risk projects and make them work. More typical is the IPA that is paid from a discounted FFS schedule and has some sort of incentive program to add dollars to the total reimbursement for the group. Such incentive plans may award a portion of any savings to physician members if the group achieves targeted utilization in areas such as pharmaceuticals and lab tests. Incentives may consist of simply a bonus, or they may be more complicated. Money may be put aside to be shared if targets are met, or a percentage increase in the fee schedule may occur if the group successfully manages its patients. The key point is that incentives are designed to encourage the group to perform at a higher level, but regardless of the success in reaching these goals, the physicians are still paid for each service provided.

Staff Model

Some medical groups or HMOs employ physicians on a straight salary basis or staff model—a model common in the late 1970s and early 1980s. Many early HMOs, such as Prudential and Humana, formulated the staff model as their primary method of caring for their members. Under the staff model, physicians employed by a care delivery organization are not distracted by concerns of generating revenue to cover practice expenses. They are able to focus on practicing medicine.

This model presents several drawbacks. One in particular is the difficulty of recruiting physicians who want to be employees. Most physicians enter medicine to practice independently, not to be under an employer's control. Despite having an employed group of doctors who theoretically have personal goals that are aligned with those of an organization, many HMOs found physician utilization to be as high and as variable as the use of physicians in private practices. The work ethic of employed physicians was a significant factor in determining the fiscal success of the staff model. Many medical directors of staff-model HMOs were frustrated by the difficulty of motivating salaried physicians to extend themselves beyond prescribed hours and tasks. As a result, the staff model withered. However, the model is still a force in California, Colorado, Georgia, Hawaii, and Ohio because of the strong presence of Kaiser Permanente, a staff-model organization. The era of the salary-based physician practice has seen better days, as noted in Exhibit 9.7.

Hospital-Based Physicians

A large cadre of physicians—hospitalists, pathologists, radiologists, and anesthesiologists, among others—practice almost exclusively within the confines of nonacademic hospitals. In the past, many were directly employed by hospitals and received a straight salary. However, these physicians have started to form professional corporations that contract with hospitals for services, often on an exclusive basis. For instance, a hospital may contract to have services provided by a group of emergency medicine physicians. This group staffs the emergency room, is paid on a contractual basis, and may even take over the administration of the unit. The basis for the contract is typically some formula that represents the billings that the unit generates, with an additional amount included for such items as administration and participation on hospital

---

EXHIBIT 9.7
Fallout from the Demise of Staff-Model Groups

For several decades, the Group Health Cooperative of Puget Sound, a staff-model HMO based in Seattle, Washington, has participated with several other HMOs in providing managed care data for public health research. The advantages of a defined population and provider group offered by Group Health Cooperative have enabled health services researchers to suggest policy improvements in care delivery. Breast cancer screening, sexually transmitted disease, adverse pharmaceutical effects, smoking mortality, and periodic health checkups illustrate areas to which health research has contributed to improved service delivery.

The HMO research network concept has been supported by staff-model groups, including the Meyers Primary Care Institute (Massachusetts), Group Health Cooperative, Harvard-Pilgrim Health Care, HealthPartners (Minnesota), Henry Ford Health System (Michigan), Kaiser, and Prudential. These groups have progressively improved their data systems to the point that large-scale collaborative investigations have been facilitated. Research has focused on both quality of care and fiscal issues.

The US healthcare industry has seen a growing transition to IPAs—network organizations where loosely affiliated physician groups do not have strong incentives to partake in research. Cost-savings concerns by IPAs further diminish the potential for research because less investment is made in data systems. Thus, the clinical fallout from the demise of staff-model groups is decreased availability of high-quality data for disease management.

committees. The same model can apply to other specialties as well. The key interaction from a reimbursement perspective occurs between the administrators of the hospital and the physicians' organization. The doctors function as independent contractors within the hospital; they are "in it" but not "of it."

The scenario changes somewhat for physicians in academic, tertiary care medical centers. Several unique aspects of these institutions must be considered. A large percentage of physicians in an academic setting are in training as residents or fellows. Their salaries are paid in large measure from Medicare reimbursements received by the medical center for the purpose of supporting graduate medical education. Thus, their salaries are not linked to their clinical performance, number of patients seen, rate of procedures performed, or other measures of productivity or quality. For staff or faculty physicians, salary is also the rule (because typically these physicians receive a straight salary that is not based on productivity), although the role of clinical activity is often figured into it.

The mission of the academic physician may be summarized as a combination of teaching, research, and patient care. With decreased reimbursements to hospitals, the need for these physicians to perform more clinical work has grown. This increase in clinical work may or may not be accompanied by an increase in salary and often depends on whether a "faculty practice plan" exists. A *faculty practice plan* is essentially a group practice that comprises the faculty of the medical center. It was created as a way to leverage the billings generated by faculty into some sort of shared distribution or at least to negotiate a higher salary for physicians who produce high clinical volumes. The amount of additional income flowing from the faculty practice plan is usually not great except for subspecialties; the principal source of income for an academic physician remains the salary from the institution. These salaries are invariably lower than those in the private-practice sector and reflect the typical differential for salaries between the academic and commercial environments.

Some physicians within the academic setting may see no patients at all and focus entirely on research. Many of them derive the bulk of their salaries from grants they secure from outside agencies; the remainder may come from the university. As a result, the longevity of a researcher in this environment may well depend on his or her skill at preparing grant applications and performing research worthy of outside support.

Locum Tenens Physicians

A growing mode of practice for physicians is working in a temporary staffing arrangement, or locum tenens. *Locum tenens physicians* are temporarily employed physicians, who are typically paid a fixed amount for services provided. This trend has been linked to the increase in female physicians, the persistence of physician shortages, the growth in the number of partially retired physicians, and the lifestyle considerations favored by new physicians (Darves

2011). Physicians move into these arrangements through personal contacts, advertisements, and assignments from a physician staffing agency. When a physician is hired through a staffing agency, payment for physician services is made directly to the agency, generally on a fee-per-day basis. The use of locum tenens physicians is likely to increase because of the flexibility this system affords to both the physician and the organization. This work arrangement is also part of a significant national trend across all industries—the use of contingent workers.

Leaders, Administrators, and Experts

Within the last decade, the number of physicians who are employed full-time as medical directors, consultants, and administrators has increased. Aside from those who work for managed care organizations, health insurers, and large provider groups, many physicians are employed by organizations that want to better understand and control the resources they devote to employee healthcare benefits. These physicians fill critical roles as internal experts on medical care and health policy. As such, they are attuned to the unique problems of their employer and are able to help benefits coordinators and HR administrators address complex employee health coverage issues. They also serve as liaisons between the benefits/HR personnel and external vendors such as health plans, provider groups, and ancillary providers.

Medical directors are also increasingly employed by state and federal agencies. As healthcare costs continue to escalate, this trend in the employment of physicians as policy experts and liaisons will likely evolve. Medical directors are typically salaried and are given the same sorts of benefits and incentives offered to executives in most companies.

Difficulties and Conflicts in Compensating Physicians

The most contentious issues that employers face with salaried physicians, whether in an academic medical center, a provider group, or a hospital system, are the same as for any other employees: benefits, perquisites, and salaries. A difficult challenge in determining physician pay is assessing the parameters based on productivity. Even for a medical group of two physicians, the potential exists for disagreements over what constitutes productivity levels. The following illustrate the complex issues behind the arguments:

- If a patient new to the practice is "counted" at a higher value than a returning patient, what defines a new patient? Someone who has never been seen before? Someone who has not been seen within a given time frame? Someone who has not been seen for a nonacute visit?
- For a procedure-based specialty, such as gastroenterology, does the physician who performs the procedure get full credit, or should partial credit go to the physician who has seen the patient most frequently over the past year?

- For an obstetric practice, should the physician who performs more vaginal deliveries (which represent more time) receive more credit than the physician who has a higher rate of cesarean section operations (which produce higher revenue)?

The details or fine points of a case may seem unimportant, but they are worth careful consideration because they are linked to a dollar value. This value can make a significant difference in overall compensation for a physician. Add elements such as seniority in the group, the number of call days taken, or outside activities such as service on hospital or medical society committees, and one can appreciate the dilemma many practices face in dividing up practice revenues.

Many medical groups have attempted to address these problems by designing formulas that incorporate multiple contributing factors to be considered when calculating compensation. By their nature, these formulas can become extremely complex in that they try to account for unrelated items that are often difficult to accurately measure. For example, a surgical group may try to include the number of patients seen with weightings based on the severity of procedures performed, coverage in the emergency room, teaching residency at the medical school, and number of holiday calls taken. Such projects take an inordinate amount of time to devise but typically end up affecting only a small fraction of the total income of the physician. A further problem is the inability of any complicated payment scheme to either reinforce behavior desired by the practice or to extinguish undesirable behavior. Problems in defining incentive pay systems are further described in Exhibit 9.8.

While employed physicians in large medical groups may not be directly affected by such productivity questions, groups are highly dependent on medical staff members for their contributions in attaining efficiency while upholding high quality of care. For many groups that went on a hiring binge in the mid-1990s, as well as hospitals that adopted practices to lock in patient referrals, the assumption often was that employed physicians would maintain the same high productivity rates they delivered when they were self-employed. However, many physicians sold their practices to reduce their workload, leading to a dramatic drop in patient volumes. As a result, healthcare organizations that employ physicians have been faced with large deficits from their staffs of providers, which have led to severe financial strains.

Future Directions for Physician Compensation

The current framework for compensating physicians has not substantially changed medical practice. The advent of capitation and the use of incentives were assumed to initiate a revolution in how physicians treat patients as well

EXHIBIT 9.8
Trends in
Physician Pay
Systems

Epstein, Lee, and Hamel (2004) cite the increasing prevalence of pay-for-performance schemes for physicians. They observe that physicians are more likely to experience schemes that encourage them to improve quality of care and patient satisfaction than utilization. Despite the relatively unsophisticated nature of these approaches (often based on questionable patient survey data), the authors conclude that the magnitude of financial incentives for physician performance is growing. They review three examples to illustrate the diversity of physician compensation approaches.

1. *Bridges to Excellence.* At its start, General Electric (GE) and other employers in Massachusetts partnered with Tufts Health Plan, the Lahey Clinic, and Partners HealthCare to create an incentive program for healthcare providers. Bridges to Excellence is a set of programs intended to reward physicians, nurse practitioners, and physician assistants who meet established performance standards. Among the Bridges to Excellence programs are those related to asthma, depression, cardiac care, diabetes, and medical home standards. The physician office systems program provides rewards for the use of evidence-based standards of care, maintenance of patient registries, the use of electronic patient records, and the interoperability of these electronic systems. Bridges to Excellence has three levels of recognition for each program, with multiple rewards such as fee schedule increases (Healthcare Incentives Improvement Institute 2014).

2. *Integrated Healthcare Association's Physician Payment Program.* Six health plans in California, known as the Integrated Healthcare Association, issue a physician performance scorecard incorporating four measurement domains: clinical quality, patient experience, meaningful use of information technology, and resource use. The program developed a common measure set totaling 62 measures recommended for payment and 48 additional measures for collection and internal reporting. Clinical quality measures focus on the six priority areas of prevention, cardiovascular, diabetes, maternity, musculoskeletal, and respiratory conditions. Participants include about 200 physician organizations representing 35,000 physicians. This incentive plan was estimated to result in the distribution of more than $500 million between 2004 and 2013 (Integrated Healthcare Association 2014).

3. *Anthem Blue Cross and Blue Shield Plan Anthem Quality-in-Sights.* This New Hampshire health plan rewards physicians on the basis of clinical quality measures related to preventive care and screening, care management, technology adoption, external recognition, and resource utilization. Clinical quality measures were developed from several sources including HEDIS (Healthcare Effectiveness Data and Information Set), National Quality Forum, and the Ambulatory Care Quality Alliance. Rewards are given based on the number of points accrued from these measures (Anthem Blue Cross and Blue Shield 2012).

as how physicians would be paid for their services. After years of continuing change in the healthcare industry, the vast majority of practicing physicians continue to be paid on some sort of FFS basis or salary plus incentive. Therefore, new compensation methods are necessary to transform patterns of medical practice. Proposed changes to medical care delivery cannot be successful unless physicians support them. This support depends on making certain that physicians are fairly and adequately compensated.

In the coming years, more opportunities for innovation will surface as the healthcare field searches for new paths to follow. These opportunities for change include the following:

- *Physicians will become more creative in defining their fee and payment structures.* Leaders in this area have been cosmetic surgeons, who have always been paid out-of-pocket for the bulk of the work they do. They were among the first physicians to make payment for services with credit cards possible and to set up payment schedules in advance of surgery. While these payment options were commonplace in the rest of the economy, in medicine they were revolutionary.

- *Reproductive endocrinologists are now asking for an up-front fee—say $30,000—to cover three cycles of in vitro fertilization.* If the patient does not conceive at the end of the third cycle, the fee is refunded except for a small amount to cover costs. Patients are thus provided with a quasi money-back guarantee. By seeking flexibility in payment, recognizing that their services are expensive, and making services more accessible to those without insurance coverage, these specialists have found new ways to secure their revenue stream.

- *Americans spend billions of dollars per year on complementary and alternative medicine modalities, such as acupuncture, massage therapy, homeopathy, and biofeedback, with much of this expenditure being paid out-of-pocket.* The public seems to have an insatiable demand for these therapies, and physicians will seek to capture some of this huge volume of care by offering more alternative medicine options within the context of traditional medical practices. Because this care occurs outside of a fee schedule negotiated with a payer, it may well come to represent a large portion of some doctors' incomes in the future.

- *For physicians who are still paid primarily by third-party payers, reimbursement will be tied to performance.* Tools for assessing outcomes of care tied to such parameters as use of various treatments and revenue generated will increase in number and utilization. However, indications from practice suggest that the complexity of physician compensation systems will moderate. Structures that incorporated patient satisfaction, committee assignments, and governance service proved to be too complex to measure and administer. Instead, report cards on doctors' practice patterns and performance will become more widely available. Just as consumers now go to a variety of sources, especially the Internet, to research the purchase of a new car or house, they will increasingly be able to do the same for selecting their physicians and hospitals. Providers who perform at a high level will be paid at a higher level than those who do not perform as well.

- *Employers will continue to reduce their role as the primary source of health insurance for their employees.* Individual patients/consumers will consequently be increasingly accountable for making the kinds of healthcare choices currently left up to benefits managers at work. Having this freedom to choose will require consumers to become more educated in managing their own health. This change will be facilitated by the creation and availability of thousands of websites devoted to medical topics as well as consumer-oriented information regarding physician quality and costs. Additionally, new business models for healthcare delivery (retail health clinics, for example) will arise in response to consumer-driven healthcare. These new business models will bring new competitive pressures to bear on some traditional physician practice settings. To succeed in an environment in which patients are more informed and discriminating consumers of healthcare services, physicians will need to provide a level of service and quality that represents superior value to patients as the ultimate payer. This ability to attract and retain patients will have a direct bearing on physician income. Physicians able to deliver superior value will see their revenues increase, while others will see their practices wither. Price will certainly be part of this value equation, and physicians will need to respond to price in ways they have never contemplated.

- *Physicians have become extremely entrepreneurial.* This change has led to a substantial increase in the number of outpatient and ambulatory centers that provide services that have traditionally been delivered in hospitals. The common scenario is that the physician has an ownership interest in the center and receives not only the professional fee for the service but also a share of the income that the facility generates. The physician also receives income from testing and diagnostics. This trend is occurring in virtually all markets in the United States and across many specialties, and it has greatly enhanced the income of entrepreneurial physicians and shifted much of the delivery of routine and complex care. As a result, for these physicians, income derived directly from patient encounters is decreasing and being replaced by the large revenues from their ambulatory center partnerships and procedures.

Summary

As pressures for control of costs and improved quality continue to drive the healthcare system, new methods of paying for health services will continue to be implemented. A key problem from the past decade of experimentation is the lack of a clear consensus on which compensation models work under different circumstances. Research is at best inconclusive, owing in part to the large variation in clinical settings and populations.

While evaluation of different compensation models will continue to be important, research in this area is difficult. Among the problems confronted in conducting valid research in compensation are developing measures of quality that are sensitive to the actions of physicians and other healthcare team members; ensuring that data to evaluate different compensation systems are valid and reliable; designing appropriate risk adjustment mechanisms; implementing research designs that have a level of consistency to enable comparisons among different clinical settings; and resolving fundamental questions about the nature of motivation and incentives. Furthermore, the ethical problems that emerge as a result of systems that reward clinical behavior and decision making through financial mechanisms will need to be considered.

Discussion Questions

1. Assume you are a manager at a low-budget healthcare setting (e.g., local health department). What will you do to recruit new staff and to motivate current employees when competitors in the area are able to pay 30 percent to 40 percent more than your organization can?

2. Assume that you are a staff nurse in a hospital that uses an incentive compensation system. Do you have an obligation to disclose the nature of the compensation arrangement to patients? If so, how should this information be communicated and by whom?

3. Regardless of your personal feelings about pay for performance, what cautions will you communicate to a team that is designing an incentive system in a healthcare organization?

4. How will you design a team-based compensation system such that free riders (or loafers) on the team cannot take advantage of the system?

5. How can job evaluation procedures be used to determine if a healthcare organization is undercompensating its female employees?

6. What are the likely roles of capitation and FFS reimbursement in the future?

7. For a four-person surgical group, what kind of formula may be devised to fairly and consistently measure and reward productivity? What changes may be needed if one surgeon decides to perform more office work and less surgery?

Experiential Exercises

Case   Mapleton Family Medicine is a physician group practice located in a small city (population 150,000) in the Midwest. Mapleton is an eight-physician practice consisting of family physicians, internists, and pediatricians. The practice is owned by two of the physicians; the other six physicians are salaried. The owners are concerned with productivity and quality in the practice. The waiting time for appointments is relatively long, and a recent chart review revealed that the percentage of children who are up-to-date with immunizations has dropped. Also, anecdotal evidence suggests that at-risk persons are not routinely receiving flu and pneumonia vaccinations. Many patients have complained about having to wait up to 90 minutes in the waiting room. At this time, however, the practice is not in a position to hire another physician.

Each physician in the practice sees an average of 25 patients per day. The owners want this number increased to 30 patients per day without sacrificing quality of care. To reach this goal, they are thinking of moving to an incentive system whereby physicians have a base salary equivalent to 75 percent of their current salary and have the opportunity to earn up to 125 percent of their base salary if they meet defined volume and quality goals. While the owners have not completely thought this system through, they want to set 30 patients per day as a base and, through the incentive system, encourage physicians to see, on average, up to 35 patients per day.

In terms of quality, the owners have considered three measures:

1. Patient satisfaction surveys
2. Child immunization audit data
3. Patient waiting times

Quality goals will be set biannually for each physician. The expectation is that physicians who achieve these goals will earn their full salary (assuming volume is adequate), and quality measures above these goals will result in bonuses according to a pay schedule.

Case Questions

1. You have been brought in to advise the owners on their proposed compensation plan. What advice will you give them before they proceed?
2. Do you see any potential negative consequences of this plan based on the information provided? If so, how will you address these concerns?
3. How do you think the physicians in the practice will react to this plan? Should they be involved in developing the plan, and if so, how should they be involved?

Project   As noted in the chapter, healthcare organizations are faced with the challenge of balancing internal equity with external competitiveness. In this exercise, compare two organizations' approaches to setting salary levels. Your first task is to identify two healthcare organizations that are similar in mission and size. For example, you may select two medical group practices, two medium-size community hospitals, or two nursing homes of similar size. You may choose two organizations in the same geographic area and labor market or two that are in different markets.

Your second task is to identify the senior HR executive or the individual most closely involved in developing and implementing the compensation program in the organization. You will interview this person, so this person will need to understand the compensation philosophy, system, design, and decision-making process. The goal of this exercise is to identify the organization's compensation strategy, including its approach to balancing competing compensation objectives.

Your third task is to summarize the compensation philosophy, policy, and practices in each organization and write a report on the similarities and differences between the two compensation systems.

Questions to Guide a Compensation Comparison

1. What is the policy of the organization on compensating employees at market rates? Does the organization have an explicit policy to pay below market, at market, or above market? Does the approach vary by the type of employee and the particular labor market?

2. Does the organization have a specific strategy for attracting, recruiting, and retaining employees in difficult-to-fill positions? If so, for which positions has the organization encountered these issues? What strategies have been used in these circumstances? Examples include (but are not limited to) sign-on bonuses, retention bonuses, paying above-market rates, and employee referral programs.

3. How does the organization evaluate jobs—that is, how does it "price" jobs? Does it conduct a formal job evaluation process? If so, how often and under what circumstances? Do any jobs exist for which the market dictates the salary, rather than the salary being the result of a job evaluation process?

4. Does the organization face any of the following problems? If so, how does the organization address them?

   – Wage compression
   – Employees "topping out" of their salary range
   – High prevalence of employee departures because of compensation-related factors
   – Perceptions among employees that aspects of the compensation system are unfair

References

Adams, J. S. 1963. "Toward an Understanding of Inequity." *Journal of Abnormal and Social Psychology* 67 (5): 422–36.

Anthem Blue Cross and Blue Shield. 2012. *2013 Quality-in-Sights Primary Care Quality Incentive Program*. Revised December. www.anthem.com/provider/noapplication/f5/s2/t0/pw_e192610.pdf.

Bardach, N. S., J. J. Wang, S. F. De Leon, S. C. Shih, W. J. Boscardin, L. E. Goldman, and A. Dudley. 2013. "Effect of Pay-for-Performance Incentives on Quality of Care in Small Practices with Electronic Health Records: A Randomized Trial." *Journal of the American Medical Association* 310 (10): 1051–59.

Beaulieu, D. 2013. "Building Compensation Plans in a Pay-for-Performance Era." *Medical Economics*. Published November 25. http://medicaleconomics. modernmedicine.com/medical-economics/content/tags/compensation/ building-compensation-plans-pay-performance-era.

Bell, R. L. 2011. "Addressing Employees' Feelings of Inequity: Capitalizing on Equity Theory in Modern Management." *Supervision* 72 (5): 3–6.

Berwick, D. M. 1995. "The Toxicity of Pay for Performance." *Quality Management in Healthcare* 4 (1): 27–33.

Bokhour, B. G., J. F. Burgess Jr., J. M. Hook, B. White, D. Berlowitz, M. R. Guldin, M. Meterko, and G. J. Young. 2006. "Incentive Implementation in Physician Practices: A Qualitative Study of Practice Executive Perspectives on Pay for Performance." *Medical Care Research and Review* 63 (1): 73S–95S.

Burchell, R. C., H. L. Smith, and N. F. Piland. 2002. *Reinventing Medical Practice: Care Delivery That Satisfies Physicians, Patients and the Bottom Line.* Denver, CO: Medical Group Management Association.

Bureau of Labor Statistics. 2014. "Employer Costs for Employee Compensation— December 2013." Economic News Release. Issued March 12. www.bls.gov/ news.release/archives/ecec_03122014.htm.

Carroll, A. E. 2014. "The Problem with 'Pay for Performance' in Medicine." *The New York Times*, July 28.

Conrad, D. A., A. M. Sales, A. Chaudhuri, S. Liang, C. Maynard, L. Pieper, L. Weinstein, D. Gans, and N. Piland. 2002. "The Impact of Financial Incentives on Physician Productivity in Medical Groups." *Health Services Research* 37 (4): 885–906.

Darves, B. 2011. "Physicians at All Stages of Their Careers Are Exploring the Flexible, Portable Practice Option." *New England Journal of Medicine* Career Center. Published October 24. www.nejmcareercenter.org/article/ locum-tenens-lifestyle-opportunities-attracting-more-physicians/.

DeCenzo, D. A., S. P. Robbins, and S. L. Verhulst. 2013. *Fundamentals of Human Resource Management*, eleventh edition. Hoboken, NJ: Wiley.

Dessler, G. 2014. *Human Resource Management*, fourteenth edition. Upper Saddle River, NJ: Prentice Hall.

Epstein, A. M., T. H. Lee, and M. B. Hamel. 2004. "Paying Physicians for High-Quality Care." *New England Journal of Medicine* 350 (4): 406–10.

Fijalkowski, N., L. L. Zheng, M. T. Henderson, A. A. Moshfeghi, M. Maltenfort, and D. M. Moshfeghi. 2013. "Academic Productivity and Its Relationship to Physician Salaries in the University of California Healthcare System." *Southern Medical Journal* 106 (7): 415–21.

Folland, S., A. C. Goodman, and M. Stano. 2012. *The Economics of Health and Health Care*, seventh edition. Boston: Pearson.

Gaynor, M., and M. V. Pauly. 1990. "Compensation and Productive Efficiency in Partnerships: Evidence from Medical Group Practice." *Journal of Political Economy* 98 (3): 544–73.

Germain, P. B., and G. G. Cummings. 2010. "The Influence of Nursing Leadership on Nurse Performance: A Systematic Literature Review." *Journal of Nursing Management* 18 (4): 425–39.

Giancola, F. L. 2009. "A Framework for Understanding New Concepts in Compensation Management." *Benefits & Compensation Digest* 46 (9): 1–16.

Gómez-Mejía, L. R., D. B. Balkin, and R. L. Cardy. 2012. *Managing Human Resources*, seventh edition. Boston: Pearson.

Gosfield, A. G. 2004. "Paying Physicians for High-Quality Care." *New England Journal of Medicine* 350 (18): 1910.

Grumbach, K., J. V. Selby, C. Damberg, A. B. Bindman, C. Quesenberry, A. Truman, and C. Uratsu. 1999. "Resolving the Gatekeeper Conundrum: What Patients Value in Primary Care and Referrals to Specialists." *Journal of the American Medical Association* 282 (3): 261–66.

Gunderman, R. B. 2004. "The Perils of Paying Academic Physicians According to the Clinical Revenue They Generate." *Medical Science Monitor* 10 (2): 15–20.

Haeberle, K. 2014. "Trying to Recruit and Motivate Generation Y? It Might Be Time for Skill-Based Pay." Integrated Healthcare Strategies. Accessed December 30. www.integratedhealthcarestrategies.com/knowledgecenter_article.aspx?article_id=479.

Harris, M. M., F. Anseel, and F. Lievens. 2008. "Keeping Up with the Joneses: A Field Study of the Relationships Among Upward, Lateral, and Downward Comparisons and Pay Level Satisfaction." *Journal of Applied Psychology* 93 (3): 665–73.

Hartmann, C. W., T. Hoff, J. A. Palmer, P. Wroe, M. M. Dutta-Linn, and G. Lee. 2012. "The Medicare Policy of Payment Adjustment for Health Care-Associated Infections: Perspectives on Potential Unintended Consequences." *Medical Care Research and Review* 69 (1): 45–61.

Healthcare Incentives Improvement Institute. 2014. "Bridges to Excellence Clinician Rewards." Accessed June 7. www.hci3.org/participate_in_bridges_to_excellence/clinicians/rewards.

Herman, B. 2014. "How Pay-for-Performance Compensation Plans Can Facilitate Physician Alignment." *Becker's Hospital Review*. Published April 7. www.beckershospitalreview.com/compensation-issues/how-pay-for-performance-compensation-plans-can-facilitate-physician-alignment.html.

Herzberg, F., B. Mausner, and B. Snyderman. 1959. *The Motivation to Work*. New York: Wiley.

Hirschkorn, C. A., T. B. West, K. S. Hill, B. L. Cleary, and P. O. Hewlett. 2010. "Experienced Nurse Retention Strategies: What Can Be Learned from Top-Performing Organizations." *The Journal of Nursing Administration* 40 (11): 463–67.

Homans, G. C. 1961. *Social Behavior: Its Elementary Forms*. New York: Harcourt, Brace and World.

Integrated Healthcare Association. 2014. "Pay for Performance (PFP) Program Fact Sheet." Published September. www.iha.org/pdfs_documents/p4p_california/P4P-Fact-Sheet-September-2014.pdf.

Kilgour, J. G. 2008. "Job Evaluation Revisited: The Point Factor Method." *Compensation and Benefits Review*, July–August, 37–46.

Lee, G. M., K. Kleinman, S. B. Soumerai, A. Tse, D. Cole, S. K. Fridkin, T. Horan, R. Platt, C. Gay, W. Kassler, D. A. Goldmann, J. Jernigan, and A. K. Jha. 2012. "Effect of Nonpayment for Preventable Infections in U.S. Hospitals." *New England Journal of Medicine* 367 (15): 1428–37.

Lindenauer, P. K., D. Remus, S. Roman, M. B. Rothberg, E. M. Benjamin, A. Ma, and D. W. Bratzler. 2007. "Public Reporting and Pay for Performance in Hospital Quality Improvement." *New England Journal of Medicine* 356 (5): 486–96.

Madden, S. 2013. "New Measures in Pay-for-Performance Programs." *Physicians Practice*. Published October 16. www.physicianspractice.com/physician-compensation/new-measures-pay-performance-programs.

Managed Care Outlook. 1999. "Florida Blues Ditch Capitation in Favor of Fee-for-Service." Accessed May 21, 2005. www.managedcaremag.com.

Martocchio, J. 2011. *Strategic Compensation*. Upper Saddle River, NJ: Pearson Education.

Maslow, A. 1970. *Motivation and Personality*, second edition. New York: Harper & Row.

Milkovich, G. T., G. Newman, and B. Gerhart. 2014. *Compensation*, eleventh edition. New York: McGraw-Hill/Irwin.

Mohr, V., J. Zinn, J. Angelelli, J. M. Teno, and S. C. Miller. 2004. "Driven to Tiers: Socioeconomic and Racial Disparities in the Quality of Nursing Home Care." *Milbank Quarterly* 82 (2): 227–56.

O'Neil, S. L. 2012. "Broadbanding." Society for Human Resource Management. Accessed June 8, 2014. www.shrm.org/hrdisciplines/compensation/articles/pages/cms_000067.aspx.

Petersen, L. A., L. D. Woodard, T. Urech, C. Daw, and S. Sookanan. 2006. "Does Pay-for-Performance Improve the Quality of Health Care?" *Annals of Internal Medicine* 145 (4): 265–72.

Pfeffer, J. 1998. "Six Dangerous Myths About Pay." *Harvard Business Review* 76 (3): 108–19.

Rangle, C. 2010. "Why Pay for Performance Does Not Work and May Impair Patient Care." KevinMD.com. Published September 1. www.kevinmd.com/blog/2010/09/pay-performance-work-impair-patient-care.html.

Rosenthal, M. B., B. E. Landon, S.-L. T. Normand, R. G. Frank, and A .M. Epstein. 2006. "Pay for Performance in Commercial HMOs." *New England Journal of Medicine* 355 (18): 1895–1902.

Starr, P. 1982. *The Social Transformation of American Medicine*. New York: Basic Books.

Van Herck, P., L. Annemans, D. De Smedt, R. Remmen, and W. Sermeus. 2011. "Pay-for-Performance Step-by-Step: Introduction to the MIMIQ Model." *Health Policy* 102 (1): 8–17.

Werner, R. M., J. T. Kolstad, E. A. Stuart, and D. Polsky. 2011. "The Effect of Pay-for-Performance in Hospitals: Lessons for Quality Improvement." *Health Affairs* 30 (4): 690–98.

Woolhandler, S., and D. Ariely. 2012. "Will Pay for Performance Backfire? Insights from Behavioral Economics." *Health Affairs Blog*. Published October 11. http://healthaffairs.org/blog/2012/10/11/will-pay-for-performance-backfire-insights-from-behavioral-economics/.

Zimbelman, J. L., S. P. Juraschek, X. Zhang, and V. W. H. Lin. 2010. "Physical Therapy Workforce in the United States: Forecasting Nationwide Shortages." *PM & R* 2 (11): 1021–29.

EMPLOYEE BENEFITS

Dolores G. Clement, Maria A. Curran, and Sharon L. Jahn

Learning Objectives

After completing this chapter, the reader should be able to

- discuss the history and trends of employee benefits management;
- explain the rationale and tax implications of offering benefits in addition to compensation and why benefits are critical to the recruitment and retention of healthcare staff;
- describe a variety of benefits that may be offered with employment, particularly healthcare benefits, and relate the management implications of offering each;
- relate the knowledge of employee benefits to selected human resources management issues and systems development; and
- make suggestions for the design and communication of benefit plans.

Introduction

Benefits are a competitive lever in recruiting and hiring employees. Employment benefits provide additional compensatory value to individuals and their families through the provision of leave time, insurance against uncertain events, and additional targeted services. The success of any healthcare organization requires a concerted investment in human capital for many reasons. Demand for experienced healthcare providers has never been greater, while competition for clinical staff, including physicians, has intensified. Nonclinical staff are in great demand as well. The availability of an adequate supply of healthcare workers is constrained by the fact that capacity at most medical, nursing, and allied health schools does not meet demand; therefore, fewer students can attend. Replacement costs and turnover costs far exceed the cost of investing wisely in human capital.

In most healthcare organizations, labor costs are the single largest line item in the operating budget. An increase in labor cost often has a correlation to the cost of employer-sponsored benefits; in fact, many fringe benefits are based on a percentage of employees' salaries. Thus, the cost of fringe benefits can be a significant line item in any operating budget. Depending on the actual benefits offered and their respective design structures, the average cost of fringe benefits in many healthcare systems can range from 20 percent to 35 percent of salary. The US Chamber of Commerce (2007) projected that, across all industries, employee benefits account for almost 40 percent of total compensation.

Early research by the University HealthSystem Consortium (2005; Bragg and Vermoch 2003) indicated that attracting and retaining clinical workforce was one of the top three concerns cited by chief executive officers (CEOs) who participated in the study. A 2013 survey of CEOs ranked the increasing costs for staff a top financial concern (American College of Healthcare Executives 2014). Personnel shortages, patient satisfaction, and quality are also in the top ten of the list. The significant workforce shortages are exacerbated by the rate of growth in healthcare jobs and the aging workforce. Therefore, offering a comprehensive fringe benefits structure is an increasingly important recruitment and retention tool. The use of the Internet and social media makes researching potential employers virtually effortless. Candidates, as well as incumbent employees, can access detailed information about employers and are often very well versed in the fringe benefits offered by various companies.

The pressure to offer a benefits package that is competitive in the marketplace is significant in healthcare. This significance is illustrated in part by the weight placed on compensation and benefits packages by organizations that are recognized as employers of choice. Benefits are an important factor to consider in an applicant's decision to accept employment. Additionally, offering a comprehensive and robust benefits package is considered an empirical domain of evidence for the prestigious designation by the American Nurses Credentialing Center (ANCC 2014) as a Magnet healthcare system. The Magnet designation is the most prestigious distinction a healthcare organization can receive for nursing excellence and quality nursing care. Organizations that achieve Magnet status are part of an esteemed group that demonstrates superior nursing practice and patient outcomes. In the time of healthcare reform, Magnet facilities are leaders in improving the care delivered to patients, families, and communities. The "Structural Empowerment" component of the Magnet model requires organizations to demonstrate that their personnel practices and programs support the professional development of nurses, and that their resources are used to support a culture of excellence and innovation (ANCC 2014).

Because of the importance of benefits to the entire employee compensation package, many tasks involved in the design, communication, and monitoring of benefit plans are the responsibility of human resources (HR) personnel. Knowledge of one's organization, the market in which it competes, and the needs of the workforce is crucial in deciding what benefits should be offered. Beyond benefits that are mandated, what other benefits should be offered to employees? To what extent should benefits be offered to different classifications of employees?

This chapter presents an overview of the most common benefits related to employment compensation, describes a variety of benefits that may be offered as well as their tax implications, explains the role of government in benefits management, and discusses key issues in the design and management of benefit plans.

Brief Historical Background

Retirement benefit programs in the United States can be traced back to the Plymouth Colony settlers' military retirement program of 1636 (Employee Benefit Research Institute [EBRI] 2013). Beyond retirement plans, health coverage benefit programs across industries are a development of the late nineteenth and early twentieth centuries in the United States. In the late 1800s, industries began to employ physicians as a result of the increasing potential for worker injury in a country that was undergoing industrialization. The railroad, mining, and lumber industries offered more extensive medical services, which were necessary because workers were helping in the expansion into areas in the West where care was not available. Companies retained a doctor and made mandatory deductions from workers' salaries to cover the cost of the medical services or the salary of the physician (Starr 1982). The rise in industrialization also led to the creation of disability insurance in the late 1800s. Although coverage was not tied to employment at that time, individuals could purchase coverage that served as assurance that they would still have income in the event of a disability.

Coverage of workers in the railroad, mining, and lumber industries was the stimulus for Justin Ford Kimball to create Baylor University's hospital prepayment plan in 1929; this plan was the precursor to the creation of Blue Cross. The initial arrangement between the university hospital and teachers in the Dallas area was simple and direct (Cunningham and Cunningham 1997). This prepayment plan (which allowed up to 21 days of care in the hospital for 50 cents per month) was different from any type of conventional insurance. Prepayments were made directly to the hospital that was providing the care with no third-party involvement.

The Great Depression, beginning in 1929, shed light on the financial problems faced by the aged, ill, and disabled populations. These concerns led to the passage of the Social Security Act in 1935 and the federal government's involvement in providing retirement income protection. By mandating salary withholding in 1935 as a contribution to the trust fund for Social Security, the act set a precedent, and other benefits coverage began to expand. Social Security provided some retirement benefits and included coverage of categorical programs but not medical coverage for the elderly or poor. Amendments to the Social Security Act in 1956 and 1965 added income protection for the disabled along with health insurance for the elderly and disabled under Medicare (EBRI 2013).

The wage freeze during World War II allowed companies to offer benefits in lieu of wage increases. Employers benefited with federal exemption of defined benefits from the companies' tax liability. Subsequent legislation that permitted preferential tax treatments gave incentives to employers to offer more private, voluntary benefits. Note that a countervailing force against increasing the number and variety of benefits is the inability of companies to subsidize offerings—more simply, providing benefits is becoming less affordable.

Federal and state governments regulate and carefully monitor the tax treatment and administration of benefits. Since the 1950s, a proliferation of legislation has established guidelines to protect individuals and employers in administering employment-related benefits and to monitor public and private benefit plans. Exhibit 10.1 lists federal legislation that affects benefits administration. Employers have the responsibility to ensure that they are in compliance with the rules and regulations governing the benefits of their employees. The following section illustrates the regulatory compliance expected of employers using four examples of the most far-reaching legislation, including the Affordable Care Act (ACA) of 2010.

Major Federal Legislation

Four major federal laws that affect benefits coverage and administration are the Employee Retirement Income Security Act of 1974 (ERISA), the Consolidated Omnibus Budget Reconciliation Act of 1986 (COBRA), the Health Insurance Portability and Accountability Act of 1996 (HIPAA), and the ACA. Each of these acts has specific implications for benefits management. Audits of compliance can be conducted, and failure to follow the provisions of these acts can subject the employer to serious penalties.

ERISA is a federal law administered by the US Department of Labor to establish minimum standards by which many pension and health plans in private industry are governed. Most nongovernmental companies in the United States are covered by ERISA, whereas state or federal agencies are not. The types of protection mandated by ERISA are primarily administrative in nature. For example, employers must maintain plan documents in accordance with applicable federal laws and ensure that definitions for plan

EXHIBIT 10.1
Legislation That Affects Employee Benefits Administration

Legislation	Major Accomplishment	Legal Citation and Web Address
Uniformed Services Employment and Reemployment Rights Act (USERRA)	Provides continuous employment and benefits for soldiers who are deployed while employed	38 U.S.C. § 4301 osc.gov/Pages/USERRA.aspx
Economic Growth and Tax Relief Reconciliation Act of 2001 (EGTRRA)	Provides greater flexibility for participants who transfer defined contribution balances at termination of employment and consistencies in deferral amounts, eligibility, and so on among defined contribution plans	P.L. 107-16 www.irs.gov/pub/irs-drop/n-02-4.pdf
Health Insurance Portability and Accountability Act of 1996 (HIPAA)	Provides for the elimination of waiting periods when participants move between group health plans; also provides regulations for privacy and security of health-related information within a company that has access to such information, and regulations for how an employer may use, store, and transmit such protected information	P.L. 104-191 aspe.hhs.gov/admnsimp/pl104191.htm
Medicare Prescription Drug, Improvement, and Modernization Act of 2003 (MMA)	Introduced Medicare Part D, prescription drug coverage, and Medicare Advantage products; allows greater choice of coverage by allowing private insurance companies to provide coverage through preferred provider organizations (PPOs), fee-for-service, medical savings accounts, and other special needs plans directly to the Medicare population	P.L. 108-173 www.gpo.gov/fdsys/pkg/PLAW-108 publ173/html/PLAW-108publ173.htm www.medicare.gov/part-d/index.html
Government Accounting Standards Board (GASB) No. 43 and No. 45	Rules that require government employers to book the accrued cost of future retiree benefits as a current liability, similar to Financial Accounting Standards Board (FASB) 106 provisions for publicly traded companies	www.gasb.org/project_pages/opeb_ summary.pdf
Pension Protection Act of 2006 (PPA)	Provides additional protection against employers that underfund defined benefit retirement plans by giving additional premiums, closing loopholes, raising caps on minimum amounts that employers must contribute, and requiring measurement of funding levels; also provides additional enhancements in the defined contribution plans; allows for easier implementation of automatic enrollment in deferred savings plans, ensuring participants have greater access to their financial investments and to professional advice	P.L. 109-280 www.dol.gov/ebsa/pensionreform. html www.gpo.gov/fdsys/pkg/PLAW-109 publ280/pdf/PLAW-109publ280.pdf
Affordable Care Act (ACA)	Provides access to quality healthcare coverage for all Americans; also establishes minimum standards of coverage required by employer-based plans, mandated benefits, removal of lifetime coverage limits and limits on coverage of preexisting conditions, access to preventive care with no out-of-pocket expenses, and a healthcare marketplace for individual purchasing of healthcare insurance	P.L. 111-148 www.gpo.gov/fdsys/pkg/PLAW-111 publ148/pdf/PLAW-111publ148.pdf www.hhs.gov/healthcare/rights/law
Defense of Marriage Act (DOMA)	Allows states to refuse to recognize same-sex marriages from other states (Section 3, ruled unconstitutional in 2013; barred legal marriages of same-sex couples for purposes of federal laws); ambiguity allows constraints on benefits to a nonemployed member of a same-sex relationship	P.L. 104-199 www.gpo.gov/fdsys/pkg/PLAW-104 publ199/html/PLAW-104publ199.htm

eligibility are not discriminatory. ERISA also includes expectations for the fiduciary aspects of administration, requiring plan administrators to appropriately manage and control the assets of the plan, to develop a process by which plan participants can obtain benefits or benefits information, and to inform participants of the right to sue for a company's breach of fiduciary responsibility. The organization must also file annual tax returns after an external audit of the plan has been conducted.

Over the years, ERISA has been amended so that health plans have greater protections. For example, COBRA provides qualifying employees and their families the right to continue to participate in employer-sponsored health coverage for a limited time after certain qualifying changes in family status, such as the loss of a job. Often, buying individual medical insurance directly is much more expensive for an employee, but COBRA helps employees and their spouses and dependents by guaranteeing them continued access to the employer's healthcare plan at the current group rate. The employee pays the full healthcare premium, which is often a less expensive option than buying an individual policy. COBRA covers any group health plan sponsored by an employer with 20 or more employees on more than 50 percent of typical business days in the previous calendar year. In addition, COBRA requires companies to provide timely notification to all covered beneficiaries in the event that a qualified family status change would make those individuals eligible for COBRA. Hefty penalties can be assessed for failure to adhere to these timely notification guidelines.

In 1996, HIPAA was enacted to protect employees and their family members who have preexisting medical conditions or who could suffer health-coverage discrimination because of health-related factors. For example, under HIPAA, an individual who changes employment may have no waiting period for coverage of a preexisting illness if the individual has less than a 63-day break in healthcare coverage from the prior employer. In addition, the confidentiality of protected health information (PHI) is specifically outlined in HIPAA. For example, details of employees' medical conditions, enrollment forms, medical claims data, or other specific health information must be filed separately from the employees' personnel files to prevent unauthorized or inappropriate access to PHI. Also, HIPAA protects the type of information that can be used in making decisions about coverage or premiums. In short, HIPAA is intended to balance access to claims information or other medical information with the need for an employer to make revenue-driven decisions. Thus, the employers' need to access claims information to make decisions about the coverage they will offer must respect individual privacy requirements. For example, employers cannot make coverage decisions that would have an adverse impact on individuals, such as eliminating coverage for a specific diagnosis because a number of employees have that diagnosis.

In many healthcare organizations, enforcing HIPAA is the responsibility of a compliance officer. Computerized medical records are also protected by HIPAA, as is the disclosure of medical information by staff. HIPAA *does not protect against accidental disclosure,* but it sets up standards that make such an incident less likely and establishes penalties if information is released in a way that does not follow the standards. For example, discussing an interesting case in the lobby of the medical center may be considered a HIPAA violation if PHI is released. The provisions of HIPAA were expanded with inclusion in the Newborns' and Mothers' Health Protection Act, the Mental Health Parity Act, and the Women's Health and Cancer Rights Act.

The ACA has affected the administration of employer-sponsored plans through coverage mandates, minimum essential coverage, removal of limits on coverage of preexisting conditions, and removal of waiting periods for employer plans. The act also mandated coverage of adult children up to age 26 regardless of their student, marital, or residency status. Employers with more than 50 employees must be in compliance with these regulations in their plans by 2015 or earlier if the plan is not a "grandfathered" plan. The ACA also established healthcare exchanges for the purchase of health insurance. These exchanges can either be public or private exchanges. The public exchanges are operated by each state, or the states can defer to the federally run exchange in lieu of running their own exchange. Health exchanges provide access to healthcare plans for individuals. The private exchanges are operated commonly by large consulting firms to provide controlled access to exchanges by employer-sponsored plans. Employer-sponsored plans must also provide access to healthcare benefits to all full-time employees. Individuals without access to an employer-sponsored plan may qualify for a subsidy for purchase of individual health insurance. Individuals who are not enrolled in an employer-sponsored plan or a plan provided through a healthcare exchange will be subject to a tax penalty. The ACA defined full-time employees as those working more than 30 hours a week. This regulation has become an employment concern for many employers in industries that have high utilization of part-time workers, such as schools, tourism, and retail.

Overview of Employment Benefits

Given the competitive nature of healthcare, administrative staff must understand the full range of benefits that the employer provides, because many, if not most, employees may not realize the richness of their organization's benefits package. For example, a registered nurse may choose to seek employment at another medical center for a modest gain in hourly rate and not realize that the benefits offered by the new employer are not as robust as those given by the current employer. In this example, the healthcare organization will have to recruit and orient a new registered nurse, when in fact the resignation may have been prevented if the individual fully understood the value of the employer's benefits package.

When educating staff about the value of the benefits package, the organization must stress the concept of total compensation. *Total compensation* is the value of the employee's base salary plus the value of the benefits package. An employer may help articulate this fact in several ways, including the following:

- Add a section on pay advices that notes the value of the employer-paid portion of health insurance.
- Provide benefits calculation tools on the company website or intranet.
- Produce customized benefits statements during the annual open enrollment process.
- Use social media to communicate benefits through a patient portal and/or interactive applications.

Communication of the worth of these benefits is essential if an employer intends them to play a part in recruitment and retention.

Following is a description of employee benefits that are mandated by law and those that are voluntary. The tax implications of each benefit are also discussed in this section; some voluntary benefits are entirely taxable, some are tax exempt, and others are tax deferred.

Mandatory Benefits
Social Security and Medicare Part A
The Federal Insurance Contributions Act (FICA) authorizes a payroll tax that funds Social Security, disability, and Medicare Part A. FICA requires Social Security payroll taxes to be collected from the employee and matched by the employer. The 2015 FICA employee contribution is 6.2 percent of wages, up to a taxable wage base of $118,500. The Medicare rate is 1.45 percent of wages, with no wage limit (Social Security Administration 2014). Employers must match each of these amounts and send the total withheld and matched amounts to the federal government. Once the taxable wage total is made, only the Medicare Part A deduction with the employer match is sent. The taxable wage base is determined annually by the Internal Revenue Service (IRS) and is subject to change.

Unemployment Compensation
Unemployment compensation is a mandatory assessment of the employer and varies by state. The intention of unemployment compensation is to protect employees who have lost their jobs under certain circumstances, such as being

laid off. Voluntary separation and termination for cause that is well documented are typically not covered. The premium amount for unemployment insurance is calculated on the basis of the types of positions in the organization as well as the company's experience with reductions in force. For example, an organization with a professional staff would likely pay more than one with a sales force because the amount of salary to supplement for a professional in the event of a layoff is likely to be higher than that of a salesperson.

Workers' Compensation

Legislation for workers' compensation was passed to protect an employer from possible litigation for workplace injuries and to provide wages and benefits, including medical expenses, to employees who are injured on the job. Each state has different rules governing its workers' compensation program. Most states mandate that employers have insurance coverage, although some states provide their own workers' compensation funds to which employers can contribute. Many organizations choose to self-insure for workers' compensation to save costs, and this option (discussed later in this chapter) can be very successful if managed well. Compliance of state workers' compensation programs with federal regulations is monitored and enforced by the Occupational Safety and Health Administration (US Department of Labor 2014a). In a healthcare setting, workers' compensation claims may result from injuries incurred from such events as lifting patients, needlesticks, and exposures to disease.

Increased emphasis on employee safety has helped healthcare organizations reduce workers' compensation expenses. For example, ensuring that staff are trained to wear personal protection equipment helps reduce exposure to blood and body fluids. Training nurses on the proper techniques to lift and position a patient, and having safe lift equipment readily available, can prevent injuries that could disable a registered nurse for life and entitle him or her to the payment of lifetime medical benefits and salary for years.

Voluntary Benefits

Most benefits that employers provide are voluntary benefits and, as such, differentiate one employer from another. Administration of some voluntary benefits may need to follow established rules and guidelines or reporting requirements, and if so, the employer is responsible for ensuring compliance. Following are the most common voluntary benefits offered by an employer.

Leave Benefits

Vacation leave is fully taxable when taken. Employers establish vacation eligibility according to employee category—salaried or hourly. Length of service usually determines the amount of vacation days that can be accrued and carried over from year to year. Employers must account for accrued vacation liability.

Sick leave allows employees to get paid during time off as a result of illness, injury, or medical appointments. As with vacation leave, employers establish sick and illness leave policies according to the category of employee.

Family and medical leave is covered by the Family and Medical Leave Act (FMLA), which applies to employers that have more than 50 employees. Under FMLA, employers must offer up to 12 weeks of unpaid leave per year for maternity or other medical needs to eligible employees (US Department of Labor 2014c). An employee can take advantage of this benefit if he or she has worked at least one year and has put in 1,250 hours of service in the 12 months before the needed leave. Individual employers may choose to pay the employee during this leave, but that decision is left to their discretion. Reasons given for FMLA leave include the birth or adoption of a child, the need to care for a family member with a serious illness, or an employee's own ailment.

The Uniformed Services Employment and Reemployment Rights Act (USERRA) expands the definition of family members to include next of kin in instances of an individual hurt in the line of duty where an immediate family member is not available. The amount of leave allowed is also extended to 26 weeks in a 12-month period for the care of a next of kin injured during active duty.

Family leave can be taken on an intermittent basis, and employers need to track the unpaid leave given that the 12-month period in which it can be taken can be based on a fixed (e.g., calendar or fiscal) year or on a rolling basis (e.g., 12 months since the first day of leave). The employer covered by the FMLA must stipulate the basis or standards for this benefit. For example, the employer may request a medical certificate if the employee requests the leave for a medical purpose.

Health and Welfare Benefits

Benefits designed to provide protections and services related to health, dental, vision, life insurance, and disability are typically categorized under health and welfare benefits.

Employer-sponsored *health insurance* is one of the most expensive items in the budget for employers as a result of escalating costs of healthcare. Although health insurance remains a "voluntary" benefit, employers—particularly larger organizations with more than 50 employees—are mandated to offer this benefit or pay a penalty under the ACA. Employers that provide health insurance can deduct their expenditures from pretax earnings. Usually, employees are offered a choice of private health insurance plans, including the traditional service benefit coverage and managed care options, and this offer extends to employees' dependents (spouse, children) as well. Exhibit 10.2 presents types of health insurance plans, and Exhibit 10.3 lists additional health and welfare benefits.

EXHIBIT 10.2

Types of Health Insurance Plans

Type	What Is Covered?	Advantages	Disadvantages
Full service	First-dollar coverage provided on all medical and hospital services up to a predetermined maximum	Members receive coverage for extensive medical and preventive care, both inpatient and outpatient	Expensive for employer because of high claims costs Complexity involved as the plans may pay physician claims and hospital claims differently
Comprehensive	Cost sharing of medical expenses at a predetermined percentage of claims (coinsurance), after an up-front deductible, up to a predetermined out-of-pocket maximum above which the plan pays 100 percent of claims	Introduced cost sharing with the member as well as other cost-control features, such as second surgical opinion, preadmission review, and full coverage for diagnostic tests	Provides no incentive to reduce overutilization and use of high-cost providers
Preferred provider organization (PPO)	Claims incurred at providers that participate in the insurance carriers' PPO network are paid at a higher level than claims incurred at nonparticipating providers	Claims costs are reduced because of negotiated discounts with the insurance carriers when members use a participating provider	Potentially substantial cost differential if care is sought at a nonparticipating medical provider Members must first determine if their provider is participating in the network
Health maintenance organization (HMO)	Only claims incurred at providers that participate in the insurance carriers' HMO network are covered; all specialty care is directed through the member's primary care physician with referrals to the appropriate provider	Primary care physicians are paid by the insurance company to be gatekeepers; this system keeps costs down as gatekeepers can manage the care received from a specialist and ensure that the specialists are part of the participating network	More limited network size, making it more difficult for members to find participating physicians All care must be directed through the gatekeeper, creating additional visits or time necessary to provide access to specialists
High-deductible health plan (HDHP)	Medical care for the member is not paid until a high deductible, typically greater than $2,000, is met; after this deductible is met, claims are paid at a predetermined cost-sharing percentage; usually provided as part of a consumer-driven health plan and supplemented with health reimbursement accounts or health savings accounts	Members are encouraged to understand the costs of medical care because they must meet a high deductible before the employer plan will pay for claims Usually, preventive care is excluded from the deductible, thus encouraging wellness	Members must pay the high-deductible amount out of their own pocket before coverage can begin; members may not have budgeted for these amounts Providers must get the billed amounts from patients instead of insurers More risk of nonpayment

EXHIBIT 10.3
Other Health and Welfare Benefits

Benefit	What Is It?	Who Pays?	Who Determines Amount?	Types of Plans
Dental	Covers a percentage of dental care up to an annual maximum	Employer and employee; generally a greater percentage of the cost is borne by the employee	Employer may choose to offer multiple plans and allow employees to elect the plan, or the employer provides a single plan	Dental indemnity; dental PPO; dental HMO; direct dental
Prescription drug coverage	Covers some amount of the cost of prescription medications	May be included in health insurance or as a separate rider to the health insurance policy	Employer may choose to offer multiple plans and allow employees to elect the plan, or the employer provides a single plan	Two-tier coverage; three-tier coverage; four-tier coverage; coverage after deductible
Vision	Covers a predetermined amount of expenses for exams, frames, lenses, contacts, and other vision needs during a specified period (annually or biannually)	May be included in health insurance or provided as voluntary supplemental coverage	Employer may choose to offer multiple plans and allow employees to elect the plan, or the employer provides a single plan	Vision PPO; vision HMO
Stop-loss coverage	Protects against catastrophic claim amounts either on a single claimant or the total claims expense	Employer pays for protection against unpredicted catastrophic claims	Employer	Specific; aggregate
Life	Provides a death benefit for the covered person payable to a pre-designated beneficiary	Employer provides a basic level of life insurance; employees may elect to purchase supplemental coverage on themselves, spouse, and/or children	Employer chooses the level of the basic coverage; employees may elect varying levels of supplemental coverage	Group term life; group universal life; group variable life; group variable universal life
Disability	Provides a level of income payable to the employee after a predetermined period out of work as a result of illness, injury, or disease	Employer provides a basic level of coverage; employees may choose to purchase supplemental coverage	Employer chooses the level of the basic coverage; employees may elect varying levels of supplemental coverage	Short-term disability; basic long-term disability; supplemental long-term disability

(continued)

EXHIBIT 10.3

Other Health and Welfare Benefits *(continued from previous page)*

Benefit	What Is It?	Who Pays?	Who Determines Amount?	Types of Plans
Flexible spending account	Allows employees to deduct a fixed, pretax amount from their paycheck over the plan year either for medical (including dental, vision, and prescription) expenses not covered by insurance or for dependent care expenses for a child under 13 years or an adult who requires care because of age or disability	Employee elects the specific payroll amount; employer has the ability to provide a matching dollar amount	Employee determines the amount based on his or her expected expenses in the respective category for the next plan year; must be elected each year, and any monies remaining after the plan year are forfeited back to the employer; the IRS determines annual contribution limits	Medical care; dependent care
Health savings account	A tax-advantaged medical savings account available to taxpayers in the United States who are enrolled in a high-deductible health plan	Employee or employer can make contributions to this plan; contributions can be either through pretax payroll deduction or directly to the financial institution and then claimed as a deduction to gross income on taxes	Amounts deposited within the plan year must not exceed the statutory limit set by the IRS; amounts remaining in the account at the end of the tax year may be rolled forward to the next year; amounts are portable when employees leave employment	Health plan only
Health reimbursement account	An employer-funded account that reimburses an employee for medical expenses	Must be funded by employer only	Employer provides funding for the account based on its own criteria—no plan requirements; funds may be used to pay individual health insurance premiums and funds may be rolled to the next plan year; portability on termination is possible with potential tax implications	Health plan only

Some employers opt to self-insure, negotiating with a private health insurance company to administer benefits to employers through an administrative services contract (self-insurance is discussed in further detail later in this chapter). Self-insured healthcare is attractive for many healthcare organizations because it typically allows greater flexibility in plan design. For example, the plan can be designed to encourage staff to use the employer's providers and facilities by providing financial incentives such as lower copayments and out-of-pocket expenses. Such a design can positively affect the cost of administering the health plan because the revenue generated may pay for the cost of paying claims. Self-insured organizations are not obligated to offer state-mandated health benefits. Other large employers are more likely to self-insure if they have experience with large claims and have the funding mechanisms to be able to handle the fluctuation in expenses. For healthcare organizations, health benefits coverage presents a unique challenge. While healthcare workers tend to use more health services than employees in other industries because of their medical knowledge and their proximity to services, the cost of providing care to them is affected by the contracts that third parties, such as managed care companies and insurance companies, have negotiated to pay healthcare providers and facilities.

Note that under the Mental Health Parity Act, mental illness is considered a medical condition, and thus employers are required to provide the same level of coverage for mental illness as they would for a physical condition. To contain costs for mental health, an employer can elect to carve out mental health and use a special behavioral health company to focus on mental health needs. Because behavioral health companies are a niche provider, they can provide economies of scale that may not be possible with a larger health insurer. An employee assistance program (EAP) is also effective in controlling mental health costs if such a program is used as a gatekeeper for access to mental health–related services. EAPs typically offer a finite number of counseling and therapy sessions with professionals in the field, and all dealings with this group are confidential. Some employers provide the option of having a manager make a mandatory referral to the EAP to address concerns about an employee's mental health. Regardless of how employees access EAPs, use of the services in these programs is typically more cost-effective than use of a psychiatrist under a healthcare benefit.

Wellness and fitness programs also fall under the category of health and welfare benefits. The adage "prevention is the best medicine" can be used by employers as a strategy to manage healthcare costs and to increase employee productivity. More and more workplace initiatives are focusing on wellness and fitness, especially in healthcare organizations. On a national level, the ACA now requires that wellness visits be provided without cost to the insured individual. Many large private employers can choose not to hire people who use tobacco products or may be overweight. The Cleveland Clinic was one of the first to announce it would not hire smokers. The trends toward onsite wellness programs, management of complex comorbid cases, and engagement of employees in their overall healthcare are likely to increase as employers encourage healthy lifestyles to help control escalating healthcare costs.

Wellness programs may be easier to implement in healthcare than in other industries for several reasons. First, many healthcare organizations require pre-employment health assessments based on the physical requirements of a position. Second, healthcare organizations typically have numerous content experts and other resources on site. Third, healthcare workers are typically more sophisticated consumers of wellness and preventive programs. Despite these reasons, many healthcare employees do not take advantage of services such as free flu shots. The low percentage of healthcare workers who get a flu vaccine has caused organizations such as The Joint Commission and the Centers for Disease Control and Prevention to bring the matter to the forefront of healthcare managers' attention. Indeed, one of The Joint Commission's goals for infection control requires hospitals and health systems to report rates of vaccination as well as identify the reasons that healthcare staff do not get flu shots and then use this information to come up with strategies to increase participation. The Centers for Medicare & Medicaid Services (CMS) now requires healthcare systems to report annual rates of participation for healthcare providers, volunteers, students, and contractors. Some organizations have mandated the flu vaccine, and others require staff who have not been vaccinated to wear masks when they have contact with patients.

The healthcare industry has shown renewed interest in providing incentives to employees to improve their health and reduce risky behaviors. Many healthcare organizations and insurance companies ask employees to complete personal health assessments to determine current and future risks based on family medical history. Others provide special payments to staff who have normal blood pressure, do not smoke, or have a healthy body mass index. Regardless of the method used to increase staff participation in wellness activities, the future will bring increased focus on prevention and fitness for duty among healthcare workers. This emphasis will stem the escalating costs of healthcare, encourage better management of chronic diseases, reduce injuries, and increase productivity. HIPAA stipulates that employers may offer these incentives to employees only if the incentive is based on participation and not on the results of the test or assessment. Employers are allowed to provide up to a 20 percent premium differential to employees to meet a health-related standard, such as nonuse of tobacco. These programs must provide an accommodation for those who are unable to meet the standard and be directly related to the promotion of good health or management of disease or chronic health conditions (US Department of Labor 2014b).

Dental insurance is sometimes offered to employees and their dependents as an addition to health insurance, although many employees expect this coverage. The cost associated with dental insurance is rising as much as the cost of health insurance. An option for a self-insured healthcare organization that is affiliated with a dental school is to contract directly with the school to provide dental care.

Vision coverage is typically an add-on to the health insurance benefit. Basic vision plans include coverage for an annual eye exam and contact lenses or glasses. A vision network frequently provides better coverage at a more affordable price.

The availability of *hearing insurance* targeted at baby boomers, who are aging yet remain in the workplace, is a recent trend. Hearing insurance is an example of a benefit that may be dependent on the changing demographics of the workforce.

Prescription drug benefits may be part of the health insurance coverage. Such coverage is costly both to the organization and to the employee even with the use of a drug formulary. Costs will continue to rise with continued acceptance of bioengineered drugs and other new lifesaving treatments. The use of a pharmacy network can control costs if the formulary is carefully constructed to encourage employees to use less costly prescriptions, such as by substituting generic drugs for brand-name drugs. The use of pharmacy benefit management companies has helped reduce pharmaceutical costs. These companies perform the normal utilization review function, manage the formulary, and negotiate the costs of drugs with pharmaceutical firms; thus, they can leverage the overall expense of providing the benefit. Intense efforts by pharmaceutical companies to advertise their premier brand-name drugs has resulted in consumers' asking their providers to prescribe these drugs. Often the consumer is not aware that an effective and less expensive generic option may be available. One strategy to help mitigate pharmaceutical costs is to implement step therapy programs. Step therapy requires the consumer to use a less costly alternative to a brand-name drug (unless the medical efficacy is not appropriate). Many plan designs have significant cost reductions if employees use mail-order services for 90-day supplies. Although expenditures for pharmaceuticals may decrease as the patents for many of the most widely used pharmaceuticals expire and generic alternatives become available, the development of designer drugs to address certain medical conditions may offset any savings.

Flexible spending accounts (FSAs) allow employees to tax defer, via payroll deduction, an amount that can be used to offset qualified expenses for medical care or dependent care. An FSA may be viewed as a "use it or lose it" benefit because of the risk it presents to the program participant who does not accurately calculate the amount of unpaid medical or dependent care expenses that will be incurred in the year ahead. The guidelines for medical and dependent care accounts differ slightly.

Medical FSAs can be used for qualified medical, dental, and vision expenses. The IRS allows employers to determine the maximum amount that employees may defer for medical spending purposes up to the IRS limit of $2,500. Employers tend to be conservative with setting the maximum because an employee can submit expenses at any time in the plan year and the employer must reimburse the employee regardless of the amount that has been deferred already. For example, an employer could elect to have $2,500 as the maximum annual limit for a health FSA. A participating employee who elected to defer the maximum could present the employer with receipts that totaled to $2,500 in January and then quit in February—long before the maximum has been deducted from the employee's paychecks. Because of this risk, employers should carefully consider their likely exposure when determining the maximum deferral allowed under a medical FSA.

The IRS has defined guidelines for what is considered a qualified expense (e.g., many cosmetic procedures are not qualified) and has allowed employers to decide whether to allow reimbursements for the cost of over-the-counter products. More and more employers are contracting with companies that provide an FSA debit card that can be used for qualified expenses. This method typically allows the employer to offer reimbursement of medical expenses, including for over-the-counter products, without requiring cumbersome paper processing and the determination of a qualifying expense by a benefits staff member.

The maximum limit for dependent care FSAs is determined by the IRS, and the employer does not have discretion to set a different limit. Current regulations allow $5,000 per household. Unlike for a medical spending account, the employee can only be reimbursed for expenses up to the amount that has actually been tax-deferred via payroll.

Medical and dependent care FSAs are popular with employers because a lowered taxable wage base means that both the employer and the employee pay less FICA tax. Further, an FSA's use-it-or-lose-it provision means that the employer can keep funds that are deferred but are not processed for reimbursement. Employers can charge administrative fees for allowing staff to use FSAs, and these fees are one way to offset the costs of processing.

Long-term disability (LTD) insurance is considered a welfare benefit because it is designed to provide employees with income in the event they become disabled and cannot work. Because of the nature of healthcare work, healthcare employees have a higher risk of disability than workers in many other industries; thus, providing this benefit may provide a competitive advantage for a healthcare organization. Physicians and nurses specifically ask about LTD coverage when comparing benefits packages between healthcare organizations.

A costly manner of providing LTD insurance is through a specialty-specific plan. This type of plan is particularly popular among physicians because the definition of a disability is that the injured person can no longer perform the duties of the specialty that the person was practicing at the time of the injury. Thus, under this definition, a surgeon who can no longer see clearly enough to perform surgery is considered disabled and as such can collect disability pay to supplement other income—say, as a general practitioner. While popular with employees, specialty-specific plans are very costly, and few insurers even offer them as an option.

LTD insurance typically becomes active after an employee has been unable to work for 180 days or more; however, this feature of the plan can be decided by the employer, and some have determined that 90 days is the elimination period. The 90-day period is more beneficial to the employee because the waiting period for eligibility is shorter. Most healthcare organizations find that LTD insurance, unlike health insurance, is too risky to self-insure because of the risk pool it requires. Healthcare employees perform physically demanding work and are often prone to injury as well as accidental exposure to diseases and infections. But because employees face such risks, LTD insurance is an attractive provision to include in a comprehensive benefits program for healthcare staff.

LTD insurance is frequently bundled with other plans that cover sickness and disability, such as paid time off, sick time accruals, and short-term disability, giving employees more coverage options in the first 90 to 180 days of disability. An organization can choose to report the amount of premiums paid on behalf of employees for LTD insurance as a taxable fringe benefit. The advantage to the employee is that in the event of disability, the income received is not taxed, and not withholding taxes means that the disability income is closer in amount to the predisability pay.

Short-term disability insurance is an optional benefit for which the employee must pay—either for the entire cost or for a significant portion of the premium. This insurance may also be an employer-paid benefit (usually in conjunction with paid-time-off benefits), where the benefits are determined according to employee tenure and salary level. With short-term disability insurance, an employee is covered from the time the illness, condition, or disability starts to the time that the elimination period for long-term disability has been satisfied. Preexisting conditions may be taken into consideration in the approval process to enroll in this type of insurance. Most plans provide 50 percent to 60 percent of salary to those who receive short-term disability.

Long-term care (LTC) insurance usually covers the cost of nursing home, home care, and assisted living. This insurance became an attractive benefit as baby boomers began to face decisions about how to care for their parents and plan for their own future. LTC insurance can include a daily allowance for care at a nursing or assisted living facility as well as in-home care. Some plans allow employees to buy inflation protection and extend coverage beyond their employment. As a result of the higher than projected costs to fund LTC claims and the failed attempt to have LTC included in the ACA, the number of insurance companies that offer LTC plans to employer groups has decreased, and those that do offer coverage may limit it because of the relatively low profit margin for employer-sponsored programs compared to individual policies.

Life insurance is frequently a base benefit offered by employers in all industries. Term group life insurance allows employers to leverage the size of their organization to purchase a more affordable plan. Although all staff who meet eligibility requirements are offered this group insurance, they are no longer covered once they leave the organization. An attractive feature of an employee-sponsored life insurance plan is its portability—that is, an employee's ability to purchase it at the group rate even after he or she resigns. Such portability is offered through a universal life insurance program, which is more expensive for the employer because its benefits extend beyond employment.

Regardless of the type of life insurance offered, the employer must adhere to current IRS regulations that require that the imputed value of policies in excess of $50,000 be calculated and reported to employees as a taxable fringe benefit. The imputed value is actuarially determined; it is not just the cost of the premiums paid by the employer for a policy with a value that is worth more than $50,000. An employer's experience rating as well as actuarial analysis of the demographics of the employee population covered can determine the cost of the plan. The employer decides the amount of the life insurance. Some companies prefer a tiered approach, where the amount is flat and is based on the employee's position level; others base the amount on the employee's salary—for example, the annual salary multiplied by two.

Supplemental life insurance is an optional benefit that many companies allow employees to purchase on behalf of their spouses and children. The ability to buy supplemental insurance at a group rate can be an attractive benefit for some employees. Again, however, portable policies are typically viewed more favorably because the employee can convert an employer-sponsored plan into an individual plan on termination or resignation from the company. Exhibit 10.4 gives brief definitions of the common types of group life insurance.

Retirement Plans

A retirement plan is often a fundamental cornerstone of a comprehensive benefits plan. The type of retirement plan offered and the amount that the employer contributes to a retirement account can be a valuable recruitment

EXHIBIT 10.4
Types of Group
Life Insurance
Plans

Insurance	What Is It?
Term	Covers all benefited employees, provided as a flat amount or multiple of salary from the date of eligibility through the length of employment
Supplemental term	May be purchased by employees to cover themselves, their spouses, and/or their dependent children
Paid up	Life coverage is paid in such a way that all or part of the coverage is fully paid up when the employee retires; as the premium is paid, the amounts of group term coverage are decreased as paid-up amount increases; this type is not commonly used anymore
Permanent	Accrues a cash value over time
Ordinary	Converts to permanent life insurance as the employee contributes to the policy over his or her employment
Variable	Premiums are level over time, but the benefits relate to the value of the assets that are behind the contract at the time the benefits are made payable
Universal	Provides both a term amount of coverage and an accumulating cash value with flexible premium amounts and timing schedules
Variable universal	Provides a guaranteed death benefit with the flexibility of universal premium schedules and the additional investment value of the assets of a variable life insurance policy
Corporate owned	Permanent life insurance purchased for key executives but owned by the organization; at the time of the insured's death, the employer will take the value of what was paid to the policy in premiums and then pay a death benefit to the executive's beneficiaries
Split dollar	Varying forms of permanent life insurance that may be purchased on key executives or company owners; these two parties split both the premium payments and/or the death benefit

tool. Further, careful plan design can create incentives that will assist retention strategies. Many organizations provide a base contribution to such plans and offer a vehicle for employees to save for their own retirement. The two main types of retirement plans are *defined contribution* and *defined benefit*. Exhibit 10.5 enumerates the differences between these two types and also presents a hybrid of the two.

The IRS further categorizes a retirement plan as either a qualified retirement plan or a nonqualified retirement plan. A *qualified retirement*

EXHIBIT 10.5

Categories of Retirement Plans

Retirement Plan	What Is It?	Types	Advantages	Disadvantages
Defined benefit	Provides a retirement benefit payable to the employee on attainment of age and years of service, based on a percentage of salary during working years; usually payable monthly for the lifetime of retiree and/or spouse	Final average salary; career average salary; dollars times years of service	Benefits based on years on the job, encouraging long-term service Benefits based on salary, usually at the highest level	Not as portable Cannot borrow against the plan Assets not directly allocated to the participant until retirement Employer must fund account based on future amounts payable Payable to retiree in either a qualified joint and survivor annuity or a life annuity
Defined contribution	Employer provides a contribution to an account based on the employee's current salary/earnings, and employee can draw on the account after retirement with reduced tax liability	Profit sharing, including 401(k) and 401(a); employee stock option plans; money purchase plans; tax-deferred savings	Employee is generally allowed to direct the investments Assets are allocated to employee such that balance is available at any time At end of employment, assets are transferable to other accounts Can be paid out in lump sum or in installments over time	Final balance in account is based on the performance of the market and the selected investments No guaranteed benefits
Hybrid	Plans that have aspects of both defined benefit and defined contribution	Cash balance; floor offset; pension equity	Balance in account is available to employee	Complex and not easily understood Although the account "balance" is available, it may not be in real dollars but may be an actuarially estimated value

plan has strict eligibility and vesting requirements and strict taxable limits. For example, at least 70 percent of employees who are not highly compensated must be eligible to participate in a qualified plan. To that end, plans that are covered by ERISA must undergo periodic nondiscrimination testing to ensure that this requirement is met. Qualified retirement plans receive more tax benefits, and typically the employee and employer are not taxed until the time a distribution is made. Most qualified plans allow employees to withdraw monies for "hardships" such as loss of home, college education for children, or excessive medical bills. The employee is taxed for a hardship withdrawal and is charged a penalty for early (before retirement age) withdrawal. *Nonqualified retirement plans* are typically designed to meet the needs of key executives and are not subject to as many government regulations. This condition allows nonqualified plans to exceed some of the limits of qualified plans. Because nonqualified plans do not come with as many restrictions, they are perceived as carrying a risk of forfeiture as creditors may attach to the plan assets.

With *defined contribution plans*, the employer contributes an amount to an employee's individual retirement account. The employer determines the rate of this contribution and has discretion over the methodology to calculate this rate. Contribution amounts vary and may be based on such factors as salary, years of service, or even a combination of age and years of service. Using age and years of service as a basis for contribution can help attract midcareer employees because the employer can contribute more to their accounts than to the plans of newer and younger staff, who may be at a stage of life in which retirement is less of a concern.

In addition, the employer can choose the vendor companies and may approve and restrict investment options for employees within these choices. Employees then determine which vendor to use and the allocation of investments they desire (e.g., maximum risk, low risk). The amount that an employee receives on retirement depends on the value that the employee initially established, continually managed, and allowed to grow over the years. The IRS determines the limits on the maximum allowable employer contributions, and these limits are adjusted annually.

Defined benefit plans are group plans, not individual accounts. The contribution amount the employer must make to such a plan is actuarially determined on the basis of the number of participants and their ages, salaries, and projected retirement dates. In theory, the funds contributed to a defined benefit plan should be sufficient to fund all retirees each year. The actual monetary benefit that the employee receives on retirement is determined formulaically and is based on the employee's years of service and salary preceding retirement. Many state-sponsored retirement plans are defined benefit plans. Other benefits of employment may continue with the payment of a cash benefit.

Tax-deferred plans are savings plans that allow staff to contribute to their own retirement. Deferred compensation results in a reduced tax liability for both the employer and the employee, thus making it a popular aspect of retirement plan design. Many organizations encourage employees to participate in tax-deferred plans by contributing a "match" to their retirement accounts.

Media coverage has touted the advantage of Roth 401(k), Roth 403(b), and other nonqualified salary deferral options. Participation by employees and/or employers in nonqualified plans should include research into their potential impacts. The total amount that can be deferred is determined by the IRS and varies annually. Further, the IRS determines the maximum allowable contributions and maximum salary (e.g., $265,000 in 2015) on which not-for-profit companies can contribute (IRS 2014a). If an employer offers multiple options, it must consider the total of all contributions. Limits are based on an aggregation of all plans offered and the actual amount of contribution by plan.

Other Voluntary Benefits

Other voluntary benefits may include programs that are offered through the employer that require participating employees to pay for the premiums. These programs can include benefits such as auto, home, or pet insurance; cancer or other specific disease coverage; supplemental hospitalization and disability payments; will preparation; and concierge services. Many healthcare organizations also offer staff uniform allowances, extensive educational and professional growth opportunities, and tuition reimbursement. Further, with a healthcare workforce that is predominantly female, organizations should consider on-site child care, a benefit offer that can make a health system more competitive from a recruitment and retention standpoint. Assistance with adult day care is another optional benefit that employers are considering.

Perquisites are benefits that may be offered to executives. Such perks may include car allowances, mobile devices, club memberships, and equipment for the home office. Other executive benefits may include cash bonuses and awards, stock options, and severance packages for full or early termination of a contract. Many of these benefits are taxable, and organizations should review their tax implications carefully.

Designing a Benefits Plan

Many factors must be considered when designing a benefits structure that meets the needs of the organization, including generational differences, demographic and economic trends, and organizational budget.

As mentioned earlier, in the US work environment, more employees from different generations are working side by side than ever before. With such a mixture of employees, employers must be aware of generational differences when designing a benefits package. For example, baby boomers may be interested in retirement plans and life insurance, whereas millennials may value paid time off and frequent bonuses. Generation Xers may share either perspective, so a range of options may need to be considered. An organization can learn these differences or preferences by using methods such as analyzing market data and garnering employee input through opinion surveys or suggestion boxes.

The demographics of the employee population can be a key determinant in benefits package design. For example, because the registered nurse workforce is predominantly female, the employer must be cognizant of the ages of employees. By analyzing the ages, the employer can determine whether programs such as prenatal care or annual mammograms are likely to drive healthcare costs and, if so, can explore more cost-effective ways to deliver these services to its registered nurses. Economic trends may affect benefit distributions. When economic downturns occur, some employees may defer retirement.

Another aspect to consider in benefits plan design is adding coverage for domestic partners. Domestic partners are not universally considered dependents. However, several states and companies have provisions that are inclusive of domestic partners. The continued debate between federal and state laws on the validity of marriage between same-sex partners has drawn more attention to the importance of considering coverage for domestic partners. The IRS has issued additional Revenue Rulings and Notices (Revenue Ruling 2013-17 [IRS 2013b], Notice 2013-61 [IRS 2013a], Notice 2014-1 [IRS 2014b]) to address these questions. Employers should consider the states in which they do business and their recruitment and retention strategies to determine whether to include domestic partners in their benefits. Employers and employees must be well informed of the possible federal and state tax implications of this decision, as well as additional obligations to provide coverage other than health insurance when domestic partners are recognized by their health plan.

Benefits program designers should be knowledgeable of the budget that has been allocated for the benefits program so that they can plan accordingly or find possible funding sources. Again, a well-rounded and comprehensive benefits program can help to attract and retain employees in a competitive market, so it must be well designed and cost-effective.

An employee is most typically aware of and concerned about the insurance premiums he or she has to pay out of pocket and the annual increases of such a deduction. Many employers pass the cost increases to employees by raising the amount deducted from employees for health insurance coverage.

This cost shifting can cause controversy if the employees are paying more than the employer or if the rate of salary raises does not absorb the cost of the benefit increases. Cost-containment strategies could range from raising out-of-pocket expenses for those who do not use the healthcare organization's facilities and providers to hiking up copayments and deductibles. Another effective cost-control strategy is to provide employees an incentive to waive coverage if they can show proof of coverage through their spouse or if they can arrange for retiree health coverage from a former employer. As discussed earlier, employers often outsource certain benefits programs such as pharmacy or mental health coverage. The option to outsource all benefits administration may be another cost-saving option. However, note that with this option the employer may lose the ability to customize the benefits package for its employees and encounter employee dissatisfaction if the customer service provided by the benefits administrator is less than ideal.

Another cost-control strategy is to use cafeteria plans or Section 125 plans, named after the section in the Internal Revenue Code that authorizes this method. These plans are popular with employers and employees alike. Employees can elect to pay through payroll deductions for certain qualifying costs on a pretax basis. Examples of qualifying costs include but are not limited to insurance premiums, certain medical expenses not covered by the employer, and expenses associated with dependent care. Also, employees can reduce their overall tax liability and thus increase their take-home pay. The advantage of a cafeteria plan for employers is that the employer match to FICA taxes is reduced and thus can save employers large amounts of money. In addition, some states reduce the employer's liability for workers' compensation.

In designing a benefits program, employers may choose to self-insure certain benefits rather than fully insure with a third party. *Self-insurance* means that the employer takes the risk to appropriately budget, underwrite, and administer a customized benefit rather than contract for a standard plan. A self-insured plan typically allows the employer greater flexibility in plan design. Self-insured health and dental plans can be structured to provide employees with incentives to seek care for themselves and their families at the facilities of the healthcare organization. If an organization chooses to self-insure, contracting with a third party for stop-loss insurance is a wise move. *Stop-loss insurance* mitigates the risk to the employer in the event of large claims in a given plan year. For example, if the employer purchases $200,000 of stop-loss insurance, then that amount is the most that the employer will pay for a given claim; all costs beyond this stop-loss amount are absorbed by the insurance vendor. Another form of stop-loss insurance is aggregate stop-loss, which covers the claims costs that exceed a certain percentage of the underwriter's projected claims costs for the plan year, typically 125 percent or 150 percent of the projected claims. Aggregate stop-loss insurance protects an employer not only from a catastrophic claim for a single participant but also from circumstances that result in multiple large claims that accumulate in excess of the aggregate stop-loss level. These tactics help employers hedge against unanticipated large claims and can significantly reduce the amount of actual claims costs as well as administrative fees associated with a self-insured plan.

Managerial Implications

Given the complexities, legalities, and fiduciary requirements associated with all of the benefits described in this chapter, assigning experienced and qualified benefits professionals to the task of designing (or assisting in) a benefits program is advisable. In particular, certified employee benefits specialists are extremely valuable in this process. Experienced benefits professionals are familiar with the requirements for accounting, audits, tax filing, and other implications of benefits administration. Further, having the benefits staff collaborate with the budget staff helps to ensure that accurate projections of changes in plan designs or premiums can be reflected in the organizational budget.

Communication is also key to the administration of a successful benefits plan. Plan administrators should use every opportunity to keep employees abreast of benefits offered. For example, employers should provide employees with regular information and updates about their total compensation, including the value of employer-sponsored benefits and salaries. During open enrollment periods, the employer must circulate detailed information because these periods are an opportune time to explain the benefits structure. Also, employers should always include a disclaimer that employer-sponsored benefits are subject to change so that staff understand the possibility that some benefits may be eliminated or reduced in the future because of economic or other operational exigencies. See Exhibit 10.6 for a listing of resources related to employee benefits.

Summary

In the competitive healthcare arena, employers are challenged to offer as comprehensive a benefits package as possible to attract and retain healthcare workers at all stages of their careers. Employers are further challenged to provide these benefits in a cost-effective manner with careful consideration to designing a structure that will meet the needs of their employees. Attention must be paid to the complex federal guidelines that govern many benefits programs so that compliance standards and fiduciary responsibilities are met.

EXHIBIT 10.6
Resources for Additional Information on Employee Benefits

Who?	Where?	What?
US Department of Labor	www.dol.gov/ebsa	Guidance and recent changes in labor laws and regulations as they pertain to employer-sponsored pensions, health plans, and other employee benefits
Internal Revenue Service Forms and Publications	www.irs.gov/formspubs/index.html	Quick access to all published forms and publications of the IRS; includes searchable database by topic or publication number
Internal Revenue Service Frequently Asked Questions and Answers	www.irs.gov/faqs/index.html	General questions and answers regarding tax regulations; includes searchable database by category or keyword
Federal Register	www.gpoaccess.gov/fr/index.html	Official daily publication for rules, proposed rules, and notices of federal agencies and organizations as well as executive orders and other presidential documents; includes an extensive search capability
Pension Benefit Guaranty Corporation	www.pbgc.gov	Federal corporation created by the Employee Retirement Income Security Act of 1974, which protects the pensions of private, single-employer, and multiemployer defined benefit pension plans
Centers for Medicare & Medicaid Services	www.cms.hhs.gov	Access to research, guidance, statistics, resources, and tools related to Medicare, Medicaid, and the Children's Health Insurance Program
Federal Health Insurance Marketplace	www.healthcare.gov	Access to health insurance coverage for individuals not covered by an employer-sponsored plan
International Foundation of Employee Benefit Plans	www.ifebp.org	A nonprofit organization dedicated to being a leading objective and independent global source of employee benefits, compensation, and financial literacy education and information in the United States and Canada
Employee Benefit News	ebn.benefitnews.com	Comprehensive, high-quality news on the benefits industry; also publishes a magazine, *Employee Benefit News*
BenefitsLink	www.benefitslink.com/index.html	Portal to news, analysis, opinions, and government documents about employee benefit plans

Discussion Questions

1. Describe the concept of total compensation. Why is it important?

2. How did the Social Security Act change the way retirement benefits were viewed?

3. In designing a benefits plan, what are the most important considerations for an employer?

4. Some industries are cutting back on benefits because of globalization and global competitiveness. Will globalization affect benefits offered in healthcare organizations, or is the benefits structure in healthcare insulated from these global pressures?

5. Employers are finding health insurance coverage more difficult to support as a benefit because it has become more costly than the tax savings for offering it. Given provisions of the ACA, should a large employer (more than 50 employees) continue to offer health insurance as a benefit or pay a penalty? What are the pros and cons of offering health insurance or letting employees go to a health insurance exchange for coverage? Note organizational, market, policy, and financial implications in your response.

Experiential Exercises

Exercise The purpose of this exercise is to give readers an opportunity to analyze the benefits provided by a healthcare organization. Begin this exercise by visiting the website (or the HR web page) of a local hospital to see how much benefits information is posted online. Then visit the organization's HR department, and answer the following questions:

1. How many total employees are in the department, and how many are assigned to handle benefits administration? How many of the staff are certified employee benefits specialists?

2. How are benefits communicated to employees at this hospital?

3. What benefits are offered to full-time, part-time, and hourly employees?

4. Do physicians receive the same benefits as other employees?

5. What perquisites are offered to executives?

6. Is the organization considering any benefits that are not currently being offered? If so, what are they and how were they identified? If not, what benefits may be added if the organization can afford to do so?

After visiting the department, write a summary of what was found. In writing the summary, make an assessment of how comprehensive the benefits package is for employees and how well it is communicated.

References

American College of Healthcare Executives. 2014. "Top Issues Confronting Hospitals: 2013." Accessed December 30. www.ache.org/PUBS/research/ceoissues.cfm.

American Nurses Credentialing Center (ANCC). 2014. "Forces of Magnetism." Accessed December 30. www.nursecredentialing.org/ForcesofMagnetism.

Bragg, D., and K. Vermoch. 2003. *Workplace of Choice Benchmarking Project Report.* Oakbrook, IL: University HealthSystem Consortium.

Cunningham, R., III, and R. M. Cunningham Jr. 1997. *The Blues: A History of the Blue Cross and Blue Shield System.* DeKalb, IL: Northern Illinois University Press.

Employee Benefit Research Institute (EBRI). 2013. *EBRI Databook on Employee Benefits.* Updated February. www.ebri.org/publications/books/?fa=databook.

Internal Revenue Service (IRS). 2014a. "COLA Increases on Dollar Limitations on Benefits and Contributions." Updated October 24. www.irs.gov/Retirement-Plans/COLA-Increases-for-Dollar-Limitations-on-Benefits-and-Contributions.

———. 2014b. "Sections 125 and 223—Cafeteria Plans, Flexible Spending Arrangements, and Health Savings Accounts—Elections and Reimbursements for Same-Sex Spouses Following the *Windsor* Supreme Court Decision." Accessed December 30. www.irs.gov/pub/irs-drop/n-14-01.pdf.

———. 2013a. "Application of *Windsor* Decision and Rev. Rul. 2013-17 to Employment Taxes and Special Administrative Procedures for Employers to Make Adjustments or Claims for Refund or Credit." Accessed December 30, 2014. www.irs.gov/pub/irs-drop/n-13-61.pdf.

———. 2013b. "Rev. Rul. 2013-17." Accessed December 30, 2014. www.irs.gov/pub/irs-drop/rr-13-17.pdf.

Social Security Administration. 2014. "Contribution and Benefit Bases, 1937–2015." Accessed December 30. www.socialsecurity.gov/OACT/COLA/cbb.html#Series.

Starr, P. 1982. *The Social Transformation of American Medicine.* New York: Basic Books.

University HealthSystem Consortium. 2005. *Member Satisfaction Survey, 2004–2005.* Oakbrook, IL: University HealthSystem Consortium.

US Chamber of Commerce. 2007. *Employee Benefits Study.* Washington, DC: US Chamber of Commerce.

US Department of Labor. 2014a. "Benefits: Workers' Compensation Programs." Accessed December 30. www.dol.gov/compliance/topics/benefits-comp.htm.

———. 2014b. "FAQs About Portability of Health Coverage and HIPAA." Accessed December 30. www.dol.gov/ebsa/faqs/faq_consumer_hipaa.html.

———. 2014c. "Wages." Accessed December 30. www.dol.gov/dol/topic/wages/.

11

ORGANIZATIONAL DEVELOPMENT AND LEARNING

Donna L. Kaye and Myron D. Fottler

Learning Objectives

After completing this chapter, the reader should be able to

- define organizational development, its role within human resources, and its contribution to the bottom line;
- identify the services offered and competencies associated with organizational development and learning;
- describe the ways organizational development and learning are organized in healthcare;
- explain the critical role of employee engagement in the overall effectiveness of the organization;
- list the steps in the process of performance improvement consultation;
- describe a basic model for diagnosing performance problems and determining root causes;
- list the steps in the process of organizational change management consultation;
- describe the types of instructional methodologies and learning management systems are that used throughout healthcare;
- describe the basic model for training development (ADDIE) and subsequent enhancements;
- express the difference between on-the-job and off-the-job training methods;
- explain the importance and key elements of new-employee onboarding;
- explain the process of succession planning; and
- describe the trends in organizational development and learning.

Introduction

An employer's strategic plans should ultimately govern the learning goals of its employees (Desmet, McGurk, and Schwartz 2010; Society for Human Resource Management 2011). As is the case with other human resources (HR) functions, the task is to identify employee behaviors required to execute the strategy and the related competencies employees will need. One survey found that establishing a link between learning and organizational performance was the number one issue facing training and organizational specialists (Wells, Swaine, and Fieldhouse 2010). *Organizational development* (OD) is one of the most significant HR activities that facilitate achievement of a healthcare organization's strategic goals.

One thing is certain in today's global workplace: It will change. According to William Roper, CEO of the University of North Carolina (UNC) Health Care System, "the health care industry is going to see more change happen more rapidly than we have seen in the history of health care" (Roper 2013). With change comes the need to bolster the organization's HR and organizational capabilities to ensure that the organization continues to meet its goals.

Facilitating change requires that healthcare organizations employ both OD and training. OD provides a systematic learning and development strategy aligned with organizational goals and may include training, but is not limited to training. In other words, organizational learning is more than the sum of all the training, lessons, and knowledge in an organization. Understanding the key constructs of effective learning is crucial to the success of OD, which is a change process through which employees formulate the required change and implement it with the assistance of trained internal and external consultants (Dodgeson 1993; Dressler 2014). It usually involves action research applying behavioral science knowledge to improve organizational effectiveness through employee empowerment, engagement, and problem solving.

Therefore, the terminology used in both the literature and actual department names has shifted from *training* to *learning*. Training is often used in association with development, but the two are not synonymous. *Training* refers to the acquisition of knowledge, skills, and abilities that are related to specific competencies needed for a job. For purposes of this chapter, the terms *training* and *learning* are used interchangeably.

More specifically, training focuses on the current job, the individual employee, the immediate time frame, and a current skill deficit. By contrast, OD focuses on both current and future jobs, the work group or organization, the long term, and future work demands (Gomez-Mejia, Balkin, and Cardy 2012). According to the Society for Human Resource Management (2014), OD is "a planned organization-wide effort to improve and increase the organization's effectiveness, productivity, return on investment and overall employee job satisfaction through planned interventions in the organization's processes." The primary goal of OD, then, is to develop the organization, not necessarily to train or develop the staff.

The OD department may have different functions in each organization, but in its classic function, OD is a planned, organization-wide effort that is managed from the top to increase organizational effectiveness and health through planned interventions in the organization's processes using behavioral science knowledge (Beckhard 1969). The field of OD has developed since the 1960s, influenced by other change-oriented movements such as quality improvement, Lean, Six Sigma, human factors, positive psychology, and even consulting firms' branding of "change management."

Organizational Development: Objectives and Services

Most often, the objectives of the OD function are the following:

- Increase the level of interpersonal trust among employees
- Increase the employees' level of satisfaction and commitment
- Confront problems instead of neglecting them
- Effectively manage conflict and increase cooperation among employees
- Increase organizational problem solving and ability to adapt to change

The services offered by an OD and learning department can vary but usually include the following:

- New-employee orientation and onboarding
- Design and delivery of leadership development programs
- Design and delivery of nonclinical professional development programs
- Promotion of employee engagement
- Leadership coaching
- Performance improvement consultation
- Cultural change management consultation
- Team development
- Succession planning
- Alignment of strategic learning
- Instructional design consultation
- Learning management systems
- Learning technology implementation and consultation (e-learning, mobile learning, webinars)

These functions are summarized in the mission statement of the Learning and Organizational Development Department at UNC Medical Center: "We enable collaborative learning, change management and development of leaders, their teams and all employees in order to create a system-wide culture of outstanding patient care and organizational effectiveness" (UNC Medical Center 2014).

Most often, the OD and learning function is part of the HR department. In an internal survey of 18 OD departments in academic medical centers conducted by University HealthSystem Consortium (UHC) members in February 2011, all but one of the organizational development departments reported to the vice president of HR (Association of American Medical Colleges 2012).

Typically, the learning function is decentralized in healthcare, with clinical education the responsibility of the nursing and the ancillary departments; information system education the responsibility of the information technology department; and the rest of education, especially leadership education, the responsibility of HR. Some organizations have moved to a more centralized learning function, with all the learning functions reporting to a chief learning officer. In the previously mentioned UHC survey from 2011, 37.5 percent of member healthcare systems responding to the inquiry had some centralized learning, though education on nursing competencies was still largely handled through the nursing division.

Competencies Needed

HR professionals who are interested in the field of OD and learning must be familiar with the competencies that employees need to be successful. An OD professional requires comprehensive knowledge of human behavior, supported by awareness of a number of intervention techniques. The Association for Talent Development (ATD; formerly the American Society for Training and Development) competency model lists six foundational competencies and ten areas of expertise (see Exhibit 11.1). This model defines the skills and knowledge required to be successful now and in the future.

Many staff members in OD departments are called OD consultants. A consultant is a person who is in a position to influence an individual, group, or organization but has no direct power to make changes or implement programs (Block 2011).

Employee Engagement

One of the major objectives of OD and learning is employee engagement. Employee engagement is a measure of employees' positive or negative emotional

EXHIBIT 11.1
ATD
Competency
Model

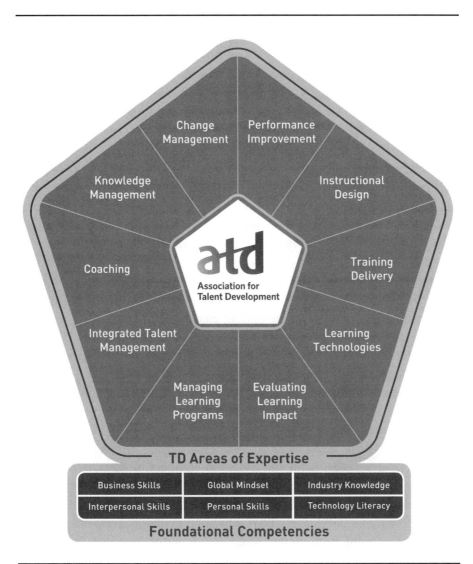

Source: Association for Talent Development (2014a).

attachment to their job, which influences their willingness to learn and perform at work. More simply stated, "an employee is engaged if he or she is willing to go above and beyond what would typically be expected in his or her role" (Effron and Ort 2010, 109). Studies have shown that engaged employees demonstrate higher levels of performance, commitment, and loyalty (BlessingWhite 2013). Evidence also suggests that higher engagement leads to better business performance. In fact, a study found that employee engagement resulted in increased financial performance over both one- and three-year periods (Towers Perrin 2009).

While actual engagement surveys are usually conducted by outside companies that can provide normative data and ensure confidentiality, the administration of the survey process, the hardwiring of processes and policies that create accountability needed to support employee engagement, and the coaching of leaders to respond to employees' needs usually are functions of the OD department.

Enhancing employee engagement is one of the challenges facing healthcare organizations. A Gallup poll found that 52 percent of all full-time workers in the United States are not involved in, enthusiastic about, or committed to their work. Another 18 percent are actually disengaged, which means that they are beyond just checking out mentally and could even be undermining their colleagues' productivity (Korn 2013). Given the negative impact of the 2008–2013 recession on healthcare employees, these general findings are likely to hold true in healthcare. The poll also found that women, managers, and employees of small organizations required higher engagement than did larger organizations. Gallup estimated that disengaged employees cost the United States $450–$550 billion a year as a result of high absenteeism and turnover (Korn 2013).

Moreover, the 2013 Nonprofit Employment Trends Survey stressed that retaining employees and motivating employees to be more engaged are the biggest problems facing nonprofit organizations (Nonprofit HR Solutions 2013). An Accenture (2012) study found that when employees are not engaged, they are more likely to leave their jobs. This study also contended that organizations can increase employee engagement by communicating the link between specific job responsibilities and organizational goals to achieve the organization's mission. Other factors related to engagement include job characteristics such as job variety, task significance, autonomy, perceived organizational support, perceived supervisor support, rewards and recognition, procedural justice, trust, empowerment, coaching, career development, and development/learning (Mone and London 2009; Word 2012).

Harter and colleagues (2013) found employee engagement to be positively and significantly related to employee performance along a number of dimensions. Engaged employees are present not only at the physical level but also at the psychological level (Rich, Lepine, and Crawford 2010). This engagement results in higher levels of attentiveness, focus, and integration. In turn, these factors enhance the employee's organizational perspective, efficiency, and effectiveness (Markos and Stridevi 2010).

A common adage is "what gets measured matters." Healthcare organizations have long measured financial performance. Now they are placing a greater emphasis on measuring clinical outcomes, patient satisfaction, and even employee satisfaction. More studies are showing a link between patient satisfaction and employee satisfaction (Fottler, Ford, and Heaton 2010; "Keeping Happy" 2004; Studer 2008).

Having a tangible measure of employee engagement gives the OD department a critical role to play in helping the organization to achieve its strategic goals. More and more healthcare organizations are including

EXHIBIT 11.2
Strategies
for Positive
Employee
Engagement

Accountability and Alignment
- Set the expectation that low employee engagement scores are not acceptable.
- Tie survey results to individual and organizational performance measures.
- Create transparency in sharing results of improvement initiatives.
- Measure results on a regular basis.
- Reassign leaders who do not achieve expected results over time.

Leadership Development
- Provide specific leadership development programs focused on employee engagement.
- Integrate employee engagement strategies into other leadership development programs.
- Assign an OD consultant staff member to coach low-performing leaders on development of improvement initiatives and engagement skills.
- Help remove any organizational barriers to success.
- Provide tools for action planning and staff involvement.

Recognition
- Recognize leaders for their strong and improved results.
- Promote staff recognition through praise, team celebrations, and acts of appreciation.
- Reevaluate rates of pay and incentive pay for key groups.

employee engagement results in their overall strategic goals and even linking them to incentive compensation (Frasch 2011b; McIlvaine 2012).

At UNC Medical Center, the increase in employee engagement has been substantial. In 2007, employee engagement, as measured by Press Ganey Associates, was at the thirty-third percentile of Press Ganey's national healthcare database—a database consisting of 350 clients representing 600 different healthcare facilities that mirror the distribution of the US healthcare labor force. In 2013, following a steady upward improvement in engagement, UNC Medical Center scored in the ninety-first percentile for employee engagement based on Press Ganey's Power Items. (Power Items are key survey items that drive engagement and commitment.) Exhibit 11.2 outlines the key strategies that contributed to the improvement in employee engagement at UNC Medical Center. These strategies can help healthcare organizations create a more engaged workforce.

Performance Improvement Consultation

To increase an organization's effectiveness, the root cause of an organizational or performance discrepancy must be diagnosed. In other words, what stands in the way of the future state that the organization desires to reach? Performance improvement consultation provides the process, methodology, and tools for analyzing human and organizational performance gaps and then closing them. The distinct phases of the consulting process are shown in Exhibit 11.3.

The better the job that the OD consultant can do in contracting with the client—agreeing on what is expected from the OD consultant and from the client and how they will work together—the more successful the performance improvement consultation will be. An example of an OD contract for coaching or consulting services is shown in Exhibit 11.4.

EXHIBIT 11.3
Performance
Improvement
Consulting
Process

Phase	Description	Goal
1. Entry	Initial contact, usually from the client	Establish credibility and build client confidence; clarify who is the ultimate client
2. Contracting	Written agreement with client about what is expected and how OD consultant and client will work together to achieve desired future state	Shared understanding of future state outcomes, roles and responsibilities of client and OD consultant, data collection methods, measurement, confidentiality, and resource needs
3. Data collection and diagnosis	Planning and implementation of tools and methods to collect pertinent information (i.e., surveys, interviews, focus groups, observation, review of already-collected data)	Greater understanding of possible root causes of performance discrepancy
4. Feedback and intervention options	Presentation (usually in writing) of the findings and interpretation of the data along with recommendations codeveloped by the consultant and client for intervention options	Client understanding of root causes and agreement on intervention options
5. Implementation	Plan for how to implement agreed-on interventions	Clarity of what, who, when, and how of intervention options as well as evaluation metrics
6. Evaluation	Measurement of the effectiveness of the intervention implemented	Determination of the effectiveness of the intervention so that adjustments can be made as needed
7. Contract renegotiation or exit	Determination, based on evaluation, if more consulting work needs to be done; renegotiation of contract if necessary or, if work is finished, provision of closure for client	Clarity about next steps; sense of completion of consulting process

Issue	Question(s) to Be Answered	Points of Agreement/ Action
Reason for coaching/consulting	What is the current state? In what area are changes desired? Why?	
Specific goal(s) of the coaching/ consulting	What specifically will the partnership try to accomplish? Why is that important for you and for the organization?	
Method/data gathering tool(s) to be used	What will be the predominant method used to achieve the goals of the partnership? What data (personal or from others) will be gathered?	
Timing	When will the coaching/consulting occur? How long? How often?	
Measurement of progress (e.g., mini-survey, employee engagement survey)	How will the parties assess progress?	
Duration/conditions of termination	At what point will the coaching/consulting relationship end?	
People to be kept informed	Who else should be informed of your/your team's progress? What method(s) will be used in sharing information, if appropriate?	
Maintaining confidentiality	Confidential/private to maximum extent possible. We are required to report • if shared information represents a threat or is perceived to be detrimental to another person, yourself, or the organization; and • if shared information requires reporting under our corporate compliance policy. Coached individual/client will be notified should it be necessary to report the above.	

EXHIBIT 11.4
Coaching/
Consulting
Contract

The meat of any performance improvement consultation is diagnosing the root cause of the performance discrepancy. Often when a client (manager, director, or executive) calls on an OD consultant to help close a performance gap, the client has predetermined a solution and simply wants the OD consultant to implement that solution—usually a particular training program. Using a performance improvement model becomes essential to make sure that the root cause of the performance discrepancy has been correctly diagnosed so that an appropriate solution can be agreed on.

Thomas Gilbert, known as the father of performance technology, applied his understanding of the process of technological improvement to human beings (Gilbert [1978] 1996). He believed that a lack of support in the environment, rather than a person's lack of knowledge or skill, was the greatest barrier to work performance. Since that time, others have adapted Gilbert's model to sort behavior influences into six categories that help OD consultants diagnose the underlying issue of a performance discrepancy (Binder 1998; Chevalier 2003). The OD consultant can gather diagnostic data by asking clients the questions in each of the categories. If the client responds "no" in some of the categories, this information can steer the consultant toward a hypothesis about the underlying cause of the performance discrepancy.

In addition to asking these diagnostic questions, the consultant can gather additional data such as employee complaints, actual performance on key organizational metrics, engagement survey results, turnover, promotion statistics, and input from focus groups. Exhibits 11.5 and 11.6 show the performance improvement diagnostic model and its interpretation. This model can be used for assessment of both consulting and training needs.

Change Management

OD consultants often help an organization adapt to change caused by shifting external business and societal forces. Whereas performance improvement consulting is concerned with closing a performance gap usually contained within a department or division, change management is concerned with responding to external forces that require the organization and its staff to think about and do their work differently.

A Google search (November 6, 2014) for the words "change management" produced 478,000,000 results, showing the proliferation of models and approaches to change management. The change management methodology in Exhibit 11.7 is a compilation of the most often cited change models (Association for Talent Development 2014a; Conner 2006; Kotter [1996] 2012; Kübler-Ross 1974; Maurer 2010).

Succession Planning

In addition to improving organizational effectiveness by closing performance gaps, OD departments can be proactive in ensuring the continuing vitality of an organization by developing potential successors for the positions identified as critical to operations.

EXHIBIT 11.5

Performance Improvement Diagnostic Model

	Information	**Instrumentation**	**Motivation**
Environmental supports	**1. Information** Have clear performance expectations and priorities been communicated? Has the critical importance of the performance expectations and priorities been explained? Are employees given specific and timely feedback regarding their performance?	**2. Resources** Do employees have the materials/equipment needed to do their jobs? Do employees have the time needed to do their jobs? Is training available to enhance knowledge and skills? Are people, information, and other resources structured to support the workflow?	**3. Incentives** Are sufficient financial incentives offered for performance? Are sufficient nonfinancial incentives (i.e., recognition) offered for performance? Are measurement and reporting systems used to track results? Are opportunities for career development provided?
Person's repertory of behavior	**4. Skills/knowledge** Do employees have the knowledge to be successful? Do employees have the skills to be successful? Do employees understand how their roles affect organizational performance?	**5. Capacity** Do employees have the ability to learn what is expected? Are employees free from any emotional or physical limitations that impede performance? Are the employee recruitment and selection processes matched to the realities of the work situation?	**6. Motives** Do employees care about the incentives offered by the job? Do the employees want to do the job to the best of their abilities? Do employees receive any rewards that reinforce poor performance or face any negative consequences for good performance? Do employees view the work environment as positive?

Note: If the answer to any of the questions in this exhibit is no, the issue shown in the corresponding box in Exhibit 11.6 may be at the root of the performance problem or gap.

EXHIBIT 11.6

Performance Improvement Diagnostic Model: Interpreting Responses to Diagnostic Questions

	Information	**Instrumentation**	**Motivation**
Environmental supports	**1. Information** Leadership communication issue	**2. Resources** Leadership and resource issue	**3. Incentives** Incentive and infrastructure issue
Person's repertory of behavior	**4. Skills/knowledge** Training and leadership communication issue	**5. Capacity** Employee motivational fit issue (wrong job for the employee)	**6. Motives** Employee motivation and satisfaction issue

EXHIBIT 11.7
Change
Management
Model

Change Management Step	Description
1. Compelling case and awareness	Make a compelling case for change to build awareness. Explain "why" before "how." Match communication style to audience preference.
2. Sponsorship	Establish sponsorship for the change with an active leadership core to guide the effort.
3. Involvement	Build involvement throughout. Identify key stakeholders and reach out to them.
4. Project management	Create a plan and project management system to keep on track.
5. Resistance management	Anticipate pushback and emotional reactions to change. Be sensitive to feelings of loss. Allow stakeholders to express emotional concerns.
6. Communication and celebration	Communicate and celebrate results along the way. Don't wait for the complete change to take place. Celebrate quick wins.
7. Cultural integration	Integrate changes into organizational culture. Hardwire the new way of doing things into key work processes and reward mechanisms.

Sources: Kotter ([1996] 2012); also Association for Talent Development (2014a); Heath and Heath (2010); and Maurer (2010).

The term *succession* contains the word *success*. In that sense, succession planning may be explained as a strategy for the organization to succeed. To some degree, succession planning has been occurring in organizations for many years. People have been groomed to take over positions through mentoring and even job-shadowing processes, but most organizations have failed to put into place a formalized structure for recognizing this tradition. "Bench strength" and "the leadership pipeline" are metaphors for the process of having replacements ready.

The purpose of *succession planning* is to provide a basis for changes such as transfers, promotions, turnovers, and retirement. The goal is to prepare for the inevitable movements of people who create holes in the hierarchy that need to be filled by qualified replacements. Such voids can be prevented by having a succession plan ready when needed. Usually healthcare organizations engage in succession planning for key positions that are crucial for the implementation of strategic organizational goals. Succession planning is most likely to occur when the OD or HR department is able to demonstrate the critical significance of such planning (Grossman 2011). The overall process of succession planning is outlined in Exhibit 11.8.

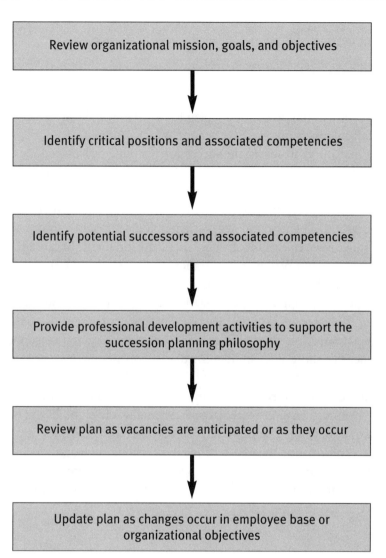

EXHIBIT 11.8
The
Succession
Planning
Process

With the fluidity of positions and people in organizations, such planning must be reviewed and revised frequently. A critical step in the succession planning model is to forecast demand and skill gaps for key positions (Blouin et al. 2006; Phillips and Gully 2012). What is a key need today is no indication of what will be needed in the future, as evidenced by the rapid changes in technology and other medical advances. Once the HR needs in key positions are identified, managers must identify and develop high-potential key employees through internal training, cross-functional experiences, job rotation, and external training (Day 2011). The final step is assessing candidates and selecting those who will actually fill the key positions.

The succession planning effort should result in the following products:

- Identification of potential vacancies in critical positions
- Identification of successors who will be ready to fill these positions with additional development

The development required and the plan for achieving it should be made clear to the staff members involved (Greer and Virick 2008).

In many organizations, the succession planning process is done only for the top executive position. That line of thinking comes with the philosophy that only "high-potential" individuals will benefit from the leadership development that supports the succession planning program (Pintar, Capuano, and Rosser 2007). This mind-set is dysfunctional. Imagine an organization facing a huge wave of employees who are near retirement. Because the organization's succession planning is designed exclusively for the top executives, no one is in line to fill the positions that these future retirees will leave vacant. That scenario will cripple the organization. Moreover, organizations need to recognize the value of exposing every employee, not just those designated as "high potential," to the training and workshops targeted to support the development of those who are identified as successors.

Keeping a list of candidates who are eligible to fill critical positions that could be vacated through retirement or other means of attrition is good practice. Doing so ensures workplace sustainability and signifies the presence of effective leadership. The candidate list may include the names of potential successors; information related to their professional preparation, including the number of years until they will be ready for the position; and the competencies necessary for the position. This list can be as simple or as sophisticated as the organization requires.

Succession planning can be a vehicle for social responsibility. Organizations can use it to give an opportunity to or advance underrepresented or protected groups. Healthcare still lags behind other industries in terms of growing leaders within the organization, a practice that was almost nonexistent in healthcare in the past. According to a 2012 study that surveyed 6,300 US hospital CEOs, 66 percent of hospitals are now utilizing succession planning in their organizations as compared with 55 percent in 2007. This increase is significant considering studies from 2005, which indicated that only 21 percent of hospitals focused on succession planning at that time (Collins et al. 2013).

Health First, located in Brevard County, Florida, addressed its succession planning needs in 2007. The organization initiated a formal mentoring process, pairing up senior executives with junior managers and directors from across the organization. To make the mentoring relationships more comfortable for participants, the paired individuals came from different business units, avoiding the conflict that can arise with direct-report relationships and allowing participants to freely express themselves (DeMarco 2007). Health First's succession planning was initiated in 2010 when CEO Michael Means announced his 2011 retirement and the Health First board of directors began a 20-month succession planning process to ensure a smooth leadership transition (Health First 2010).

In the future, the bench strength of an organization will continue to play an important part in organizational vitality. The most important benefits of formal succession planning include establishing a supply of highly qualified individuals ready for future job openings, providing career opportunities and employee incentives for retention, ensuring adequate staffing as the organization changes over time, and enhancing the branding of the company as a desirable place to work (Ketter 2009). Formalized succession planning is typically found in larger healthcare organizations.

Common succession planning mistakes include not linking the process to the strategic plan, focusing only on CEO and top management succession, starting only after openings are present, allowing the CEO to direct the process and make all succession decisions, and looking only internally for succession candidates (Ketter 2009).

Learning Goals

Many organizations have some mandatory or required training for all employees as well as specified training requirements for particular positions that may involve licensing or certification and annual or periodic renewals. Healthcare personnel, for example, may need to obtain a certain number of training hours per year in their field to maintain professional licensure. Healthcare organizations also undergo an accreditation process every few years to ensure patient safety and quality of services.

Training for evolving job roles enables employees to perform their jobs better. It allows for the continuing updating of skills and knowledge as roles change over time. Interpersonal and problem-solving training addresses both operational and interpersonal problems by focusing on interpersonal communication, managerial and supervisory skills, and conflict resolution (Frasch 2011a). Finally, developmental and career training provides a longer-term focus on both individual and organizational capabilities for the future. (See Exhibit 11.9.)

The Joint Commission (2014) is the major accrediting organization in the healthcare industry, and its qualifying process requires healthcare professionals and staff to have education and training. The Joint Commission standards for compliance and patient safety must be met, including tracking and documentation. Documentation at the minimum includes the name of the training or intervention, the participant's name, and the date of completion of training.

Training represents a significant expenditure for most employers. However, it is often viewed tactically rather than strategically. In other words,

Dimension of Training	Typical Topics
Legal or management mandated	Antiharassment Diversity Disaster preparedness Quality improvement New-employee orientation Employee licensing/certification requirements Safety compliance Benefits enrollment
Position-specific topics	Patient safety Understanding organ donation Patient-centered care In-service learning Record keeping Information technology systems
Interpersonal problem solving	Customer service Building high-performing teams Dealing with difficult people Coaching for excellence Embracing change Conflict resolution
Developmental and career	Healthcare trends Leadership Change management Career planning Strategic thinking

many employers view it as a short-term activity that can be stopped and started periodically rather than an activity that has long-term implications for organizational effectiveness. As a result, management frequently supports training in words rather than in action. Training is among the first expenses to be cut in challenging economic times (Schramm 2011).

The pace of change in healthcare is such that if staff are not continuously trained, they may fall behind and the organization may become less competitive. Continuous training allows healthcare organizations to develop staff members with the knowledge, skills, and abilities needed to achieve competitive advantage (Sum 2011).

Training can also positively influence organizational competitiveness by enhancing employee retention. A major reason many employees leave healthcare organizations is a shortage of career training and development opportunities. Employers who invest in training and developing their employees generally enhance their retention efforts (Davis 2012).

Designing Training for Sustainability

Not all training is effective. In a McKinsey survey, only one quarter of employers said that their training programs measurably improve their organization's performance, and most did not measure the programs' effectiveness. The most common evaluation method was simply to ask participants if they liked the training or not (DeSmet, McGurk, and Schwartz 2010). Those who view training as a strategic investment align training with long-term organizational goals in order to provide value.

To ensure that organizational learning is effective, a systematic approach is prescribed as a best practice. The consistency of planning, execution, and metrics gives credibility and power to the OD process.

Training can come in many formats, including in-person classes, e-learning, online asynchronous or synchronous courses, self-paced videos, and even videoconferencing. Training may be defined by its delivery mode (e.g., online, self-directed), but *training design* is the unifying thread of all training modes. Changes in technology and advances in healthcare influence not only the operation of an organization but also its processes, necessitating new training and education and thus new training designs. Quality assurance reports may be helpful in identifying areas in which deficiencies exist and training is needed. Several training design models exist, and all of them are based on the primary necessity of an effective training initiative. After all, who wants to train for the sake of training? In today's business climate, no organization or department can afford to be frivolous—at least not if it wants to survive.

One ubiquitous model used for instructional system design is the ADDIE model (analysis, design, development, implementation, and evaluation). The ADDIE model ensures that the how, what, why, where, who, and when of training are addressed. Furthermore, this approach constantly evaluates the training initiative for compatibility with and proficiency in the changing workplace. Exhibit 11.10 depicts the five steps in this model that are integral to good training design.

The ADDIE model has come under criticism because of its inflexibility and failure to address iterative processes. The book *Leaving ADDIE for SAM* (Allen and Sites 2012) explains how newer methods of training design and development foster more creativity and more effective stakeholder involvement. This book introduces two concepts—the successive approximation model (SAM) and the Savvy Start. Together, they incorporate contemporary design processes that simplify training design and development (see Exhibit 11.11). This combination yields a more energetic and effective learning experience. In this method, prototypes promote brainstorming and creative problem solving, help the team determine what is and is not important, and help align the team's values (Allen and Sites 2012).

EXHIBIT 11.10
ADDIE Training
Design Process
Overview

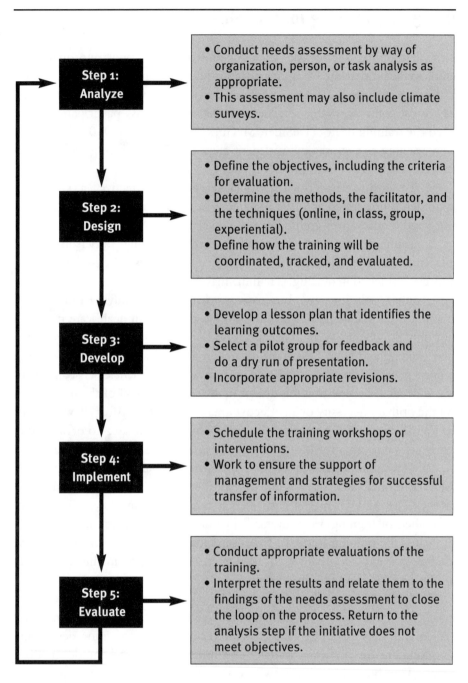

Step 1: Analyze	• Conduct needs assessment by way of organization, person, or task analysis as appropriate. • This assessment may also include climate surveys.
Step 2: Design	• Define the objectives, including the criteria for evaluation. • Determine the methods, the facilitator, and the techniques (online, in class, group, experiential). • Define how the training will be coordinated, tracked, and evaluated.
Step 3: Develop	• Develop a lesson plan that identifies the learning outcomes. • Select a pilot group for feedback and do a dry run of presentation. • Incorporate appropriate revisions.
Step 4: Implement	• Schedule the training workshops or interventions. • Work to ensure the support of management and strategies for successful transfer of information.
Step 5: Evaluate	• Conduct appropriate evaluations of the training. • Interpret the results and relate them to the findings of the needs assessment to close the loop on the process. Return to the analysis step if the initiative does not meet objectives.

An effective training design plan must be detailed and include updated timelines, but the plan must also be flexible enough to change with organizational requirements as they evolve. In dynamic healthcare environments, OD departments must be visionary and respond to the needs for learning experiences that are propagated by constant institutional changes (Mailloux 1998). The organizational structure should facilitate, not detract from, the success of a training initiative.

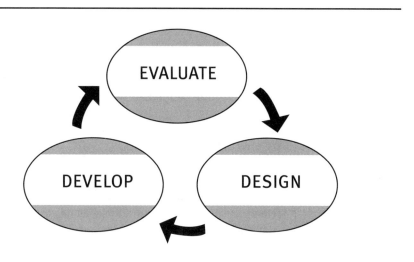

EXHIBIT 11.11
Basic Iterative
Design

Source: Allen and Sites (2012).

Decisions about the training method and the involved personnel should follow a systematic assessment. For example, an employer may be tempted to choose a facilitator before even assessing the need for training. This action may jeopardize the effectiveness of the training and may add pressure to the process, reducing the purpose of the training to "make it fit" rather than to provide value. Simply, the needs assessment and design phase should drive the training initiative. Sometimes, a needs assessment will reveal that training is not the proper remedy for the problem. For example, lack of employee motivation or poor staff morale cannot be rectified by offering training. Numerous companies have spent thousands of dollars on a training initiative that did not meet its intended objectives.

The following six-step training design process incorporates the structure of the ADDIE process with the flexibility of SAM. Step 1 of the training design process is an *organizational needs analysis*, in which facts are collected to determine the intervention necessary, if any. It involves an assessment of short- and long-term development needs based on the organization's business strategy, its culture, and expected changes in its external environment (Brown and Sitzman 2011). Needs assessment is the heart of this phase, serving as a tool to gather information on whether gaps exist in the desired and actual levels of performance according to organizational requirements or performance standards. Exhibit 11.12 provides basic questions that should be asked during the needs assessment phase as well as specific questions that should be answered before embarking on any type of training.

Training needs can be determined by analyzing current organizational outcomes and future organizational needs. In other words, what knowledge, skills, and abilities will be needed now, as well as in the future, as both jobs and organizations change? Answering this question requires analyzing the

EXHIBIT 11.12
Questions to
Consider for
Training Needs
Assessment

Basic Questions	Specific Questions
Why?	• Does a performance deficiency exist anywhere in the organization? • What data is this deficiency tied to (e.g., absenteeism, medical errors, poor customer service, grievances)? • Are any changes (e.g., legislative or regulatory changes, downsizing, new processes, new technology) expected to affect performance?
Who?	• Who is involved in addressing a performance deficiency or expected changes in the workplace?
How?	• How can the performance deficiency be corrected? • Can the skill or knowledge deficiency that created the problem be ameliorated by training?
What?	• What is the best way (based on interviews, observations, and standards of performance) to perform the specific job task? • Do the staff have the skills and knowledge to perform the most critical tasks?
When?	• When should training occur to provide the most benefit to staff with the least impact on business operations? • What format (e.g., classroom, experiential, online) is most effective? • What else is needed to make the training most effective?

Source: Adapted from Cekada (2011).

technical deficiencies of current employees and the inadequately educated labor force from which new workers may be drawn. Data relevant to training needs assessment come from measures of organizational performance such as turnover, customer complaints, grievance rates, high absenteeism, poor performance, and other staff deficiencies.

A needs assessment can be performed in many ways. Mailloux (1998) found that to determine learning needs, nursing educators use methods that include reviewing job performance data, customer complaint data, supervisors' performance appraisals, and critical incident reports; directly observing employees; conducting attitude surveys with questionnaires; and interviewing employees and their supervisors. Methods that involve the direct feedback of staff, such as surveys, can be administered with an instruction to respondents to either identify themselves or answer anonymously

Step 2 of the process consists of *job task analysis*. By comparing the job requirements with the knowledge, skills, and abilities of current staff, training needs can be identified (Dolezalek 2009). Other ways to determine training gaps include surveying employees, having them anonymously evaluate the skill levels of themselves and other employees. A training needs survey may take the form of questionnaires or interviews with supervisors and employees either individually or in groups. Many healthcare facilities face the possibility of miscommunication or accidents in areas where a high percentage of employees speak a primary language other than English. Such data would suggest the need for language training for some employees. A final way to determine training needs is to include managerial and nonmanagerial input on what types of training are needed. Individuals can often identify their own training needs (Buck and Martin 2012).

Step 3 of the process is *establishment of training priorities and objectives*, in which the grand plan is established, the timelines are set, and the overall project outline is created. In keeping with good business protocol, developing options to keep the plan flexible is advisable. The critical tasks in this phase are to accurately outline the objectives, communicate them to all involved, and ensure that they are thoroughly understood. Training objectives and priorities can be established by gap analysis, which indicates the distance between employee capabilities and the skills necessary to achieve a particular objective. Training objectives and priorities can then be determined to close the gap in areas such as employee attitudes, employee knowledge, and employee skills (Parker 2011).

At this point, consider the answer to the number one question of people who attend training: What's in it for me? This question must always be at the forefront of training design because it reminds the designer that participants must be kept engaged, and engagement is mostly based on what lessons and experiences participants can take away from the training.

Step 4 of the process requires *development of a training plan*, in which the tangibles take shape. Deliverables include the curriculum, the learning outcomes, and a dry run, in which feedback is crucial to determine whether revisions or midcourse corrections are needed. Training has evolved from the days of the presenter standing in front of a room dumping massive amounts of information on the participants (also known as the "sit and soak" method). Today's trainer serves as the facilitator of ideas and thought, involving the participants so that their transformation can begin even before they walk out the door. During this step, the curriculum is molded and sharpened to guide and enhance the facilitation.

For training to be successful, trainees must be willing and able to learn. Therefore, they must have the ability to learn, be motivated to learn, have confidence in their ability to learn, see value in the learning, and have a learning style that fits the training. Malcolm Knowles's previous work on adult learners suggests five principles related to training design (Knowles, Holton, and Swanson 2011). According to these principles, learners need to

- know why they are learning something,
- have a need that is self-directed,
- bring work-related experiences into the process,
- begin the experience with a problem-centered approach, and
- have a motive to learn for both extrinsic and intrinsic reasons.

Step 5 of the process is *implementation*, in which the rollout occurs and evaluation data are collected for future analysis. At this time, the flexibility built into the plan helps because user or participant feedback may dictate design revisions to ensure training quality. Thus, retaining this flexibility is prudent. To help employees and supervisors manage their time appropriately, make the training schedule available early and hold multiple sessions on different days and times to accommodate individual needs.

Several factors influence the effectiveness of training (Blume 2010). Among the most significant are offering employees an overview of the training content and its relationship to the organization's strategy, having the training mirror the job context as much as possible, encouraging supervisors to support trainees in using their new skills, giving trainees the opportunity to use the training, and holding the trainees accountable for transferring the training from the classroom to the job site (Burke and Saks 2009; Martin 2010).

Step 6 is *evaluation*, in which the information is reviewed to determine whether objectives were met. Kilpatrick (2010) identified four levels at which training can be evaluated: reaction, learning, behavioral change, and organizational results. Organizations evaluate trainee reaction by conducting trainee interviews or questionnaires. Typically, trainees are asked to rate the value of the training, the style of the instructors, the usefulness of the training, and their general reaction to the overall experience. Learning levels are evaluated by measuring how well trainees have acquired facts, ideas, concepts, theories, and attitudes. Tests are given before and after training to determine the incremental learning. Behavioral change can be measured by evaluating job performance before and after the training. This evaluation is typically done by supervisor observation. Finally, employers can evaluate organizational results by measuring changes in productivity, turnover, quality of care, and costs. Such an evaluation is done by comparing records before and after training.

The difficulty with this level of evaluation is pinpointing whether changes are a result of training or other factors. Having a control group that takes the pretest and posttest without going through the training is one way of determining the effect on organizational results. If the test group shows a greater improvement than the control group, then the business case for such training may be strengthened. However, this setup is not possible in every situation.

If, according to the evaluation, the OD department fell short on the training objectives and the training did not address or improve the situation at hand, the design process goes back to step 1. With objectives sometimes shifting with organizational changes, the design process often needs to be iterative. Many OD departments run this cycle on their training programs to maintain quality and to ensure that the objectives continue to be met.

Instructional Methods

Instructional methods involve the development of curriculum content and learning outcomes. Instructional methods should incorporate principles of learning, active participation in the learning process, rewards for incremental mastery, trainee feedback, an opportunity to use newly developed skills, and responsiveness to the cultural backgrounds of the participants (Carter and Beier 2010; Day 2010; Mesmer-Mangus and Viswesvaran 2010).

Because the main training objective is for the information to be transferable or applicable to the work of the learner, the following sections examine the most common methods for accomplishing that goal. The instructional method should match the learning objective appropriately. Selecting the proper method will optimize the quality and usefulness of the training and will increase the likelihood of accomplishing the objective. Sometimes the best method is a combination of two or three techniques.

Internal Approaches

Instructional methods may be either internal to the organization or external to the organization. Internal options include lecture, group discussion, role playing, case study, simulation, job shadowing, coaching, mentoring, and cross-training.

A *lecture* usually consists of a verbal presentation by an instructor, and it is effective with large groups and when the dissemination of information is the goal. On the other hand, *group discussion* may include a lecture but also affords participants an opportunity to inject their own ideas and thoughts into the training. It is very effective for small groups and where idea generation is needed or is a desired outcome, but the discussions need to be well facilitated to ensure that the group stays on track.

Role playing is very applicable and transferable back to the workplace because it involves creating a realistic scenario, with the learners taking on roles and practicing the skill sets necessary to accomplish the task. Although the problem-solving arena is the context in which role playing occurs, the development of skills is the main objective for the learner. The role-playing technique is an excellent way to teach feedback (giving and receiving), coaching, and conflict resolution skills.

Use of the *case study* is another way to build practicality and workplace transferability into the training experience. When a written description of a real-world incident or issue is presented to a group for discussion and formulation of strategies or solutions, the discussion can be lively and encourages the learner to think critically. The case study method may demonstrate the viability of many possibilities for resolving the incident as well as serve as a way for group members to practice other skills, including communication, decision making, and even negotiation.

Simulation, like the case study method, can be an efficient means of providing practical experience to learners. During a simulation, learners are briefed about a fictitious or real (their own) organization, given information about that organization's culture, and presented with an actual or imagined situation. Learners are then divided into groups to discuss and make a decision about the simulated problem; the work of each group is then evaluated by the other groups. Debriefing by the other groups is a valuable way to demonstrate the practical learning that can be applied or transferred back to the workplace. Simulation is also an excellent teaching tool within departments. For example, a simulation is suitable for training emergency room employees in disaster response and management.

Job shadowing is used to show an employee what a colleague or a supervisor actually does on a daily basis. Common job-shadowing activities include attending meetings, sitting in on decision-making sessions, and literally following in the footsteps of the person being shadowed. This method works best when a transfer of knowledge (e.g., from a departing employee to a trainee) must occur quickly and when a position is complex. The effectiveness of the method depends on the ability of the person being shadowed and the willingness of the learner.

Coaching is another type of on-the-job training. Although coaching requires patience and an understanding of how to effectively give feedback, it provides timely information or correction that is highly individualized. This method usually demands a high degree of trust between the coach and the learner to ensure that the experience is valuable and that feedback can be freely given.

Formal *mentoring* involves a more experienced staff member who guides a less experienced protégé. Typically, supervisors guide the development of their subordinates as a normal part of their job. However, with formalized mentoring both understand that they are engaging in activities intended for the long-term benefit of the employee. The goal is to enhance the protégé's competencies, achievements, and overall understanding of the organization (Dragoni et al. 2009). Mentors usually counsel their protégés by providing personal advice and information on how to network and advance in the organization (O'Brien et al. 2010).

Cross-training occurs when an individual is trained in more than one job to fill in when needed. For an employer, the advantages of cross-training are flexibility and lower costs (Lee 2011). While some organizations have a culture that encourages cross-training, others do not (Bokhorst 2011). Learning bonuses awarded for successful cross-training might mitigate such situations.

External Approaches

External training options include formal courses, certificate/degree programs, simulations, business games, training delivered by a third party at an outside location, Web conferences, podcasts, educational leave, and teleconferencing. A popular option for employers is to use vendors and suppliers to train employees (Lalla 2010). Many suppliers host user conferences in which employees from different firms and organizations receive detailed training on how to use products and services that are new to them. Some vendors also conduct training at the organization site if a sufficient number of employees need such training.

The reasons that outside training is not more widely used may include cost concerns as well as an emphasis on linking training to organizational strategies. In other words, the knowledge provided by external training may not transfer well to the workplace (Lee 2009; Saks and Belacort 2006).

Paid and unpaid *internships* are another external training method. Internships give students hands-on experience of the day-to-day tasks of their intended career goal. To be most effective, internships should be structured to achieve student learning goals (Beenen and Rousseau 2010).

Employee Onboarding

Even before most job candidates arrive for the interview, they have already researched the organization through websites, company literature, or conversations with current or former employees. The interview process, then, adds to the candidates' knowledge, allowing them to piece together an overall picture and to figure out how they will fit into the larger organizational scheme. Therefore, when the new employee reports to the job for the first time, his or her socialization wheel has already been set in motion.

The formal orientation process provides a huge opportunity to engage the new employee in formulating expectations for a future with the organization. If a formal orientation process is not provided, the employee will go through an informal process that involves indoctrination by other employees. Certainly an orientation by peers is valuable, but it is not sufficient. When left with only an informal orientation, the new employee will receive inaccurate, incomplete, and even biased information. This situation will cause frustration for the new employee.

The *new-employee orientation* is a process by which the organization answers many employee-centered questions. This orientation is the opportunity for the organization to explain and educate new employees on workplace structure; policies, processes, and practices; and related information, standards, and expectations that will assist the newcomers in their development and success with the organization. During the orientation, the employee should be exposed to a balance of job-specific and organization-related information.

Content

Because each organization is unique, the new-employee orientation should be customized, not generic. On the other hand, many topics are found in nearly every organization's orientation program, such as compensation, benefits, work hours, and career planning. Exhibit 11.13 lists the areas that are commonly covered in new-employee orientations. Orientations provide new employees with basic background information they need to perform their jobs. In contrast, *onboarding* helps to socialize the employee with the attitudes, standards, values, and patterns of behavior that their organization expects.

Appreciating the organization's culture and values distinguishes onboarding from traditional orientation. One example of onboarding is the Mayo Clinic's "heritage and culture" programs, which emphasize core values such as teamwork, personal responsibility, and mutual respect (Hicks, Peters, and Smith 2006; Mayo Clinic 2012).

Logistics

As today's world continues to expose us to huge amounts of knowledge, and as we try to accommodate all or much of that information in our busy lives, we have developed fast-paced ways to learn. This trend in short-length learning has been adopted in orientation programs as well. In the usual healthcare workplace situation, the supervisor feels the pinch of an unfilled position. The usual management response to the situation is to get the new hire initiated quickly so that person can attack the learning curve.

One of the best approaches to orienting a new employee is the "eating of the apple" method—one bite at a time. In the workplace, this method translates into breaking up the orientation into brief sessions over days or weeks. The employee remembers much more because the integration of information takes place as he or she adjusts to the new work surroundings, with the information presented in "bites" that the employee can digest thoroughly. This arrangement translates into a win for the organization as well because the employee is given a chance to stay connected to the process, which in turn may lead to the employee's satisfaction with work and to a greater probability of retention.

Employee-Centered Information	Organization-Specific Information
Compensation, including pay rates, deductions, overtime, and holiday pay	Overview of organization, including mission, history, structure, services, and customs/traditions
Benefits, including insurance, holidays, leave, and retirement	Safety, including precautions and accident-reporting procedures
Facilities, including food services/cafeteria, parking, restrooms, security, first aid, security, and badges/name tags	Employee relations, including reporting sick leave, length of probationary period and limitations of activities associated with that, expectations and disciplinary practices, and grievance processes
Details of job duties, including work hours, job description, and performance criteria	
	Policies and procedures
Department tour, including workspace/office, entrances/exits, supervisor's location, water fountains, and smoking areas	Where to find resources and who to call to report discrimination or illegal activities
Career planning, including development opportunities and resources for growth	Community activities and sponsored events

EXHIBIT 11.13
Types of Information Conveyed in an Orientation

Best-Practice Ideas

Many organizations have successfully revamped or renewed their new-employee orientation process. The Mayo Clinic in Rochester, Minnesota, welcomes new employees with balloons, upbeat music, and breakfast. The organization strives to provide a positive, lasting first impression and to keep that momentum going through the orientation process (Hicks, Peters, and Smith 2006; Mayo Clinic 2012).

Trends in Organizational Development and Learning

One trend has been to brand OD as part of the talent management function. *Talent management* is the science of using strategic HR to improve business value and encompasses everything that is done to recruit, retain, develop, reward, and promote people. Talent management increased in popularity after McKinsey's research and subsequent book *The War for Talent* (Michaels, Handfield-Jones, and Axelrod 2001). Talent management is based on the principle that a business is only as good as its people. It is the goal-oriented and integrated process of planning, recruiting, developing, managing, and compensating the best employees (Dressler 2014, 88). In response to this trend, some HR departments have been rebranded as talent acquisition departments, and integrated HR information systems are commonly branded as talent management systems. The American Society for Training and Development (ASTD), a premier professional society for learning and OD professionals, changed its name to the Association for Talent Development in 2014 "to meet the growing needs of a dynamic, global profession" (Association for Talent Development 2014b).

In a review of the employment website Monster.com (November 6, 2014), almost twice as many job opportunities were listed under "talent development" (30) than under "organizational development" (17), yet the jobs listed under these two different titles were very similar. OD jobs in healthcare have not been as quick to brand the department with the "talent" nomenclature. In fact, many of the OD departments in UHC member organizations still have the title "Education" or "Human Resource Development."

What will the future bring for OD and training? Will instructor-led, in-class workshops be just a memory in the next few years? How will workplace learning look in the ever-shifting business climate?

For now, organizational learning is at the "head of the table." In this time of extreme competition and globalization, organizations rely on workplace learning strategies to develop highly skilled workers, who are then expected to drive productivity and quality. This practice will likely remain constant. In the past, OD departments have been the first to march to the chopping block, but that outcome has become less common as organizations have increasingly relied on strategic training to drive performance. According to the ATD, the trend shows an acceleration of initiatives toward employee learning, capitalizing on the development of knowledge and skills that are at the heart of organizational impact (Ketter 2006).

The trends in learning delivery are pointing to more use of electronic media, a benefit of prior investments in technology-based delivery such as online learning or e-learning. A fast-growing technological innovation is *m-learning*, or mobile learning. With this delivery medium, learning can take place through smartphones and tablets. In this way, learning becomes easy to access and flexible enough to accommodate just about any schedule. M-learning has expanded rapidly since 2009.

Online learning offers the advantages of lower costs and the ability to provide training content to more people at one time than traditional training. It also reduces lost work hours and travel/hotel costs (Engebretson 2010). Almost 30 percent of learning hours today are technology based, and e-learning is preferred by workers under the age of 30 (Udell 2012). Most companies today use technology testing and knowledge as part of work and classroom instruction (Rossett and Marsh 2010). However, training staff in complex skills or concepts is better accomplished through interaction with experienced people.

Gamification is the application of typical elements of game playing (i.e., point scoring, competition with others, rules of play) to nongame activities such as OD and learning. The purpose is to move toward a goal or to ensure engagement with a product or service. Gamification is most often applied in online and mobile applications and is used in social applications that put users in friendly competition with each other. Alternatively, it can provide incentives for users to share content with others (Rosenthal 2014). Healthcare organizations are exploring how gamification can be applied to online learning. One example might be a leader board, which shows which department within an organization has the highest number of training course completions.

Other available technology-based learning methods include videoconferencing, instant messaging, online meetings, and webinars. *Webinars*—the term combines *Web* and *seminars*—have proliferated quickly within the business-to-business sales area because they are able to deliver on-demand training through a live or video-recorded broadcast on the Internet. This medium allows both the presenters and the training participants to sit in their own offices or be in different cities or even countries.

More and more in-house training departments and organizations with employees at different or remote sites are relying on webinars, which help prevent the high costs of training widely dispersed staff in a single location. Instant messaging (IM) holds promise as an avenue for training in real time, offering quick responses to real-time on-the-job needs by employees. With slow response times, e-mail does not offer promptness of information. IM, on the other hand, can provide constant and instant accessibility. A trainer can establish a schedule for IM accessibility as a way to enhance conventional training methods or as an adjunct to a general workshop, a coaching session, or nurse education.

Examination of the cost to exclusively deliver training in electronic format is prudent. Because so much of an organization's training content is customized according to the organization's needs, relying fully on electronic delivery may not be practical because the costs multiply when customization is involved. These costs are not solely monetary. The most important cost may be that the quality of training in some areas (e.g., interpersonal skills) is not high. The results manifest in the workplace in the form of conflict or poor service, which adversely affects the bottom line.

For example, "soft skills"—team building, conflict resolution, coaching, giving feedback—are based on interaction with others. Thus, training in this area is very difficult to deliver effectively outside of a physical classroom. However, with so much business conducted in the virtual world, the development of effective soft-skills training in the online environment is surely on the horizon.

Healthcare organizations are increasingly recognizing the importance of meeting and exceeding customer expectations (Fottler, Ford, and Heaton

2010). Toward that end, they are providing customer service training to give staff the skills they need to exceed customer expectations. Such service skills can significantly influence job satisfaction, retention, customer loyalty, and market share. These skills are particularly important for frontline employees (Beatson, Gudergan, and Lings 2008).

A final trend is an increase in ethics training for all staff members. Unethical practices can defeat the best efforts in healthcare organizations. Such behavior takes many forms, including cutting corners, engaging in unsafe practices, bullying others, and stealing from the organization. When such behavior is allowed to continue, employee satisfaction and productivity can suffer. Ethics training can provide staff with the skills they need to challenge unethical behavior. This training is best done by developing relevant communication skills, using role playing that incorporates strategies to challenge an offender, and providing feedback on performance (Kurtz and Kucsan 2009).

Summary

OD is part of the changing healthcare landscape. The challenge is for OD to remain flexible enough to respond to the educational and training needs of the organization and its employees, yet stable enough to deliver learning that will power up the enterprise as a whole. Sustained organizational learning depends on the ability of OD departments to facilitate, coach, and guide training toward the desired goals and objectives.

Finding the proper training methods that will help build a productive, highly functioning workforce is not easy. Adaptability, innovation, and continual pursuit of best practices are some ways to ensure sustainable results. An OD department that serves as a strategic partner to executive management allows the organization to adapt to the constantly shifting environment. Together, this partnership creates a systematic perspective that yields positive responses to OD initiatives.

This chapter provides an overview of the important role of OD and practical applications for development of a successful training initiative, from the needs assessment to the actual program delivery and evaluation. It summarizes important OD processes that begin as new employees are hired, socialized, and managed through career and performance development. Various methods of organizational sustainability are examined, including employee onboarding, employee engagement, the succession planning process, and current and future trends in organizational development and learning.

Discussion Questions

1. Using the ADDIE model, design a training program that addresses the customer service expectations of walk-in patients in the emergency department. Include an evaluation process that answers the following questions:

   a. What method will you use to evaluate the training program?

   b. How will you know whether you met your training objective?

2. Your healthcare facility assigned you to explore succession planning as a possible strategy for organizational sustainability. What will you do? To obtain information that will help you with this assignment, research two organizations that have adopted a succession planning strategy, and compare and contrast their programs and the outcomes.

3. Describe an example of a successful new-employee orientation. Why are both employee needs and organizational needs important to consider?

4. Why is it important to engage senior management early on in the process when preparing for a learning initiative?

5. What is employee engagement, why is it important, and how can it be enhanced in a healthcare organization?

Experiential Exercises

Case 1   Argosy Medical Center, a 400-bed critical care facility located in the Northeast, has been in operation for more than 18 years. Its mission is to provide quality healthcare services with the highest standard of excellence from employees who are dedicated to caring and patient satisfaction.

At one time, staff were really excited to be part of the Argosy family, and the patients noticed this attitude and enthusiasm. Argosy became the hospital of choice because the patients felt that the staff really cared about them, which made the patients' experience positive regardless of their health status. Patient exit surveys were excellent, and patients frequently wrote glowing comments about the staff's genuine concern and about what a wonderful employer the hospital must be to have such a dedicated workforce.

In the last couple of years, however, the employees seem to have lost their passion. This change has resulted in higher patient complaints of poor customer service. Management has attributed this deteriorated employee attitude to higher workloads and burnout. Training was instituted. Employees are required to attend a refresher course every year in an effort to keep them motivated and in tune with the hospital mission and to reenergize them about the workplace. The course includes a review of the hospital values, mission, and standards of service that everyone is expected to follow. Because the course is only for one hour, participants do not get to interact, ask questions, or give feedback afterward. In fact, since the refresher course was implemented, employees have not been surveyed to get their feedback or insights. Because the staff are constantly busy, they have had no opportunity to talk among themselves, with their managers, or in focus groups about the decline in employee morale and the poor customer service. Everyone knows the problem is there, but no time has been put aside to address it, other than an organizational reminder to give good customer service regardless of the situation.

Argosy's CEO has summoned you, the director of the OD department, to come up with a way to address the problem that is affecting absenteeism, turnover, and the hospital bottom line.

1. Using the performance improvement diagnostic model in Exhibits 11.5 and 11.6, discuss the factors that might be at the root of the performance problem of low patient satisfaction scores. What questions would you want to ask the client?

2. What additional data would you want to collect?

3. With that analysis in mind, what interventions would you recommend? Come up with two options.

Case 2 Over the past two years, an academic medical center has purchased four community hospitals across the state with bed sizes ranging from 26 to 500. In trying to act on the organization's strategic goals of providing greater economic and process efficiencies and increasing brand identification and market share, the chief HR officer has asked you to come up with a proposal for how to change the new-employee orientation and onboarding process to meet the following goals:

- Reduce costs of new-employee onboarding
- Promote a sense of system or brand identification, while still maintaining the culture of the community hospital where it is valuable

Currently each hospital has its own separate two-day new-employee orientation program and onboarding process, which the HR department at each of the hospitals is responsible for.

Using the change management model in Exhibit 11.7 and your knowledge of the use of learning technology, answer the following questions:

1. Who would you suggest sponsor this change and be your active leadership core guiding this change?

2. What data would you want to collect?

3. What efficiencies would you expect to gain, and how would you realize them?

4. What resistance would you anticipate? How would you address it?

5. How would you go about getting buy-in for this change?

Case 3 A new director of pharmacy services began work in her position six months ago. She faces a situation in which the employee engagement scores in most of the departments within the pharmacy have been low for the past two years. She has asked to meet with you to help her figure out how best to work with her management team to improve staff engagement and morale.

1. What performance improvement consulting phase(s) should you be focused on at this point?

2. How would you build rapport and credibility with this client to establish a sound consultant–client relationship?

3. What do you anticipate will be the easiest part of the coaching/consulting contract (see Exhibit 11.4) to complete? What will be the most difficult?

4. How would you suggest to measure progress?

5. How would you close this meeting?

References

Accenture. 2012. *Increasing Employee Engagement in the Nonprofit Sector: How to Engage Employees for High Performance*. Published May 11. www.accenture.com/us-en/Pages/insight-increasing-employee-engagement-nonprofit-sector.aspx.

Allen, M. W., and R. H. Sites. 2012. *Leaving ADDIE for SAM: An Agile Model for Developing the Best Learning Experiences*. Alexandria, VA: American Society for Training & Development.

Association for Talent Development. 2014a. "The ATD Competency Model." Accessed December 23. www.astd.org/Certification/Competency-Model.

———. 2014b. Homepage. Accessed December 23. www.astd.org.

Association of American Medical Colleges. 2012. *CME and Its Evolution in the Academic Medical Center: The 2011 AAMC/SACME Harrison Survey*. Washington, DC: AAMC Press.

Beatson, A. L., S. Gundergan, and I. Lings. 2008. "Service Staff Attitudes, Organisational Practices and Performance Drivers." *Journal of Management and Organization* 14 (3): 168–79.

Beckhard, R. 1969. *Organizational Development: Strategies and Models*. Reading, MA: Addison-Wesley.

Beenen, G., and D. M. Rousseau. 2010. "Getting the Most from MBA Internships: Promoting Intern Learning and Job Acceptance." *Human Resource Management* 49 (1): 3–22.

Binder, C. 1998. "The Six Boxes: A Descendant of Gilbert's Behavior Engineering Model." Binder Riha Associates. Accessed December 23, 2014. www.binder-riha.com/sixboxes.html.

BlessingWhite. 2013. *Employee Engagement Research Update—January 2013.* Published January. http://blessingwhite.com/research-report/employee-engagement-research-report-update-jan-2013/.

Block, P. 2011. *Flawless Consulting: A Guide to Getting Your Expertise Used.* San Francisco: Pfeiffer.

Blouin, A., K. McDonagh, A. Neistadt, and B. Helfand. 2006. "Leading Tomorrow's Healthcare Organizations: Strategies and Tactics for Effective Succession Planning." *Journal of Nursing Administration* 36 (6): 325–30.

Blume, B. D. 2010. "Transfer of Training: A Meta-analytic Review." *Journal of Management* 36 (4): 1065–102.

Bokhorst, J. C. 2011. "The Impact of the Amount of Work in Process on the Use of Cross Training." *International Journal of Production* 49 (11): 3171–90.

Brown, K. G., and T. Sitzman. 2011. "Training and Employee Development for Improved Performance." In *APA Handbook of Industrial and Organizational Psychology.* Vol. 2, *Selecting and Developing Members for the Organization,* edited by S. Zedeck, 469–503. Washington, DC: American Psychological Association.

Buck, M., and M. Martin. 2012. "Leaders Teaching Leaders." *Employee Benefit News,* September, 60–62.

Burke, L. M., and A. M. Saks. 2009. "Accountability in Training Transfer: Adapting Schlenker's Model of Responsibility to a Persistent But Solvable Problem." *Human Resource Development Review* 8 (3): 382–402.

Carter, M., and M. E. Beier. 2010. "The Effectiveness of Error Management Training with Working-Aged Adults." *Personnel Psychology* 63 (3): 641–75.

Cekada, T. L. 2011. "Need Training: Conducting an Effective Needs Assessment." *Professional Safety* 56 (12): 28–34.

Chevalier, R. 2003. "Updating the Behavior Engineering Model." *Performance Improvement* 42 (5): 8–14.

Collins, S. K., R. C. McKinnies, E. Matthews, and K. S. Collins. 2013. "Succession Planning: Trends Regarding the Perspectives of Chief Executive Officers in US Hospitals." *The Health Care Manager* 32 (3): 233–38.

Conner, D. 2006. *Managing at the Speed of Change: How Resilient Managers Succeed and Prosper Where Others Fail.* New York: Random House.

Davis, A. 2012. "Back to School." *Employee Benefit News,* September 15, 26–28.

Day, D. V. 2011. *Developing Leadership Talent.* Alexandria, VA: SHRM Foundation.

———. 2010. "The Difficulties of Learning from Experience and the Need for Deliberate Practice." *Industrial and Organizational Psychology* 3 (1): 41–44.

DeMarco, J. M. 2007. "Homegrown Leaders." *Modern Healthcare* 37 (33): 23.

DeSmet, A., M. McGurk, and E. Schwartz. 2010. "Getting More from Your Training Programs." *McKinsey Quarterly,* October, 1–6.

Dodgeson, M. 1993. "Organizational Learning: A Review of Some Literature." *Organization Studies* 24 (3): 375–94.

Dolezalek, H. 2009. "Best Practices Deconstructed." *Training,* June, 50–52.

Dragoni, L., J. E. Tesluk, A. Russell, and I. Oh. 2009. "Understanding Managerial Development: Integrating Developmental Assignments, Learning Orientation, and Access to Developmental Opportunities in Predicting Managerial Competencies." *Academy of Management Journal* 52 (4): 731–43.

Dressler, G. 2014. *Human Resource Management,* fourteenth edition. Upper Saddle River, NJ: Pearson.

Effron, M., and M. Ort. 2010. *One Page Talent Management: Eliminating Complexity, Adding Value.* Boston: Harvard Business School Publishing.

Engebretson, J. 2010. "Economy Drives Shift to Online Training." *SDM: Security Distributing & Marketing* 40 (10): 176.

Fottler, M. D., R. Ford, and C. Heaton. 2010. *Achieving Service Excellence,* second edition. Chicago: Health Administration Press.

Frasch, K. B. 2011a. "Defining Global Leadership Competencies." *Human Resource Executive Online.* Published August 5. www.hreonline.com/HRE/view/story.jhtml?id=533340461.

———. 2011b. "The 'Virtuous Cycle' of Engagement and Productivity." *Human Resource Executive Online.* Published August 22. www.hreonline.com/HRE/view/story.jhtml?id=533340647.

Gilbert, T. F. (1978) 1996. *Human Competence: Engineering Worthy Performance.* New York: McGraw-Hill. Tribute edition, Washington, DC: HRD Press and ISPI Publications.

Gomez-Mejia, L. R., D. B. Balkin, and R. L. Cardy. 2012. *Managing Human Resources,* seventh edition. Upper Saddle River, NJ: Pearson Education.

Greer, C. R., and M. Virick. 2008. "Diverse Succession Planning: Lessons from the Industry Leaders." *Human Resource Management* 47 (2): 351–67.

Grossman, R. 2011. "Rough Road to Succession." *HR Magazine* 56 (6): 47–51.

Harter, J. K., F. L. Schmidt, S. Agrawal, and S. K. Plowman. 2013. *The Relationship Between Engagement at Work and Organizational Outcomes: 2012 Q12 Meta-analysis.* Omaha, NE: Gallup.

Health First. 2010. "Health First President/CEO Announces Retirement." Accessed December 23, 2014. www.health-first.org/news_and_events/hf_health_first_ceo_announces_retirement_2010.cfm.

Heath, C., and D. Heath. 2010. *Switch: How to Change When Change Is Hard.* New York: Random House.

Hicks, S., M. Peters, and M. Smith. 2006. "Orientation Redesign." *T+D* 60 (7): 43–47.

Joint Commission. 2014. "Facts About The Joint Commission." www.jointcommission.org/about_us/fact_sheets.aspx.

Ketter, P. 2009. "Sounding Succession Alarms." *T+D* 63 (1): 20.

———. 2006. "Investing in Learning: Looking for Performance." *T+D* 60 (12): 30–34.

Kilpatrick, D. 2010. "The Four Levels Are Still Relevant." *T+D* 64 (9): 16.

Knowles, M. S., F. H. Holton, and A. R. Swanson. 2011. *The Adult Learner*, seventh edition. New York: Elsevier.

Korn, M. 2013. "Employed, but Not Engaged on the Job." *Wall Street Journal.* Published June 11. www.wsj.com/news/articles/SB100014241278873234 95604578539712058327862.

Kotter, J. (1996) 2012. *Leading Change.* Boston: Harvard Business Review Press.

Kübler-Ross, E. 1997. *On Death and Dying.* New York: Scribner.

Kurtz, L., and R. Kucsan. 2009. "Close Encounters: Using Scenario Training to Handle Difficult Employees." *T+D* 63 (8): 28.

Lalla, S. 2010. "Tips to Outsource Training." *Training*, October 1, 7.

Lee, K. 2011. "Reinforce Training." *Training* 48 (3): 24.

———. 2009. "Implement Training Successfully." *Training* 46 (5): 16.

Mailloux, J. P. 1998. "Learning Needs Assessments: Definitions, Techniques, and Self-Perceived Abilities of the Hospital-Based Nurse Educator." *Journal of Continuing Education in Nursing* 29 (1): 40–45.

Marketing Health Services. 2004. "Keeping Happy." *Marketing Health Services* 24 (1): 6.

Markos, S., and M. S. Stridevi. 2010. "Employee Engagement: The Key to Improving Performance." *International Journal of Business Management* 5 (12): 89–95.

Martin, J. H. 2010. "Workplace Climate and Peer Support as Determinants of Training Transfer." *Human Resource Development Quarterly* 21 (1): 87–104.

Maurer, R. 2010. *Beyond the Wall of Resistance: Why 70% of All Changes Still Fail—and What You Can Do About It*, revised edition. Austin, TX: Bard Press.

Mayo Clinic. 2012. "Welcome to Mayo Clinic Health System." Accessed December 23, 2014. www.mayoclinichealthsystem.org/~/media/local-files/eau-claire/documents/careers/eau-claire-orientation-2014.pdf.

McIlvaine, A. R. 2012. "The Engagement Factor." *Human Resource Executive Online.* Published June 13. www.hreonline.com/HRE/view/story.jhtml?id=533348424.

Mesmer-Magnus, J., and C. Viswesvaran. 2010. "The Role of Pre-training Interventions in Learning: A Meta-analysis and Integrative Review." *Human Resource Management Review* 20 (4): 261–82.

Michaels, E., H. Handfield-Jones, and B. Axelrod. 2001. *The War for Talent.* Boston: Harvard Business School Press.

Mone, E. M., and M. London. 2009. *Employee Engagement Through Effective Performance Management.* New York: Routledge.

Nonprofit HR Solutions. 2013. *Nonprofit Employment Trends Survey.* Accessed March 7, 2015. www.nonprofithr.com/wp-content/uploads/2013/03/2013-Employment-Trends-Survey-Report.pdf.

O'Brien, K. E., A. Biga, S. R. Kessler, and T. D. Allen. 2010. "A Meta-analytic Investigation of Gender Differences in Mentoring." *Journal of Management* 36 (2): 537–54.

Parker, A. 2011. "Soft Skills: A Case for Higher Education and Workplace Training." *T+D* 65 (11): 16.

Phillips, J., and S. Gully. 2012. *Strategic Staffing*. Upper Saddle River, NJ: Pearson Education.

Pintar, K., T. Capuano, and G. Rosser. 2007. "Developing Clinical Leadership Capability." *Journal of Continuing Education in Nursing* 38 (3): 115–21.

Rich, B. L., J. A. Lepine, and A. R. Crawford. 2010. "Job Engagement: Antecedents and Effects on Job Performance." *Academy of Management Journal* 53 (3): 617–35.

Roper, W. 2013. "Address to All Leadership Session." Presented at the University of North Carolina at Chapel Hill.

Rosenthal, D. 2014. "Gamification." Health Care Compliance Strategies. Published February 1. www.hccs.com/newslettersarticle.php?nID=78.

Rossett, A., and J. Marsh. 2010. "E-Learning: What's Old Is New Again." *T+D* 64 (1): 34–38.

Saks, A. M., and J. M. Belcourt. 2006. "An Investigation of Training Activities and Transfer of Training in Organizations." *Human Resource Management* 45 (4): 629–48.

Schramm, J. 2011. "Undereducated." *HR Magazine* 56 (9): 136.

Society for Human Resource Management. 2014. "HR Terms." Accessed September 30. www.shrm.org/templatestools/glossaries/hrterms/pages/default.aspx.

Studer, Q. 2008. *Results That Last: Hardwiring Behaviors That Will Take Your Company to the Top*. Hoboken, NJ: Wiley.

Sum, V. 2011. "Integrating Training in Business Strategies Means Greater Impact of Training on the Firm's Competitiveness." *Research in Business and Economics Journal* 4 (August): 1–19.

Towers Perrin. 2009. *Closing the Engagement Gap: A Roadmap for Driving Superior Business Results*. Stamford, CT: Towers Perrin.

Udell, C. 2012. *Learning Everywhere: How Mobile Content Strategies Are Transforming Training*. Alexandria, VA: ASTD Press.

UNC Medical Center. 2014. "Learning and Organizational Development Department." Intranet site. Accessed November 1. http://hr.intranet.unchealthcare.org/hr/LOD/index.html.

Wells, A., D. Swain, and L. Fieldhouse. 2010. "How Support Staff Can Be Helped to Challenge Unacceptable Practice." *Nursing Management* 16 (9): 24–27.

Word, J. 2012. "Head and Heart: Employee Engagement in the Nonprofit Sector." Paper presented at the annual meeting of the ARNOVA Annual Conference, Indianapolis, IN, November 14, 2012.

Web Resources

- The Joint Commission is the accreditation body for healthcare organizations. According to its website (see www.jointcommission.org), it "accredits and certifies more than 20,500 health care organizations and programs in the United States." The website is a rich resource for understanding standards and improvements in healthcare, which often drive training and education for those who seek to meet or maintain certification and who strive for excellence.

- The Society for Human Resource Management is an association for HR professionals. Its website (see www.shrm.org) has a very active organizational development and learning area. The site also contains information on student organizations and memberships. The Society for Human Resource Management produces *HR Magazine* and other HR publications.

- The Association for Talent Development (ATD), formerly the American Society for Training and Development (ASTD), is an organization dedicated to workplace learning and training professionals. For more information, go to www.astd.org. ATD publishes *TD* magazine.

- The Organization Development Network (OD Network) is "an international, professional association whose members are committed to practicing organization development intentionally and rigorously as an applied behavioral science" (see www.odnetwork.org). OD Network has an e-mail discussion list that serves as a forum for dialogue on issues of interest to OD professionals in the field of healthcare. The e-mail list provides information on trends, best practices, and networking opportunities.

- University HealthSystem Consortium (UHC), formed in 1984, is an alliance of 117 national academic medical centers and more than 300 affiliated hospitals. The mission of UHC is "to create knowledge, foster collaboration, and promote innovation to help members succeed." For more information, see www.uhc.edu.

MANAGING WITH ORGANIZED LABOR

Donna Malvey and Amanda Raffenaud

Learning Objectives

After completing this chapter, the reader should be able to

- address the relationship of organized labor and management in healthcare,
- distinguish the different phases of the labor relations process,
- describe the evolving role of unions in the healthcare workforce,
- examine legislative and judicial rulings that affect management of organized labor in healthcare settings,
- review emerging healthcare labor trends, and
- consider the potential impact of the Internet on the labor–management relationship.

Introduction

The *labor relations process* occurs when management (as the representative for the employer) and the union (as the exclusive bargaining representative for the employees) jointly determine and administer the rules of the workplace. A *union* is an organization formed by employees for the purpose of acting as a single unit when dealing with management about workplace issues, and hence the term *organized labor*. Unions are not present in every organization because employees must authorize a union to represent them. Unions typically are viewed as threats by management because they interfere with management's ability to make and implement decisions. Once a union is present, management may no longer unilaterally make decisions about the terms and conditions of work. Instead, management must negotiate these decisions with the union. Similarly, employees may no longer communicate directly with management about work issues but instead must go through the union. Thus, the union functions as a middleman, which is relatively expensive to maintain for both parties. Employees pay union dues, and management incurs additional costs for such things as contract negotiations and any increases in salaries and benefits negotiated by the union (Freeman and Medoff 1984).

In healthcare, because labor costs generally account for 70 percent to 80 percent of expenditures, controlling labor costs is critically important. Thus, if a union negotiates even a minor wage or benefit increase, it will result in a significant increase in total costs. Consequently, management has a strong incentive to keep unions out of the organization (Scott and Seers 1996). However, given the trends of unionization in healthcare, managers are increasingly forced to work with unions. This chapter examines the phenomenon of healthcare unionization and provides direction for managing with organized labor. In addition, it discusses the possible behaviors and strategies that constitute the labor–management relationship; explains the generic labor relations process of organizing, negotiating, and administering contracts; explores developments in organizing a relatively unorganized healthcare workforce; considers the impact of labor laws, amendments, and rulings on human resources (HR) strategies and goals; and considers the potential impact of the Internet on the labor–management relationship.

Managing with organized labor involves the application and maintenance of a positive labor relations program within the organization. A productive and positive labor–management relationship can only be accomplished through integration with other HR functions. For example, employees expect management to provide environments that are clean and safe from workplace hazards and health-related concerns, such as AIDS and hepatitis B. If management allows the environment to deteriorate, union organizers will focus on these issues (Becker and Rowe 1989; Fennell 1987). In addition, the labor relations process occurs across all levels of the organization and involves all levels of management. Upper-level management will develop objectives and strategies regarding wage rates and staffing ratios while mid-level managers and first-line supervisors will implement these objectives.

Developing strategies and goals to implement a positive labor relations program in healthcare requires an understanding of the generic labor relations process of organizing, negotiating, and administering contracts with a union as well as specific knowledge of emerging healthcare labor trends. A productive and positive labor–management relationship involves compromise by both parties because of the adversarial nature of the relationship. Just because a union has won the right to represent employees does not mean that management has to accept all of its terms. All parties—management, unions, and employees—have a vested interest in the success and survival of the organization; yet they also have opposing or conflicting interests. For example, unions will look toward improving the benefits package for employees, while management, faced with budget cutbacks and declining reimbursements, will have concerns about containing costs. Thus, the challenge for management is working with the union to reconcile differences in a fair and consistent manner.

As Exhibit 12.1 suggests, the labor–management relationship reflects a continuum of possible behaviors and strategies, ranging from the most positive or collaborative (in which management and the union share common goals oriented toward the organization's success) to the most negative or oppositional and self-serving. Even if the relationship is neutral and both parties cooperate to maintain the status quo, a variety of factors can cause the relationship to shift in either direction. For instance, restructuring, such as a merger, may create uncertainty for both the union and management and, as a result, may reposition their relationship along the continuum. However, the direction in which the relationship moves will depend largely on the knowledge and understanding of the labor relations process on both sides of the issue.

Overview of Unionization

Union membership has been declining steadily for decades. In the 1950s to 1970s, union membership represented 25 percent to 30 percent of the US workforce. During the 1980s and 1990s, organized labor's influence and bargaining power declined and weakened as the nature of US industries shifted from factories and traditional union strongholds to service and technologies (Fottler et al. 1999). This trend appears to have continued, as evidenced by the fact that organized labor has been unable to make any

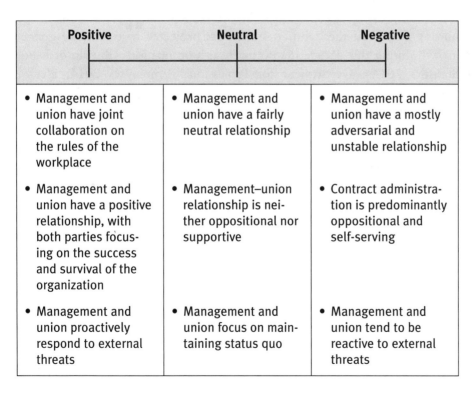

Positive	Neutral	Negative
• Management and union have joint collaboration on the rules of the workplace	• Management and union have a fairly neutral relationship	• Management and union have a mostly adversarial and unstable relationship
• Management and union have a positive relationship, with both parties focusing on the success and survival of the organization	• Management–union relationship is neither oppositional nor supportive	• Contract administration is predominantly oppositional and self-serving
• Management and union proactively respond to external threats	• Management and union focus on maintaining status quo	• Management and union tend to be reactive to external threats

EXHIBIT 12.1
Ranges of the Labor–Management Relationship in Healthcare

net gains in membership despite downward pressure on wages, increasing healthcare insurance costs, and outsourcing of service and manufacturing jobs overseas (*Christian Science Monitor* 2004).

The union membership rate has steadily decreased from 20.1 percent in 1983, the first year for which comparable union data are available, to 11.3 percent in both 2012 and 2013. In 2013, the total number of employees belonging to a union was approximately 14.5 million. Unions appear to be more successful in organizing workers in the public sector than in the private sector and more successful in healthcare than in other industries. The union rate for government or public-sector workers has held steady at approximately 35.3 percent since 1983, while the rate for private-sector workers has fallen to 6.7 percent. Within the public sector, however, local government workers had the highest union membership rate—40.8 percent. This group reflects several heavily unionized occupations such as teachers, firefighters, and police officers (Bureau of Labor Statistics 2000a, 2000b, 2004, 2006a, 2006b, 2014b; Scott and Lowery 1994).

The healthcare workforce comprises an estimated 16.4 million workers and represents one of the largest pools of unorganized workers in the United States and a prime target for union organizers. Only 7.2 percent of the healthcare workforce was affiliated with union membership in 2013 (Bureau of Labor Statistics 2014b). Unions in the healthcare sector, other than the hospital segment, have consistently won a greater percentage of their elections than those in other industries (Scott and Seers 1996). Many of the fastest-growing occupations are health related, and registered nurses and nursing aides, orderlies, and attendants are projected to experience greater growth during this decade than other health occupations (Bureau of Labor Statistics 2014a; Department for Professional Employees 2014; Hecker 2004). One-third of the projected job growth from 2012 to 2022 will occur in the healthcare field (Bureau of Labor Statistics 2013). Even though labor surveys indicate that the demand for unions exists, healthcare unions have not yet realized significant membership increases (Kearney 2003; *Christian Science Monitor* 2004). Nevertheless, some labor experts believe that healthcare unions represent one of the few areas in which organized labor has been showing some energy. Healthcare unions are reported to have invested heavily in recruiting members and helping members gain influence (Evans 2006).

The Labor Relations Process

In an attempt to protect workers' rights to unionize, the US Congress passed the National Labor Relations Act (NLRA) in 1935. This act serves as the legal framework for the labor relations process. Although the NLRA has been amended over the years, it remains the only legislation that governs federal labor relations. The law contains significant provisions intended to protect workers' rights to form and join unions and to engage in collective bargaining. The law also defines unfair labor practices, which restrict both unions and employers from interfering with the labor relations process. The NLRA delegates to the National Labor Relations Board (NLRB) the responsibility for overseeing implementation of the NLRA and for investigating and remedying unfair labor practices. NLRB rule making occurs on a case-by-case basis.

Key participants in the labor relations process include (1) management officials, who serve as surrogates for the owners or employers of the organization; (2) union officials, who are usually elected by members; (3) the government, which participates through executive, legislative, and judicial branches occurring at federal, state, and local levels; and (4) neutral third parties such as arbitrators. The process also involves three phases that are equally essential: the recognition phase, the negotiation phase, and the administration phase.

Recognition Phase

During this phase, unions attempt to organize employees and gain representation through either voluntary recognition of the union or a representation election, which certifies that the union has the authority to act on behalf of employees in negotiating a collective bargaining agreement. In rare cases, the NLRB may direct an employer to recognize and bargain with the union if evidence exists that a fair and impartial election would be impossible. Since the early 1990s management strategies and tactics have become more aggressive during the recognition phase as management has endeavored to keep unions from becoming the employees' representative. For example, management may institute unfair labor practices such as filing for bankruptcy, illegally firing union supporters, and relocating the company. Although unions may file grievances with the NLRB over these practices and the use of any illegal or union-busting tactics, legal resolution usually occurs years after the fact and long after union elections have been held. Thus, both unions and management understand that the battle lines are drawn in the recognition phase, and both sides will be fervently engaged in shoring up support.

The desire to unionize is believed to result from three issues: wages, benefits, and employee perceptions about the workplace. Because ascertaining the desires of employees is difficult, management must rely on signals or indicators in the workplace. Exhibit 12.2 summarizes some of the behaviors that may indicate organizing activities or the potential for organizing employees. For example, high turnover of 20 percent or greater, depending on nursing specialty, characterizes healthcare institutions such as hospitals (NSI Nursing Solutions Inc. 2014). However, when employees are leaving their jobs for a local competitor, management must investigate the underlying reasons for turnover. Even simple issues, such as an increase in requests for information on policies and procedures, can indicate problems and should not be discounted.

EXHIBIT 12.2
Warning Indicators for Healthcare Organizations

Item	Increase/ Decrease	Comment
Turnover— especially to competitors	Increase	Turnover in healthcare organizations typically is much higher than in organizations in other industries because of enhanced mobility from licensing and standardization; however, if employees are moving to competing organizations in the local area, such movement may indicate dissatisfaction rather than career opportunities.
Employee- generated incidents	Increase	Staff members are fighting among themselves; theft or damage of the organization's property occurs; insubordination occurs in response to routine requests by supervisors.
Grievances	Increase	More grievances are being filed with the HR office compared with informal settlements of supervisors and employees.
Communication	Decrease	Staff members are reluctant to provide feedback and generally become quiet when management enters the room; suggestion boxes are empty and employees are less willing to avail themselves of "open-door" systems or other mechanisms to air dissatisfaction or problems.
HR office informational requests	Increase	Employees are interested in policies, procedures, and other matters related to the terms and conditions of employment, and they want this information in writing; verbal responses no longer satisfy them.
Off-site meetings	Increase	Employees appear to be congregating more at off-site premises.
Grapevine activity	Increase	Rumors increase in number and intensity.
Absenteeism or tardiness	Increase	Employees are engaging in union-organizing activities prior to and during work hours.
Social media activity	Increase	Employee postings on Facebook and other social networking websites trend negative about the employer.

During the recognition phase, the union solicits signed authorization cards that designate the union to act as the employees' collective bargaining representative. When at least 30 percent of employees in the bargaining unit have signed their cards, the union requests that employers voluntarily recognize the union. Voluntary recognition is rarely granted by employers, however, and occurs less than 2 percent of the time in healthcare organizations (NLRB 2005). When employers refuse voluntary recognition of the union, the union is then eligible to petition the NLRB for a representation election. In response to the petition, the NLRB verifies the authenticity of the signatures collected by the union, determines the appropriate bargaining unit, and sets a date for a secret-ballot election. Healthcare workers represent a significant number of all workers participating in NLRB elections. According to NLRB annual reporting, about 16 percent of the 1,639 NLRB elections held involved healthcare workers, and these workers were more likely to vote for a union compared with all other industries (NLRB 2009).

In the past decade, unions have supported legislative efforts that would amend existing labor laws to eliminate secret-ballot elections. Such efforts are perceived to be part of organized labor's strategy to target the union election process itself. Under existing labor law, the period leading up to the election can take several months to a year, during which employers are permitted to contest eligibility of workers to vote in a unit. Subsequent hearings and appeals can further extend the process. Even though it is illegal for employers to intimidate workers during this period, unions allege such tactics. Unions also claim that by the time the election is actually held, workers are too afraid to vote for the union as their representative (Kaira 2005). Although legislative attempts to eliminate secret-ballot elections have been unsuccessful, they reflect the continuing determination of unions to revise the organizing process in their favor.

In 2011, two board members of the NLRB voted to make a number of changes to the election process, including what became known as the "quickie elections" rule. This rule, which was later invalidated by the US District Court for the District of Columbia in *Chamber of Commerce of the United States of Am. v. NLRB*, No. 1:11-cv-02262 (D.D.C., May 14, 2012), would have reduced the average time between filing of an election petition and actual voting from 38 days to 25 days (Brown and DeLarco 2012).

Bargaining Units

The NLRB determines which employees are eligible to be in a bargaining unit and thereby eligible to vote in the election. Currently, the NLRB permits a total of eight bargaining units in healthcare settings. The implications of this number and some historical perspective are provided in the section of this chapter that summarizes legislative and judicial rulings. Although the NLRB has modified its criteria over the years, it has not changed its outlook on managerial or supervisory employees, who are ineligible for membership in a bargaining unit. Under a provision of the NLRA (29 U.S.C. § 15(11)), an employee is a "supervisor" if the employee has the authority, in the interest of the employer, to engage in specific activities, including responsible direction of other employees, where exercise of such authority requires the use of independent judgment. In a landmark 2006 ruling, the NLRB clarified and set forth guidelines for determining whether an individual is a supervisor under the NLRA. The NLRB ruled that charge nurses were supervisors, thereby making them and certain other nurses like them ineligible for bargaining unit representation. This ruling represents an opportunity to reclassify many nurses as management and thereby potentially decreases the union's ability to recruit new members.

Generally, the union election is scheduled to occur on workplace premises during work hours. The union is permitted to conduct a pre-election campaign in accordance with solicitation rules that are prescribed for both unions and management. For example, patient care areas such as treatment rooms, waiting areas used by patients, and elevators and stairs used in transporting patients are off limits, but kitchens, supply rooms, business areas, and employee lounges are permissible locations. During the campaign, management may not make threats or announce reprisals regarding the outcome of the election, such as telling nurses that layoffs will result if the union is elected or that pay raises will be given if the union loses. Management also may not directly ask employees about their attitudes or voting intentions or those of other employees. Management is allowed, however, to conduct captive-audience speeches, which are meetings during work time to inform employees about the changes that certifying a union will mean for the organization and to persuade employees to give management another chance.

To win the election and be certified by the NLRB as representing the bargaining unit, the union must achieve a simple majority, or 50 percent plus 1 of those voting. Consequently, if voter turnout is low, the decision to be unionized will be decided by less than a majority of employees eligible to vote. When the union wins the election, it assumes the duties of the exclusive bargaining agent for all employees in the unit even if those employees choose not to join the union and pay membership dues. Similarly, any negotiated agreements will cover all employees in the bargaining unit. If the union loses, however, it can continue to maintain contact with employees and provide certain representational services such as informing them of their rights. The union may lose the right to represent employees in the bargaining unit through a decertification election.

Rulings by what appears to be an activist and pro-union NLRB have affected bargaining unit composition. In the NLRB's decision in *Specialty Healthcare and Rehabilitation Center of Mobile*, 357 NLRB No. 83 (August 26, 2011), the NLRB overruled a 20-year-old case that had established clear categories of appropriate units for non-acute care facilities. In doing so, the NLRB opened up possibilities of micro-organizing activity for healthcare employers that are not acute care hospitals. That is, these employers are expected to confront union organizing efforts for small groups of employees. Because healthcare employers typically have many classes of employees, this decision can be particularly problematic for management (Brown and DeLarco 2012).

Negotiation Phase

After winning the election, the union will begin to negotiate a contract on behalf of the employees in the bargaining unit. Federal labor laws encourage collective bargaining on the theory that employees and their employers are best able to reach agreement on issues such as wages, hours, and conditions of employment by negotiating their differences. The process of negotiating this contract is referred to as *collective bargaining*. The NLRA (§ 8(d), 1935) defines collective bargaining as

> the performance of the mutual obligation of the employer and the representative of the employees to meet at reasonable times and confer in good faith with respect to wages, hours, and terms and conditions of employment, or the negotiation of an agreement or any question arising thereunder, and the execution of a written contract incorporating any agreement reached if requested by either party, but such obligation does not compel either party to agree to a proposal or require the making of a concession.

The NLRA requires an employer to recognize and bargain in good faith with a certified union, but it does not force the employer to agree with the union or make any concessions. The key to satisfying the duty to bargain in good faith is approaching the bargaining table with an open mind and negotiating with the intention of reaching final agreement.

Issues for bargaining have evolved as the result of NLRB and court decisions. Bargaining issues are categorized as illegal, mandatory, or voluntary (permissive). Illegal subjects, such as age-discrimination employment clauses, may not be considered for bargaining. Mandatory bargaining issues are related to wages, hours, and other conditions of employment; Exhibit 12.3 provides a partial list of these issues. Mandatory subjects must be bargained if they are introduced for negotiation. Voluntary, or permissive, bargaining issues carry no similar restriction. Examples of voluntary issues include strike insurance and benefits for retired employees.

Prior to bargaining, management will formulate a range for each issue, which is similar to an opening offer, followed by a series of benchmarks that represent expected levels of settlement. Of course, management must calculate a resistance point beyond which it will cease negotiations. Fisher and Ury

EXHIBIT 12.3

Mandatory
Bargaining
Issues

- Wages
- Arbitration
- Duration of agreement
- Reinstatement of economic strikers
- Work rules
- Lunch periods
- Bonus payments
- Promotions
- Transfers
- Plant reopening
- Bargaining over "bar list"
- Arrangement for negotiation
- Plant closedown and relocation
- Overtime pay
- Company houses
- Union-imposed production ceiling
- No-strike clause
- Workloads
- Cancellation of security upon relocation of plant
- Employer's insistence on clause giving arbitrator right to enforce award
- Severance pay
- Safety
- Checkoff
- Hours
- Holidays (paid)
- Grievance procedure

- Change of payment (hourly to salary)
- Merit wage increase
- Pension plan
- Price of company meals
- Seniority
- Plant closing
- Employee physical examination
- Truck rentals
- Change in insurance carrier/benefits
- Profit-sharing plan
- Agency shop
- Subcontracting
- Most-favored-nation clause
- Piece rates
- Change of employee status to independent contractor
- Discounts on company's products
- Clause providing for supervisors' keeping seniority in unit
- Nondiscriminatory hiring hall
- Prohibition against supervisors doing unit work
- Partial plant closing
- Discharge
- Vacations (paid)
- Layoff plan
- Union security and checkoff

- Work schedule
- Retirement age
- Group insurance (health, life, and accident)
- Layoffs
- Job-posting procedures
- Union security
- Musician price list
- Change in operations resulting in reclassifying workers from incentive to straight time, cut workforce, or installation of cost-saving machine
- Motor carrier union agreement
- Sick leave
- Discriminatory racial policies
- Work assignments and transfers
- Stock-purchase plan
- Management rights clause
- Shift differentials
- Procedures for income tax withholding
- Plant rules
- Superseniority for union stewards
- Hunting on employer forest preserve where previously granted

Note: This is a list of major items for bargaining; the list does not include subcategories.

(1981) developed a principled method of negotiation based on the merits or principles of the issues. The following four basic points are involved:

1. *People.* Separate the people from the problem.
2. *Interests.* Focus on interests, not the positions that people hold.

3. *Options.* Generate a variety of alternative possibilities.

4. *Criteria.* Insist that solutions be evaluated using objective standards.

According to this method, management will formulate a best alternative to a negotiated agreement for each issue. In this manner, negotiators evaluate whether the type of agreement that can be reached is better than no agreement at all. By considering mutual options for gain, the negotiator offers a more flexible approach toward bargaining and increases the likelihood of achieving creative solutions.

Collective bargaining is a laborious and time-consuming endeavor. Bargaining requires not only listening to others but attempting to understand the motivational force behind the dialogue. Successful negotiators make every effort to understand fully what truly underlies bargaining positions and why these positions are so fiercely held. Also, negotiators must be receptive to any signals that are being communicated, including nonverbal communication such as body language (Fisher and Ury 1981). Bargaining, as depicted in Exhibit 12.4, can be conceptualized as a continuum of behaviors and strategies. At one end of the continuum is *concessionary bargaining*, in which the employer asks the union to eliminate, limit, or reduce wages and other commitments in response to financial constraints. This type of bargaining is likely to occur when the organization is in financial jeopardy and is struggling to survive. At the opposite end is *integrative bargaining*, which seeks win-win situations and solutions that creatively respond to both parties' needs. This type of bargaining requires the trust and cooperation of both parties. In the center is *distributive bargaining*, which is a win-lose type in which each party gives up something to gain something else. This type of bargaining is likely when negotiations are contentious and full of conflict.

Even when both parties negotiate in good faith and fulfill the covenants of the NLRA, an agreement still may not be reached. When this happens, parties are said to have reached an impasse. To resolve an impasse, a variety of techniques may be implemented. These techniques involve third parties and include mediation, in which a mediator evaluates the dispute and then issues nonbinding recommendations. If either party rejects the mediator's recommendations, arbitration is an alternative. Similar to mediators,

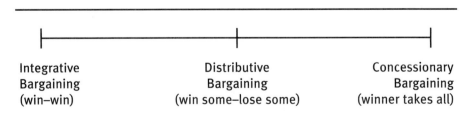

EXHIBIT 12.4
Collective
Bargaining
Continuum

arbitrators are neutral third parties, but their decisions are legally binding. For example, arbitrators may recommend that either party's position be accepted as a final offer, or they can attempt to split the differences between the two parties' positions.

If these techniques fail to resolve the impasse, employers or the union can initiate work stoppages that may take the form of lockouts or strikes. A lockout occurs when the employer shuts down operations either during or prior to a dispute. A strike, on the other hand, is employee initiated. Lockouts or strikes can occur during negotiations and also during the life of the contract. Special provisions for these work stoppages in healthcare settings are discussed in the section on the history of judicial and legislative rulings later in this chapter.

In addition, no-strike and no-lockout clauses can be negotiated in the agreement. No-strike clauses essentially prohibit strikes, either unconditionally or with conditions. An unconditional no-strike clause means that the union and its members will not engage in either a strike or a work slowdown while the contract is in effect. A conditional no-strike clause bans strikes and slowdowns except in certain situations and under specific conditions, which are delineated in detail in the agreement. Comparable clauses for lockouts exist for employers.

Administration Phase

When an agreement between the union and the employer is reached, it must be recorded in writing and executed in good faith, which means that the terms and conditions of the agreement must be applied and enforced. This agreement will include disciplinary, grievance, and arbitration procedures. The collective bargaining agreement imposes limitations on the disciplinary actions that management may take. The right to discharge, suspend, or discipline is clearly enunciated in contractual clauses and in the adoption of rules and procedures that may or may not be incorporated into the agreement.

Management may discipline employees through discharge only for sufficient and appropriate reasons and must base all procedures on due process. The union's role in the process is to defend employees and to determine the propriety of management action. The burden of proof rests with management to prove that whatever action was taken was proper and consistent with progressive discipline procedures. If the grievance proceeds to arbitration, arbitrators will usually support management if they find evidence of progressive discipline and evidence that employees were fully aware of the standards against which their behavior was to be measured. These standards include very basic rules and regulations that outline offenses for which employees will be subject to disciplinary action and the extent of such action.

The heart of administering the collective bargaining agreement is the *grievance procedure*. This procedure is a useful and productive management tool that allows implementation and interpretation of the contract. A grievance must be well defined and restricted to violations of the terms and conditions of the agreement. However, other conditions may give rise to a grievance, including violations of the law or company rules, a change in working conditions or past company practices, or violations of health and safety standards.

The grievance process usually contains a series of steps. The first step always involves the presentation of the grievance by the employee (or representative) to the immediate, first-line supervisor. If the grievance is not resolved at this step, broader action is taken. Because most grievances involve an action by the immediate supervisor, the second step necessarily must occur outside the department and at a higher level; thus, the second step will involve the employee (or representative) and a department head or other administrator. Prior to this meeting the grievance will be written out, dated, and signed by the employee and the union representative. The written grievance will document the events as the employee perceived them, cite the appropriate contract provisions that allegedly were violated, and indicate the desired resolution or settlement prospects. If the grievance is unresolved at this point, a third step that involves an in-house review by top management becomes necessary. A grievance that remains unresolved at the conclusion of the third step may go to arbitration if provided for in the contract and if the union is in agreement.

Most collective bargaining agreements restrict the arbitrator's decision to the application and interpretation of the agreement and make the decision final and binding on both parties. Most agreements also specify methods for selecting arbitrators. If the union agrees to arbitration, it must notify management, and an arbitrator is jointly selected. In evaluating the grievance, arbitrators focus on a variety of criteria, including the actual nature of the offense, the past record of the grieving employee, warnings, knowledge of rules, past practices, and discriminatory treatment. Thus, a large number of factors interact, making arbitration a complex process.

An arbitration hearing gives each side an opportunity to present its case. As in a court hearing, witnesses, cross-examinations, transcripts, and legal counsel may be used. Like a court hearing, arbitration is adversarial. Thus, cases may be lost because of poor preparation and presentation. Generally, the courts will enforce an arbitrator's decision unless it is shown to be unreasonable, unsound, or capricious relative to the issues under consideration. Also, if an arbitrator has exceeded his or her authority or issued an order that violates existing state or federal law, the decision may be vacated. Consistent and fair adjudication of grievances is the hallmark of a sound labor–management relationship.

In healthcare settings, the strike is the most severe form of a labor–management dispute. A critical part of planning for negotiations is an honest assessment of strike potential. This involves identifying strike issues that are likely to be critical for all parties. Although estimating the impact of possible strikes, including economic pressures from lost wages and revenues, is essential, the key to a successful strike from the perspective of the union is to impose enough pressure on management to expedite movement toward a compromise. Pressure may be psychological as well as economic. In healthcare settings, the real losers in a strike are the patients and their families. During a strike, patients may be denied services or forced to postpone treatment, be relocated to another institution, or even be discharged prematurely.

Management must be aware of critical factors that affect its ability and willingness to withstand a strike. When attempting to estimate the impact of these factors, managers will evaluate several key indicators, including revenue losses, timing of the strike, and availability of replacements for striking workers. However, management must also contemplate factors that affect the union, such as the question of whether striking employees will be entitled to strike benefits, especially health benefits. If so, for how long? Both parties must also consider the impact of outside assistance to avoid or settle a strike.

A Review of Legislative and Judicial Rulings

Exhibit 12.5 summarizes important legislative and judicial rulings and their impact on healthcare settings. As the exhibit indicates, in the late twentieth century, significant rulings have centered primarily on organizing issues. In 2004, the focus appeared to shift to financial issues such as changes to the Fair Labor Standards Act, which exempted most nurses from overtime pay. Unions were also affected by changes to the Labor-Management Reporting and Disclosure Act of 1959. Stricter reporting requirements that aimed at increased transparency and accountability for how unions spend dues money were instituted (*Harvard Law Review* 2004). In 2006, attention was directed toward organizing issues, specifically the determination of who is a nursing supervisor; a supervisor, after all, is excluded from the bargaining unit. With the election of President Obama, who openly supported unions and also enjoyed their support, especially in gaining passage of the Affordable Care Act (ACA), a more activist NLRB emerged. The NLRB has issued a number of rulings favoring unions, some of which have been invalidated by the courts. However, the NLRB's ruling on bargaining units for non-acute care hospital employers has opened up the potential for what has come to be known as micro-bargaining, or bargaining with smaller units.

As management structures have grown increasingly flat and less hierarchical, many jobs have assumed expanded duties that include a managerial component. Accordingly, determining who is a supervisor has become challenging, especially with regard to health professionals who operate with some autonomy (Von Bergen 2006). Of particular significance for healthcare employers are two decisions that concern supervisory status. The first is the US Supreme Court decision in the case of the *NLRB v. Kentucky River*

Year	Legislation or Judicial Ruling	Impact on Healthcare Organizations
1947	Taft-Hartley amendments to NLRA	Exempted not-for-profit hospitals from NLRA coverage, including collective bargaining
1962	Executive Order #10988	Permitted federally supported hospitals to bargain collectively
1974	Healthcare amendments to NLRA	Extended NLRA coverage to private, not-for-profit hospitals and healthcare institutions; special provisions for strikes, pickets, and impasses
1976	NLRB ruling: *Cedars-Sinai Medical Center* (Los Angeles)	Ruled that medical residents, interns, and fellows (house staff) are students and excluded from collective bargaining
1989/ 1991	NLRB ruling/Supreme Court affirmation on multiple bargaining units: P.L. 93-360	Expanded the number of bargaining units in acute care hospitals from three to eight
1999	NLRB ruling: *Boston Medical Center Corporation*	Reversed Cedars-Sinai Medical Center decision and ruled that house staff are employees, not students, and can therefore be included in collective bargaining
2001	Supreme Court decision regarding nurse supervisors: *NLRB v. Kentucky River Community Care, Inc.*	Court ruled that registered nurses who use independent judgment in directing employees are supervisors Impact of the ruling: Limits unions' ability to organize nurses
2003	US Department of Labor adopted a rule that increases union financial reporting requirements (19 C.F.R. 403 and 408) to provide for transparency of union financial structures and accountability of how unions spend their dues	
2004	US Department of Labor issued new rules that make most nurses ineligible for overtime pay under part 541 of the Fair Labor Standards Act	

EXHIBIT 12.5
Summary of Important Legislative and Judicial Rulings

(continued)

Year	Legislation or Judicial Ruling	Impact on Healthcare Organizations
2006	NLRB ruling: *Oakwood Healthcare Inc.* (Taylor, Michigan)	NLRB addressed supervisory status in response to the Supreme Court's decision in the *Kentucky River* case; issued guidelines for determining whether an individual is a supervisor under the NLRA; and reclassified certain nurses (charge nurses) as management, thus making them ineligible to join unions
		Impact of the ruling: Reduces potential for union recruitment and could permit employers to challenge existing contracts and remove nurses from bargaining units
2011–2013	In *Specialty Healthcare*, 357 NLRB No. 83, the NLRB redefined the "appropriate unit" standard to allow for smaller bargaining units. This ruling was later appealed, and in 2013, the US Court of Appeals for the Sixth Circuit granted the right to enforce the original ruling.	Bargaining units that consist of one department or one classification (e.g., certified nursing assistants) rather than "wall-to-wall" units are permitted. This ruling does not apply to employers that are acute care hospitals.

Community Care, Inc., 532 U.S. 706 (2001). The Supreme Court criticized the NLRB's lack of clarity in its interpretation of the term *independent judgment* to determine supervisory status. Subsequently, the NLRB addressed its definition of supervisory status. In a landmark case, *Oakwood Healthcare, Inc.*, 348 NLRB No. 37 (September 29, 2006), the NLRB ruled that permanent charge nurses employed by Oakwood Heritage Hospital in Taylor, Michigan, an acute care hospital, exercised supervisory authority in assigning employees within the meaning of section 2(11) of the NLRA. In this ruling, the NLRB reexamined and clarified its interpretations of the terms *independent judgment*, *assign*, and *responsibility to direct*. At issue was whether nurses at Oakwood assigned and directed other nurses using their own judgment rather than following written instructions or orders from a supervisor. The NLRB held that charge nurses who usually assign work and monitor care during a shift were supervisors and hence excluded from the bargaining unit. Nurses who handled such responsibilities on a part-time basis were not considered to be supervisors and therefore would remain eligible for union membership (Evans 2006; *PR Newswire* 2006).

The impact of this ruling was consequential for union membership because the ruling substantially limited the ability of unions to recruit nurses. Also, this ruling made organizing a union in a hospital or other healthcare facility more difficult because fewer workers were eligible. However, healthcare employers can challenge union elections and attempt to decertify nurses who are no longer protected by the collective bargaining agreements (Harrell 2006). Further, because of the ruling's impact, employers may also face union challenges and may be called on to demonstrate that supervisory assignments were consistent with the NLRB guidelines. Because the definition of a charge nurse varies from hospital to hospital, gray areas are left to be settled. These gray areas are what unions will ultimately challenge (Alexander 2006; Evans 2006). In addition, unions will likely fight for contract provisions to keep supervisory nurses in the union.

The Taft-Hartley Act amended the NLRA in 1947. The primary intent of these amendments was to strike a balance in the NLRA because most of its protections and rights applied to workers and employers needed a means for redress. The Taft-Hartley Act also gave states federal permission to enact right-to-work laws, which essentially prohibit employees from being forced to join unions as a condition of employment. Twenty-four states, mostly in the South and West, have enacted such laws (National Right to Work Legal Defense Foundation 2014). Unions oppose right-to-work laws in part because under the NLRA, unions are responsible for representing all employees in the bargaining unit, even members who choose not to join the union and consequently pay no union dues. (Nonunion members of the bargaining unit are often referred to as "free riders" because they acquire all of the benefits of union membership without any cost. Meanwhile, proponents of right-to-work laws maintain that no one should be forced to join a private organization, especially if that organization is using dues money to support causes that contravene an individual's moral or religious beliefs.)

Although the NLRA, as it was initially enacted in 1935, did not exempt healthcare employees explicitly, court interpretations tended to exclude healthcare workers from its regulations until later amendments asserted jurisdiction over a variety of healthcare institutions. The Taft-Hartley Act had a significant impact on healthcare workers because section 2(2) specifically excluded private, not-for-profit hospitals and healthcare institutions from the definition of "employer." However, the NLRB asserted jurisdiction over proprietary hospitals and nursing homes, and the 1974 Health Care Amendments, P.L. 93-360, brought the private, not-for-profit healthcare industry within the jurisdiction of federal labor law.

Approximately 2 million additional healthcare workers became eligible for representation with the 1974 Health Care Amendments (Stickler 1990). These amendments afforded stringent protections regarding work stoppages to safeguard patient care. Exhibit 12.6 summarizes the provisions for strikes and pickets as well as impasse requirements. In drafting the 1974 amendments, the congressional committee specifically included a ten-day strike and picket notice provision, a requirement that had not been applied to other industries. The committee did so to ensure that healthcare institutions would have sufficient advance notice of a strike. Furthermore, the committee report of the amendments held that a union is in violation if it has a strike at a facility more than 72 hours after the designated notice time, unless the parties agreed to a new time or the union issued a new ten-day notice. In addition, if the union does not begin the strike or other job action at the time designated in the initial ten-day notice, it must provide the healthcare facility with at least 12 hours' notice before the actual beginning of the action. Thus, the

EXHIBIT 12.6
Comparison of Provisions for Strike or Picket Notification and Impasse Requirements

1974 Health Care Amendments to the Taft-Hartley Act	General NLRA Provisions
30-day "reasonable" time to picket following which a representation petition must be filed by the union with NLRB.	Similar requirement
90-day notice for modifying an existing collective bargaining agreement.	60-day requirement
60-day notice to FMCS of impending expiration of existing collective bargaining agreement.	30-day requirement
Following FMCS notification, contract must remain in effect for 60 days without any strikes or lockouts.	30-day requirement
30-day notice of a dispute must be given to FMCS and appropriate state agency during initial negotiations.	No similar requirement
The director of FMCS is authorized to appoint a board of inquiry in the event of a threatened or actual work stoppage.	No similar authority
10-day written notice to employer and FMCS of strikes or pickets required of healthcare unions. (This notice cannot occur before either (1) the end of the 90-day notice to modify the existing contract or (2) the 30-day notice in the case of an impasse during negotiations of the new contract.)	No similar requirement
A new section 19 provides for an alternative, a contribution to designated 501(c)(3) charities, to the payment of union dues for persons with religious convictions against making such payments.	No similar requirement

Note: FMCS = Federal Mediation and Conciliation Service.

12-hour "warning" must fall completely within the 72-hour notice period. Repeatedly serving ten-day notices on the employer also constitutes evidence of a refusal to bargain in good faith and is a violation of the NLRA.

The reprisals for violating the ten-day notice are substantial. For example, workers engaged in work stoppage in violation of the strike notice lose their status as employees and are subsequently unprotected by the NLRA provisions. Exceptions to the requirements for unions to provide notices are provided as well. If the employer has committed a flagrant or serious unfair labor practice, notices are not required. In addition, the employer may not use the ten-day notice period to essentially undermine the bargaining relationship that otherwise exists. For example, the facility can receive supplies, but it is not free to stockpile supplies for an unduly extended period. Similarly, the facility cannot bring in large numbers of personnel from other facilities for the purpose of replacing striking workers (Metzger, Ferentino, and Kruger 1984).

In 1989, an NLRB ruling established eight units for the purpose of collective bargaining in acute care hospitals: (1) physicians, (2) nurses, (3) all other professionals, (4) technical employees, (5) business office clerical employees, (6) skilled maintenance employees, (7) guards, and (8) all other nonprofessionals. As with all bargaining unit determinations, supervisors are excluded from unit membership. The American Hospital Association (1991) strongly opposed the ruling and appealed to the US Supreme Court, protesting that the eight units would lead to a proliferation of bargaining units in the hospital, further fragmenting healthcare collective bargaining, increasing bargaining costs, making implementation of hospitalwide policies more difficult, and ultimately inflating the cost of healthcare, thereby rendering the bargaining process more complicated, lengthy, and subject to legal appeals and challenges. The Supreme Court disagreed, affirming the NLRB's ruling in 1991. Although little empirical evidence specifically evaluates the impact of the eight-unit ruling (Hirsch and Schumacher 1998), election activity and the union win rate within these eight units have increased. Exhibit 12.7 presents information on election activity in health services elections. Healthcare and social service assistance industries represent a significant number of all union elections. In 2010, one in six NLRB union elections were healthcare related (NLRB 2010).

Finally, despite lobbying campaigns, unions have failed consistently in their attempts to eliminate secret-ballot NLRB elections. As discussed earlier in this chapter, unions prefer to revise the organizing process in their favor by calling for a card-check method instead of an election. An example of such an effort is the Employee Free Choice legislation, including Senator Ted Kennedy's Employee Free Choice Act of 2007 (Senate Bill 1041). This act sought to amend labor laws to eliminate elections for certification. Although unions have not yet achieved legislative success, they are likely to continue to push for change.

Meanwhile, in the first decade of the twenty-first century, the NLRB has reportedly engaged in obvious union-friendly changes that significantly

EXHIBIT 12.7
Summary of
Election Activity
in Health Ser-
vices Elections,
1995–1999,
2009

Year	Total Elections	Union Wins
1995	291	156
1996	370	205
1997	407	258
1998	486	290
1999	517	333
2009	268	188

Source: Industrial Distribution of Representation Elections Held in Cases Closed, FY 1995–1999. Annual reports of the NLRB; NLRB (2009).

affect healthcare employers. Examples of changes include actions such as changing the requirements for bargaining units to encourage the proliferation of micro-bargaining units, as discussed previously.

Developments in Organizing Healthcare Workers

Unions

The union landscape shifted dramatically in 2005, when the SEIU (Service Employees International Union) ended its relationship with the AFL-CIO (American Federation of Labor and Congress of Industrial Organizations) because of a failure to pursue aggressive strategies to recruit new members. The SEIU subsequently aligned itself with the Change to Win federation, joining six other former AFL-CIO affiliates that similarly chose to sever ties. The SEIU action was consequential because it reduced the AFL-CIO membership of 13 million by about a third. In 2007, the SEIU, which reportedly represented 1.9 million members, announced the formation of a separate national healthcare union—SEIU Healthcare—that focused exclusively on healthcare workers. The SEIU visibly supported efforts to expand nurse–patient ratios and efforts to organize physicians. In addition to its focus on hospital, nursing, and long-term care workers, SEIU Healthcare targeted employees in ambulatory surgery centers, laboratories, clinics, and other healthcare areas (SEIU 2007; Siderius 2005). The local unions of SEIU Healthcare have been visibly active in recruitment and bargaining. In 2007, SEIU Healthcare successfully negotiated one of the largest labor contracts with HCA, a private-sector hospital chain. The contract covered six facilities and 4,000 workers across HCA hospitals in Florida and included a wage increase (Dorschner 2007). SEIU represents more than 10,000 healthcare workers at 19 HCA-owned hospitals throughout Florida and continues to organize hospitals in Florida and the West (SEIU 2014).

In 2009, the National Union of Healthcare Workers (NUHW) formed in response to troublesome practices regarding the management of healthcare unions. After a split from the SEIU over organizing philosophy, the NUHW aims to maintain complete transparency in establishing better working conditions and giving its members a stronger voice in the workplace. In 2013, the NUHW teamed up with the California Nurses Association (CNA), which represented 85,000 nurses in 2013 and proved to be a politically large partner for the NUHW. The NUHW represented 10,000 healthcare workers in 2013, compared to the SEIU Healthcare arm, which represented more than 1 million healthcare workers (Maher 2013).

Physicians

Historically, physicians resisted union organizing for professional and philosophical reasons. In fact, much of the American Medical Association (AMA) membership generally views unionism as antithetical to professionalism and sees unions as economic devices that extract benefits for their members at the expense of patient trust and confidence. In addition, organizing of physicians presented legal challenges because the majority of physicians are independent contractors and thus are technically ineligible for union membership. Only physicians who are technically employees, including those employed in academic settings, are authorized to bargain collectively. Physicians who practice as independent contractors are restricted from collective bargaining by the Sherman Antitrust Act of 1890, which prohibits business combinations that restrain free trade. Therefore, these physicians cannot legally talk with one another about prices of service. Independent contractors who engage in collective bargaining with entities such as health plans and insurers risk exposure to federal antitrust suits (Anthony and Erf 2000; Association of American Medical Colleges Executive Council 1999; Cohen 1999).

Nonetheless, the growth of "tight" managed care in the 1990s provided a powerful incentive for the rise of the physician union movement in the United States. The vast majority of physician complaints and efforts to unionize derived from corporate interference in medical decision making and coercive practices of managed care organizations (Anawis 2002; Luepke 1999). At its annual meeting in June 1999, the AMA House of Delegates approved a controversial resolution, creating a national bargaining unit for physicians. The bargaining unit—Physicians for Responsible Negotiations (PRN)—permitted employed physicians to bargain with health plans and insurers. The resolution was controversial because the AMA, which previously had opposed physician unions, reversed its position. In so doing, the AMA recognized collective bargaining as an acceptable professional mechanism for interacting with government and other third-party payers. Federal and state legislation also was proposed in support of amending antitrust laws to permit independent physicians to unionize. However, this legislation did not gain widespread support and was subsequently abandoned.

The PRN struggled for survival and recruited few members. In 2002, the AMA reduced its financial support for the PRN, only guaranteeing the union's survival through 2003. In March 2004, the AMA, with little press attention, severed its relationship with the PRN. In June 2004, the PRN partnered with the SEIU and its two other affiliated doctors' unions—the Doctors Council and the National Doctors Alliance. This affiliation represented the largest collection of unionized physicians in the United States, including approximately 20,000 members made up of salaried and private-practice physicians as well as medical residents and interns (Michels 2004; Romano 2004). Although little evidence exists to explain why the PRN was not well supported by physicians, the loosening of managed care was likely a dominant factor. Increases in consumer choice and open access effectively reduced many of the physician complaints and problems that previously substantiated interest in unionizing. For example, by the late 1990s, specialty physicians were regaining status as revenue and profit generators. Still, physicians also likely recognized the potential for obtaining judicial relief when they filed and won a class-action suit for reimbursement disputes against Aetna (Casalino, Pham, and Bazzoli 2004; Martinez 2003).

With the advent of the ACA and accountable care organizations (ACOs) and hospitals' trend toward employing physicians, physician unions could resurface because physicians are increasingly becoming employees rather than self-employed. In 2012, approximately half of physicians were already employed by large healthcare entities, and some industry experts predict that this number could reach 80 percent of all physicians (Leffell 2013). In addition, these numbers may have a generational component because younger physicians appear to be willing to give up income for a better quality of life, which means more regular working hours and less responsibility for patients after hours. Regardless of its reasons, the trend toward employment of physicians opens up possibilities for physicians at the bargaining table (Leffell 2013).

House Staff (Medical Residents, Interns, and Fellows) and Medical Students

In 1999, the NLRB ruled that house staff at Boston Medical Center were employees, not students. The impact of this ruling is that house staff in private hospitals are legally entitled to bargain collectively. This determination was a reversal of a 1976 ruling for Cedars-Sinai Medical Center in Los Angeles in which house staff were classified as students (Yacht 2000). In 2001, medical residents at 525-bed Brookdale University Hospital and Medical Center in New York became the first private-sector hospital physicians in the United States to ratify a collective bargaining agreement since that right was affirmed by the NLRB (*Modern Healthcare* 2001). Opponents of house staff unionization suggest that union activity will create adversarial relationships between house staff and instructors. For example, unions can negotiate resident promotions and fight against disciplinary actions and dismissal of poorly performing house staff (Levenson 1999).

Nurses

Nurses are predominantly employed in hospitals, where they represent the largest service and thus a significant labor cost. Nurses play a key role in patient care, providing care 24 hours a day, seven days a week. Historically, nurses have struggled with conflict among their obligation to their patients, their profession, and union representation. Approximately 2.7 million registered nurses (RNs) work in the United States, and despite uneven salary levels across the profession and widespread, persistent discontent with working conditions, the majority of these nurses do not belong to a union. Approximately 18 percent of RNs are unionized (Bureau of Labor Statistics 2006a; Leung 1999; Maher 2013; NLRB 2010). In addition, because of a 2006 NLRB landmark ruling concerning supervisory status, many nurses are no longer eligible for union membership (see Exhibit 12.5).

Unlike physicians, whose workplace problems and needs are often addressed without the help of unions, nurses have a different experience. As a nurse activist explains in the interview later in this chapter, nurse–management relationships are strained. National nurse shortages and pressures on hospitals to trim labor costs have increased nursing workloads and hours and thus the potential for nurses to commit errors during long shifts. Nurses often speak out in protest against cost-reducing measures that negatively affect patient care (Malvey 2010). In 2010 protests outside Tufts Medical Center and Boston Medical Center, nurses took a stand against plans to increase patient loads (Malvey 2010). In Massachusetts, work hours are a contentious nursing issue and have led to work stoppages and strike threats during contract negotiations (Kowalczyk 2004; Rowland 2006). Research affirms that for nurses to vote in favor of a union, they must believe that joining a union will help them gain greater control over patient care (Clark et al. 2000). Thus, patient care issues appear to have motivated many nurses to unionize (DeMoro 2002; Meier 2000).

Nurse activism remains ongoing and widespread. From informational pickets and protests to threats of strikes, nurses appear prepared to take action to ensure patient safety, adequate staffing, wages, and benefits. For example, in December 2006, nurses filed a class-action antitrust lawsuit against hospitals and health systems in the Detroit area. The suit alleged a collusion among these facilities to fix wages at below-market levels, and it is only one among similar class-action cases filed on behalf of nurses in other states, including Arizona, Illinois, New York, Tennessee, and Texas (Taylor 2006). In May

2007, judges allowed the nurse class-action case in Tennessee to continue despite attempts by the employing hospitals to have the case dismissed. The judge ruled that the nurses had facts that are sufficient to support claims of a conspiracy to depress nurses' wages (Evans 2007).

Patient care issues often remain top priorities for nurses and are addressed through protests and threats of strikes. In February 2014, 200 Kaiser RNs protested against the "downgrading of care" that they claimed would accompany the opening of its new facility in Oakland, California (Burger 2014). The RNs described proposed cuts and short staffing, despite 95,000 new enrollees in Kaiser health insurance plans through the ACA's insurance exchanges. Additionally, Kaiser RNs citied 1,400 reports to management regarding unsafe patient care, which reflects how patient care has suffered as a result of RN staffing cuts (Burger 2014). In March 2014, the CNA reported that the registered nurses at St. Rose Hospital in Hayward, California, authorized a strike centered on issues that are fundamental to quality patient care. Failure to provide adequate RN training, chronic short staffing in hospital units, and required overtime shifts were priority issues for St. Rose Hospital's RNs (California Nurses Association 2014). Nurses remain committed to their patients and their profession, and this commitment often requires activist activities in order to be heard.

By joining and becoming active in unions, nurses are exercising their voice and using tools of unionism such as election petitions, contract negotiations, and work stoppages such as sick-outs and strikes. Nurses are capturing the public's attention and using their influence to obtain community support (see the interview with a nurse activist later in this chapter). However, aggression and activism have yielded mixed results. Nurses' efforts to influence patient safety and quality-of-care legislation have been successful at the state level but not at the federal level. For example, California enacted the first law that establishes nurse-to-patient staffing ratios. This law, in effect, requires hospitals to reduce nurse workloads and improve patient safety by guaranteeing minimum nurse-to-patient ratios. It also serves as a framework for mandates in other states and at the federal level (Benko 2004). Similarly, nursing unions have achieved success at the state level with mandatory overtime legislation. State laws prohibiting or limiting mandatory overtime have been enacted in at least five states—Maine, Minnesota, New Jersey, Oregon, and Washington. However, corresponding federal legislation has not been enacted despite heavy union opposition to mandatory overtime. Nursing unions also failed to stop revisions to the Fair Labor Standards Act, which effectively exempts most nurses from overtime pay (see Exhibit 12.5).

Nurses are among the most stressed workers, with 80 percent reporting in a 2013 *Nursing Times* survey that they were under more pressure than the previous year and were experiencing physical ailments as a result (MacDonald 2013). The survey also reported the following:

- Nearly half (46 percent) said that they worked noticeably longer hours than they did at the same time in the previous year.

- Seventy-three percent said that they had suffered the side effects of work-related stress, such as physical or mental health problems, in the past year.

- More than a third (37 percent) had taken more sick leave in the past 12 months than they normally would.

- Seventy-four percent said that they had felt pressure from their organization to come to work when they were feeling ill that year (MacDonald 2013).

Nurses have become increasingly aggressive in having their voices heard through unionization, and the emergence of large and powerful nursing unions indicates that nurses will continue to be heard in the workplace.

Interview with a Nurse Activist

This interview was conducted on May 25, 2004, with the cochair of the nurses' union at a large, urban hospital in the northeast. She has more than 30 years of experience as a nurse and considers herself a nurse activist. Although the interview was conducted in 2004, the issues discussed are still relevant. Nurses are still concerned with patient safety and care. They are also still concerned with the undue stress associated with working long shifts and working with fewer nurses on those shifts and the impact of that stress on their ability to care for patients.

The nurse activist explained that nurses cannot trust management because managers will tell nurses anything just to get what they want. In her opinion, even nurses who are promoted to management cannot be trusted. "Management lies," she said. She explained that, at the end of a recent negotiation, management and union representatives did not even shake hands. Respect has been lost on both sides. At a time when management and nursing need to work together, a chasm of mistrust separates them. The main issues are not money, but human resources—that is, staffing, mandatory overtime, and workloads. Nurses are working harder and longer shifts; the potential for error increases in such environments. Patient safety and quality of care are at stake. According to the nurse activist, she was eight months pregnant and coming off of an eight-hour shift when she was ordered to work an additional four hours. "We are playing a game with patient safety," she said. "Management should be held accountable for what

(continued)

(continued from previous page)

they are doing." As a result, nurses are going to the bargaining table to hold management responsible for the staffing decisions that are threatening patient care.

Nurses are also taking their case to the public. The nurse activist routinely appears on local television and radio shows to gather support for nurses. The community is a key stakeholder. After all, she explained, patients make up the community, and they recall who actually cared for them during hospital visits: the nurse with the bedpan at 2 a.m., or the nurse giving comfort to the parents of a sick child. It was not management. With issues of patient safety and medication errors, nurses find it straightforward to get the community on their side in demands for staffing and work hours.

Peter Drucker, who invented the field of management study, may agree with this nurse activist. In an interview with the *Wall Street Journal*, he chided management for not treating nurses as professionals who know their jobs. Although he acknowledged that management is under financial pressure, Drucker said that instead of telling nurses what to do, management should invite nurses to find solutions to the problems (Petzinger 1999).

The Impact of the Internet

The role of the Internet in union organizing and solicitation campaigns and in collective bargaining and contract administration is receiving increasing attention. The Internet has become an influential tool for unions, as it has for many other causes. Union websites offer up-to-date information on union activities and developments and promote membership benefits. Because unions must observe specific rules about visiting work premises to solicit during union recognition campaigns, the Internet offers unprecedented opportunities to communicate with employees without time and place restrictions.

With e-mail, social networking websites, and blogs, unions are equipped with communication channels that can reach prospective members without alerting their employers. Some websites, such as the CNA's, offer sample contracts for nurses to use in bargaining with employers. Similarly, employers have the ability to disseminate information via the Internet. Furthermore, websites and blogs are dedicated to sharing negative information about unions, such as the number of complaints of unfair labor practices filed against unions for coercive or intimidating behavior exhibited toward employees. Enhanced communication also means transparency, and the Internet offers both employers and unions unprecedented insight and information regarding each other's efforts.

For example, when the SEIU began efforts to organize at teaching hospitals in Boston, it sent a letter to some trustees of Beth Israel Deaconess Medical Center, a teaching hospital, alleging that the hospital had potentially misrepresented its charity care in financial statements (Strom 2008). In response, the CEO of Beth Israel Deaconess Medical Center used his widely read blog to accuse the union of unfair tactics, such as attacking the reputation of teaching hospitals, their senior management, and their trustees. The SEIU's response to the CEO's blog was posted on its website and was e-mailed (Cooney 2007). Judging from this example alone, the Internet seems to have enhanced the ability of all parties (employees, employers, and unions) to communicate about the labor relations process. How the Internet will affect the labor–management relationship remains to be seen.

Experts suggest that "Facebook and other social networking websites may be the new 'water cooler,'" and employers will need to figure out how to both react to and prevent disruptive online activity (Brown and DeLarco 2012). NLRB reports regarding employee use of social networking websites suggest that employees who post negative information about their employers on Facebook are often engaged in activity protected by the NLRA. For example, if the post relates to wages, benefits, work hours, discipline, or similar topics, it is likely to be considered protected activity. The NLRB reporting also raises issues concerning the ability of employers to terminate or discipline employees who engage in inappropriate social media activity as well as the ability of employers to promote social media policies for their employees (Brown and DeLarco 2012).

The Impact of the Affordable Care Act

The impact of the ACA is still very much uncertain, and it is too early to determine the policy's effects on healthcare union activity. Union activity may be delayed in response to this policy intervention until organizations fully understand the policy's outcomes.

Even though unions were among the key institutional supporters of the ACA, they have become quite vocal in their overall disappointment with the ACA and its potential disruption of the health benefits of union members. In particular, unions believe that the ACA may incentivize businesses to reduce employees' hours to avoid the costs of providing ACA-mandated health benefits (Roy 2013).

A key ACA provision includes the formation of ACOs. ACOs consist of hospitals, physician groups, and other providers that join together to improve quality and patient outcomes, while reducing provider costs. Providers can obtain significant financial incentives for performing well, and these incentives can put pressure on providers, especially underperforming ones. Because the ACO acts as a "joint employer," hospitals should avoid interfering with other ACO members' employment decisions to avoid potential liability. ACOs must be set up and administered in a way that promotes compliance with collective bargaining agreements (Punke 2013).

The ACA may ultimately lead to changes in the nature of physician employment as physicians increasingly become employed by large healthcare entities. When the majority of physicians in the United States are no longer self-employed, and when their new employed status affords them the right to collective bargaining, the impact on labor–management relations will be unprecedented. Physicians provide a service that cannot be outsourced, and the emergence of this powerful group could put additional pressure on hospitals that are already confronting strike threats from nursing unions (Leffell 2013).

The Impact of the Marijuana Industry

The use of medical marijuana is legal in 23 states and Washington, DC. Medical marijuana is prescribed as an analgesic for people with many medical conditions. The United Food and Commercial Workers International Union (UFCW), the largest retail union, is in agreements with many medical marijuana dispensaries. The cannabis industry employs 3,000 UFCW members, and the industry has serious potential for growth. As the industry expands, it will likely increase union membership within the UFCW. The UFCW and other retail unions are fighting for fair wages and an increase in full-time employment opportunities; these two factors have been on the decline among retail employees for decades. Nevertheless, many marijuana retailers are openly inviting the UFCW into their shops in hopes that the union will assist in establishing the legitimacy of their businesses, navigating the difficult legal climate, and providing support against competition (Jacobs and Dobuzinskis 2013).

Management Guidelines

The following are six key points to remember about labor relations.

1. *Whether a healthcare organization is union or nonunion, it should have a policy on unionism, and this policy should be communicated to current and prospective employees.* A positive labor–management relationship begins with the screening process. All prospective employees should be given information about the institution's position toward unions as well as its goals and strategies of fair and consistent dealings with unions. Employee handbooks and orientation represent other opportunities to communicate management's commitment to provide equitable treatment

to all employees concerning wages, benefits, hours, and conditions of employment. Furthermore, management must also communicate that each employee is important and deserves respect and that adequate funds and management time have been designated to maintain effective employee relations (Rutkowski and Rutkowski 1984).

2. *Management not only must have effective policies and procedures for selection of new employees but also must ensure proper fit of personnel with specific jobs.* Job analyses, job descriptions, and job evaluations, as well as fair wage and salary programs, are essential in establishing a fundamental basis for fair representation. Management must not make promises that cannot be fulfilled; at the same time, it should strive to do whatever is possible to improve employee relations. Monitoring employee attitudes through surveys is essential; otherwise, management is dependent on the union for communicating worker problems or change in attitudes.

3. *Management must fulfill its roles and responsibilities to employees by providing necessary training, especially for first-line supervisors who are instrumental in determining how policies are implemented and in serving as liaisons between management and employees.* If supervisors are not properly trained, grievances are less likely to be settled quickly and are more likely to escalate into substantive formal disputes. Training is especially critical in healthcare settings because of constant and rapid changes in technology and workplace safety issues. Management's commitment to training must be consistent with fair and honest treatment of employees. Similarly, if management fails to establish objective performance policies or does not ensure that such policies are followed routinely, the labor–management relationship is affected. Employees may perceive inequities and unfairness and experience problems of declining morale and productivity if rewards are not matched with performance.

4. *Inconsistent and unfair application of disciplinary policies and procedures can create unnecessary grievance problems.* At a minimum, the principle of just cause should guide the disciplinary process. When employees file grievances, they expect prompt attention to their requests. Delaying a response or ignoring complaints sends a clear signal to employees that management does not care about their problems and thus cannot be trusted. Furthermore, management's credibility with employees will then deteriorate, creating an imbalance in the labor–management relationship that leads to employees' perception that the union's position is the most honest.

5. *The phases of the labor relations process are interrelated, and each phase can affect the outcome of the others.* For example, if the union is able to

obtain representation through voluntary recognition, the negotiations for a collective bargaining agreement will likely be less adversarial than a representation election. Similarly, if the negotiations for a collective bargaining agreement are contentious, difficulties may occur in administering the contract. Thus, having a full understanding of each phase and its potential to enhance or impede the overall process of labor relations is essential.

6. *Management must ensure that all employee documents, including handbooks and policy statements, are routinely updated and made available to all employees.* Management must ensure that a social media policy is available to guide both supervisors and employees with regard to permissible use of social networking websites. Employees as well as managers must consider whether a post is protected and concerted, especially when the post could lead to disciplinary action or even termination (Brown and DeLarco 2012).

Summary

Managing with organized labor is challenging. Even though unionism has been declining nationally for decades, the relatively unorganized healthcare workforce has continued to grow and has become a serious target for unions. With one-third of the projected job growth from 2012 to 2022 occurring in the healthcare field, new jobs will require a wide range of personnel, from home health aides to nurses, technicians, and physicians (Bureau of Labor Statistics 2013). Because union membership and election activity have increased in healthcare settings, managers must devote high-level attention to the application and maintenance of a positive labor relations program that integrates HR functions and includes social media networking sites and other Internet-based communication tools.

The rise of claims of unfair labor practices and the increase in threats of strikes, walkouts, and other work stoppages suggest that the labor–management relationship in healthcare is strained. Pressure from the shrinking economy and healthcare reform have led to widespread layoffs and reimbursement cuts. The growth in the number of employed physicians could mean significantly more pressure on employers at the bargaining table and rising costs to meet physicians' demands. And the dissatisfaction expressed by nurses and their willingness to organize cannot be ignored. Management must be prepared to deal with these challenges.

Discussion Questions

1. Why should management have a policy on unionism? What purpose does such a policy serve?

2. Describe the three phases of the labor relations process. Why are all phases equally important?

3. What are some of the behaviors that may indicate to managers that organizing activities are occurring?

4. Explain the potential far-reaching impact of the NLRB ruling on nursing supervisors. Will this ruling have a chilling effect on nursing unions?

5. How might the advent of social media tools be a positive force for union activity, including union formation? How might the increased use of social media tools present a challenge for both unions and employers?

Experiential Exercises

Case 1   The CEO of a midsize urban hospital was working late one Friday evening when he took a shortcut that caused him to walk by the employee lounge. He looked inside and shook his head. With all the problems of budget cuts and trying to make ends meet, he realized that little money had been available for upkeep of nonpatient areas such as the employee lounge. The carpet was dirty and worn, the coffee mugs were chipped, the wallpaper was torn, and the refrigerator groaned as it cycled on and off. The CEO decided enough was enough. The employees had worked hard and should at least have an employee lounge that was inviting and pleasant.

He marched back to his office and called the chief operating officer (COO) to instruct her to create a weekend miracle by calling in the work crews to update and refurbish the employee lounge. He ordered new carpets, new wallpaper, and new appliances, and he wanted it all done by Monday. The CEO told the COO, "I keep telling the employees how much I appreciate their help, especially in these financially tight times, but now I am going to show them. And be sure to replace those old, chipped coffee mugs." Early on Monday morning, the CEO walked by the employee lounge. It looked terrific, and someone had already made coffee. He made a note to himself to tell the COO what a great job she had done.

When he got to his office, he found the union steward sitting on the couch. "I need to have a word with you," the union steward said. He had several words, as it turned out: He said that the CEO had violated the collective bargaining contract and that refurbishing the employee lounge should have been discussed with the union. The union steward spent 20 minutes complaining about violations and procedures. After he left, the CEO called the COO and told her to put the lounge back the way it was, including the chipped coffee mugs. Then the CEO muttered to himself, "That is the last time I try to do anything nice for anyone around here. I have learned my lesson."

Case Questions

1. What is the problem in this case?
2. If you were the CEO, would you respond in the same way? Why, or why not?

3. What, if anything, can be done at this point?

Case 2   Rollins, a physician, was an exemplary employee at a midsized suburban hospital. He had been on staff at the hospital and was well respected by those with whom he worked as well as his patients and their families. But one Saturday evening, everything changed. Rollins, who was on call, had been alerted to an incoming patient who had been in a serious automobile accident. Without delay, Rollins left a restaurant where he had been dining with friends and headed toward the hospital. Once there, he was directed to the operating room where the surgical team was about to operate on the accident victim. Four hours later, the surgery was completed, and Rollins headed to the changing area. While in the changing area, Rollins updated his Facebook page for his friends. In that update, he posted how he had saved a life that night and described in some detail the condition of the patient, including details of the automobile accident. Within a few days, Rollins received a notice of termination. The hospital informed him that he had violated the hospital's social media policy. Rollins was perplexed. He didn't know what he had done wrong. Moreover, he wasn't aware that the hospital had such a policy.

Case Questions

1. What could hospital management have done to prevent this situation?
2. How can management best communicate its social media policy to hospital staff?
3. Is termination too severe a punishment for a first-time violation of a social media policy?

Exercise 1   Think of a healthcare facility in your community. Consider its nursing situation. Then answer the following questions:

1. Are the nurses treated as professionals? Why, or why not?
2. If given the opportunity, do you think these nurses are likely or unlikely to join a labor union in the future? Why, or why not?

Exercise 2   Refer to Exhibit 12.2. Using the indicators listed in the exhibit, conduct an audit of a hospital or a healthcare organization. Determine if the organization has experienced an increase or a decrease in any of the indicators. Then explain the possible reasons for these increases or decreases.

Exercise 3 Using Exhibit 12.1 as a guide, complete the chart in Exhibit 12.8 by listing specific goals for the union and the organization. Once you have completed the chart, answer the following:

1. Which goals are similar?
2. Which goals have the potential for conflict?

Goal Areas	Union Goals	Organization Goals
Survival		
Growth		
Profitability		
Competitiveness		
Recruitment and retention of employees		
Motivation of employees		
Flexibility		
Decision making		
Effective use of human resources		

EXHIBIT 12.8
Union and Organization Goal Worksheet

References

Alexander, A. 2006. "Charge Nurses Can Take Part in Vote to Unionize." *Knight Ridder Tribune Business News*. Accessed September 17, 2007. ABI/Inform Global Database, www.proquest.com.

American Hospital Association. 1991. "Legal Memorandum Number 16: Collective Bargaining Units in the Health Care Industry." Chicago: American Hospital Association.

Anawis, M. A. 2002. "The Ethics of Physician Unionization: What Will Happen If Your Doctor Becomes a Teamster?" *DePaul Journal of Health Care Law* 6 (1): 83–110.

Anthony, M. F., and S. Erf. 2000. "Can Physician Unionization Succeed?" *Healthcare Executive* 15 (2): 50–51.

Association of American Medical Colleges Executive Council. 1999. "AAMC Statement on Negotiating Units for Physicians." *AAMC Reporter* 9 (2): 7.

Becker, W. L., and A. M. Rowe. 1989. "Update on Union Organization in Health Care." *Review of Federation of American Health Systems* 22 (5): 11–12, 14–16.

Benko, L. B. 2004. "Workforce Report 2004: Ratio Fight Goes National." *Modern Healthcare* 34 (24): 23, 30.

Brown, S. J., and M. E. DeLarco. 2012. "Health Care Institutions and Recent NLRB Activity: Preventative Action Is the Best Medicine." Bloomberg BNA. Published July 12. www.bna.com/health-care-institutions-and-nlrb/.

Bureau of Labor Statistics. 2014a. "Fastest Growing Occupations." Published January 8. www.bls.gov/ooh/fastest-growing.htm.

———. 2014b. "Union Members Summary." Published January 24. www.bls.gov/news.release/union2.nr0.htm.

———. 2013. "Industry Employment and Output Projections to 2022." *Monthly Labor Review*. Published December. www.bls.gov/opub/mlr/2013/article/industry-employment-and-output-projections-to-2022-1.htm.

———. 2006a. "Current Population Survey (CPS), Table 3, Union Affiliation of Employed Wage and Salary Workers by Occupation and Industry." Accessed October 29, 2007. www.bls.gov/news.release/union2.t03.htm.

———. 2006b. "Union Members in 2006." Accessed August 15, 2007. www.bls.gov/news.release/union2.nr0.htm.

———. 2004. "Union Members in 2003." Accessed July 6. www.bls.gov/news.release/union2.nr0.htm.

———. 2000a. "Union Membership Edges Up but Share Continues to Fall." Accessed December 5, 2001. http://stats.bls.gov/opub/ted.

———. 2000b. "Unpublished Tabulations from Current Population Surveys, Union Membership Tables, 1999 Annual Averages." Washington, DC: US Government Printing Office.

Burger, D. 2014. "200 Kaiser RNs Rally to Protest Downgrading of Care for New Oakland Hospital." National Nurses United. Published February 27. www.nationalnursesunited.org/blog/entry/200-kaiser-rns-rally-to-protest-downgrading-of-care-for-new-oakland-hospita/.

California Nurses Association. 2014. "St. Rose Hospital RNs in Hayward Ready to Strike to Stop Erosion in Patient Care Standards." National Nurses United. Published March 24. www.nationalnursesunited.org/press/entry/st.-rose-hospital-rns-in-hayward-ready-to-strike-to-stop-erosion-in-patient/.

Casalino, L. P., H. Pham, and G. Bazzoli. 2004. "Growth of Single-Specialty Medical Groups." *Health Affairs* 23 (2): 82–90.

Christian Science Monitor. 2004. "A Worker–Union Disconnect." *Christian Science Monitor* 96 (83): 8.

Clark, D. A., P. F. Clark, D. Day, and D. Shea. 2000. "The Relationship Between Health Care Reform and Nurses' Interest in Union Representation: The Role of Workplace Climate." *Journal of Professional Nursing* 16 (2): 92–96.

Cohen, J. J. 1999. "Unions Are Bad Medicine for Doctors." *Academic Medicine* 74 (8): 905.

Cooney, E. 2007. "Beth Israel Deaconess CEO and Union Lock Horns." Published August 1. www.boston.com/yourlife/health/blog/2007/08/levy_and_seiu_l.html.

DeMoro, R. A. 2002. "What California Has Started: Staffing Ratios, Union Activism Are National Solutions to the Nurse Shortage." *Modern Healthcare* 32 (13): 26.

Department for Professional Employees. 2014. "Nursing: A Profile of the Profession." Published April. http://dpeaflcio.org/programs-publications/issue-fact-sheets/nursing-a-profile-of-the-profession/.

Dorschner, J. 2007. "Union Strikes a Bargain with 6 Hospitals in Chain: Six Hospitals Agree to a Union Contract That Will Increase Wages and May Increase Nurse-Patient Ratios." *Knight Ridder Tribune Business News*. Accessed September 17, 2007. ABI/Inform Global Database, www.proquest.com.

Evans, M. 2007. "Judge Lets Nurses' Class-Action Case Continue." *Modern Healthcare*'s Daily Dose. Published May 21. www.modernhealthcare.com/article/20070521/NEWS/305210020.

————. 2006. "Nurses Ready to Fight Back." *Modern Healthcare* 6 (40): 6–9.

Fennell, K. S. 1987. "The Unionization of the Healthcare Industry: General Trends and Emerging Issues." *Journal of Health in Human Resources Administration* 10 (1): 66–81.

Fisher, R., and W. Ury. 1981. "Getting to Yes—Negotiating an Agreement Without Giving In." In *Harvard Negotiation Project*, edited by B. Patton, 21–53. Boston: Houghton Mifflin.

Fottler, M. D., R. A. Johnson, K. J. McGlown, and E. W. Ford. 1999. "Attitudes of Organized Labor Officials Toward Health Care Issues: An Exploratory Survey of Alabama Labor Officials." *Health Care Management Review* 24 (2): 71–82.

Freeman, R. B., and J. L. Medoff. 1984. *What Do Unions Do?* New York: Basic Books.

Harrell, J. 2006. "National Labor Relations Board to Send Labor Up the River." *Long Island Business News Ronkonkoma*. Accessed July 28. ABI/Inform Global Database, www.proquest.com.

Harvard Law Review. 2004. "Labor Law: Department of Labor Increases Union Financial Reporting Requirements." *Harvard Law Review* 117 (5): 1734–40.

Hecker, D. E. 2004. "Occupational Employment Projections to 2012." *Monthly Labor Review* 127 (2): 80–105.

Hirsch, B. T., and E. J. Schumacher. 1998. "Union Wages, Rents and Skills in Health Care Labor Markets." *Journal of Labor Research* 19 (1): 125–47.

Jacobs, S., and A. Dobuzinskis. 2013. "Insight: Shrinking U.S. Labor Unions See Relief in Marijuana Industry." *Reuters*. Published February 6. www.reuters.com/article/2013/02/06/us-usa-marijuana-unions-idUSBRE91507E20130206.

Kaira, R. 2005. "Labor Paints a Target on Union-Election Law." *Knight Ridder Tribune Business News.* Accessed June 14. ABI/Inform Global Database, www.proquest.com.

Kearney, R. C. 2003. "Patterns of Union Decline and Growth: An Organizational Ecology Perspective." *Journal of Labor Research* 24 (4): 561–78.

Kowalczyk, L. 2004. "University of Pennsylvania Study Links Long Hours, Nurse Errors." *Knight Ridder Tribune Business News,* July 7, 1.

Leffell, D. J. 2013. "The Doctor's Office as Union Shop." *Wall Street Journal.* Published January 29. http://online.wsj.com/news/articles/SB1000142412787323337520457827040113873997 8.

Leung, S. 1999. "More Nurses Join Unions Across State." *Wall Street Journal,* September 15.

Levenson, D. 1999. "Private Hospitals Worry NLRB Ruling Will Spark Intern, Resident Disputes." *AHA News* 35 (47): 1–2.

Luepke, E. 1999. "White Coat, Blue Collar: Physician Unionization and Managed Care." *Annals of Health Law* (8): 275–98.

MacDonald, I. 2013. "Survey: Nurses Overworked, Understaffed and Stressed." *Fiercehealthcare.* Published October 1. www.fiercehealthcare.com/story/survey-nurses-overworked-understaffed-and-stressed/2013-10-01.

Maher, K. 2013. "Health-Care Unions Will Join Forces." *Wall Street Journal,* January 3.

Malvey, D. 2010. "Unionization in Healthcare: Background and Trends." *Journal of Healthcare Management* 55 (3): 154–57.

Martinez, B. 2003. "Aetna to Announce Settlement with Physicians." *Wall Street Journal,* May 22, A3.

Meier, E. 2000. "Is Unionization the Answer for Nurses and Nursing?" *Nursing Economics* 18 (1): 36–38.

Metzger, N., J. Ferentino, and K. Kruger. 1984. *When Health Care Employees Strike.* Rockville, MD: Aspen.

Michels, T. J. 2004. "Three Doctors' Unions Form Partnership to Unite Resident, Salaried, and Private Practice Physicians." Service Employees International Union press release. Accessed October 24, 2007. www.seiu.org/media/pressreleases.

Modern Healthcare. 2001. "The Labor Picture." *Modern Healthcare* 31 (22): 12.

National Labor Relations Board (NLRB). 2010. *Annual Report.* Washington, DC: National Labor Relations Board.

———. 2009. *Annual Report.* Washington, DC: National Labor Relations Board.

———. 2005. *Annual Report.* Washington, DC: National Labor Relations Board.

National Right to Work Legal Defense Foundation. 2014. "Right to Work States." Accessed December 30. www.nrtw.org/rtws.htm.

NSI Nursing Solutions Inc. 2014. *2014 National Healthcare and RN Retention Report.* Published March. www.nsinursingsolutions.com/Files/assets/

library/retention-institute/NationalHealthcareRNRetentionReport2014. pdf.

Petzinger, T. Jr. 1999. "Talking About Tomorrow—Peter Drucker: The 'Arch-Guru of Capitalism' Argues That We Need a New Economic Theory and New Management Model." *Wall Street Journal* Eastern Edition, December 31, R34.

PR Newswire. 2006. "NLRB Issues Lead Case Addressing Supervisory Status in Response to Supreme Court's Decision in Kentucky River." *PR Newswire.* Accessed September 17, 2007. ABI/Inform Global Database, www.proquest. com.

Punke, H. 2013. "What ACOs Mean for Hospital Labor Relations." *Becker's Hospital Review.* Published December 6. www.beckershospitalreview.com/accountable-care-organizations/what-acos-mean-for-hospital-labor-relations.html.

Romano, M. 2004. "Labor Union Didn't Work." *Modern Healthcare* 34 (22): 32–34.

Rowland, C. 2006. "Nurses Union Flexing Clout in Contract Talks." *Knight Ridder Tribune Business News.* Accessed September 17, 2007. ABI/Inform Global Database, www.proquest.com.

Roy, A. 2013. "Labor Unions: Obamacare Will 'Shatter' Our Health Benefits, Cause 'Nightmare Scenarios.'" *Forbes.* Published July 15. www.forbes.com/sites/theapothecary/2013/07/15/labor-leaders-obamacare-will-shatter-their-health-benefits-cause-nightmare-scenarios/.

Rutkowski, A. D., and B. L. Rutkowski. 1984. *Labor Relations in Hospitals.* Rockville, MD: Aspen.

Scott, C., and C. M. Lowery. 1994. "Union Election Activity in the Health Care Industry." *Health Care Management Review* 19 (1): 18–27.

Scott, C., and A. Seers. 1996. "Determinants of Union Election Outcomes in the Non-Hospital Health Care Industry." *Journal of Labor Research* 17 (4): 701–15.

Service Employees International Union (SEIU). 2014. "Fast Facts." Accessed December 30. www.1199seiu.org/hca.

———. 2007. "SEIU Plans to Form Healthcare Unit." *FierceHealthcare.* Published January 30. www.fiercehealthcare.com/story/seiu-plans-to-form-healthcare-unit/2007-01-31.

Siderius, C. 2005. "Union Official Rallies Nurses at Swedish." *Seattle Times.* Published August 15. http://community.seattletimes.nwsource.com/archive/?date=20050815&slug=seiu15m.

Stickler, K. B. 1990. "Union Organizing Will Be Divisive and Costly." *Hospitals,* July 5, 68–70.

Strom, S. 2008. "Hospital's Accounting Is Under Fire by a Union." *New York Times.* Published February 20. www.nytimes.com/2008/02/20/us/20hosp. html?ref=us.

Taylor, M. 2006. "Nurses Sue Detroit-Area Hospitals." *Modern Healthcare*'s Daily Dose. Published December 20. www.modernhealthcare.com/article/ 20061220/news/61220011/.

Von Bergen, J. M. 2006. "Testing Unions' Clout: Pivotal Cases: For Some Employees, Their Union Status Hinges on an NLRB Decision That Will Define the Word Supervisor." *Knight Ridder Tribune Business News.* Accessed September 17, 2007. ABI/Inform Global Database, www.proquest.com.

Yacht, A. C. 2000. "Unionization of House Officers: The Experience at One Medical Center." *New England Journal of Medicine* 342 (6): 429–31.

Web Resources

- Online listings of private-sector and public-sector agreements (collective bargaining agreements) are available at the website of the US Department of Labor's Office of Labor-Management Standards (go to www.dol.gov/olms/regs/compliance/cba/index.htm). For example, agreements for Kaiser Permanente facilities can be found under "K" in the list of private-sector agreements.

- The website for the California Nurses Association contains model RN contracts. The website also provides a listing of salaries and differentials, benefits, working conditions, staffing and professional practices, and performance committees, among other information. Sample contracts are also available for downloading, and these contracts will be updated per current bargaining. Because this source is a union website, the information posted here will likely change over time. Visit www.nationalnursesunited.org/site/entry/cna-facilities.

- Up-to-date healthcare workforce and union information can be found on the National Union of Healthcare Workers website at nuhw.org. Click on "News & Press" for timely information.

- SEIU Healthcare union news can be found at www.seiu.org/ seiuhealthcare/.

WORKFORCE PLANNING IN A RAPIDLY CHANGING HEALTHCARE SYSTEM

Erin P. Fraher and Marisa Morrison

Learning Objectives

After completing this chapter, the reader should be able to

- describe the importance of workforce planning in a rapidly changing healthcare system;
- describe the methods used to project workforce supply and estimate the demand for healthcare workers;
- understand the challenges in determining the right number and mix of workers needed to meet patients' demand for healthcare services;
- apply workforce planning methods to real-world issues facing healthcare workforce planners; and
- interpret the results of workforce planning models and determine their implications for human resource planners in a healthcare organization.

The Link Between Macro-Level Policy and Micro-Level Healthcare Workforce Outcomes

The goal of healthcare workforce planning is to "provide the right number of healthcare workers with the right knowledge, skills, attitudes and qualifications, performing the right tasks in the right place at the right time" (International Centre for Human Resources in Nursing 2008, 1). If that were not lofty enough an ambition, healthcare workforce planners must accomplish this goal while achieving the "triple aim" of healthcare—lower costs, higher patient satisfaction, and improved health outcomes for populations (Berwick, Nolan, and Whittington 2008). The US healthcare system is undergoing transformative change, and at the heart of this transformation is the workforce who staff the nation's hospitals, physician offices, nursing facilities, walk-in clinics, drugstores, and other settings.

To respond to changes in the healthcare delivery system, hospitals and health systems are increasingly turning to healthcare workforce planning as a critical element of organizational strategy. From an organizational perspective, taking a strategic and proactive approach to healthcare workforce planning can help the organization do the following:

- *Improve care delivery for patients* by ensuring that the organization has the right number and skill mix of healthcare workers needed to deliver care at the highest possible levels of quality and patient satisfaction and with the lowest costs.
- *Reduce costs for payers and the healthcare organization itself* by lowering the cost of recruitment, turnover, and training of healthcare workers. A well-designed healthcare workforce team can improve staff productivity, morale, and retention, which in turn increase efficiencies in the care delivery process.
- *Improve employee engagement,* which is beneficial because organizations with higher levels of employee engagement have 37 percent less absenteeism, have 41 percent fewer safety incidents, and are 21 percent more productive and 22 percent more profitable than organizations with lower levels of employment engagement (Gallup 2013).
- *Achieve efficiencies for employers and health systems* because more strategic and long-range healthcare workforce planning that is linked to the organization's mission leads to better operational and financial outcomes as a result of better utilization of human resources.

Many of the chapters in this book view human resources (HR) management from the perspective of the healthcare organization. Chapters focus on such topics as job design, recruitment and retention, and evaluation of individual performance. However, organizations are affected by the larger external environment in which they deliver healthcare services. External factors such as workforce policy and the labor market affect an organization's ability to attract and retain employees. An organization may have a well-designed and sound recruitment program for nurses, but if sufficient numbers of nurses are not being trained in the national healthcare system or nurses are not being trained with the skills they need to practice, the organization's nurse recruitment efforts will likely prove unsuccessful. This chapter's focus is unique among the chapters of this book because it addresses workforce planning from a macro policy perspective. It explores the methods used to ensure the United States has the "right" workforce in place, rather than focusing on the needs of a particular organization.

Macro-level policy changes that influence the number of health professionals trained affect the overall supply of workers available in the labor pool. Regulations that govern workers' scope of practice determine the types of services they can provide to patients. How health professionals are paid affects which careers they choose to enter, and not surprisingly, individuals often choose higher-paying jobs in specialty care rather than lower-paid positions in primary care. The gap between the two is striking. The median annual salary for a family physician in 2012 was $164,168, while the median cardiovascular surgeon earned $444,025 (Medical Group Management Association 2012). Payment also affects the volume and type of services provided, with procedural services such as cardiovascular procedures generating more revenue than preventative care services delivered by family physicians.

The Importance of Healthcare Workforce Planning in a Rapidly Changing System

With an estimated 18 million workers employed in the health sector in the United States (Bureau of Labor Statistics 2014), the magnitude and importance of healthcare workforce planning is clear. Nurses are the largest single component of the healthcare workforce, with an estimated 2.8 million nurses in active practice, but the number of unlicensed or paraprofessional healthcare workers such as home health aides and nursing assistants is large and projected to grow even faster than the number of licensed health professionals such as doctors and nurses (Bureau of Labor Statistics 2013).

Of the $2.6 trillion spent in the United States in 2010 on healthcare, 56 percent was wages for healthcare workers (Kocher and Sahni 2011). As a nation's wealth increases, so do its appetite for healthcare services and its per capita supply of physicians (Cooper, Getzen, and Laud 2003). As Exhibit 13.1 shows, the share of the US gross domestic product (GDP) spent on health increased from 5 percent in 1960 to 17.2 percent in 2012 (Centers for Medicare & Medicaid Services 2014). Evidence suggests that the growth in healthcare spending is slowing (Altarum Institute 2014; Martin et al. 2014). This trend likely reflects the impact of the economic recession that hit in 2008 (Dranove, Garthwaite, and Ody 2014) but also a consensus that the current system is unsustainable. Calls to "bend the cost curve" (Antos et al. 2009) in health spending have employers, health systems, the federal government, and other stakeholders looking for more efficient ways to deploy the healthcare workforce.

Without systematic and ongoing workforce planning, the healthcare system lurches from oversupply to shortage (Fraher, Harden, and Kimball 2011). Insufficient numbers of health professionals lead to staffing shortages that result in long wait times or the inability to access needed care. Geographic maldistribution of providers causes disparities in access to healthcare

EXHIBIT 13.1
US National
Health
Expenditures as
a Percentage of
GDP, 1960–2012

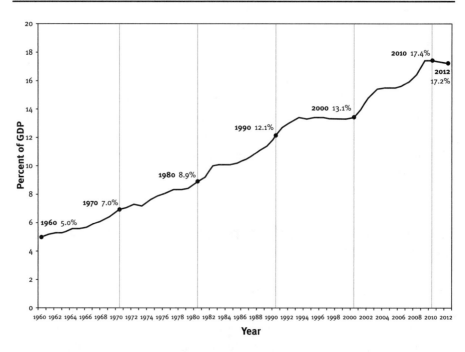

Source: Centers for Medicare & Medicaid Services (2014), using data from Centers for Medicare & Medicaid Services, Office of the Actuary, National Health Statistics Group; US Department of Commerce, Bureau of Economic Analysis; and US Bureau of the Census.

services, particularly in rural and underserved communities where fewer providers are available and where patients often have higher healthcare needs and poorer health outcomes. Inadequate training of health professionals or a poorly designed skill mix of providers within an organization can affect the distribution of tasks among staff. This problem leads some staff to be overqualified for the tasks they perform and other staff to be underqualified to take on the tasks assigned to them. For example, some observers suggest that nurses are often not allowed to work "to the full extent of their education and training," leading to higher costs, lower staff morale, higher turnover, and lower productivity (Institute of Medicine 2011, 4). On the other end of the spectrum are worries that inappropriate use of medical assistants—unlicensed staff who may have a high school diploma and on-the-job training—to undertake tasks for which they are not adequately trained may lead to lower quality of care and medical errors (Hull et al. 2013).

The Strengths and Weaknesses of Workforce Models

Healthcare workforce planning relies on forecasting models to estimate the future supply of and demand for healthcare workers. Workforce models are important tools for policymakers, health professionals, employers, and other stakeholders to understand current trends and plan for how many healthcare workers to train or hire in the future. Traditional workforce models have sought to estimate one "right" answer of how many health professionals will be needed, but more recent models include the ability to model the outcome of "what if" scenarios. Scenarios allow planners to analyze how changes at the macro (policy) level or the micro (organizational) level may affect workforce supply and demand and to understand how long interventions will take to have an effect.

Scenarios often show surprising results that can be used to educate stakeholders about how different policy changes will affect the workforce. For example, as the nation debates whether we have a shortage of physicians or just a maldistribution of providers, models can help stakeholders see that training more physicians will not affect overall supply for about seven years because of the long training pathway to becoming a doctor. Scenarios show that bigger and more immediate changes in the effective supply of physicians result from changing the behavior of health professionals already in the workforce, for example, by increasing the number of hours worked or delaying retirement rates (Cecil G. Sheps Center for Health Services Research 2014). On the demand side, model scenarios allow policymakers to compare the effects that different demographic and policy changes will have on the use of healthcare services. For example, scenarios show that demographic shifts such as the aging of the population have a much bigger and longer-term effect (e.g., increase) on healthcare utilization than macro policy changes such as insurance expansions (Cecil G. Sheps Center for Health Services Research 2014; Spetz 2014).

Healthcare workforce models are useful, but they are not perfect predictors of the future healthcare system. Models are based on data and assumptions derived from current patterns of healthcare delivery. Even if the model includes scenarios for plausible changes that might occur in the healthcare system, they cannot account for unexpected outcomes. For example, policymakers who have expanded health insurance coverage to the uninsured hope that it will, among other things, shift how and where patients seek healthcare services. In theory, patients who have insurance should seek more primary and preventative care delivered in physician offices instead of accessing their care through more expensive emergency departments. However, when Oregon expanded Medicaid coverage to low-income, previously uninsured patients, the newly insured individuals increased their use of emergency rooms (Taubman et al. 2014).

Workforce models are a simplification of reality. Powell and Baker (2009, 1) define modeling as the "process of creating a simplified representation of reality and working with this representation in order to understand or control some aspect of the world." Healthcare workforce modeling uses simplifying assumptions and data to project trends about whether the supply of healthcare workers for a defined geographic area will be adequate to meet the demand for healthcare services in 5, 10, 15, or more years. The next section of this chapter describes the basic methods for developing supply and demand projections.

Estimating the Supply of Healthcare Workers

Exhibit 13.2 outlines the basic approach to modeling the current and future supply of healthcare workers.[1] The process starts by developing an inventory of the current workforce and then examines inflows and outflows of workers to estimate the size of the future workforce.

Current Workforce

An estimate of what healthcare workforce needs might be in the future first requires a baseline assessment of the current workforce. A good inventory includes the age distribution of the workforce so that retirements can be planned for and workers replaced. The distribution of health professionals by specialty, geography, and employment setting is also needed to understand the type of services provided in different areas. A key challenge in this first step is determining the unit of geography for the analysis, and the geography selected depends heavily on data availability. The smaller the unit of geography, the harder it is to find reliable data. While the number of nurses in the US workforce, and even the number in a particular state, might be known, it is often hard to get the number of nurses in a particular county or region that are actively providing patient care and to determine in what settings they

EXHIBIT 13.2
Healthcare
Workforce
Supply Inflows
and Outflows

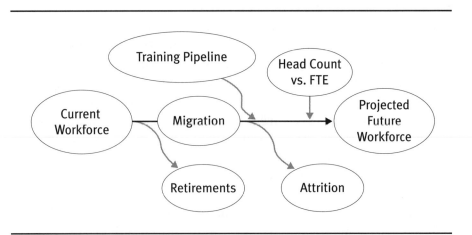

Note: FTE = full-time equivalent.

are working. The unit of geography also depends on the catchment area for services: Do patients receive care in the county where they live, or do they travel to another county? The catchment area might depend on the type of healthcare services for which the workforce plan is being developed. Primary care services are often available locally, but patients needing more specialized heart or cancer care might need to travel to a regional hospital or center of excellence.

Head Count Versus Full-Time Equivalent

The supply of healthcare workers can be measured in two ways: as a head count of the number of individuals in practice or by the amount of time they spend delivering direct patient care. Measuring full-time equivalent (FTE) hours in direct patient care is a more accurate reflection of effective workforce supply than a simple head count is. Practitioners may, for many reasons and over different parts of their careers, decide to work more or fewer hours. From a modeling perspective, the fact that not all practitioners work what would be considered full-time means that meeting the demand for healthcare services will require more practitioners than indicated by a simple head count. Models must also account for the fact that hours worked vary by age and by gender. Exhibit 13.3 shows that male physicians tend to work more hours than female physicians at all ages and especially during the childbearing years but that both male and female physicians begin to reduce their hours in their mid-50s. Hours in patient care also vary by specialty. The data in Exhibit 13.3 also reflect that female physicians are more likely to select specialties (e.g., pediatrics, family medicine) in which physicians work fewer hours than in male-dominated specialties (e.g., orthopedic surgery, neurosurgery), in which physicians tend to work more hours.

Training Pipeline

Projecting the future growth in supply depends on how many new workers will enter the workforce and how this number is likely to change in the future. For example, the numbers of graduates from nurse practitioner (NP) and physician assistant (PA) programs have seen rapid growth in the United States in the last decade. In 2001, NP programs graduated 7,261 students, but by 2013 this number had jumped 121 percent to 16,031. Similarly, the number of graduates from pharmacy school increased 75 percent from 7,260 graduates in 2000 to 12,719 in 2012. These dramatic increases have some workforce analysts wondering if education programs have expanded too rapidly—and not just for NPs, PAs, and pharmacists (Salsberg 2014). Similar trends are evident in the number of graduates from registered nurse programs. If these trends continue, the nation may soon have an oversupply of some types of providers, but much will depend on how the healthcare system

EXHIBIT 13.3

Average Weekly
Hours Worked
in Patient Care
by Male and
Female
Physicians in
North Carolina,
2011

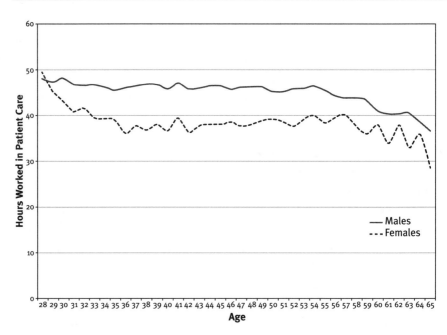

EXHIBIT 13.3
Average Weekly Hours Worked in Patient Care by Male and Female Physicians in North Carolina, 2011

Source: North Carolina Health Professions Data System, Cecil G. Sheps Center for Health Services Research, University of North Carolina at Chapel Hill.

reorganizes care and changes payment incentives to reward team-based models of care that incorporate more NPs, PAs, pharmacists, registered nurses, and other healthcare providers into patient care models.

Attrition

Because of the relatively steady and large number of workers retiring each year from the workforce, projections are highly sensitive to the assumptions made about retirement. The challenge is that retirement ages are constantly shifting, and data on when practitioners actually exit the workforce are limited. Past retirement rates tell us only about the behavior of past generations, which may not reflect the workforce behavior of younger generations. Analysts sometimes try to account for this potential difference by asking about the retirement plans of younger generations still in the workforce. But practitioners completing such surveys tend to report that they will retire at an earlier age than they actually do (Konrad 2014).

Retirement rates are also highly dependent on the economy. Practitioners often delay retirement when the economy is weak because their spouse is unemployed or because they want to allow their retirement savings plans to recover. Another complicating factor is the phenomenon of serial retirement, in which practitioners retire from their full-time job but return to work part-time. Serial retirement is an increasing issue for baby boomers, who face longer lifespans, rising healthcare costs, and shrinking pension plans. To deal with the uncertainty around retirement, it is helpful to model the future under at least three different sets of assumptions: The workforce will retire at the same rate as previous generations, the workforce will retire at later ages than previous generations, and the workforce will retire at earlier ages than previous generations.

While most workforce attrition comes from retirement, workers also drop out of the workforce for other reasons, including death and time taken off to raise children, to care for elderly family members, or to pursue additional training. Sometimes this break becomes permanent, but many return to the workforce. Like retirement decisions, workforce retention rates are often cyclical with the economy. For example, nurses tend to stay in the workforce during economic downturns, presumably to offset a decline in earnings by their spouses (Staiger, Auerbach, and Buerhaus 2012). Nurse workforce retention rates have also been shown to be sensitive to changes in wages. As wages increase, workforce participation rates increase (Buerhaus, Auerbach, and Staiger 2007). Modeling attrition from the workforce due to economic factors is difficult because economic conditions cannot be anticipated. To overcome this difficulty, analysts often assume an average attrition rate that evens out boom and bust cycles over the projection period.

Developing Subnational Projections and Accounting for Migration

One of the critiques of past workforce models is that they have only provided projections at the national level, yet the situation in Idaho may look very different than that in New York. New York trains more physicians than Idaho. Idaho has more family physicians per capita, but New York has more cardiologists per capita (Cecil G. Sheps Center for Health Services Research 2014). This variation is likely due to differences in the healthcare needs of the populations in the two states (Centers for Disease Control and Prevention 2012). But even if patient needs were the same in the two places, variation would still exist in how the workforce is configured. This variation stems from differences in the availability of various types of providers and because models of care differ. Different types of healthcare workers in different specialties or different professions can meet the same types of healthcare needs. This concept, known as *plasticity*, is explained in greater detail later in this chapter, in the section that discusses how supply and demand models come together to estimate workforce needs.

Models must also account for the migration of health professionals between different places. Like the general population, the healthcare workforce is mobile, so workforce models need to be able to account for the migration of health professionals from one geographic location to another.

About 20 percent of the active employed physician workforce will relocate to another county within a five-year period, with the average move being 146 miles. Older, male, and urban physicians are less likely to move. Surgeons and primary care physicians are less likely to move relative to those in other specialties (Ricketts 2013). When they do move, surgeons are more likely to move to places with other surgeons and to areas with a better overall economic environment (Ricketts 2010). By contrast, nurses are less mobile: 52.5 percent work within 40 miles of where they attended high school (Kovner, Corcoran, and Brewer 2011). Health professionals with higher levels of education and more specialized training (physicians) are more likely to move than are health professionals graduating from a local community college (ultrasound technicians) or those who might enter the workforce directly after high school (medical assistants).

Estimating the Demand for Healthcare Services

For the purpose of estimating the amount of care patients will require in the future, it is important to clarify that the demand for healthcare services is different than patients' need for or utilization of care. To determine what, and how many, services are *needed* to address the population's burden of illness is a subjective and difficult process that requires asking health professionals how many and which types of healthcare services patients should have and when they should have them. However, while fully meeting patients' needs for care might be ideal, many patients may have unmet needs because they do not have insurance, because they do not see the importance of preventative and primary care, or because other care-seeking barriers exist. Therefore, workforce planners more often try to measure the demand for healthcare services, or the healthcare services patients are willing to pay for at different prices. When patients are insured, the demand for healthcare closely approximates the actual utilization of healthcare services observed in the market. This situation makes measuring demand easier and more practical than measuring need. The remainder of this section focuses on the demand for healthcare services, recognizing that the demand may not reflect patients' actual utilization or need for care.

Estimating demand is complex, and the main drivers are (1) demography; (2) epidemiology; (3) healthcare delivery models, including technology; and (4) economic factors.

Demography
The demographic characteristics of the population are an important predictor of patients' demand for care. As shown in Exhibit 13.4, the overall utilization

of physician, PA, and NP services for primary care is highest among people aged 0–5 years, is relatively low among people aged 6–44 years, and then increases with age. Not surprisingly, people aged 0–5 years see more pediatricians, while the elderly, who have more comorbidities such as diabetes and high blood pressure, see more internal medicine physicians and family practitioners. Demand models use the type of information in Exhibit 13.4 to project how changes in the size, age, race/ethnicity, and gender of the population will affect future use of healthcare services and, in turn, the demand for different types of healthcare providers.

Epidemiology

Healthcare demand models must also take into account the prevalence of risk factors including obesity, smoking, diabetes, hypertension, and other factors known to increase the utilization of healthcare services. Healthcare workforce projections try to account for how changes that might occur in the distribution of these risk factors among the population will affect the future demand for healthcare services. Estimating these rates can be difficult because it is hard to determine how the rising prevalence of some conditions (e.g., increased chronic disease among the elderly) might be offset by reduction in others (e.g., declining smoking rates).

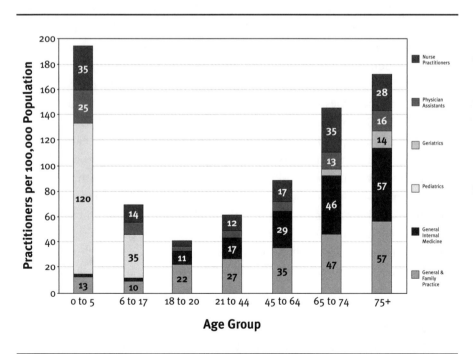

EXHIBIT 13.4
Estimated Use of Primary Care Practitioners (Full-Time Equivalents) per 100,000 Persons Within Each Age Group, 2010

Source: US Department of Health and Human Services, Health Resources and Services Administration (2013). Colors and legend placement have been modified slightly to be more readable in black and white.

Healthcare Delivery Models

How healthcare is organized and delivered is a key driver of demand. In different employment settings and geographies, work may be divided among healthcare professionals in different ways. Some organizations make greater use of physicians to deliver care, while other organizations rely more on NPs, PAs, and other nonphysician clinicians in team-based models of care. Skill-mix configurations also differ among employment settings. Hospitals make greater use of specialists, and outpatient settings tend to contain more generalists, such as family physicians, pediatricians, and other primary care providers.

Much attention has been paid to new and emerging models of healthcare designed to lower costs and improve the quality of healthcare. Public and private healthcare payers nationwide are moving toward patient-centered medical home (PCMH) models that emphasize primary and preventative care as the cornerstone of the US healthcare system. PCMHs strive to reorganize care to be more patient centered, accessible, coordinated, and comprehensive. Preliminary evidence indicates that PCMH practices have different workforce configurations than non-PCMH practices (Peikes et al. 2014). Compared to non-PCMH practices, PCMH practices are more likely to employ care managers and care coordinators (41.7 percent of PCMH practices compared to 11.6 percent of non-PCMH practices), pharmacists (9.3 percent vs. 5.5 percent), social workers (7.4 percent vs. 3.4 percent), and nutritionists (5.9 percent vs. 2.7 percent). One challenge facing workforce planners is determining if, and how, the widespread adoption of PCMHs, accountable care organizations, and integrated delivery systems will affect the numbers and types of healthcare providers needed in the future (Auerbach et al. 2013; Bodenheimer and Smith 2013; Cooper 2013; Everett et al. 2013; Smith, Bates, and Bodenheimer 2013). Much of this research points to the potential of team-based models of care to result in a more efficient and effective distribution of tasks among health professionals, with nonphysician clinicians working to the "top of their license" and physicians taking on only more complex tasks that require their advanced training and skills. The degree to which this result will occur remains unclear because of the way that health professionals are paid and regulated but also because of "turf protection" by health professionals who are unwilling to delegate the tasks that they have traditionally performed.

Economic Factors

Household income and health insurance coverage are related factors that drive healthcare use. Nonelderly individuals who live in higher-income households are more likely to have health insurance coverage, and having health insurance coverage increases the use of healthcare services. In 2012, approximately one-third of individuals in households with annual incomes below $20,000 were uninsured, compared to just 8 percent of individuals in households with annual incomes above $40,000 (Kaiser Commission on Medicaid and the Uninsured 2013). Yet even when low-income individuals have health insurance coverage, they have trouble paying for medical expenses that their insurer will not cover. As a result, low-income individuals with health insurance coverage may postpone or skip using healthcare services as a result of concerns about cost (Schoen et al. 2014). In 2012, 72 percent of individuals in households with annual incomes below $40,000—but only 38 percent of individuals in households with annual incomes above $90,000—put off using healthcare because of the cost of those services (Kaiser Family Foundation 2012).

While individuals with insurance use healthcare services at higher rates than uninsured individuals, the evidence is mixed about whether health insurance coverage causes individuals to seek more care in all healthcare settings. Evidence from Oregon, where previously uninsured adults were randomly assigned to Medicaid coverage through a lottery system, suggests that newly Medicaid-covered enrollees were more likely to use outpatient, inpatient, and emergency department services compared to their uninsured peers (Finkelstein et al. 2012; Taubman et al. 2014). By contrast, the near-universal expansion of health insurance coverage in Massachusetts in 2006 increased the use of ambulatory care according to some research (Miller 2012b) but had no change (Kolstad and Kowalski 2012; Miller 2012b) or resulted in lower rates of hospital and emergency department visits in other studies (Miller 2012a).

Dealing with Uncertainty in Projections

Determining the timeline for a projection is important. Projections become more uncertain the further the model projects into the future. This uncertainty is due to both cyclical factors (e.g., economic downturns) and structural factors (e.g., changes in payment policy or technology) that can dramatically shift the outcome of the projection. Known as "black swans" (Taleb 2010), these events are changes that are unexpected yet can significantly affect the supply or demand for healthcare workers. One way to conceptualize the amount of uncertainty associated with workforce projections is to think of them as analogous to a hurricane forecast (Exhibit 13.5). The exact trajectory of a hurricane is unknown and depends on factors such as water temperature and winds, the effects of which are able to be more precisely determined the closer the hurricane is to landfall. For this reason, workforce projections sometimes contain confidence intervals, which become broader further into the future.

Changes in technology and clinical practice innovations are constantly changing the demand for healthcare services and changing the skill sets

EXHIBIT 13.5
Increasing
Uncertainty
of Estimates
Further into the
Future

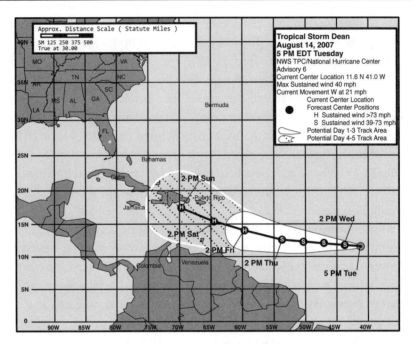

Hurricane Forecast

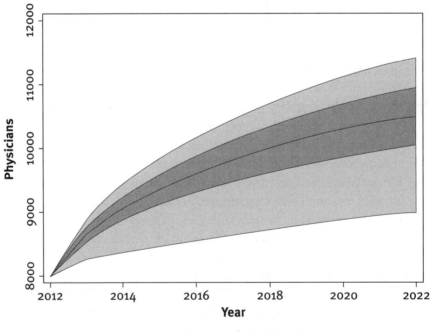

Physician Supply Forecast

Source: Upper image courtesy of the National Oceanic and Atmospheric Administration (adapted for clarity).

needed to provide services. For example, laparoscopic surgery has reduced the need for large incisions for gallbladder, urologic, orthopedic, abdominal, and other surgeries, resulting in quicker, less painful operations that can be done on an outpatient rather than inpatient basis. The use of stents to restore blood flow in blocked arteries has reduced the demand for cardiothoracic surgeons to perform coronary artery bypass surgeries. The emergence of new imaging technologies, such as computed tomography (CT) and magnetic resonance imaging (MRI), has dramatically changed the work of radiologists. Before CT and MRI technology, radiologists made assessments from a single film image, which was difficult and more susceptible to misdiagnoses. The use of CTs and MRIs has enabled radiologists to make assessments based on three-dimensional images that are generated by combining hundreds of different views of the patient. Therefore, the technological innovation has improved diagnosis but now requires more work to arrive at that diagnosis. The electronic health record (EHR) is yet another technological innovation that has altered healthcare delivery and organization in large and small organizations alike. EHRs are used for billing, ordering, and documentation, and they house large amounts of data about patients. Physicians and other professionals need informatics skills to use these data to better understand care delivery patterns and improve population health. The adoption of EHRs has also created a new healthcare professional—the scribe—an unlicensed professional who helps input patient data into EHRs (American Health Information Management Association 2012).

Beyond the adoption of EHRs, fundamental changes to healthcare delivery that are underway will change the types of care patients receive, the kinds of providers needed, and the locations where healthcare services are delivered. These changes are motivated by a desire to control rising healthcare costs while improving patients' experience of care. Both healthcare cost containment and healthcare delivery reform likely will magnify the current trend of shifting patient care from expensive hospital to less expensive outpatient settings.

The move toward patient-centered care is one example of a type of healthcare delivery reform that could change healthcare roles and healthcare, complicating workforce projections. Patient-centered care—a term used to describe care in which a patient actively participates (Epstein and Street 2011; Rickert 2012)—has created the need to help patients and their families navigate the complexities of the healthcare system. Sometimes physicians, nurses, and existing health professionals take on this function, but increasingly healthcare organizations are creating new jobs for care coordinators, patient navigators, care managers, patient educators, and health coaches. When these new roles are included in healthcare delivery interventions, they have the potential to reduce patient demand for expensive hospital and emergency department care. For example, emerging evidence suggests that interventions to provide transitional care for patients newly discharged from the hospital reduce hospital readmissions, lower healthcare costs (Allen et al. 2014; Naylor et al. 2011), and improve patient satisfaction with care (Allen et al. 2014). Despite the potential of patient-centered reforms such as transitional care, such reforms have not yet been widely implemented, so the broad impact of these reforms on healthcare workforce supply and demand is challenging to estimate.

Healthcare workforce planning is a complicated task that is fraught with uncertainties and challenges. Issuing a hurricane forecast and then not updating the public about how the forecast has changed is unthinkable, yet workforce projections are often released and then not updated. The rapid pace of health system change, the emergence of new technology, and the changing demographics of the population and the physician workforce require that supply and demand projections be reviewed at least annually. The review should include a "backcast" that attempts to compare what actually happened and what was projected to understand why the forecast was wrong and how future forecasts might be improved. But more importantly, stakeholders need to be made aware that the forecast has changed so that they can alter plans and policies put in place. For example, if the United States is going to face a surplus of nurse practitioners, pharmacists, and physician assistants, educators may want to ramp down production of new graduates. These changes can then be included in subsequent forecasts so that over- or undercorrections are not made and the supply does not lurch from surplus to shortage and back again.

Matching Supply to Demand

After estimating the supply and demand for healthcare workers, the next step is to use this information to determine how many healthcare workers will be needed in the future. This step requires careful consideration of what is affordable and what is likely to happen to supply and demand under different scenarios. Workforce planners use different methods to determine if supply will be adequate to meet demand, including population-based and benchmarking approaches.

Population-based approaches plan by using normative ratios of providers to population. These ratios are not always generated from epidemiological analysis or careful study of productivity and utilization. Often they are based on observations of current and past ratios. For example, in the United States, the process to designate a location as a Health Professional Shortage Area views a ratio of one FTE primary care physician for every 3,500 people as an indicator of a severe level of need. A ratio of one physician to 3,000 people accompanied by elevated population-risk indicators, such as high infant mortality and a high proportion of people older than 65 years, in a rational service area also signals high need, making the area or population eligible for a shortage designation.

Many ratios have been suggested as indicative of an "ideal" or "adequate" ratio of providers to population, but these ratios vary considerably. The wide variation in ratios points to inherent weaknesses in population-based approaches. Variability can be the result of differences in assumptions concerning the productivity of practitioners, differences in the needs for services in the population, and even miscalculations caused by poor data about how many physicians are in active practice in the workforce. Nevertheless, analysts and planners persist in using ratios as standard indicators of desired staffing or as guides to their studies of professional supply.

Population approaches produce silo-based estimates of the numbers of different health professionals needed for specific health professional groups and specialties. These types of projections are popularly expressed as needs such as "45,000 primary care physicians and 46,000 surgeons and specialists by 2020" (*New York Times* 2014). A new approach relies on the concept of plasticity. The term *plasticity* describes the idea that multiple configurations of healthcare providers are able to meet a community's use of healthcare services because health professionals in different professions and different specialties have overlapping scopes of service provision (Holmes et al. 2013). For example, multiple physician specialties—such as cardiologists, family physicians, and internists—manage circulatory conditions. Calculating plasticity requires matching services to the types of healthcare professionals—such as physicians of different specialties—who provide those services. Such data allow the analyst to develop a matrix that looks like a more complex version of Exhibit 13.6.

The rows in Exhibit 13.6 show the types of patient visits handled in a given specialty, while the columns show how the demand for different types of healthcare services are met by different specialties. For example, the cell in the last row and second column shows that while 26 percent of all outpatient circulatory visits are to internists, 54 percent of all internal medicine visits in the outpatient setting are related to circulatory conditions. To calculate whether a specific geographic area has an adequate healthcare professional supply to meet healthcare demand, one has to "translate" whether the local healthcare professional supply is sufficient to meet demand using the matrix. If healthcare professional capacity to deliver certain services is equivalent to local demand for those services, then demand and capacity are in balance in that geographic area. If demand exceeds capacity, a shortage exists, and if capacity exceeds demand, a surplus exists. Relative capacity can be calculated at both the state and substate levels for multiple types of services. Therefore,

EXHIBIT 13.6
Sample
Plasticity
Matrix

Healthcare Services Demand (ambulatory visits)

Physician Specialties	Cancer Visits	Circulatory Visits	Respiratory Visits	Pregnancy and Childbirth Visits
Cardiology	145,802	34% 23,684,068	593,326	898
Dermatology	11,913,249	<1% 154,326	187,179	16,234
Family medicine	1,772,218	38% 26,485,370	19,943,025	1,264,0030
Obstetrics/ gynecology	2,575,715	1% 496,124	17,533	29,821,750
Internal medicine	1,545,030 4%	26% 18,097,752 54%	5,496,049 40%	32,315 3%

relative capacity at a higher geographic level—for example, at the state level—will mask variations in relative capacity within smaller geographic units, such as at the county level. Also, relative capacity in any geographic area is likely to differ for different service types.

Real-World Applications

Shrinking budgets mean that policymakers and health system executives are facing cost pressures to reconfigure the workforce. Payment and new care delivery reforms are creating new roles for healthcare professionals. Increasing evidence points to "vertical" integration (e.g., shifting tasks from physicians to nurse practitioners and physician assistants) and "horizontal" integration (e.g., shifting work from specialists to generalist practitioners). The most advanced projection models are beginning to use plasticity methods to project the needs for different configurations of providers to meet patients' need for care. These models examine how tasks can be reallocated within a healthcare team to allow maximal use of everyone's skills.

HR management for healthcare workers is more complex than in other industries because of barriers to enter the healthcare workforce in the form of long training periods and regulatory limitations on who can do what to the patient. Given these constraints, what can organizations do to address workforce imbalances?

As Exhibit 13.7 indicates, healthcare workforce planners at the organizational level have several options for dealing with healthcare shortages or surpluses. If they face a shortage, they can hire additional workers, although this approach may be challenging if the organization is competing with other organizations for these same workers. If they are unable to hire new workers, they might try to increase the number of hours the existing workforce spends providing patient care. This approach could be accomplished by providing financial incentives, such as overtime pay or salary increases, to workers who work longer hours. Or they can increase the amount of time that the healthcare workforce spends in patient care by decreasing the amount of time workers spend on non–patient care tasks, such as administration.

Another option for reducing healthcare workforce shortages at the organizational level is to use financial and nonfinancial incentives to try to reduce the rate at which workers leave the organization. For example, a salary increase may convince some workers to delay retirement. When facing shortages of workers with specific types of skills, organizations can opt not only to hire workers from outside the organization but also to develop the skills of workers already within the organization. Other chapters in this book address in more detail many of these strategies, including retention, internal promotions, and training.

In the case of persistent oversupply of healthcare workers, reducing the number of employees or the number of hours that employees work may be inevitable. However, in the short term, healthcare workforce planners may be able to reduce oversupply by retraining workers to fill different roles within the organization or by moving workers to different settings or locations within that organization. For example, a health system could redeploy employees from an oversupplied hospital to an undersupplied clinic in a different location.

Healthcare Workforce Condition	Organizational Options
Shortage	• Hire new workers • Increase the amount of time that workers provide patient care • Retain workers who would have otherwise retired or left the organization • Develop skills of workers within organization
Surplus	• Lay off workers • Retrain existing workers to fill new roles • Redeploy workers to different settings or to different roles

EXHIBIT 13.7
Organizational Options for Healthcare Workforce Shortages and Surpluses

Summary

As this chapter's introduction emphasized, healthcare workforce shortages and surpluses at an organization level are often related to shortages and surpluses at local and national levels. Therefore, one organizational strategy to prevent shortages or surpluses is to participate in healthcare workforce policy debates at the local, state, and national levels. The healthcare workforce modeling techniques described in this chapter can help organizations not only conduct healthcare workforce planning but also understand how they might contribute to healthcare workforce policy development.

Discussion Questions

1. Assume that you work for the US Department of Health and Human Services (DHHS). DHHS is considering ways to increase the number of dentists participating in the National Health Service Corps loan repayment assistance program. Through this program, healthcare workers receive loan repayment assistance in exchange for practicing in areas that the US government designates as Health Professional Shortage Areas. How could a health workforce model help guide decision making on this potential change to the loan repayment program? What kinds of supply data might you gather for your model of dentist supply? In this case, at what geographic level would you model dentist supply?

2. Assume that you are a planner within a large healthcare system in a state that is participating in the Affordable Care Act's expansion of Medicaid coverage. You want to project the demand for healthcare services over the next ten years in the counties in which your healthcare system operates. What data will you need to model demand for healthcare services? Assume that the model you produce projects a significant increase in demand for ambulatory care visits over the next ten years. How should the healthcare system respond to these projections?

3. The nursing school at a public university is considering increasing the class size of its nurse practitioner (NP) program to address shortages in primary care capacity in certain regions of your state. How could you use healthcare workforce modeling to show whether increasing the enrollment within the NP program at the university will have the intended effect? Taking into consideration the factors that affect healthcare workforce supply, why might increasing NP class size at the university *not* reduce the primary care capacity shortages within your state? (Hint: Use Exhibit 13.2 to think about factors that could affect the future supply of NPs.)

4. What types of scenarios could you develop to model how health workforce supply will respond to changes in the economy? What factors in Exhibit 13.2

are likely to be affected and in what direction?

5. Why might the local supply of health professions look very different than state or national supply? Which types of health professionals would you expect to see in most counties, and which types of health professionals would you see clustered in certain regions of each state?

6. Assume you are an HR manager in a large hospital facing a shortage of nurses. What measures might you take to address the shortfall?

7. How will the aging of the population affect both the supply of health professionals and the demand for healthcare services?

8. The healthcare system at which you work is considering implementing a medical home model within the primary care practices that it owns. How could you use scenarios to model the effect that the implementation of medical homes will have on each of the following?

   a. The demand for healthcare services among patients who visit the healthcare system's primary care practices

   b. The system's healthcare workforce— in terms of both the number of workers and the types of workers— needed to support the medical home model in the primary care practices

Experiential Exercise

The objective of this exercise is to use workforce data to develop a supply model for the physician workforce in the United States.[2] This exercise uses a simple Microsoft Excel model. Double-clicking on cells within the Excel spreadsheet will reveal the formulas used to fill in those cells. Students may access the live spreadsheet model at ache.org/books/HRHealthcare4.

Step 1: Current Workforce
1. Open the template Excel model.
2. Note the head count and FTE of the current physician workforce in cells E6 and E7. What are some reasons that the FTE is lower than the head count?
3. The FTE/head count ratio is 0.6, which means that the effective number of physicians delivering care is about

60 percent of the head count. Why is this important to know? Do you expect male or female physicians to work more hours? Which other factors might affect the FTE/head count ratio?

Step 2: Retirees and Leavers
4. In cells E12 through E20, enter the age distribution of the workforce shown in Exhibit 13.8.
5. The model will automatically generate an age distribution in cells L12 through L41.
6. Enter a typical retirement age of 68 into cell H13.
7. The model will automatically generate an annual retirement estimate in cells O12 through O29.

EXHIBIT 13.8
Age Distribution of the Workforce

All Ages	700,000
< 35	73,224
35 to 39	96,316
40 to 44	102,258
45 to 49	99,715
50 to 54	103,640
55 to 59	95,285
60 to 64	65,373
65 & over	64,189

Step 3: Training Pipeline

8. After medical school, physicians enter a residency training program. Once these individuals complete residency training, they become part of the physician workforce. The table in Exhibit 13.9 shows the number of residents entering training in each year in the model.

EXHIBIT 13.9
Number of Residents Entering Training

Year	Number
2014	25,000
2015	25,000
2016	25,000
2017	25,000

This modeling exercise makes the following assumptions about the residency training pipeline:

- Residents have a 10 percent attrition rate—that is, 10 percent of residents who begin residency programs do not complete their programs and therefore do not enter the physician workforce.
- The number of trainees entering residency remains unchanged between 2014 and 2031.

Using these data and assumptions about attrition and residency supply, populate the residency training pipeline in cells D46 through D63 with the number of residents completing training in each year. How many residents complete training in 2020?

Step 4: FTE/Head Count Participation

9. Cells D69 through E81 contain data on physician head counts and FTEs between 2001 and 2013.
10. Cells F69 through F81 show the physician FTE/head count ratio for the years 2001 through 2013.
11. Cells F82 through F99 show the estimated physician FTE/head count ratio for the years 2014 through 2031. (In this simple model, the FTE/head count ratio for these years is calculated using the Excel TREND function.)

Step 5: Forecast

12. The model uses Excel's SUM function to calculate the annual head count forecast for physicians in cells D115 through D132. The model calculates each year's estimated physician head count by subtracting retirements and adding the number of new

residents entering the workforce to the previous year's estimated physician head count.

13. The model calculates annual physician FTE forecasts using the FTE/head count ratio. Cells E115 through E132 show the FTE forecasts.

14. The preceding steps produce a line graph similar to the one in Exhibit 13.10.

If you do not get the same display, unhide the "Possible Solution" worksheet to see how this forecast can be created.[3]

Step 6: Evaluation

15. Does this forecast seem reasonable to you? How might you improve it?

16. What happens to the head count and FTE forecasts if all physicians retire at the age of 65?

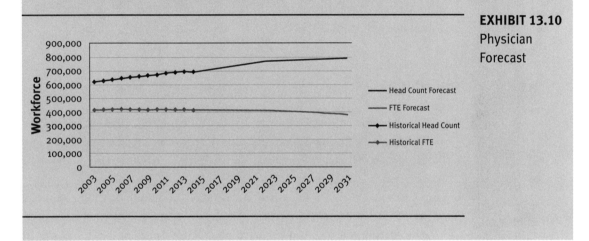

EXHIBIT 13.10
Physician
Forecast

Notes

1. Exhibit 13.2 is a simplified workforce supply model that does not include all factors. One such factor, the in-migration of foreign-trained health professionals to fill supply gaps, can be significant in some professions and can accelerate in response to shortages or decelerate in response to downturns in the economy. For example, the number of foreign-trained registered nurses who entered the US workforce increased prior to the 2008 recession. With the subsequent increase in US nursing school graduates, the percentage of nurses that are foreign trained is declining (Budden et al. 2013). The authors of this chapter are indebted to Katie Gaul, research associate at the Cecil G. Sheps Center for Health Services Research at the University of North Carolina, for her assistance in designing the exhibits.

2. The authors would like to acknowledge Andy Knapton, director of Strategic Modelling Analysis & Planning (SMAP) Ltd. in the United Kingdom, for his substantial contributions and suggestions to improve this chapter. We drew on his significant expertise in workforce modeling and adapted the experiential exercise from one he uses when teaching workforce planning in the United Kingdom.

3. See Microsoft Office support for instructions on how to unhide a worksheet in Microsoft Excel 2013: http://office.microsoft.com/en-us/excel-help/unhide-sheet-is-under-home-hide-unhide-HT103308166.aspx?CTT=1. For information on how to unhide a worksheet in Microsoft Excel for Mac 2011, see "Show or Hide Sheets" on the Microsoft website at https://support.office.com/en-us/article/Show-or-hide-sheets-01437b75-ac7a-4267-b365-f8f76da79cc8.

References

Allen, J., A. M. Hutchinson, R. Brown, and P. M. Livingston. 2014. "Quality Care Outcomes Following Transitional Care Interventions for Older People from Hospital to Home: A Systematic Review." *BMC Health Services Research* 14 (1): 346.

Altarum Institute. 2014. "Anticipated Acceleration in Health Spending Appears to Be Delayed." *Spending Brief.* Published August 7. www.altarum.org/sites/default/files/uploaded-related-files/CSHS-Spending-Brief_August%202014.pdf.

American Health Information Management Association. 2012. "Using Medical Scribes in a Physician Practice." *Journal of AHIMA* 83 (11): 64–69 [expanded online version]. Accessed January 27, 2015. http://library.ahima.org/xpedio/groups/public/documents/ahima/bok1_049807.hcsp?dDocName=bok1_049807.

Antos, J., J. Bertko, M. Chernew, D. Cutler, D. Goldman, M. McClellan, E. McGlynn, M. Pauly, L. Schaeffer, and S. Shortell. 2009. "Bending the Curve: Effective Steps to Address Long-Term Healthcare Spending Growth." *American Journal of Managed Care* 15 (10): 676–80.

Auerbach, D. I., P. G. Chen, M. W. Friedberg, R. Reid, C. Lau, P. I. Buerhaus, and A. Mehrotra. 2013. "Nurse-Managed Health Centers and Patient-Centered Medical Homes Could Mitigate Expected Primary Care Physician Shortage." *Health Affairs* 32 (11): 1933–41.

Berwick, D. M., T. W. Nolan, and J. Whittington. 2008. "The Triple Aim: Care, Health, and Cost." *Health Affairs* 27 (3): 759–69.

Bodenheimer, T. S., and M. D. Smith. 2013. "Primary Care: Proposed Solutions to the Physician Shortage Without Training More Physicians." *Health Affairs* 32 (11): 1881–86.

Budden, J. S., E. H. Zhong, P. Moulton, and J. P. Cimiotti. 2013. "Highlights of the National Workforce Survey of Registered Nurses." *Journal of Nursing Regulation* 4 (2): 5–14.

Buerhaus, P. I., D. I. Auerbach, and D. O. Staiger. 2007. "Recent Trends in the Registered Nurse Labor Market in the U.S.: Short-Run Swings on Top of Long-Term Trends." *Nursing Economic$* 25 (2): 59–66.

Bureau of Labor Statistics. 2014. "Health Care and Social Assistance: NAICS 62." Data extracted August 8. www.bls.gov/iag/tgs/iag62.htm.

———. 2013. "Table 1.2: Employment by Detailed Occupation, 2012 and Projected 2022." Last modified December 19. www.bls.gov/emp/ep_table_102.htm.

Cecil G. Sheps Center for Health Services Research. 2014. "FutureDocs Forecasting Tool." Accessed October 9. www2.shepscenter.unc.edu/workforce/model.php.

Centers for Disease Control and Prevention. 2012. "Chronic Disease Indicators: United States Compared with Idaho, New York." Last reviewed February. http://apps.nccd.cdc.gov/cdi/SearchResults.aspx?IndicatorIds=0,26,1,33,37,2,15,3,4,6,5,9,35,11,22,64,29,7,8,126,76,73,59,57,45,51,63,70,58,53,47,41,65,69,72,75,48,42,23,18,27,25,13,20,62,56,52,46,40,78,68,28,39,32,12,61,34,31,24,19,38,127,128,129,130,131,132,133,134,36,50,44,136,135,55,16,122,123,124,54,49,10,14,74,77,43,30,17,21,60,&StateIds=46,13,33&StateNames=United%20States,Idaho,New%20York&FromPage=HomePage.

Centers for Medicare & Medicaid Services. 2014. *National Health Expenditures; Aggregate and Per Capita Amounts, Annual Percent Change and Percent Distribution: Selected Calendar Years 1960–2012*. Published January. www.cms.gov/Research-Statistics-Data-and-Systems/Statistics-Trends-and-Reports/NationalHealthExpendData/Downloads/tables.pdf.

Cooper, R. A. 2013. "Unraveling the Physician Supply Dilemma." *Journal of the American Medical Association* 310 (18): 1931–32.

Cooper, R. A., T. E. Getzen, and P. Laud. 2003. "Economic Expansion Is a Major Determinant of Physician Supply and Utilization." *Health Services Research* 38 (2): 675–96.

Dranove, D., C. Garthwaite, and C. Ody. 2014. "Health Spending Slowdown Is Mostly Due to Economic Factors, Not Structural Change in the Health Care Sector." *Health Affairs* 33 (8): 1399–1406.

Epstein, R. M., and R. L. Street Jr. 2011. "The Values and Value of Patient-Centered Care." *Annals of Family Medicine* 9 (2): 100–103.

Everett, C., C. Thorpe, M. Palta, P. Carayon, C. Bartels, and M. A. Smith. 2013. "Physician Assistants and Nurse Practitioners Perform Effective Roles on Teams Caring for Medicare Patients with Diabetes." *Health Affairs* 32 (11): 1942–48.

Finkelstein, A., S. Taubman, B. Wright, M. Bernstein, J. Grubera, J. P. Newhouse, H. Allen, K. Baicker, and the Oregon Health Study Group. 2012. "The Oregon Health Insurance Experiment: Evidence from the First Year." *Quarterly Journal of Economics* 127 (3): 1057–1106.

Fraher, E. P., B. Harden, and M. C. Kimball. 2011. "An International Call to Arms to Improve Allied Health Workforce Planning." *Journal of Allied Health* 40 (1): 43–49.

Gallup. 2013. *State of the American Workplace: Employee Engagement Insights for U.S. Business Leaders*. Accessed January 27, 2015. www.gallup.com/strategic consulting/163007/state-american-workplace.aspx.

Holmes, G. M., M. Morrison, D. E. Pathman, and E. Fraher. 2013. "The Contribution of 'Plasticity' to Modeling How a Community's Need for Health Care Services Can Be Met by Different Configurations of Physicians." *Academic Medicine* 88 (12): 1877–82.

Hull, T., P. Taylor, E. Turo, J. Kramer, S. Crocetti, and M. McGuire. 2013. "Implementation of a Training and Structured Skills Program for Medical Assistants in a Primary Care Setting." *Journal of Healthcare Quality* 35 (4): 50–60.

Institute of Medicine. 2011. *The Future of Nursing: Leading Change, Advancing Health*. Washington, DC: National Academies Press.

International Centre for Human Resources in Nursing. 2008. *Health Human Resources Planning*. Published June. www.ordemenfermeiros.pt/relacoesinter nacionais/gri_documentacao/ICN_FolhasInformativas_vsINGePT/FI_ versao_ING/Human_Resources_Planning_Development/2g_FS-Health_ Human_Resources_Planning.pdf.

Kaiser Commission on Medicaid and the Uninsured. 2013. *The Uninsured: A Primer—Key Facts About Health Insurance on the Eve of Coverage Expansions*. Kaiser Family Foundation. Published October 23. http://kff.org/report-section/the-uninsured-a-primer-2013-1-how-did-most-americans-obtain-health-insurance-in-2012/.

Kaiser Family Foundation. 2012. "Health Security Watch." *Kaiser Public Opinion*. Published June. http://kaiserfamilyfoundation.files.wordpress. com/2013/05/8322_hsw-may2012-update.pdf.

Kocher, R., and N. R. Sahni. 2011. "Rethinking Health Care Labor." *New England Journal of Medicine* 365 (15): 1370–72.

Kolstad, J. T., and A. E. Kowalski. 2012. "The Impact of Health Care Reform on Hospital and Preventive Care: Evidence from Massachusetts." *Journal of Public Economics* 96 (11): 909–29.

Konrad, T. R. 2014. Personal correspondence, July.

Kovner, C. T., S. P. Corcoran, and C. S. Brewer. 2011. "The Relative Geographic Immobility of New Registered Nurses Calls for New Strategies to Augment That Workforce." *Health Affairs* 30 (12): 2293–300.

Martin, A. B., M. Hartman, L. Whittle, A. Catlin, and National Health Expenditure Accounts Team. 2014. "National Health Spending in 2012: Rate of Health Spending Growth Remained Low for the Fourth Consecutive Year." *Health Affairs* 33 (1): 67–77.

Medical Group Management Association. 2012. *Physician Compensation and Production Survey: 2012 Report Based on 2011 Data.* Englewood, CO: Medical Group Management Association.

Miller, S. 2012a. "The Effect of Insurance on Emergency Room Visits: An Analysis of the 2006 Massachusetts Health Reform." *Journal of Public Economics* 96 (11): 893–908.

———. 2012b. "The Effect of the Massachusetts Reform on Health Care Utilization." *Inquiry* 49 (4): 317–26.

Naylor, M. D., L. H. Aiken, E. T. Kurtzman, D. M. Olds, and K. B. Hirschman. 2011. "The Care Span: The Importance of Transitional Care in Achieving Health Reform." *Health Affairs* 30 (4): 746–54.

New York Times. 2014. "Bottlenecks in Training Doctors." Published July 19. www.nytimes.com/2014/07/20/opinion/sunday/bottlenecks-in-training-doctors.html.

Peikes, D. N., R. J. Reid, T. J. Day, D. D. Cornwell, S. B. Dale, R. J. Baron, R. S. Brown, and R. J. Shapiro. 2014. "Staffing Patterns of Primary Care Practices in the Comprehensive Primary Care Initiative." *Annals of Family Medicine* 12 (2): 142–49.

Powell, S. G., and K. R. Baker. 2009. *Management Science: The Art of Modeling with Spreadsheets.* Hoboken, NJ: Wiley.

Rickert, J. 2012. "Patient-Centered Care: What It Means and How to Get There." *Health Affairs Blog.* Published January 24. http://healthaffairs.org/blog/2012/01/24/patient-centered-care-what-it-means-and-how-to-get-there/.

Ricketts, T. C. 2013. "The Migration of Physicians and the Local Supply of Practitioners: A Five-Year Comparison." *Academic Medicine* 88 (12): 1913–18.

———. 2010. "The Migration of Surgeons." *Annals of Surgery* 251 (2): 363–67.

Salsberg, E. 2014. "Sharp Increases in the Clinician Pipeline: Opportunity and Danger." *Health Affairs Blog.* Published June 9. http://healthaffairs.org/blog/2014/06/09/sharp-increases-in-the-clinician-pipeline-opportunity-and-danger.

Schoen, C., S. L. Hayes, S. R. Collins, J. Lippa, and D. Radley. 2014. *America's Underinsured: A State-by-State Look at Health Insurance Affordability Prior to the New Coverage Expansions.* Published March. www.commonwealthfund.org/~/media/files/publications/fund-report/2014/mar/1736_schoen_americas_underinsured.pdf.

Smith, M., D. W. Bates, and T. S. Bodenheimer. 2013. "Pharmacists Belong in Accountable Care Organizations and Integrated Care Teams." *Health Affairs* 32 (11): 1963–70.

Spetz, J. 2014. "How Will Health Reform Affect Demand for RNs?" *Nursing Economic$* 32 (1): 42–44.

Staiger, D. O., D. I. Auerbach, and P. I. Buerhaus. 2012. "Registered Nurse Labor Supply and the Recession—Are We in a Bubble?" *New England Journal of Medicine* 366 (16): 1463–65.

Taleb, N. N. 2010. *The Black Swan: The Impact of the Highly Improbable*, second edition. New York: Random House.

Taubman, S. L., H. L. Allen, B. J. Wright, K. Baicker, and A. N. Finkelstein. 2014. "Medicaid Increases Emergency-Department Use: Evidence from Oregon's Health Insurance Experiment." *Science* 343 (6168): 263–68.

US Department of Health and Human Services, Health Resources and Services Administration. 2013. *Projecting the Supply and Demand for Primary Care Practitioners Through 2020*. National Center for Health Workforce Analysis report. Published November. http://bhpr.hrsa.gov/healthworkforce/supplydemand/usworkforce/primarycare/.

14

THE NURSE WORKFORCE IN HEALTHCARE ORGANIZATIONS

Cheryl B. Jones, George H. Pink, and Lindsay T. Munn

Learning Objectives

After completing this chapter, the reader should be able to

- describe the factors that affect nurse workload and staffing;
- discuss the influence of nursing shortages on the deployment of nursing staff and on the ability of a healthcare organization to deliver quality patient care;
- compare and contrast the terms *nurse workload* and *nurse staffing*;
- recognize the types of licensed and unlicensed nursing personnel employed in patient care delivery, and describe how different types of personnel affect nurse workload and staffing decisions;
- identify three reasons for measuring nurse workload;
- explain how an organization's philosophy influences nurse workload and staffing decisions, and be aware of stakeholder perspectives on staffing and workload issues;
- understand how patient classification systems are used in calculating nurse workload, and discuss the strengths and weaknesses of these systems;
- determine the types of information needed to calculate nursing full-time equivalents and the process for acquiring and using this information; and
- address the impact of nurse workload and staffing on nurse stress and burnout and on the quality of patient care.

Introduction

Nurses are a constant in healthcare organizations. They are on the front line and at the point of care, 24 hours a day, seven days a week. They are the most visible faces in these highly complex organizations, where outcomes are critical and services are often provided under difficult and unpredictable conditions. Nurses provide a critical surveillance function, particularly in hospitals, by monitoring care and safeguarding patients; thus, the availability and work of nurses affect the quality and safety of care that patients receive (Needleman and Hassmiller 2009). Nurses are also a primary determinant of patient satisfaction (Kutney-Lee et al. 2009)—an outcome that takes high priority in a highly competitive healthcare environment that has shifted toward value-based purchasing. Clearly, a well-trained, motivated, and appropriately deployed nursing staff has a strong influence on a healthcare organization's ability to provide effective and efficient patient care.

A critical problem for healthcare managers is how best to deploy nursing staff while considering the quality and costs of care. This challenge is complicated by recurring nursing shortages and by the fierce competition for these professionals. During shortages, healthcare managers must often take extraordinary steps (such as closing beds or hiring temporary nurses) to ensure that sufficient numbers of nurses are available to care for patients, and these steps are often taken under constrained budgets and without knowing the specific impact on patient outcomes. Managers must be aware of the implications of nurse workload and staffing decisions, particularly during times of nurse shortages, because such decisions may affect staff morale and increase turnover. A basic understanding of nurse workload and staffing issues allows managers to meet day-to-day patient care requirements as well as cope with changing patient care demands, personnel, reimbursement policies, and regulations.

This chapter provides an overview of nurse staffing, workload, and measurement and the issues that pertain to nurse workload. An understanding of these issues and how to address them is essential for managers who oversee the planning, staffing, budgeting, and evaluation of patient care delivery on units and in departments. Also, in this chapter, the types of nursing professionals are discussed, the terms *nurse workload* and *nurse staffing* are defined, the approaches used in different healthcare settings to measure nurse workload are examined, the perspectives of different stakeholders on workload measurement are provided, and nurse staffing metrics are presented along with examples of staffing calculations.

Types of Nursing Personnel

In the United States, licensed and unlicensed nursing personnel differ in terms of education; knowledge, skills, and abilities; and patient care responsibilities. These differences must be taken into account when planning nurse workload and staffing.

Licensed nursing personnel include those who work under a specific scope of practice set by state and/or national regulatory requirements (Bureau of Labor Statistics 2014). The two types of licensed nurses are registered nurses (RNs) and licensed practical nurses (LPNs).[1] Each type has its own educational, licensure, and practice requirements, and healthcare organizations require proof of licensure from both types. Unlicensed nursing personnel, such as nursing assistants, provide support services to licensed nurses and other healthcare professionals. Characteristics of licensed and unlicensed nursing personnel are summarized in Exhibit 14.1.

Healthcare organizations employ a mix of nursing and other personnel to meet patient care needs. Decisions about the numbers and types of nursing personnel hired reflect an organization's philosophy about the role and importance of nursing; patient safety and satisfaction; quality of care; and the job satisfaction, perceived value, and safety of nurses and other nursing staff. In short, nurse staffing decisions represent the value that the unit, department, or organization places on nursing practice and on patient care delivery (Welton 2011). This value then is the foundation on which nurse workload and resource allocation decisions are based.

Definitions and Measurement

The terms *nurse workload* and *nurse staffing* are often used interchangeably and inconsistently. For the purposes of this chapter, the following definitions will be used:

- *Nurse workload* means (1) the number of patients or patient days for which nursing care is required on a unit or within a department or organization or (2) the number of patients cared for by an individual nurse (often referred to as the *nurse-to-patient ratio*).
- *Nurse staffing* means (1) the number of nurses deployed (also called *staffing level*) or (2) the process by which the appropriate number and type of nursing personnel are deployed to satisfy nurse workload requirements.

A review of the literature reveals that researchers define and measure nurse staffing in different ways. These ways include (1) the number of nursing personnel, by type of nurse; (2) the hours of a type of nursing personnel (e.g., RN hours) as a percentage of total nursing care hours; (3) the number of personnel (i.e., head count) as a percentage of total nursing staff; (4) the number of full-time equivalents (FTEs) for specific nursing personnel; and (5) the percentage of total nursing FTEs, by type of nurse (e.g., RN FTEs) (Harless and Mark 2010; Mark, Hughes, and Jones 2004; Seago 2001).

EXHIBIT 14.1
Description of Licensed and Unlicensed Nursing Staff

	Licensed Nursing Personnel		Unlicensed Nursing Personnel[a]
	RNs	**LPNs**	
Educational preparation	Three-year diploma (hospital-based program[b]); two-year associate degree; four-year baccalaureate degree.[c] (Some master's and doctoral programs also provide entry-level preparation.)	One to two years of training at a technical or vocational school.	Varies; some healthcare organizations have mandatory training requirements and certification requirements; some states have a registry of certified individuals.
Licensure required	Issued by states; examination required.	Issued by states; examination required.	Certification by an accrediting body may or may not be required.
Duties	Provide complex nursing care to promote patient health, prevent disease, and help patients cope with illness. Observe, assess, and evaluate patient conditions. Work with patients, families, and other healthcare professionals to coordinate, develop, and manage patient plans of care. May function independently; often work in collaboration with physicians and other healthcare professionals. May supervise other licensed and unlicensed nursing personnel.	Provide routine nursing care, which may include taking patient vital signs, administering medications as regulated by the state and/or agency of practice, monitoring patient reactions to routine medications and treatments, assisting with personal hygiene and activities of daily living, collecting patient samples, performing routine lab tests, teaching simple tasks to patients and families, and performing some clerical duties. In skilled nursing facilities, may evaluate patient needs.	Provide support services to licensed nurses and other healthcare professionals. Provide routine assistive care to patients, such as answering call lights, serving meals, assisting in patient feeding and hygiene care, taking patient vital signs, preparing equipment for patient procedures and treatment, assisting with certain procedures, stocking patient supplies, and performing some clerical duties. In skilled nursing facilities, develop relationships with patients and families.
Supervision	May function independently within scope of practice, or may be supervised by other RNs and in some cases physicians.	Supervised by RN and/or physician; may also supervise other LPNs and/or unlicensed nursing personnel.	Supervised by RN and/or physician; sometimes supervised by LPN.

Source: Bureau of Labor Statistics (2014).

[a] Unlicensed nursing personnel include nursing aides, nursing assistants, patient care assistants, and orderlies.

[b] Since the early 1980s, both the number of diploma programs and the number of graduates have been in decline (Health Resources and Services Administration 2010).

[c] Advanced practice nurses (i.e., clinical nurse specialist, nurse practitioner, nurse midwife, nurse anesthetist) require a master's or higher-level degree and/or certification in nursing.

As discussed later in this chapter, studies have documented the relationship between nurse staffing and adverse patient events (see, for example, integrative reviews conducted by Kane et al. 2007; Lankshear, Sheldon, and Maynard 2005; Thungjaroenkul, Cummings, and Embleton 2007; West et al. 2009). However, comparing the findings from these studies is difficult because of the inconsistencies and variation in the definition and measurement used.

In addition, disagreement abounds in the nursing field about how to best ensure that staffing levels are adequate to meet patient care demands and to keep patients safe. According to the American Nurses Association (2013), three general approaches have been used to address the appropriateness of nurse staffing levels. The first requires hospitals to use nurse-led staffing committees to establish and implement staffing plans based on patient need and other nursing-related criteria. The second is a legislative approach, whereby specific nurse staffing ratios are mandated by state law. The third requires healthcare organizations to report nurse staffing levels to regulatory agencies and/or the public.

In 1999, California was the first state to pass nurse staffing legislation for hospitals, setting a minimum nurse-to-patient ratio of 1:6 beginning in 2004, with the ratio declining to 1:5 in 2005. These ratios were established on the assumption that higher nurse staffing levels would lead to improved patient care. However, little evidence exists to support the specific ratios selected, and disagreement about whether or not nurse staffing levels should be legislated still exists. Recognizing these arguments, California followed the 1999 staffing legislation with other bills that call for the evaluation of the mandated ratios and the development of staffing plans in hospitals. In 2005, California's governor attempted to halt implementation of the legislated nurse-to-patient ratio of 1:5, but this suspension was later overturned by the courts. Other states have taken similar actions by introducing legislation to mandate the development and implementation of specific nurse staffing plans, minimum staffing ratios, or some combination of both (Aiken et al. 2010; American Nurses Association 2014). While studies have indicated that significant increases in nurse staffing levels followed the implementation of staffing legislation (Aiken et al. 2010; Mark et al. 2013; Serratt et al. 2011), the evidence is inconsistent regarding whether increased staffing levels have resulted in significant improvements in the overall quality of care provided to patients. For example, Aiken and colleagues (2010) reported that mandated staffing levels in California were associated with lower mortality rates, but others (Mark et al. 2013; Spetz et al. 2013) have suggested that improvements in quality of care resulting from increased nurse staffing levels in California were marginal.

Although nurse staffing legislation influences administrative decision making in some states, these laws do not cover all nursing personnel or patient care situations. In most states, nurse staffing legislation does not exist. As a result, managers still struggle with several important questions:

- What numbers of nursing staff are needed to provide care for patients?
- What types of nursing staff are needed to provide care for patients?
- What mix of nursing staff is needed to provide quality care and ensure patient safety?
- What numbers, types, and mix of nursing staff can the organization afford?
- How does the mix of nursing staff vary by patient care area?

Finkler, Jones, and Kovner (2013) define nurse workload as the volume of work required to deliver nursing care for a patient care unit or department.[2] To facilitate the calculation of nurse workload, unidimensional metrics, such as patients or patient days, are used. However, in using this approach, the manager should appreciate that these metrics do not always capture the complexity of nursing "work," which is multifaceted, requires specialized knowledge and skills, and entails more than the amount of time spent with patients. Electronic tools to capture the complexities of nursing work have been designed; an example is the Clinical Demand Index reported by Harper (2012), which determines how nurses spend their time through the use of data mining techniques to abstract key terms and concepts and identify key variables. Until such systems are widespread, however, unit managers must take the complexity of nurses' work into account when determining nurse staffing and strive for a "balance of [nursing] job demands with sufficient resources (adequate staffing, time available to plan and carry out work)" (Koehoorn et al. 2002, 6).

Exhibit 14.2 presents four scenarios to illustrate the basic components of average nurse workload. Scenario 1 shows that, given a constant nurse workload (number of patients), a decrease in nurse staffing (the number of nurses) increases the average workload (the number of patients per nurse). Scenario 2 shows that, given constant nurse staffing, an increase in nurse workload also increases the average workload. Scenario 3 shows that average nurse workload does not change if the number of patients and the number of staff change at the same rate. Scenario 4 shows that the average nurse workload increases if the number of patients increases at a faster rate than the number of staff. These scenarios illustrate the following points: (1) An increase in the average nurse workload may be the result of more patients, fewer nurses, or both and (2) the average nurse workload is not reduced by an increase in nurse staffing if the workload (number of patients) increases at a faster rate. Of course, in the real world, nurse workload is seldom constant, and the work of an individual nurse usually fluctuates as patient numbers and

Scenario	Nurse Workload (No. of Patients)	Nurse Staffing (No. of Nurses)	Average Nurse Workload (No. of Patients per Nurse)
1. Constant number of patients, decreasing number of nurses	25 25 25	6 5 4	4.2 5.0 6.3
2. Increasing number of patients, constant number of nurses	20 25 30	5 5 5	4.0 5.0 6.0
3. Increasing number of patients and nurses with same rate of change	20 25 30	4 5 6	5.0 5.0 5.0
4. Increasing number of patients and nurses with different rates of change	20 25 30	4 4.5 5	5.0 5.6 6.0

EXHIBIT 14.2
Basic Components of the Average Nursing Workload

conditions change. Nevertheless, the average nurse workload may be considered a crude measure of the adequacy of nurse staffing.

Most healthcare organizations use formal nurse staffing processes to reasonably, fairly, and safely address nurse workload issues. These processes include the use of committees with nursing representatives; the development and implementation of staffing policies and procedures, including standards for the number and skill mix of nursing staff; and the determination of hours-of-care requirements for different types of patients. In addition, nurse staffing issues are usually part of the collective bargaining agreement between employers and nurse unions.

Use of Measures

Nurse workload is measured for three primary reasons: (1) to inform the budgeting process; (2) to meet regulatory and accreditation standards; and (3) to inform the development, implementation, and evaluation of staffing plans. The budgeting process necessitates the calculation of nurse workload to prepare an organization's operating budget and, specifically, to determine nursing personnel requirements and costs (Finkler, Jones, and Kovner 2013). The budgeting process involves decision making about the level and mix of nurse staffing, the workload that nurses will assume, and the allocation of resources. Regulatory requirements and accreditation standards necessitate that healthcare organizations comply with regulations of the Centers for Medicare & Medicaid Services and with the standards of The Joint Commission (2014). For example, in 2002, The Joint Commission instituted a staffing effectiveness requirement for hospital accreditation. Nurse workload systems may be used to gather staffing and outcomes data to document compliance with this requirement.

Nurse staffing plans, on the other hand, are blueprints for meeting specific patient care and regulatory requirements and for deploying nursing personnel efficiently and effectively. Staffing plans also enable managers to develop policies for determining reasonable work schedules, which promote a positive work environment, and for accommodating operational uncertainties and contingencies.

Nurse workload measures differ across types of healthcare settings. For example, nurse workload can be measured in terms of the number of patients or number of patient days in hospitals, the number of residents or resident days in long-term-care facilities, the number of clinic visits in ambulatory clinics, the number of home visits in home health care services, the number of deliveries in maternity wards, and the number of procedures in outpatient surgery or operating rooms (Finkler, Jones, and Kovner 2013). Measurement systems have been developed to assess nurse workload in these different settings. These systems (usually electronic) capture the variable nature of nursing care requirements across different types of patients and healthcare settings, and they are used to determine the number of nurses required to care for different types of patients (Fasoli and Haddock 2010; Harper 2012). In short, these systems provide critical information that aids in decision making and in nursing resource allocation (Jennings 2008).

Perspectives of Stakeholders

Patients and their families want to be assured that a sufficient number of nurses are available and appropriate nurse-to-patient ratios are in place so that they can receive individualized care and timely, relevant communications about their condition and treatment (O'Brien et al. 2002). Patients' perceptions are therefore important to healthcare organizations. However, nurse workload measures or systems do not take into account consumers' preferences and desires.

Healthcare managers, including patient care unit or nursing managers, are concerned about nurse workload measurement for several reasons.

First, they are responsible for allocating nursing resources—a decision that ensures patient care needs are met. For example, on a day-to-day basis, nurse managers[3] must modify staffing levels as necessary to meet nurse workload requirements. This responsibility may mean using agency or per diem nursing staff to cover for permanent staff who call in sick or are on vacation, to cover ongoing position vacancies that result from turnover or the development of new staffing plans or programs, or to respond to unexpected variations in patient care requirements. Second, they have to balance the costs of delivering nursing care with organizational reimbursements. If the nursing staff is too large (i.e., too few patients per nurse), the costs of providing nursing services may be unnecessarily high. On the other hand, if the nursing staff is too small (i.e., too many patients per nurse), costs may be lower in the short run; however, the work under this condition may increase nursing errors, stress, burnout, dissatisfaction, absenteeism, and turnover, which likely will lead to higher costs over the long run. Thus, managers must ensure that nurse workloads are reasonable and fair, allowing nurses to deliver the level of nursing care needed by patients.

Insurer and payer perspectives have a financial basis as well. In some cases, an increase in charges as a result of nurse workload and staffing can increase reimbursements. An increase in overall healthcare costs because of workload and staffing also increases the costs of coverage, which are then passed along to consumers. In turn, employers and consumers need to make a decision about whether to retain coverage with the insurer, and if so, whether to keep the same level of coverage.

Policymakers view nurse workload in terms of ensuring that nursing resources are sufficient in providing safe, effective care to communities and in meeting changing patient care demands. For example, the aging US population means that, in the future, more nursing resources will be needed to care for the elderly and long-standing nursing shortages in many geographic areas will increase the gap between supply and demand. Policymakers must see to it that government and industry workforce policies recognize changing demographics and support human resources (HR) adjustments, such as providing incentives to nurses and other healthcare providers to enter the geriatric care field and educating nurses and other caregivers about long-term care. In addition, policymakers must develop guidelines to ensure that nurse staffing levels are safe and do not place patients at risk of harm or injury.

Nurses view many aspects of workload and staffing in terms of how they are directly affected. These aspects include volume of work; responsibility to their patients, themselves, and their unit; multiple, concurrent, and often competing demands on their time; their feelings of overload and inability to complete work; the need to deal with unexpected events or interruptions; their familiarity with and support of work requirements; the abilities of other caregivers with whom they work; the degree to which the workload spills into their personal lives; their level of emotional and physical exhaustion from work; and their lack of control over the workload (Gaudine 2000; Hayes, Bonner, and Pryor 2010).

Determining Nurse Staffing Requirements

Nurse staffing involves determining the numbers and types of nursing personnel employed on a patient care unit in a hospital, long-term-care facility, emergency department, ambulatory clinic, or community health center. Decisions about the numbers and types of nurses employed on a patient care unit are based on (1) the patient population, (2) nurses' characteristics, and (3) the organization's philosophy about nursing and patient care delivery.

Patient Population Data

An important source of workload data is information about the patient population. This information is maintained in the *patient classification system* or *acuity system*. Patient classification systems are typically maintained electronically and used to categorize individual patient demands and nursing care requirements (Fasoli and Haddock 2010) based on the patient's acuity or severity of illness,[4] not on the patient's diagnostic category. The literature review by Fasoli and Haddock (2010) indicates that common variables considered in patient classification systems are patient characteristics (e.g., care needs, complexity of care required), nursing characteristics (e.g., education and experience of staff, as well as skill mix), and organizational characteristics (e.g., volume of services, patient turnover).

These systems provide a standard measure of nursing care for classes of patients (generally measured in hours of nursing care required per patient day) and provide a way of matching patient needs with nursing requirements. Commercial makers of patient classification systems include GRASP Systems and QuadraMed, and some of their products can be customized by organizations to meet their needs and integrate with other management information systems. Individual organizations also create their own patient classification systems.

The potential of patient classification systems is great because they can be used to project nurse staffing needs, develop unit budgets, establish costs for nursing services, and inform risk management and quality improvement initiatives (DeGroot 1989; Fasoli and Haddock 2010; Seago 2001; Van Slyck 2000). Unfortunately, patient classification systems are often not used to their potential, are generally distrusted by nurses and managers as not reliable or valid, and consequently are often not employed in decision making. More specifically, some variables in patient classification scores are based on nurses' ratings, such as patients' characteristics, their severity of illness, and the required number and complexity of treatment interventions (Fasoli and Haddock 2010). Because of the way in which patient scores are obtained, some claim that nurses may actually inflate patient ratings (which is also known as *acuity creep* or *classification creep*) to increase unit staffing (hence reducing nurse workload) or to prevent staff from being pulled[5] to work on another unit that may be understaffed (Malloch and Conovaloff 1999). On the other hand, some nurses believe that managers are not responsive and do not increase the number of staff when ratings suggest that more nurses are needed. Patient classification systems generally do not take into account the nurses' educational level, years of experience, or knowledge and cannot match the skills of individual nurses with the needs of individual patients. Thus, while these systems may be commonly used to estimate staffing and workload, they do not replace a manager's judgment and staff input for day-to-day or shift-to-shift staffing (Jennings 2008).

Historical Data

Historical data, such as the following, help reveal variations in patient care on a unit:

- *Utilization data*
  - Average daily census (the average number of patients cared for per day over a defined period) helps in determining a staffing standard for numbers and mix of nursing personnel by shift.
  - Occupancy rate (average daily census or average number of patient days divided by the number of beds on the unit) aids in examining the extent to which unit capacity is reached.
  - Admissions, discharges, and transfers and information on short-stay patients provide insight into patient turnover and work requirements.
  - Temporal variations in care reveal factors that may affect patient admissions and requirements. For example, the flu season may increase admissions on certain units, especially on units that provide geriatric care.
- *Payroll data*
  - Data on productive and nonproductive time paid assist in determining paid hours per patient day.
- *HR data*
  - Staffing vacancies or the number of open positions help in estimating future staffing needs.
  - Nurse turnover rates, or the number of nursing staff who leave over a defined period, facilitate estimates of the percentage of productive hours and determine budget adjustments for the given period.

- Collective agreements account for personnel contract changes.
- Numbers of new and experienced nurses aid in identifying productivity differences between new and experienced staff.

Key Issues in Managing Nurse Staffing and Workload

When organizations face financial pressure, labor—the largest expense for most healthcare organizations—often becomes a target of budget cuts. Organizations have engaged in strategies such as implementing nurse staffing plans that reduce the number of nurses, increase nurse workloads, or increase the number of hours worked by nurses (including overtime). In the short run, these strategies may solve immediate nurse staffing problems. However, in the long run, they may be counterproductive and may negatively affect a manager's ability to appropriately staff a unit.

Managers should consider several issues as they reconcile budgetary and staffing issues, which are outlined in Exhibit 14.3 and discussed in greater detail in the following sections. Healthcare managers, especially first-line patient care unit or nurse managers, should be aware of such issues and the impact of staffing decisions on nurses and nurse perceptions as well as on patients, care delivery, and overall organizational performance.

Nurses' Workload, Stress, and Burnout

Workload is one of the most significant predictors of negative health outcomes, stress, decreased job satisfaction, and burnout. Burke (2003) studied the relationship between changing nurse-to-patient ratios and nurse perceptions of workload, job satisfaction, psychological well-being, and effectiveness of their institutions. According to this study, as the number of patients nurses were assigned to care for increased, nurses reported heavier workloads,

EXHIBIT 14.3
Key Issues in
Managing Nurse
Staffing

- Workload stress and staff burnout
- Staff turnover, recruitment, and retention
- Aging of the nursing workforce
- The nature of nursing work
- Union versus nonunion environment
- Nurse–physician relationship
- Nurse–nurse conflict
- Workforce diversity
- Balancing quality and costs of care

lower job satisfaction, poorer psychological health, and a decreased view of hospital effectiveness. This study suggests that when nurses perceive excessive workloads (that is, they feel they have too much work to complete during work hours), they experience stress and burnout, which, in turn, lead to feelings of anger. Nurses in this situation may be more likely to call in sick or leave the organization altogether. High nurse workloads also have been associated with higher 30-day patient mortality and increased levels of nurse burnout and dissatisfaction (Aiken et al. 2002; Gabriel et al. 2013); high levels of nurse burnout and emotional exhaustion have been linked to low levels of patient satisfaction (McHugh et al. 2011).

Healthcare managers must be sensitive to the potential effects of nurse workload stress and burnout. They must design staffing strategies that minimize potential lapses in patient care quality and patient satisfaction. Following are a few simple approaches to address staff concerns about workload and overload (Gaudine 2000; Hayes, Bonner, and Pryor 2010; Prescott and Soeken 1996):

- Involve nurses in unit decision making, including the establishment of appropriate workloads.
- Engage nurses in contingency planning to deal with sudden changes in patient care needs or conditions and to manage fluctuations in staffing (e.g., callouts, vacations, educational leaves).
- Be aware of changes in clinical practice and provider policies that can affect nurse workload.
- Examine workload and quality data to help make a case for adequate nursing resource allocation.
- Provide adequate support staff (e.g., clerks) to assist nurses in carrying out non-nursing tasks and thus relieve nurses to care for patients.
- Develop strategies to give nurses as much control as possible over their workload. For example, ask nurses for input on the timing of patient admissions, the temporary closing of beds, and approaches to staffing and scheduling.

Staff Turnover, Recruitment, and Retention

Staff retention and turnover become a primary concern for unit managers during times of staff shortages. When staff are in short supply, more job-change opportunities are available within and outside the organization. But if turnover becomes excessive, it may bring about additional turnover as staff lose colleagues, work teams become disrupted, and staff reflect more on their work environment and wages relative to those provided by competitors in the market (Jones 2004). High levels of turnover can also make recruiting new staff into a work unit difficult. When an organization has many vacancies, working conditions suffer and this information is communicated into the market through social and professional networks.

A more important issue, however, is that turnover is costly (Li and Jones 2013), with some estimates indicating costs per nurse turnover of more than $60,000 (Advisory Board Company 1999; Jones 2005) or 1.3 times a departing nurse's salary (Jones 2005). In addition to its quantifiable costs, turnover also presents qualitative costs, such as those that affect quality of care and patient safety as staff leave and enter patient care teams. For example, a nurse who leaves takes with him or her valuable human capital in the form of knowledge, skills, and experiences that are specific to the work unit and the patient populations served by the organization. This loss then affects the work of the entire team until or unless a comparable replacement is hired. While aspects of this human capital loss are quantifiable (e.g., the costs of advertising for a replacement), other elements are harder to put a dollar figure on—that is, we cannot measure the cost of losing an individual's knowledge, skills, and experiences.

Following are several steps that healthcare managers can take to deal with staff turnover:

1. *Become familiar with organizational systems for tracking nurse turnover.* These systems are often monitored by the HR department, but line managers typically receive ongoing reports that compare their unit's turnover rate with that of other units and even other organizations.

2. *Establish a unit-level database with more detailed nurse turnover information that can be used in managing existing staff, looking for appropriate replacements, and identifying opportunities for growth.* Organizational systems to monitor staff turnover rarely contain fine-grained data, such as the level of expertise that is lost when a particular staff member leaves.

3. *Create a process for tracking retention and determining a retention rate.* This process is different from tracking turnover. Examining retention requires that the manager follow individuals (or cohorts of individuals) over time, beginning at their initial employment date (Waldman and Arora 2004).

4. *Establish a mechanism for gathering ongoing feedback about why nurses leave, why they stay, and their perceptions of the work environment.* This feedback will help the manager understand staff concerns, examine trends over time, and identify areas for future improvement.

Aging of the Nursing Workforce

A great deal has been written about the aging of the nursing workforce, highlighting the fact that the number of younger nurses is insufficient to replace those who will retire over the next 20 years. According to a nationally representative sample of US nurses in a 2008 study, the average age of RNs was 47, with 44.8 percent age 50 or older and only 9.4 percent under age 30 (Health Resources and Services Administration 2010). These numbers reflect a dramatic shift in the nursing workforce since 1980, when only 25 percent were older than 50 years and 25 percent were younger than 30 years. In fact, aging of the nursing workforce has been cited as a reason that the current nursing shortage is different and perhaps more severe than past shortages (Buerhaus, Auerbach, and Staiger 2009).

For the first time in nursing history, four generations of nurses are working side by side: millennials (or generation Y), born after 1980; generation X, born between 1965 and 1980; baby boomers, born between 1946 and 1964; and veterans, born between 1925 and 1945 (Hendricks and Cope 2013). Members of each generation have different needs and desires that drive their expectations about work and the workplace. They also have different perspectives on and degrees of comfort with technology. Some simply use e-mail or other electronic systems during the process of routine activities, while others tote tablets and specific pieces of equipment in caring for patients. In turn, these generational differences in needs, desires, and expectations may create conditions that bring out intergenerational conflicts (Hendricks and Cope 2013).

Age and generational issues, combined with changes in healthcare organizations and patient populations, require special attention from the manager. For example, patients today are sicker, have shorter lengths of stay, and require more intensive nursing care than patients in the past. This change in patient needs is the result of many factors, including technological capabilities that enable the delivery of more complex care; an increase in obesity rate, which leads to health problems; and a longer life expectancy, which typically means additional health concerns. These and other factors combine to exert more physical stress and strain on nurses and put them at risk for physical injury.

Creating a positive work environment for nurses requires sensitivity to generational needs. Following are some strategies toward that end (Greene 2005; Hendricks and Cope 2013; Swearingen and Lieberman 2004):

- Conduct an ergonomic evaluation of the work environment and address necessary concerns.
- Give adequate support in terms of patient transportation, lifting, and moving.
- Offer adequate training on the multitude of technological devices and equipment used on the unit.
- Provide adequate staffing so that meals and mental breaks can be taken from the sometimes relentless cognitive and physical demands.

- Put a process in place to stay in touch with generational perceptions and expectations of nurses pertaining to such issues as types of rewards and recognition, job satisfaction, and organizational commitment (Kovner et al. 2006).

The Nature of Nursing Work

Nurses' work has been characterized as complex, fragmented, and unpredictable (Tucker and Spear 2006); ambiguous and dangerous (Philbin 2007); and physically demanding (Barker and Nussbaum 2011). Potter and colleagues (2004) combined qualitative and human factors methods to examine the work of nursing. They reported that nurses often traverse long and repetitive distances, even when based on a single patient care unit. Nurses' work is also intellectually, emotionally, and psychologically demanding because of its composition and context. For example, the work environment is often chaotic, requiring nurses to perform at an intense cognitive level and to make numerous judgments about patients' conditions, many of which are of an urgent nature and must be made under pressure. Some nursing judgments entail actions that must be taken on behalf of patients, while other judgments involve contacting and interacting with physicians and other care providers to respond to changing patient conditions. According to Potter and colleagues, nurses' work is nonlinear and is plagued with numerous interruptions, which these researchers determined through the use of cognitive mapping. Nurses juggle numerous competing priorities during a shift, and the order of priorities can change quickly as patients' conditions change. In fact, Wolf and colleagues (2006) used human factors engineering and qualitative methods to study the nature of nursing work and reported that nurses often "stack" up to ten or more tasks at one time and experience more than three interruptions per hour. Such practices create conditions that are conducive to mistakes and omissions in care.

Others studies report on the effects of work strains that prevent nurses from recovering from work and gaining sufficient rest. Winwood and Lushington (2006) found that the high-paced work environment exacerbates nurses' psychological strains, which inhibit their ability to sleep and potentially lead to long-term health problems and withdrawal from the workforce. Other studies observed that nurses' work hours (frequently 12-hour shifts or longer) and the subsequent fatigue jeopardize quality of care, patient safety, and patient satisfaction and can contribute to nurse burnout (Dean, Scott, and Rogers 2006; Rogers et al. 2004; Scott et al. 2006; Stimpfel, Sloane, and Aiken 2012).

To address the complexity of nurses' work, managers can engage nurses in a dialogue to gain insights into current processes and systems that support or impede nurses' ability to do their job. This dialogue can be used to identify strategies to reduce the number of interruptions that nurses experience and to give nurses the tools to minimize the cognitive stacking of tasks and priorities. Many nurses do not get meal breaks or short breaks during their shift, or they skip breaks to complete their work. Strategies can be developed to ensure that sufficient staff is available to cover breaks and mealtimes so that nurses can get a mental respite and better focus on meeting patient needs.

Union Versus Nonunion Environment

Approximately 23 percent of the US nursing labor market is covered by a union agreement, and union density in hospitals is 14.3 percent, compared to 6.9 percent in the nonhealthcare sector (Buerhaus 2010; Moody 2014). Nursing unions are not without detractors, who claim that nurses' participation in union activities is unprofessional and associated with decreased job satisfaction and morale (Fitzpatrick 2001; Seago and Ash 2002). However, the following concerns converged in the late 1990s and have continued to bring about nurses' renewed interest in unions: declining nurse staffing levels, growing nursing shortage, increasing patient acuity, decreasing patient lengths of stay, proliferation of managed care, decreasing reimbursements, and widespread layoffs (Buerhaus 2010; Forman and Davis 2002; Lovell 2006; Moody 2014; Schraeder and Friedman 2002; Steltzer 2001). For a detailed discussion of unionization in healthcare, see Chapter 12.

Several interesting observations have been made about unionization of nursing. Lovell (2006) reported that the presence of unions increased wages for both union and nonunion nurses in certain geographic markets. Lovell's study indicated that nurses who worked in the most unionized states earned roughly 28 percent more than nurses who worked in the least unionized states. However, evidence about wage differences is somewhat contradictory, as Spetz and colleagues (2011) reported that the pay structure between union and nonunion hospitals does not significantly differ in most circumstances.

Lovell (2006) also suggested that the presence of unions increases nurse staffing, with approximately 18 percent more nurses working in the most unionized cities than in the least unionized cities, and in turn improves the quality of care. Seago and Ash (2002) examined the relationship between the presence of a union and the outcomes of hospitalized patients with acute myocardial infarction in California. According to that study, patients cared for in unionized hospitals had a 5.7 percent lower mortality rate than patients cared for in nonunion hospitals, after controlling for risk factors. The authors further suggested that the mechanisms through which patient outcomes may be affected include staff stability, staff autonomy, and nurse–physician relationships, all of which improve the work environment and ultimately care delivery. However, some evidence suggests that strikes in hospitals have a significant negative effect on patients' morbidity and mortality (Gruber and Kleiner 2012).

Unionization is typically viewed as the result of an adversarial relationship or irreconcilable differences between management and staff. Unfortunately, as Forman and Davis (2002, 377) report, nurses have "identified their manager as their greatest source of stress—even greater than heavy patient loads." Managers, whether in a union organization or not, should realize that nurses typically seek unions when they believe that they do not have a voice in issues that pertain directly to their work and the delivery of patient care (Clark and Clark 2009; Forman and Davis 2002; Schraeder and Friedman 2002). In fact, many staffing concerns are focused on issues that pertain to communication, such as lack of input into decision making, workers' feeling undervalued, and perceptions of fear and intimidation from organizational leaders (Clark and Clark 2009; Fitzpatrick 2001).

Managers in unionized hospitals must obviously understand the collective bargaining process and the terms and conditions of the specific agreement at their organization. They also need to develop a strong relationship with the HR department and consult with its personnel to address staff questions that pertain to the agreement. Managers must be knowledgeable about dispute resolution and grievance and disciplinary processes, and they must be comfortable with addressing disagreements that may arise between the organization and the union (Forman and Davis 2002). In the worst case, if disputes cannot be resolved and a strike ensues, managers should have a contingency staffing plan in place.

Time and again, frontline managers have been found to play a critical role in shaping nurse satisfaction and retention. The most important step that frontline managers can take, regardless of whether their hospital is under a union agreement, is to maintain open, honest, and consistent dialogue with the nursing staff (Schraeder and Friedman 2002). This simple strategy alone may avoid union disagreements, strikes, or union organizing activities. Managers who do not work in unionized hospitals should be aware of organizing activities in the event that nurses initiate a union campaign within the institution (Forman and Powell 2003). The bottom line is to keep the lines of communication open; to focus on patient care, protecting the safety, security, and well-being of patients and nurses; and to always take the high road by using factual data and acting in a professional manner (Block and Jamerson 2005). Porter-O'Grady (2001) recommends that managers view the union as a partner instead of an adversary and work from the mutual understanding that both sides can achieve positive outcomes and benefits. By doing so, managers and their organizations can take advantage of what nurses actually seek through unionization activities—namely, improving the work environment, nurse staffing levels, and the quality of care received by patients.

Nurse–Physician Relationships

The nurse–physician relationship is a key ingredient in sustaining a healthy work environment but is one of the greatest impediments to an improved workplace. When nurse–physician relationships are collegial, collaborative, and founded on open communication, nurses tend to be more satisfied with their work environment and are more likely to remain in their positions (Jansky 2004; O'Brien-Pallas et al. 2005; Schmalenberg and Kramer 2009). When nurse–physician relationships are not collegial, nurses become dissatisfied, demoralized, undervalued, and burned out—feelings that may cause them to leave their jobs (Gabriel et al. 2013). In the long run, patient care may suffer.

Because both nurses and physicians work for the good of the patients and to promote quality care, one would expect their relationships to be positive. However, nurse–physician relationships, in general, have been characterized as dysfunctional and in some cases pathologic (Stein 1967). A strong and inverse relationship exists between nurse–physician collaboration and nurse job stress (right behind nurse job satisfaction) (Zangaro and Soeken 2007). Schmalenberg and colleagues (2005) argue that, although both nurses and physicians rate their relationship as important, literature on the topic has appeared primarily in nursing journals. Another study of nurses and physicians reported that both groups acknowledged the presence of disruptive physician behavior in their organization (Rosenstein 2002). However, in a follow-up study conducted in 50 hospitals, nurses were reported to misbehave almost as often as physicians, and respondents believed that poor nurse–physician relationships caused stress, frustration, and burnout and had a negative impact on concentration, communication, collaboration, information transfer, and workplace relationships (Rosenstein and O'Daniel 2005).

Nurse–physician relationships also are purported to influence nurses' perceptions of staffing adequacy (Laschinger and Leiter 2006; O'Brien-Pallas et al. 2005). Specifically, nurses perceive work overload when they are frequently involved in negative and emotionally draining interactions with physicians. Poor nurse–physician relationships are a burden on both nurses and physicians, often requiring additional communications, unnecessary follow-up, and sometimes disciplinary actions for those who may already feel fragmented and stretched because of increased patient demands or short staffing. Poor nurse–physician relationships may also be linked to difficulties in recruiting new staff to the unit during times of shortage. For example, if nurse–physician relationships on a particular unit are known to be poor, other units likely know about it; as this information spreads, potential new hires may be deterred from working on the unit.

In addition to the negative effect on individual nurses and physicians, a poor relationship affects the quality of patient care. Rosenstein and O'Daniel (2005) report that nurses and physicians perceived that negative relationships potentially affect patient care and outcomes, resulting in adverse events, medical errors, compromised patient safety, increased patient mortality, and lowered patient satisfaction. Other studies have found a link between good relationships and high patient satisfaction, lower patient mortalities, fewer ICU readmissions, decreased length of stay, lower costs, and perception of higher quality of care (O'Brien-Pallas et al. 2005; Schmalenberg et al. 2005).

Following are important recommendations for managers seeking to improve nurse–physician relationships on their unit or in their organization:

- Conduct training workshops on interdisciplinary collaboration, communication, and coordination (O'Brien-Pallas et al. 2005).
- Hold joint, interdisciplinary staff meetings, rounds, and/or case reviews (O'Brien-Pallas et al. 2005; Schmalenberg et al. 2005).
- Articulate expectations clearly regarding nurse–physician relationships (Matthews and Lankshear 2003; Schmalenberg et al. 2005).
- Facilitate the development of joint critical pathways and protocols (Schmalenberg et al. 2005).
- Develop and articulate clear processes for conflict resolution (Schmalenberg et al. 2005).
- Manage conflicts in a positive manner when they occur (Schmalenberg et al. 2005).
- Highlight strong, positive relationships that exist between nurse and medical leaders (Schmalenberg et al. 2005).
- Foster nurse competence through educational offerings (Schmalenberg et al. 2005).
- Create a positive culture that puts patients first, empowers nurses and builds their confidence, values teamwork and collegiality, builds trust, and respects each individual (Schmalenberg et al. 2005).

Walking rounds by the manager will also provide opportunities to observe nurse–physician interactions and to address concerns that may affect the work environment. Above all, managers play a fundamental role in fostering positive nurse–physician relationships, which in turn affects patients and potentially future unit staffing.

Nurse–Nurse Conflict

Within healthcare organizations, negative interaction between nurses, often referred to as nurse–nurse conflict, is a problem that affects nursing morale, retention, and patient outcomes (Purpora and Blegen 2012; Townsend 2012). The phenomenon of nurse–nurse conflict is often described as lateral or horizontal violence (i.e., as occurring among nurses in similar positions, or between nurses in different position levels of power), bullying, or nurses "eating their young" (Sheridan-Leos 2008). The problem has become so serious that in 2009, The Joint Commission, one of the primary accrediting bodies for US hospitals, released a new standard to address such inappropriate and disruptive behavior (Pontus 2011). Evidence suggests that the following interventions are successful when managers and healthcare organizational leaders implement policies to address lateral violence among nurses (Coursey et al. 2013):

- Aim to change behaviors of staff in a way that supports policies on lateral violence.
  - Managers should provide feedback to nurses and other employees in a mutually respectful manner.
  - Managers must raise awareness of nurse–nurse conflict through open dialogue and the provision of education on lateral violence to nursing staff.
- Managers should be involved in any matters of lateral violence.
- Managers must work to intentionally change the environment so that culture does not support or tolerate lateral violence among nurses.

Although conflict among employees can occur among any type or level of employee, when conflicts and poor relationships have the potential to affect the quality and safety of care at the point of delivery, managers need the skills and knowledge to work with others to remedy the situation in the short run, and change the work environment over the long run.

Workforce Diversity

One of many recommendations for addressing the nursing shortage has been to increase diversity in the nursing workforce (American Association of Colleges of Nursing 2014; Joint Commission 2002). Consensus exists among all national nursing organizations, hospital associations, and important stakeholder groups in the healthcare sector that recruitment of diverse, underrepresented groups into the nursing profession is a priority of the future. The Joint Commission (2002, 24) recommended diversifying the nursing workforce as a means of addressing the nursing shortage "to broaden the base of potential workers and to improve patient safety and health care quality for patients of all origins and backgrounds." Unfortunately, nursing's progress toward achieving this goal has been characterized as "slow, sporadic, and overdue" (Lowe and Archibald 2009, 17).

Nursing always has been and still is predominantly composed of white females. About 6.6 percent of the nursing workforce is made up of males (Health Resources and Services Administration 2010). While this figure represents a 38 percent increase in male nurses since 2000 (and an approximate 349 percent increase since the National Sample Survey of Registered Nurses was conducted in 1980), males still represent a very small percentage of the nursing workforce overall. Additionally, approximately 16.8 percent of the nursing workforce is made up of nonwhite or Hispanic nurses (Health Resources and Services Administration 2010). Similar to the percentage of males in nursing, nurses of diverse racial and ethnic backgrounds still represent a very small proportion of the overall nursing workforce, which does not mirror the composition of the US population at large.

Literature on the effects of workforce diversity on nurse staffing is largely absent. However, growing evidence suggests that individuals prefer to receive care from healthcare professionals who share their racial background and that healthcare professionals are more sensitive to the values and beliefs of patients from their own racial background (American Association of Colleges of Nursing 2014; Institute of Medicine 2004). Although the composition of the nursing workforce is changing, progress in achieving diversity in the last 20 years has been slow when compared to changes in the US population; however, data indicate that, overall, graduates of health occupation educational programs are generally more diverse than the workforce at large (Frogner and Spetz 2013). The continued movement to enhance diversity in the nursing workforce will require efforts that improve the nursing work environment and salaries for nursing personnel in general, and then more specific strategies that provide attractive employment opportunities to individuals from diverse backgrounds, including sensitivity to their cultural beliefs and embracing cultural competence in the healthcare workplace. Little has been done to examine the effectiveness of specific strategies to attract individuals from diverse backgrounds; thus, this area is ripe for research.

Several documents offer recommendations for healthcare leaders and managers on building a more diverse workplace (American Organization of Nurse Executives 2011; Institute of Medicine 2010):

- Create diversity and cultural competence through educational programs and standards.
- Provide opportunities for individuals of diverse racial and ethnic backgrounds to receive mentoring and guidance from leaders of similar and different backgrounds.
- Recognize the value of diversity on the patient care team, and promote diversity through hiring practices.
- Engage staff in developing a unit-based diversity plan.
- Seek information from nurses of diverse backgrounds to target recruitment and retention programs to diverse populations.
- Involve staff in recruitment and hiring decisions.
- Create leadership career paths for nurses from diverse backgrounds.

Unit and Organizational Knowledge

Efficient nurse staffing hinges on unit and organizational knowledge. First, knowledge of clinical policies is critical. For example, a manager who is staffing an oncology unit must be aware of the unit's clinical policy about patients on certain chemotherapeutic agents, the type of nursing personnel required to observe patients during treatment, the number of patients who typically receive these medications and treatments during a period of time, and the associated risks of the treatment. Second, knowledge of internal organizational changes in care delivery is needed to estimate the effect of changes in programs, procedures, or treatment protocols on staffing requirements. For example, if a new clinical guideline is developed regarding treatment of a particular type of oncology patient, the manager must understand the implications of the guideline's implementation on the numbers and types of staff required as well as their educational needs.

Third, knowledge of collective agreements is needed to ensure that staffing is in compliance with provisions agreed on. For example, if staff on the oncology unit can work no more than 60 hours per week and the unit has staffing vacancies, the manager will need to develop a plan in accordance with policy that covers shifts when unit needs exceed the supply and availability of existing staff. Fourth, knowledge of the internal and external organizational environment, such as anticipated structural changes or policy developments, is important. For example, if a second oncology unit will be opening to provide care to a specific group of patients, a plan must be in place to transition relevant existing staff to the new unit, cover the original unit, and hire additional staff as needed. Each of these pieces of information should be taken into account when calculating nurse staffing needs. The supplement to this chapter provides a detailed example of FTE and nurse staffing calculations.

Full-Time Equivalent Calculations

The metric for determining the numbers and types of nurses is the full-time equivalent or FTE. Nursing FTE calculations are used to determine unit and departmental staffing needs and are the key input to the budgeting process. An FTE is based on the concept of one individual working full time (40 hours a week) for a year, or 2,080 hours over a 52-week period (Finkler, Jones, and Kovner 2013).[6] FTE calculations include both productive and nonproductive time. Strasen (1987) defines *productive time* as time spent providing care to patients and *nonproductive time* as time spent not giving care. Nonproductive time includes sick, vacation, holiday, orientation, and professional development days as well as other paid time off that is part of the employment benefit (Klaus et al. 2013). The amount of nonproductive time for different types of personnel is based on organizational policy and may be associated with the individual's length of service to the organization. Although the amount of nonproductive time paid varies by organization, only productive time is used in calculating the amount of nurse workload available to deliver care to patients. See Exhibit 14.4 for an example.

The following data are needed to determine nursing FTEs and staffing (Finkler, Jones, and Kovner 2013):

- *Projected patient days.* A patient day is an accounting term that represents the concept of one patient who is cared for during a 24-hour period. Projected patient days are an estimate of future workload needs.
- *Nursing care hours (productive time) per patient day.* This is time spent delivering care to patients during a 24-hour period and is generally reported as a monthly average.
- *Staffing mix.* This is the proportion of RNs, LPNs, and unlicensed nursing personnel used to provide care in a 24-hour period.

EXHIBIT 14.4
Calculating FTEs

If organizational policy indicates that 90 percent of nurses' paid time is considered productive, and 10 percent is vacation, sick time, professional development, and non-patient-care time, then the organization has 0.90 × 2,080 hours paid per FTE = 1,872 productive hours per FTE.

Today, 12-hour shifts and other flexible schedules are commonplace. Under these arrangements, nurses may actually work less or more than 40 hours per week (Strasen 1987). Thus, the number of hours worked must be considered along with the policy regarding paid hours (i.e., total hours, both productive and nonproductive), and the number of productive hours per FTE must be taken into account when calculating unit FTEs (Finkler, Jones, and Kovner 2013). Nurse staffing calculations must take into account the fact that not all nursing personnel work full time. Many nurses work part time, providing managers with some degree of flexibility in staffing a patient care unit. On any particular patient care unit, FTEs may be composed of full-time staff only, part-time staff only, or most likely a mix of full-time and part-time staff. For example, on a patient care unit where full-time nurses work 7 days of 12-hour shifts in a 2-week pay period, the time per position exceeds 1 FTE:

12 hours per day × 7 days = 84 hours
84 hours in 2 weeks ÷ 80 hours in 2 weeks = 1.05 FTE

Alternatively, if full-time nurses on a patient care unit work 6 days of 12-hour shifts in a 2-week pay period, the time per position is less than 1 FTE:

12 hours per day × 6 days = 72 hours
72 hours in 2 weeks ÷ 80 hours in 2 weeks = 0.90 FTE

For illustration purposes, consider the example in Exhibit 14.5.

Balancing Quality and Costs of Care

Healthcare organizations are feeling increasing pressure to improve the quality of care while operating under a constrained financial environment. Also, during times when organizational revenues fall short of expenditures or healthcare costs rise, labor often becomes the target of budget cuts. This cost-cutting measure puts pressure on nurses because they are typically the largest group of professionals in the organization. Nurse staffing often comes under scrutiny in cases when the organization is considering whether the number of nurses can be reduced or whether the nurse workload and work hours can be increased.

Nurse staffing has received a great deal of attention because of society's increasing concerns about patient safety and the high-profile reports that document the relationship between low nurse-staffing levels and adverse patient events (Aiken et al. 2002; Aiken et al. 2003; Kovner and Gergen 1998; Kovner et al. 2002; Mark, Harless, and Berman 2007; Mark et al. 2004; McGillis Hall et al. 2003; McGillis Hall, Doran, and Pink 2004; Needleman et al. 2002, 2006, 2011). For example, Aiken and colleagues (2003) document that higher ratios of patients cared for per nurse are associated with a higher risk of mortality and failure to rescue among surgical patients. Specifically, the risk of death is 14 percent higher in hospitals where workloads or ratios are six or more patients per nurse, and this risk is 31 percent higher in hospitals with workloads of eight or more patients per nurse, relative to hospitals where

---

EXHIBIT 14.5
Calculating
Nursing Hours

A patient care unit that averages 25 patients per day during a 30-day month pays for 6,000 RN hours. Of these 6,000 RN hours, 90 percent are considered productive. What are the paid nursing hours per day and per patient day? How many nursing care hours per patient day are involved? Here are the calculations:

- *Paid nursing hours*
  6,000 nursing hours paid per month ÷ 30 days in the month = 200 paid nursing hours per day
  200 hours of nursing care per day ÷ 25 patients per day = 8.0 nursing hours paid per patient per day
- *Nursing care hours*
  6,000 nursing hours paid per month × 90 percent productive = 5,400 nursing care hours per month
  5,400 nursing care hours per month ÷ 30 days in the month = 180 nursing care hours per day
  180 hours of nursing care per day ÷ 25 patients per day = 7.2 nursing care hours per patient per day

nurse workloads are four or fewer patients per nurse. This study also found that hospitals that employ higher numbers of nurses with a baccalaureate (or higher) degree have lower patient mortality rates than hospitals that employ fewer nurses with a baccalaureate (or higher) degree.

Pay-for-performance programs, which strive to compensate healthcare providers on the basis of their achieving certain patient outcomes, are becoming commonplace in the US healthcare system. This approach evolved in an attempt to better align patient safety and quality of care with the payments rendered for the care actually received by patients. Payments to healthcare organizations are based on required outcomes data submitted on certain quality and patient safety metrics so that the public—including patients, insurers, and providers—is aware of the performance of specific organizations. The Centers for Medicare & Medicaid Services (CMS) and Hospital Quality Alliance (HQA) first required the public reporting of 30-day mortality measures for acute myocardial infarction and heart failure in June 2007, followed by rates of pneumonia in June 2008 (CMS 2014). The list of CMS-required publicly reported outcome measures also includes 30-day readmission rates for these same conditions, plus complications and readmission data for hip or knee replacements, in-hospital adverse events, and mortality. As noted on the CMS website, the public reporting of these measures "increases the transparency of hospital care, provides useful information for consumers choosing care, and assists hospitals in their quality improvement efforts" (CMS 2014). Using claims and administrative data, CMS makes outcome measures available on an annual basis to the public via its Hospital Compare website (www.hospitalcompare.org). Conflicting evidence exists regarding the effectiveness of pay for performance, but given that influential private groups, such as the Leapfrog Group, also reimburse providers based on pay-for-performance systems, this payment scheme will likely become the standard for reimbursing hospitals in the future.

Evidence is growing that suggests that the lowest-cost mix of nursing staff may not be the best option to improve quality of care and patient outcomes. In fact, Needleman and colleagues (2006) provide what they call an "unequivocal" business case for nurse staffing. Using existing data, they conducted three different nurse staffing simulations to determine associated costs: (1) increasing the proportion of RN nursing care hours per day to the 75th percentile for hospitals below that level; (2) increasing the number of nursing care hours per day to the 75th percentile for both RNs and LPNs, again for hospitals below that percentile; and (3) using a combination of the first two options. The results of these simulations indicated that increasing nurse staffing under the first option provided the greatest return on investment. That is, increasing RN hours only without increasing the total hours of licensed nursing staff was associated with a net reduction in costs.

Given that a richer RN staff has been documented to improve quality and to save money, changing nurse staffing to improve or sustain good patient outcomes may well be one of the best solutions for a unit or hospital to consider when examining ways to improve quality scores and in turn increase reimbursements. As Litvak and colleagues (2005) suggest, if one considers all of the patient safety measures being implemented, none of them can substitute for adequate nurse staffing. To ensure adequate staffing, managers can take several steps:

- Managers should stay up-to-date on current research to be familiar with evidence that can help build their case for justifying changes or modifications in nurse staffing.
- Managers should work with financial staff to develop and put in place a process for evaluating staffing costs relative to patient outcomes and quality. This kind of evaluation can be used to determine returns on investments made in modifying staffing levels and to develop a business case for modifying nurse staffing levels. It will also help managers understand how variations in staffing may affect patient and organizational outcomes.
- Managers must involve staff in any attempts to address quality of care or cost concerns through modifications in nurse staffing. By involving staff in decisions regarding changes in the numbers or types of unit-based staff, the manager will gain insights from frontline caregivers regarding how potential staff changes may affect patient care and staff. The net result likely will be an improved overall staffing strategy for the unit.

Looking to the Future

The Nursing Workforce of the Future

Two important policy events that occurred in 2010 are likely to significantly influence the direction of the nursing workforce in this country: The Affordable Care Act (ACA) was signed into law, and the Institute of Medicine released its report *The Future of Nursing: Leading Change, Advancing Health*.

The ACA (Public Law 111-148) was signed into law on March 23, 2010. The aim of the law was to expand insurance coverage, thus reducing the significant number of uninsured and underinsured Americans, as well as to reduce the rising cost of healthcare in this country (Finkler, Jones, and Kovner 2013). The ACA is expected to further stimulate the already growing healthcare economy in the United States (Frogner and Spetz 2013).

Workforce projections predict a 26 percent increase in nursing jobs by 2020, with one-third of the projected increases resulting from the ACA (Frogner and Spetz 2013; Spetz 2014). The majority of nursing jobs derived from the ACA are likely to be in the outpatient setting rather than in acute care settings (Auerbach, Buerhaus, and Staiger 2014; Spetz 2014). The skills required of nurses are likely to include care coordination, patient education, and case management, which may require additional education through continuing education or formal degree programs (Auerbach, Buerhaus, and Staiger 2014; Spetz 2014).

The Institute of Medicine report titled *The Future of Nursing: Leading Change, Advancing Health* identified four areas in which efforts are needed to advance nursing in the future (Institute of Medicine 2010, 4):

1. Barriers should be removed so that nurses have the ability to practice to the full scope of their education and training.
2. Nurses should obtain progressively higher levels of education and training in an improved educational system that promotes seamless academic progression (i.e., from undergraduate through graduate training).
3. Nurses should be full partners with physicians and other healthcare professionals in redesigning US healthcare.
4. Better data collection and improved information infrastructure support are needed to more effectively plan and inform policies aimed at improving the healthcare workforce.

The Future of Nursing: Leading Change, Advancing Health can help healthcare leaders and managers to embrace changes in their external environment created by the ACA by positioning nurses as leaders in meeting the needs of patients (Caramenico 2013; Ellerbe and Regen 2012):

- Leaders should clarify and support the role of the nurse so that nurses are empowered and enabled to practice to the full extent of their licenses (Ellerbe and Regen 2012).
- Schools of nursing throughout the country must work to efficiently and effectively train a nursing workforce that is prepared for the changing needs of the healthcare sector, particularly in the areas of patient care coordination, case management, and more complex roles in healthcare systems of the future (Auerbach, Buerhaus, and Staiger 2014).
- To better facilitate the Institute of Medicine's recommendation of seamless transition through the academic setting, healthcare leaders and managers should encourage educational advancement among nurses

by providing tuition reimbursement and other educational incentives (Ellerbe and Regen 2012).

- To encourage nurses' involvement in the redesign of the healthcare system, healthcare leaders and managers should encourage nurses' involvement in local, state, and national nursing organizations that represent nurses' perspectives in the shaping of an improved healthcare system (Ellerbe and Regen 2012).

- Finally, healthcare organizations collect a wealth of information on quality and safety indicators within their hospitals. By participating in national databases such as the National Database of Nursing Quality Indicators, organizations can contribute to a better data collection infrastructure (Ellerbe and Regen 2012).

The Nurse Workforce and Information Technology

Technology is changing all areas of our world, and the healthcare industry is no exception (Huston 2013). Advances in information technology (IT) affect care delivery and enable managers to capture the costs and quality indicators associated with care delivery (Vlasses and Smeltzer 2007). Three specific areas where IT is likely to affect the nurse workforce are electronic health records (EHRs), computerized physician/provider order entry (CPOE) systems, and administrative information systems that improve organizational performance and decision making, including nurse staffing technologies.

EHRs have changed the way that nurses document their patients' health and the care they receive (Huston 2013). When President George W. Bush was in office, he set the national goal of moving toward EHRs for all patients by 2014, and President Barack Obama continued the same support for widespread adoption with financial assistance for hospitals to implement EHRs (Huston 2013). While tremendous strides have been made in the adoption of EHRs in healthcare organizations in the United States, significant challenges in full-scale adoption remain. One particular hurdle is the capacity to share the EHR with patients; only 10.4 percent of hospitals have that capability (Millman 2014).

CPOE systems allow providers to write orders for patients electronically rather than on paper (Spaulding and Raghu 2013). This technology is in widespread use in hospitals and is considered an important safeguard in providing safe, high-quality care to patients (Spaulding and Raghu 2013). The increased utilization of CPOE systems has affected how nurses perform their work. In particular, a study on the effects of CPOE systems on the work of nursing found that the use of CPOE created gaps in nurses' knowledge about their patients, particularly information about the psychosocial aspects of patient care (Zhou, Ackerman, and Zheng 2010).

Measuring nurse workload and staffing and acting on the results are issues that have occupied healthcare managers and researchers for decades. As Edwardson and Giovannetti (1994) suggest, many thought that patient classification systems would identify the right numbers of staff to provide care for certain patients. However, these systems proved to be problematic, especially in terms of their reliability and validity, leaving managers with the need to establish nurse workloads and calculate nurse staffing needs for their units. Also, healthcare organizations lack the ability to completely free nurses from many non-nursing tasks (e.g., retrieving medications from the pharmacy in some hospitals) that further increase nurse workloads but do not require specific nursing knowledge to carry out (Moody 2004).

Moody (2004) advocated a nurse workload approach that is grounded in human capital theory. This approach uses a nursing productivity index that takes into account nurses' knowledge, skills, and abilities (i.e., human capital) and the needs of patients for whom they provide care. Moody's model captures data on patient intensity, nurse staffing, infection and error rates, organizational resources (financial and human), patient outcomes, patients' ability to provide self-care, and provider outcomes. This idea of valuing nurses' work on the basis of knowledge, skills, and abilities is intuitively appealing and is aligned with computerized systems such as the Clinical Demand Index noted earlier in this chapter, which estimates the intensity of nursing on the basis of how nurses spend their time, data mining techniques, and data on variables that reflect these metrics (Harper 2012).

Computerized nurse workload and staffing systems that take into account short-term staffing contingencies and variability in patient demand, improve the deployment of nursing personnel, and facilitate the development of long-term staffing plans are needed. Queuing theory and other operations management techniques can be used to understand and manage variability, smooth the extremes of demand, and reduce stress on the system (Litvak et al. 2005). By eliminating or minimizing controllable variability (e.g., appropriate use of block scheduling for physicians' operating room time, more coordinated discharge planning), healthcare organizations can then better staff for uncontrollable or patient-driven demand, and minimize the use of necessary and unnecessary resources and dollars spent on healthcare delivery.

Pickard and Warner (2007) discussed the use of a demand management model to support staffing that is based on patient outcomes, measured in real time, and used to project future short-term patient demand (i.e., days). These requirements are embedded in a decision-support system that uses electronically captured data. This approach forecasts demand for controllable (provider-imposed, including scheduling of elective surgeries and patient discharges) and uncontrollable (patient- and disease-driven, such as patient admissions through the emergency department) variability by incorporating progress patterns for different types of patients; scheduled and predictable unscheduled admissions (based on staff input and historical data); and staffing information to help identify demand by unit, by day, and by hour and shift, which can then be used in making short-term staffing projections. Staffing is continuously updated on the basis of patient outcomes and progress.

Although electronic systems such as the demand management model are becoming more commonplace, they are not a substitute for the critical judgment of managers, who possess unique knowledge of nurse workload measurement, the work of nurses, clinical care processes, and the patients whom nurses serve. Healthcare managers can contribute unique insights into nurse staffing to proactively plan and ensure that (1) nurses are involved in decisions that affect unit operations and nurse workloads, (2) adequate nursing resources are available to provide patient care, and (3) adequate support services are in place to support nurses and relieve them of performing nonessential tasks (Burke 2003).

As new and emerging technologies are implemented in healthcare organizations, the following recommendations may be helpful to leaders (Huston 2013; Kutney-Lee and Kelly 2011):

- Healthcare leaders and managers need to champion the appropriate use of EHRs to staff as a means of improving the quality and safety of care that patients receive.

- Staff should be reminded regularly to avoid allowing technology to inhibit face-to-face communication. Losing sight of the patient can be easy as technology takes a more important role in patient care.

- Healthcare leaders and managers must understand the fundamentals of nurse staffing and workload, and ensure that nurses are engaged in developing relevant staffing parameters.

- Adequate education must be provided and sufficient resources must be allocated for the implementation and ongoing training required to achieve staff comfort and competence in the use of healthcare IT.

Nurses and Value-Based Purchasing

As discussed earlier in this chapter, the US healthcare environment is shaped by an ever-increasing focus on both the cost and the quality of care provided to patients. Along with the ACA's goal of expanding insurance coverage is a focus on containing the rising costs of healthcare. As the healthcare industry transitions from a fee-for-service pay structure to a value-based purchasing or pay-for-performance model, healthcare organizations will look to nursing for improvements in care delivery and, in turn, a reduction in costs.

Value-based purchasing is based on six domains of performance: patient safety, care coordination, clinical processes and outcomes, population and community health, efficiency and cost reduction, and patient- and caregiver-centered experience (Blumenthal and Jena 2012, 274). Nurses have a significant influence on each of these domains and will be key players in improving hospital performance in these areas. For example, Wolosin, Ayala, and Fulton (2012) demonstrated that the largest determinant of patient satisfaction scores is nursing care. Results from another study indicated that higher nurse retention rates in nursing homes were associated with lower 30-day rehospitalization rates (Thomas et al. 2013). An additional study in a pediatric intensive care unit showed significant reductions in healthcare-acquired infections after three different interventions were implemented with significant buy-in from nursing staff (Harris et al. 2011).

In 2008, key leaders from practice, research, and professional organizations held a staffing summit to identify best practices in nurse staffing and to develop a model of staffing excellence that would inform future work in the field. After years of work, review, and revisions, the Data-Driven Model for Excellence in Staffing (Anderson et al. 2014) has evolved as a way of conceptualizing nurse staffing to span the settings where nurses work (beyond hospitals) and the continuum of service-research-innovation to value nurses' contributions to care delivery. This evidence-based model addresses five core concepts: healthcare users and patients; healthcare providers; the environments where care is delivered; the delivery of care; and quality, safety, and outcomes of care. This model builds on the changes proposed in both the ACA (e.g., prevention, new models of care delivery across the care continuum, new payment structures) and the Institute of Medicine's *Future of Nursing* report (removal of barriers to allow nurses to practice to their full scope of education, advancement of education and training, partnership in leading healthcare change, improved data collection and infrastructure to support workforce planning). The intent of this project is to serve as a catalyst for improving nurse staffing by examining best practices, fostering future research and dissemination, translating relevant research findings into practice, and removing barriers that impede nurse staffing innovations.

These studies and others demonstrate the important influence nurses have on performance outcomes, which ultimately influence the bottom line of healthcare organizations. More important, however, is the valuable role nurses play in improving the quality and safety of care delivered to patients. Healthcare leaders and managers must look to nurses as they seek to improve performance in value-based purchasing domains. They must also provide leadership by embracing changes in future nurse staffing practices and taking bold steps to recognize the important role that nurses play by adding value in care delivery.

Summary

Nurses are key members of the healthcare team. Understanding how best to deploy nurses while balancing quality and costs is an important ongoing function for healthcare managers that may be especially challenging during periods of nursing shortage, in which adequate numbers and types of nurses to ensure the delivery of safe, high-quality care may be in short supply. Even when nursing resources are in greater supply, understanding the fundamentals of allocating nursing resources is essential. This chapter provides an overview and examples of important tools and techniques that can be used to calculate nurse workload. Use of these tools and techniques aids in the routine planning of patient care delivery, development of unit and organizational budgets, and the equitable distribution of nursing staff. More importantly, however, use of these practices will foster the creation of an environment that increases nurse job satisfaction and well-being and that decreases the stress and burnout often associated with high workloads and inadequate staffing. Over the long run, sensitivity to nurse workload and staffing issues will contribute to the delivery of high-quality patient care, the formation of high-performing patient care teams, greater financial returns, and improvements in overall organizational performance.

Discussion Questions

1. What are the elements that compose nurse workload?

2. How is nurse workload related to nurse staffing?

3. What critical data are necessary to assemble before calculating nurse staffing needs?

4. How is organizational philosophy reflected in the measurement of nurse workload?

5. What other workforce issues may affect nurse staffing? How and why do these issues relate to nurse staffing and workload?

Experiential Exercises

Exercise 1 Needleman and colleagues (2006) examine different nurse staffing arrangements in a *Health Affairs* article titled "Nurse Staffing in Hospitals: Is There a Business Case for Quality?" In this study, the authors used nurse staffing and patient discharge data from 799 US hospitals to simulate three different nurse staffing approaches and to determine which of these options produced the greatest cost savings. Read this article, and then answer the following questions.

Questions

1. Assume that you are the manager of a 30-bed general medical-surgical unit at a 200-bed community hospital. How can you use the findings from this article to help make staffing decisions on your unit?

2. What other important data sources will you examine before making a decision to increase or decrease the nurse-to-patient ratio?

Exercise 2   The Joint Commission's staffing effectiveness standard requires that hospitals provide written reports annually on "all system or process failures, the number and type of sentinel event, information provided to families/patients about the events, and actions taken to improve patient safety" (see Phillion 2010). In turn, these undesirable events must be examined relative to staffing; if negative staff trends are observed, a report must be filed with the organization's leadership. Most healthcare organizations must meet this requirement to receive Joint Commission accreditation, and that accreditation is paramount to the ability of hospitals to operate and receive reimbursement.

Questions

Visit two patient care units at a local hospital, and talk to the manager of each one. Ask the following questions of each manager:

Exercise 3   Susan is the nurse manager in charge of a 25-bed medical unit at St. Eligius Hospital. She is preparing the nurse staffing plan for the next fiscal year. Hospital management has provided all nurse managers with a list of assumptions for staff planning, most of

3. Now consider that you are the chief executive officer at a large academic health hospital in an urban setting. Over the next two years, the nurse staffing ratio on the general medical-surgical units in your facility is projected to decrease from one nurse per six patients to one nurse per four patients. How will you estimate the costs and savings of such a change? Be sure to consider the organization's philosophy of care in your evaluation plan.

1. How has your unit interpreted The Joint Commission's staffing effectiveness standards?

2. How have unit operations changed as a result of this standard?

3. How has this implementation affected the quality of care delivered to patients on your unit?

4. How has the nursing staff on your unit responded to this implementation?

Following the interviews, compare and contrast the two managers' approaches for meeting the required staffing effectiveness standards. Is one approach better than the other? How can you use the experiences of these two unit managers to inform your own nurse workload and staffing decisions in the future?

which are to use last year's numbers as first estimates for next year. Susan has assembled the following data for last year:

- The percentage of productive nursing hours was 83 percent.

- Fifty-two percent of nursing staff worked days, and 48 percent worked nights.
- The nursing staff was made up of 74 percent RNs, 16 percent LPNs, and 10 percent unlicensed nursing personnel (NAs).

- At St. Eligius Hospital, 1.0 FTE = 2,080 hours.

Susan also assembled information from the hospital's patient classification system for last year (see Exhibit 14.6).

Patient Classification Level	Historical Patient Days	Historical Average Care Hours per Patient Day	Historical Total Unit Workload
1	1,000	4	4,000
2	2,000	6	12,000
3	3,000	10	30,000
4	2,000	14	28,000
5	1,000	18	18,000
Total	9,000		92,000

EXHIBIT 14.6
Patient Classification Data

Susan is an experienced manager and is aware of several changes that will affect the nursing unit in the next year. More specifically, Dr. Smith, a senior physician who accounted for a large proportion of the unit's admissions, has just retired. In recent years, Dr. Smith has limited his practice to simpler medical cases, referring more complex cases to specialists who do not admit to the medical unit.

Dr. Jones just started at the hospital; she was recruited to replace Dr. Smith. Dr. Jones is a recent graduate who intends to care for many of the complex patients whom Dr. Smith previously referred to other specialists. Although the hospital projects that the unit's patient days will not differ from historical patient days, Susan is projecting a change in the mix of patients because of the arrival of Dr. Jones: 500 level 1 patient days, 1,500 level 2 days, 3,000 level 3 days, 2,500 level 4 days, and 1,500 level 5 days. Susan also knows that Dr. Jones plans to do more complex treatments during the day, which will (1) increase the percentage of nursing staff who work days to 57 percent and reduce the percentage who work nights to 43 percent and (2) increase the percentage of nursing staff who are RNs to 78 percent, decrease LPNs to 14 percent, and decrease NAs to 8 percent.

Questions

1. Based on Susan's projection of patient days, what is the projected total unit workload by patient classification level? What differences do you notice between the projected and the historic total unit workload?

2. Calculate the historical number of FTEs by staff type and by shift. On the basis of Susan's projection of patient days, calculate the projected number of FTEs by staff type and shift. What differences do you notice between the projected and historic FTEs?

Notes

1. LPNs are known as licensed vocational nurses (LVNs) in California and Texas (Bureau of Labor Statistics 2014).
2. For budgeting purposes, the patient care unit or department represents a cost center or entity for which nursing workload is determined.
3. Nurse managers oversee the day-to-day operations of patient care units. Other healthcare managers may serve in this capacity as well. However, nurse managers commonly fill this role because they understand clinical care processes, the implications of nursing practice, and the scope of practice for different types of nursing personnel at the point of care delivery.
4. Patient needs and care requirements vary, even within the same disease category or classification.
5. The practice of pulling nurses from their regularly assigned unit to work on another understaffed unit is often referred to as *floating*.
6. In a two-week pay period, 1 FTE equals 80 hours.

References

Advisory Board Company. 1999. "A Misplaced Focus: Reexamining the Recruiting/Retention Trade-Off." *Nursing Watch* 11: 1–14.

Aiken, L. H., S. P. Clarke, R. B. Cheung, D. M. Sloane, and J. H. Silber. 2003. "Educational Levels of Hospital Nurses and Surgical Patient Mortality." *Journal of the American Medical Association* 290 (12): 1617–23.

Aiken, L. H., S. P. Clarke, D. M. Sloane, J. Sochalski, and J. H. Silber. 2002. "Hospital Nurse Staffing and Patient Mortality, Nurse Burnout, and Job Dissatisfaction." *Journal of the American Medical Association* 288 (16): 1987–93.

Aiken, L. H., D. M. Sloane, J. P. Cimiotti, S. P. Clarke, L. Flynn, J. A. Seago, J. Spetz, and H. L. Smith. 2010. "Implications of the California Staffing Mandate for Other States." *Health Services Research* 45 (4): 904–21.

American Association of Colleges of Nursing. 2014. "Enhancing Diversity in the Workforce." Updated January 21. www.aacn.nche.edu/media-relations/fact-sheets/enhancing-diversity.

American Nurses Association. 2014. "Nurse Staffing Plans and Ratios." Updated December. www.nursingworld.org/MainMenuCategories/Policy-Advocacy/State/Legislative-Agenda-Reports/State-StaffingPlansRatios.

American Organization of Nurse Executives. 2011. *AONE Guiding Principles for Diversity in Health Care Organizations.* Accessed January 9, 2015. www.aone.org/resources/PDFs/AONE_GP_Diversity.pdf.

Anderson, R., S. Ellerbe, S. Haas, K. Kerfoot, K. Kirby, and D. Nickitas. 2014. "Excellence and Evidence in Staffing: A Data-Driven Model for Excellence in Staffing (2nd Edition)." *Nursing Economic$* 32 (3 suppl.): 1–36.

Auerbach, D. I., P. I. Buerhaus, and D. O. Staiger. 2014. "Registered Nurses Are Delaying Retirement, a Shift That Has Contributed to Recent Growth in the Nurse Workforce." *Health Affairs* 33 (8): 1474–80.

Barker, L. M, and M. A. Nussbaum. 2011. "Fatigue, Performance and the Work Environment: A Survey of Registered Nurses." *Journal of Advanced Nursing* 67 (6): 1370–82.

Block, V. J., and P. A. Jamerson. 2005. "Running a Successful Campaign Against Unionization." *Journal of Nursing Administration* 35 (1): 29–34.

Blumenthal, D., and A. B. Jena. 2012. "Hospital Value-Based Purchasing." *Journal of Hospital Medicine* 8 (5): 271–77.

Buerhaus, P. I. 2010. "It's Time to Stop the Regulation of Hospital Nursing Staff Dead in Its Tracks." *Nursing Economic$* 28 (2): 110–13.

Buerhaus, P., D. Auerbach, and D. Staiger. 2009. "The Recent Surge in Nurse Employment: Causes and Implications." *Health Affairs* 28 (4): w657–w668.

Bureau of Labor Statistics. 2014. *Occupational Outlook Handbook, 2014–15 Edition.* US Department of Labor. Published January 8. www.bls.gov/oco/.

Burke, R. J. 2003. "Hospital Restructuring, Workload, and Nursing Staff Satisfaction and Work Experiences." *Health Care Manager* 22 (2): 99–107.

Caramenico, A. 2013. "How Healthcare Reform Affects Nurses." *FierceHealthcare.* Published October 24. www.fiercehealthcare.com/story/how-healthcare-reforms-affect-nurses/2013-10-24.

Centers for Medicare & Medicaid Services (CMS). 2014. "Outcome Measures." Modified October 31. www.cms.gov/Medicare/Quality-Initiatives-Patient-Assessment-Instruments/HospitalQualityInits/OutcomeMeasures.html.

Clark, P. F., and D. Clark. 2009. "Nurses' Unions Efforts to Give RNs a Greater Voice in Patient Care." *LERA 61st Annual Proceedings.* Accessed January 9, 2015. http://assets.conferencespot.org/fileserver/file/120650/filename/2009_357.pdf.

Coursey, J. H., R. E. Rodriguez, L. S. Dieckmann, and P. N. Austin. 2013. "Successful Implementation of Policies Addressing Lateral Violence." *AORN Journal* 97 (1): 101–9.

Dean, G. E., L. D. Scott, and A. E. Rogers. 2006. "Infants at Risk: When Nurse Fatigue Jeopardizes Quality Care." *Advances in Neonatal Care* 6 (3): 120–26.

DeGroot, H. A. 1989. "Patient Classification System Evaluation: Part 2, System Selection and Implementation." *Journal of Nursing Administration* 19 (7): 24–30.

Edwardson, S. R., and P. B. Giovannetti. 1994. "Nursing Workload Measurement Systems." *Annual Review of Nursing Research* 12 (1): 95–123.

Ellerbe, S., and D. Regen. 2012. "Responding to Health Care Reform by Addressing the Institute of Medicine Report on the Future of Nursing." *Nursing Administration Quarterly* 36 (3): 210–16.

Fasoli, D. R., and S. Haddock. 2010. "Results of an Integrative Review of Patient Classification Systems." *Annual Review of Nursing Research* 28 (1): 295–316.

Finkler, S. A., C. B. Jones, and C. T. Kovner. 2013. *Financial Management for Nurse Managers and Executives,* fourth edition. Philadelphia, PA: W. B. Saunders.

Fitzpatrick, M. A. 2001. "Collective Bargaining, Part 1: A Vulnerability Assessment." *Nursing Management* 32 (2): 41–42.

Forman, H., and G. A. Davis. 2002. "The Rising Tide of Healthcare Labor Unions in Nursing." *Journal of Nursing Administration* 32 (7/8): 376–78.

Forman, H., and T. A. Powell. 2003. "Managing During an Employee Walkout." *Journal of Nursing Administration* 33 (9): 430–33.

Frogner, B., and J. Spetz. 2013. *Affordable Care Act of 2010: Creating Job Opportunities for Racially and Ethnically Diverse Populations.* Joint Center for Political and Economic Studies. Published October. http://jointcenter.org/sites/default/files/Affordable%20Care%20Act%20of%202010_0.pdf.

Gabriel, A. S., R. J. Erickson, C. M. Moran, J. M. Diefendorff, and G. E. Bromley. 2013. "A Multilevel Analysis of the Effects of the Practice Environment Scale of the Nursing Work Index on Nurse Outcomes." *Research in Nursing & Health* 36 (6): 567–81.

Gaudine, A. P. 2000. "What Do Nurses Mean by Workload and Work Overload?" *Canadian Journal of Nursing Leadership* 13 (2): 22–27.

Greene, J. 2005. "What Nurses Want: Different Generations. Different Expectations." *Hospitals and Health Networks* 79 (3): 34–38, 40–42.

Gruber, J., and S. A. Kleiner. 2012. "Do Strikes Kill? Evidence from New York State." *American Economic Journal: Economic Policy* 4 (1): 127–57.

Harless, D. W., and B. A. Mark. 2010. "Nurse Staffing and Quality of Care with Direct Measurement of Inpatient Staffing." *Medical Care* 48 (7): 659–63.

Harper, E. M. 2012. "Staffing Based on Evidence: Can Health Information Technology Make It Possible?" *Nursing Economic$* 30 (5): 262–67, 281.

Harris, B. D., C. Hanson, C. Christy, T. Adams, A. Banks, T. S. Willis, and M. L. Maciejewski. 2011. "Strict Hand Hygiene and Other Practices Shortened Stays and Cut Costs and Mortality in a Pediatric Intensive Care Unit." *Health Affairs* 30 (9): 1751–61.

Hayes, B., A. Bonner, and J. Pryor. 2010. "Factors Contributing to Nurse Job Satisfaction in the Acute Hospital Setting: A Review of Recent Literature." *Journal of Nursing Management* 18 (7): 804–14.

Health Resources and Services Administration. 2010. *The Registered Nurse Population: Findings from the 2008 National Sample Survey of Registered Nurses.* Published September. http://bhpr.hrsa.gov/healthworkforce/rnsurveys/rnsurveyfinal.pdf.

Hendricks, J. M., and V. C. Cope. 2013. "Generational Diversity: What Nurse Managers Need to Know." *Journal of Advanced Nursing* 69 (3): 717–25.

Huston, C. 2013. "The Impact of Emerging Technology on Nursing Care: Warp Speed Ahead." *Online Journal of Issues in Nursing* 18 (2): Manuscript 1. Published May 31. http://nursingworld.org/MainMenuCategories/ANA Marketplace/ANAPeriodicals/OJIN/TableofContents/Vol-18-2013/No2-May-2013/Impact-of-Emerging-Technology.html.

Institute of Medicine. 2010. *The Future of Nursing: Leading Change, Advancing Health.* Washington, DC: National Academies Press.

———. 2004. *In the Nation's Compelling Interest: Ensuring Diversity in the Health Care Workforce.* Washington, DC: National Academies Press.

Jansky, S. 2004. "The Nurse–Physician Relationship: Is Collaboration the Answer?" *Journal of Practical Nursing* 54 (2): 28–30.

Jennings, B. M. 2008. "Patient Acuity." In *Patient Safety and Quality: An Evidence-Based Handbook for Nurses,* edited by R. G. Hughes, 1–8. Rockville, MD: Agency for Healthcare Research and Quality.

Joint Commission. 2014. "CMS Renews Joint Commission Hospital Accreditation Deeming Authority." Published June 30. www.jointcommission.org/cms_renews_joint_commission_hospital_accreditation_deeming_authority/.

———. 2002. *Health Care at the Crossroads: Strategies for Addressing the Evolving Nursing Crisis.* Accessed January 9, 2015. www.jointcommission.org/assets/1/18/health_care_at_the_crossroads.pdf.

Jones, C. B. 2005. "The Costs of Nursing Turnover, Part 2: Application of the Nursing Turnover Cost Calculation Methodology." *Journal of Nursing Administration* 35 (1): 41–49.

———. 2004. "The Costs of Nursing Turnover, Part 1: An Economic Perspective." *Journal of Nursing Administration* 34 (12): 562–70.

Kane, R. L., T. Shamliyan, C. Mueller, S. Duval, and T. Wilt. 2007. *Nursing Staffing and Quality of Patient Care.* Evidence Report/Technology Assessment No. 151. AHRQ Publication No. 07-E005. Rockville, MD: Agency for Healthcare Research and Quality.

Klaus, S. F., N. Dunton, B. Gajewski, and C. Potter. 2013. "Reliability of the Nursing Care Hour Measure: A Descriptive Study." *International Journal of Nursing Studies* 50 (7): 924–32.

Koehoorn, M., G. S. Lowe, K. V. Rondeau, G. S. Schellenberg, and T. H. Wagar. 2002. *Creating High-Quality Health Care Workplaces.* Ottawa, Canada: Canadian Policy Research Networks and Canadian Health Services Research Foundation.

Kovner, C. T., C. Brewer, Y. Wu, Y. Cheng, and M. Suzuki. 2006. "Factors Associated with Work Satisfaction of Registered Nurses." *Journal of Nursing Scholarship* 38 (1): 71–79.

Kovner, C. T., and P. J. Gergen. 1998. "Nurse Staffing Levels and Adverse Events Following Surgery in U.S. Hospitals." *Image: Journal of Nursing Scholarship* 30 (4): 315–21.

Kovner, C. T., C. B. Jones, C. Zahn, P. Gergen, and J. Basu. 2002. "Nurse Staffing and Post-Surgical Adverse Events: An Analysis of Administrative Data from a Sample of U.S. Hospitals, 1990–1996." *Health Services Research* 37 (3): 611–29.

Kutney-Lee, A., and D. Kelly. 2011. "The Effect of Hospital Electronic Health Record Adoption on Nurse-Assessed Quality of Care and Patient Safety." *Journal of Nursing Administration* 41 (11): 466–72.

Kutney-Lee, A., M. D. McHugh, D. M. Sloane, J. P. Cimiotti, L. Flynn, D. F. Neff, and L. H. Aiken. 2009. "Nursing: A Key to Patient Satisfaction." *Health Affairs* 28 (4): w669–w677.

Lankshear, A. J., T. A. Sheldon, and A. Maynard. 2005. "Nurse Staffing and Healthcare Outcomes: A Systematic Review of the International Research Evidence." *Advances in Nursing Science* 28 (2): 163–74.

Laschinger, H. K. S., and M. P. Leiter. 2006. "The Impact of Nursing Work Environments on Patient Safety Outcomes: The Mediating Role of Burnout/Engagement." *Journal of Nursing Administration* 36 (5): 259–67.

Li, Y., and C. B. Jones. 2013. "A Literature Review of Nursing Turnover Costs." *Journal of Nursing Management* 21 (3): 405–18.

Litvak, E., P. I. Buerhaus, F. Davidof, M. C. Long, M. L. McManus, and D. M. Berwick. 2005. "Managing Unnecessary Variability in Patient Demand to Reduce Nursing Stress and Improve Patient Safety." *Journal of Quality and Patient Safety* 31 (6): 330–38.

Lovell, V. 2006. *Solving the Nursing Shortage Through Higher Wages*. Institute for Women's Policy Research. Accessed January 9, 2015. www.iwpr.org/publications/pubs/solving-the-nursing-shortage-through-higher-wages/at_download/file.

Lowe, J., and C. Archibald. 2009. "Cultural Diversity: The Intention of Nursing." *Nursing Forum* 44 (1): 11–18.

Malloch, K., and A. Conovaloff. 1999. "Patient Classification Systems, Part 1: The Third Generation." *Journal of Nursing Administration* 29 (7/8): 49–56.

Mark, B. A., D. W. Harless, and W. F. Berman. 2007. "Nurse Staffing and Adverse Events in Hospitalized Children." *Policy, Politics and Nursing Practice* 8 (2): 83–92.

Mark, B. A., D. W. Harless, M. McCue, and Y. Xu. 2004. "A Longitudinal Examination of Hospital Registered Nurse Staffing and Quality of Care." *Health Services Research* 39 (2): 279–300.

Mark, B. A., D. W. Harless, J. Spetz, K. L. Reiter, and G. H. Pink. 2013. "California's Minimum Nurse Staffing Legislation: Results from a Natural Experiment." *Health Services Research* 48 (2, pt. 1): 435–54.

Mark, B. A., L. C. Hughes, and C. B. Jones. 2004. "The Role of Theory in Improving Patient Safety and Quality Health Care." *Nursing Outlook* 52 (1): 11–16.

Matthews, S., and S. Lankshear. 2003. "Describing the Essential Elements of a Professional Practice Structure." *Canadian Journal of Nursing Leadership* 16 (2): 63–73.

McGillis Hall, L., D. Doran, G. R. Baker, G. H. Pink, S. Sidani, L. O'Brien-Pallas, and G. J. Donner. 2003. "Nurse Staffing Models as Predictors of Patient Outcomes." *Medical Care* 41 (9): 1096–109.

McGillis Hall, L., D. Doran, and G. H. Pink. 2004. "Nurse Staffing Models, Nursing Hours, and Patient Safety Outcomes." *Journal of Nursing Administration* 34 (1): 41–45.

McHugh, M. D., A. Kutney-Lee, J. P. Cimiotti, D. M. Sloane, and L. H. Aiken. 2011. "Nurses' Widespread Job Dissatisfaction, Burnout, and Frustration with Health Benefits Signal Problems for Patient Care." *Health Affairs* 30 (2): 202–10.

Millman, J. 2014. "Electronic Health Records Were Supposed to Be Everywhere This Year. They're Not—but It's Okay." *Washington Post.* Published August 7. www.washingtonpost.com/blogs/wonkblog/wp/2014/08/07/electronic-health-records-were-supposed-to-be-everywhere-this-year-theyre-not-but-its-okay/.

Moody, K. 2014. "Competition and Conflict: Union Growth in the U.S. Hospital Industry." *Economic and Industrial Democracy* 35 (1): 5–25.

Moody, R. C. 2004. "Nurse Productivity Measures for the 21st Century." *Health Care Management Review* 29 (2): 98–106.

Needleman, J., P. Buerhaus, S. Mattke, M. Stewart, and K. Zelevinsky. 2002. "Nurse-Staffing Levels and the Quality of Care in Hospitals." *New England Journal of Medicine* 346 (22): 1715–22.

Needleman, J., P. Buerhaus, S. Pankratz, C. Leibson, S. R. Stevens, and M. Harris. 2011. "Nurse Staffing and Inpatient Hospital Mortality." *New England Journal of Medicine* 364 (11): 1037–45.

Needleman, J., P. I. Buerhaus, M. Stewart, K. Zelevinsky, and S. Mattke. 2006. "Nurse Staffing in Hospitals: Is There a Business Case for Quality?" *Health Affairs* 25 (1): 204–11.

Needleman, J., and S. Hassmiller. 2009. "The Role of Nurses in Improving Hospital Quality and Efficiency: Real-World Results." *Health Affairs* 28 (4): w625–w633.

O'Brien, A. J., M. Abas, J. Christensen, T. H. Nicholls, T. L. Prou, A. Hekau, and J. Vanderpyl. 2002. *Nursing Workload Measurement in Acute Mental Health Inpatient Units: A Report for the Mental Health Research and Development Strategy.* Auckland, New Zealand: Health Research Council of New Zealand.

O'Brien-Pallas, L., J. Hiroz, A. Cook, and B. Mildon. 2005. *Nurse–Physician Relationships: Solutions & Recommendations for Change.* Toronto, ON, Canada: Nursing Health Services Research Unit.

Philbin, S. 2007. "Managing Ambiguity and Danger in an Intensive Therapy Unit: Ritual Practices and Sequestration." *Nursing Inquiry* 14 (1): 51–59.

Phillion, M. 2010. "Joint Commission Issues Interim Staffing Effectiveness Standards." *Health Leaders Media*. Published February 10. www.healthleaders media.com/print/HR-246346/Joint-Commission-Issues-Interim-Staffing-Effectiveness-Standards.

Pickard, B., and M. Warner. 2007. "Demand Management: A Methodology for Outcomes-Driven Staffing and Patient Flow Management." *Nurse Leader* 4 (2): 30–34.

Pontus, C. 2011. "Is It Lateral Violence, Bullying or Workplace Harassment?" *Massachusetts Nurse Newsletter*. Published April 15. www.massnurses.org/news-and-events/archive/2011/p/openItem/6082.

Porter-O'Grady, T. 2001. "Collective Bargaining, Part 3: The Union as Partner." *Nursing Management* 32 (6): 30–32.

Potter, P., S. Boxerman, L. Wolf, J. Marshall, D. Grayson, J. Sledge, and B. Evanoff. 2004. "Mapping the Nursing Process: A New Approach for Understanding the Work of Nursing." *Journal of Nursing Administration* 34 (2): 101–9.

Prescott, P. A., and K. L. Soeken. 1996. "Measuring Nursing Intensity in Ambulatory Care, Part I: Approaches to and Uses of Patient Classification Systems." *Nursing Economic$* 14 (1): 14–21, 33.

Purpora, C., and M. A. Blegen. 2012. "Horizontal Violence and the Quality and Safety of Patient Care: A Conceptual Model." *Nursing Research and Practice* 28 (5): 306–14.

Rogers, A. E., W. T. Hwang, L. D. Scott, L. H. Aiken, and D. F. Dinges. 2004. "The Working Hours of Hospital Staff Nurses and Patient Safety." *Health Affairs* 23 (4): 202–12.

Rosenstein, A. H. 2002. "Nurse–Physician Relationships: Impact on Nurse Satisfaction and Retention." *American Journal of Nursing* 102 (6): 26–34.

Rosenstein, A. H., and M. O'Daniel. 2005. "Disruptive Behavior and Clinical Outcomes: Perceptions of Nurses and Physicians." *American Journal of Nursing* 105 (1): 54–64.

Schmalenberg, C., and M. Kramer. 2009. "Nurse-Physician Relationships in Hospitals: 20,000 Nurses Tell Their Story." *Critical Care Nurse* 29 (1): 74–83.

Schmalenberg, C., M. Kramer, C. R. King, M. Krugman, C. Lund, D. Poduska, and D. Rapp. 2005. "Excellence Through Evidence: Securing Collegial/Collaborative Nurse–Physician Relationships, Part 1." *Journal of Nursing Administration* 35 (10): 450–58.

Schraeder, M., and L. H. Friedman. 2002. "Collective Bargaining in the Nursing Profession: Salient Issues and Recent Developments in Healthcare Reform." *Hospital Topics* 80 (3): 21–24.

Scott, L. D., A. E. Rogers, W. T. Hwang, and Y. Zhang. 2006. "Effects of Critical Care Nurses' Work Hours on Vigilance and Patients' Safety." *American Journal of Critical Care* 15 (1): 30–37.

Seago, J. A. 2001. "Nurse Staffing, Models of Care Delivery, and Interventions." In *Making Health Care Safer: A Critical Analysis of Patient Safety Practices*, edited by K. G. Shojania, B. W. Duncan, K. M. McDonald, and R. M. Wachter, 423–46. Evidence Report/Technology Assessment No. 43. AHRQ Publication No. 01-E058. Rockville, MD: Agency for Healthcare Research and Quality.

Seago, J., and M. Ash. 2002. "Registered Nurse Unions and Patient Outcomes." *Journal of Nursing Administration* 32 (3): 143–51.

Serratt, T., C. Harrington, J. Spetz, and M. Blegen. 2011. "Staffing Changes Before and After Mandated Nurse-to-Patient Ratios in California's Hospitals." *Policy, Politics and Nursing Practice* 12 (3): 133–40.

Sheridan-Leos, N. 2008. "Understanding Lateral Violence in Nursing." *Journal of Oncology Nursing* 12 (3): 399–403.

Spaulding, T. J., and T. S. Raghu. 2013. "Impact of CPOE Usage on Medication Management Process Costs and Quality Outcomes." *Inquiry* 50 (3): 229–47.

Spetz, J. 2014. "How Will Health Reform Affect Demand for RNs?" *Nursing Economic$* 32 (1): 42–44.

Spetz, J., M. Ash, C. Konstantinidis, and C. Herrera. 2011. "The Effect of Unions on the Distribution of Wages of Hospital-Employed Registered Nurses in the United States." *Journal of Clinical Nursing* 20 (1–2): 60–67.

Spetz, J., D. Harless, C. N. Herrera, and B. A. Mark. 2013. "Using Minimum Nurse Staffing Regulations to Measure the Relationship Between Nursing and Hospital Quality of Care." *Medical Care Research and Review* 70 (4): 380–99.

Stein, L. I. 1967. "The Doctor–Nurse Game." *Archives of General Psychiatry* 16 (6): 699–703.

Steltzer, T. M. 2001. "Collective Bargaining, Part 2: A Wake-Up Call." *Nursing Management* 32 (4): 35–48.

Stimpfel, A. W., D. M. Sloane, and L. H. Aiken. 2012. "The Longer the Shifts for Hospital Nurses, the Higher the Levels of Burnout and Patient Dissatisfaction." *Health Affairs* 31 (11): 2501–9.

Strasen, L. 1987. *Key Business Skills for Nurse Managers*. Philadelphia, PA: Lippincott.

Swearingen, S., and A. Lieberman. 2004. "Nursing Generations: An Expanded Look at the Emergence of Conflict and Its Resolution." *Health Care Manager* 23 (1): 54–64.

Thomas, K. S., V. Mor, D. A. Tyler, and K. Hyer. 2013. "The Relationships Among Licensed Nurse Turnover, Retention, and Rehospitalization of Nursing Home Residents." *Gerontologist* 53 (2): 211–21.

Thungjaroenkul, P., G. G. Cummings, and A. Embleton. 2007. "The Impact of Nurse Staffing on Hospital Costs and Patient Length of Stay: A Systematic Review." *Nursing Economic$* 25 (5): 255–67.

Townsend, T. 2012. "Break the Bullying Cycle." *American Nurse Today* 7 (1). Published January. www.americannursetoday.com/break-the-bullying-cycle/.

Tucker, A. L., and S. J. Spear. 2006. "Operational Failures and Interruptions in Hospital Nursing." *Health Services Research* 41 (3, pt. 1): 643–62.

Van Slyck, A. 2000. "Patient Classification Systems: Not a Proxy for Nurse 'Busyness.'" *Nursing Administration Quarterly* 24 (4): 60–65.

Vlasses, F. R., and C. H. Smeltzer. 2007. "Toward a New Future for Healthcare and Nursing Practice." *Journal of Nursing Administration* 37 (9): 375–80.

Waldman, J. D., and S. Arora. 2004. "Measuring Retention Rather Than Turnover: A Different and Complementary HR Calculus." *Human Resource Planning* 27 (3): 6–9.

Welton, J. M. 2011. "Nurse Staffing and Inpatient Mortality: Is the Question Outcomes or Nursing Value?" *Medical Care* 49 (12): 1045–46.

West, E., N. Mays, A. M. Rafferty, K. Rowan, and C. Sanderson. 2009. "Nursing Resources and Patient Outcomes in Intensive Care: A Systematic Review of the Literature." *International Journal of Nursing Studies* 46 (7): 993–1011.

Winwood, P. C., and K. Lushington. 2006. "Disentangling the Effects of Psychological and Physical Work Demands on Sleep, Recovery and Maladaptive Chronic Stress Outcomes Within a Large Sample of Australian Nurses." *Journal of Advanced Nursing* 56 (6): 679–89.

Wolf, L. D., P. Potter, J. A. Sledge, S. B. Boxerman, D. Grayson, and B. Evanoff. 2006. "Describing Nurses' Work: Combining Quantitative and Qualitative Analysis." *Human Factors* 48 (1): 5–15.

Wolosin, R., L. Ayala, and B. Fulton. 2012. "Nursing Care, Inpatient Satisfaction, and Value-Based Purchasing: Vital Connections." *Journal of Nursing Administration* 42 (6): 321–25.

Zangaro, G. A., and K. L. Soeken. 2007. "A Meta-Analysis of Studies of Nurses' Job Satisfaction." *Research in Nursing and Health* 30 (4): 445–58.

Zhou, X., M. S. Ackerman, and K. Zheng. 2010. "Computerization and Information Assembling Process: Nursing Work and CPOE Adoption." In *Proceedings of the 1st ACM International Health Informatics Symposium (IHI '10)*, edited by T. Veinot, 36–45. New York: Association for Computing Machinery. Accessed January 9, 2015. http://web.eecs.umich.edu/~ackerm/pub/10b61/ihi10-workarounds.pdf.

Supplement: An Example of Full-Time Equivalent and Nurse Staffing Calculations

Consider the annual nurse staffing needs for a busy, 30-bed inpatient pediatric unit at an academic health center. The nurse manager for the unit must determine the total unit workload, or nursing care hours, for the coming year using patient classification system data and patient days projected from historical data. The total workload for this unit is shown in Exhibit 14.7.

Patient Classification Rating	Average Care Hours (ACH) per Patient Day	Projected Patient Days (PD)	Total Unit Workload (ACH × PD)
1	3.5	1,500	5,250
2	5	2,500	12,500
3	9	3,000	27,000
4	13	2,100	27,300
5	17.5	1,100	19,250
Total		10,200	91,300

EXHIBIT 14.7
Total Unit Workload for a 30-Bed Inpatient Unit

The number of FTEs required to staff the unit over a year must be calculated and then distributed across the day shift and the night shift. FTEs must also be further divided according to the types of nurses required for each shift. The nurse manager also knows the following:

- 1.0 FTE = 2,080 hours paid.
- The percentage of productive nursing hours on the unit is 85 percent (an average of 1,768 productive hours per FTE).
- Work schedules for nursing personnel on this unit are based on a staffing standard of 55 percent for the day shift and 45 percent for the night shift.
- The staff mix is 75 percent RNs, 15 percent LPNs, and 10 percent unlicensed nursing personnel (NAs).

The overall number of FTEs required to staff this unit is determined as follows:

91,300 total hours of care required per year ÷ 1,768 productive hours per FTE

= 51.6 FTEs for year-round nursing care coverage

The number of nursing FTEs required to staff day and night shifts for the year (shown in Exhibit 14.8) is calculated as follows:

- Day shift coverage (annual projections)
  - 51.6 FTEs × 55% × 75% RNs = 21.3 RN FTEs
  - 51.6 FTEs × 55% × 15% LPNs = 4.3 LPN FTEs
  - 51.6 FTEs × 55% × 10% NAs = 2.8 NA FTEs
  - 51.6 FTEs × 55% = 28.4 total FTEs

EXHIBIT 14.8
Full-Time
Equivalent
Calculations

Staff	Days	Nights	Total
RNs	21.3	17.4	38.7
LPNs	4.3	3.5	7.7
NAs	2.8	2.3	5.2
Total FTEs	28.4	23.2	51.6

Note: Due to rounding, totals may not be exact.

- Night shift coverage (annual projections)
  - 51.6 FTEs × 45% × 75% RNs = 17.4 RN FTEs
  - 51.6 FTEs × 45% × 15% LPN = 3.5 LPN FTEs
  - 51.6 FTEs × 45% × 10% NAs = 2.3 NA FTEs
  - 51.6 FTEs × 45% = 23.2 total FTEs

The 51.6 FTEs are scheduled such that nursing and shift requirements are met. Over time, if patient classification data reflect a change in nursing care requirements, the FTE and scheduling requirements may change. The total number of FTEs needed on this unit is known, but the actual number of shifts and types of personnel needed must still be determined (shown in Exhibit 14.9). Furthermore, considering the number of allocated FTEs, managers must make decisions about the actual number of people to schedule to meet ongoing requirements within budget constraints. The number of shifts by type of personnel is calculated as follows:

- Days
  - 20.8 shifts per day × 55% day shift × 75% RNs = 8.6 RN shifts
  - 20.8 shifts per day × 55% day shift × 15% LPNs = 1.7 LPN shifts
  - 20.8 shifts per day × 55% day shift × 10% NAs = 1.1 NA shifts
- Nights
  - 20.8 shifts per day × 45% night shift × 75% RNs = 7.0 RN shifts
  - 20.8 shifts per day × 45% night shift × 15% LPNs = 1.4 LPN shifts
  - 20.8 shifts per day × 45% night shift × 10% NAs = 0.9 NA shifts

Different approaches can be used to achieve staffing needs, as determined in this example. One manager may decide to staff for 9 RNs on days and 7 on nights, 2 LPNs on days and 1 on nights, and 1 NA on days and nights. Another manager may staff for 8 RNs on days and 6 on nights, 2 LPNs on days and nights, and 1 NA on days and 2 NAs on nights. These

Staff	Days	Nights	Total
RNs	8.6	7.0	15.6
LPNs	1.7	1.4	3.1
NAs	1.1	0.9	2.1
Total shifts per day	11.4	9.4	20.8

EXHIBIT 14.9
Shift Calculations

Note: Due to rounding, totals may not be exact.

decisions should be based on a manager's understanding of patient needs, staff availability, and organizational policy.

FTEs are likely to be filled with combinations of full-time and part-time personnel. For example, the 21.3 RN FTEs may be made up of 22 full-time RNs or 18 full-time RNs and 7 part-time RNs, and so forth. These decisions are necessary to determine the actual number of nursing positions that will staff the unit and, in turn, meet the unit personnel budget requirements.

Nursing care requirements may vary by day of the week. Fewer nurses may be needed on the weekends because certain services for patient care testing and procedures are available only on weekdays. For example, the 145.6 nursing shifts per week (20.8 nursing shifts per day × 7 days per week—see Exhibit 14.10) can be distributed so that there are fewer than 20.8 nursing shifts per day on weekends and greater numbers on weekdays (Finkler, Jones, and Kovner 2013), depending on unit operations.

If patient census on the unit changes over time, nurse staffing requirements may change too. In this case, the manager may need to advocate for additional permanent or temporary nursing personnel (from unit or in-house staffing pools or outside agencies), decrease permanent FTE requirements, or ask unit staff to take vacation time and work fewer shifts. In both of these cases, the perspective and judgment of the nurse or unit manager are critical.

Returning to the example in Exhibit 14.10, if we divide the 51.6 FTEs required to staff the unit over a year by the 20.8 daily nursing shifts, we see that 2.48 FTEs are needed to fill each nursing shift for the year. Therefore, approximately 2.5 nursing staff must be hired full-time (or a greater number must be hired if some work part-time) to cover a 12-hour shift for 365 days (4,380 hours). The difference between hours paid to 2.48 FTEs (5,158 hours = 2.48 × 2,080 hours) and patient care hours required (4,380) takes into account the personnel needed to cover for staff days off, sick time, holidays, vacations, and so forth (Finkler, Jones, and Kovner 2013).

Finally, in the example in Exhibit 14.10, 8.58 RN shifts (21.3 RN FTEs) are required to cover days, and 7.02 RN shifts (17.4 RN FTEs) are

EXHIBIT 14.10

Sample Staffing
Calculations for
a 30-Bed
Inpatient
Pediatric Unit

Determine the following:

1. Nursing care hours required each day
2. Number of nursing shifts per day and per week
3. Number of nursing personnel required on day and night shifts
4. Breakdown of RN/LPN/NA staffing for day and night shifts
5. Ratio of FTEs to shifts

Solutions:

1. An average daily nursing care requirement = 91,300 nursing care hours per year ÷ 365 days per year = 250 nursing care hours per day
2. 250 nursing care hours per day, with 12-hour shifts = 20.8 nursing shifts per 24-hour day (250 hours ÷ 12 hours per shift)

   20.8 nursing shifts per day × 7 days per week = 145.6 nursing shifts per week

3. Using the 55 percent/45 percent standard:

   20.8 shifts × 55% = 11.44 nursing shifts on days

   20.8 shifts × 45% = 9.36 nursing shifts on nights

4. Days: 8.58 RN shifts (11.44 × 75%), 1.72 LPN shifts (11.44 × 15%), and 1.14 NA shifts (11.44 × 10%). Nights: 7.02 RN shifts (9.36 × 75%), 1.40 LPN shifts (9.36 × 15%), and 0.94 nursing assistant shifts (9.36 × 10%).
5. 2.48 FTEs are required to cover one shift for the entire year (28.4 nurse FTEs are required to staff 11.44 nursing shifts during days, 23.2 nurse FTEs are required to staff 9.36 nursing shifts during nights, etc.). Therefore, 2.48 full-time nurses must be hired to cover one 12-hour shift, 365 days of the year.

required to cover nights, with a census of 25 patients. Dividing the shift results by the patient census yields an average workload of approximately 2.9 patients per RN for the day shift and 3.6 patients per RN for the night shift.

HUMAN RESOURCES MANAGEMENT PRACTICES FOR QUALITY AND PATIENT SAFETY

Jordan Albritton and Bruce J. Fried

Learning Objectives

After completing this chapter, the reader should be able to

- describe the history of quality improvement and its role in healthcare;
- understand the value of quality improvement methods, including key features and tools;
- discuss human resources management considerations for implementing and sustaining a quality improvement effort;
- explain how team effectiveness contributes to quality improvement success; and
- describe the role managers can play in improving and maintaining team effectiveness.

Introduction

Measuring and improving quality have become imperative for healthcare organizations. Beyond the moral obligation to provide high-quality health services, financial incentives are clearly coming into line with quality. Federal guidelines, such as the Physician Quality Reporting System, provide incentive payments to providers who report on quality measures for services covered under Medicare Part B. Medicare physician fee schedules will be linked to a value-based payment modifier, which is based on physician performance. Physician practices participating in the Medicare electronic health record (EHR) incentive program are rewarded for practices that achieve meaningful use of EHRs. Accountable care organizations are also moving in the direction of rewarding quality, and commercial payers are encouraging healthcare organizations to participate in quality improvement (QI) efforts (Watkins 2014). In sum, attentiveness to quality, value, and quality improvement is here to stay.

Chapter 1 addressed the topic of strategic human resources management, and evidence is cited supporting the link between effective human resources (HR) practices and profitability, productivity, growth, and other positive organizational outcomes. The subject of this chapter is the connection between HR practices and quality. A QI-oriented culture is a requirement for organizations wishing to provide high-quality services. Furthermore, organizations pursuing a QI strategy—a category that includes virtually all healthcare organizations—must review and modify their HR practices to ensure alignment between QI goals and HR practices. The QI enterprise is built on the twin pillars of data and measurement, the application of human capital to define and address quality problems, and the design and implementation of meaningful changes. As the QI movement has progressed, much attention has been given to the accuracy and precision of measurement, yet the human side of QI has not kept pace with the measurement side. Little has been written about how to recruit and train people to engage in QI activities or how QI teams can more effectively mobilize their human capital to make meaningful and sustainable organizational changes. The goal of this chapter is to help HR managers move toward parity between measurement and human engagement.

Defining Quality

In a discussion of quality and QI, clarifying the meaning of quality is important. At the most basic level, *quality* refers to ensuring that every patient receives the appropriate care at the appropriate time. The Institute of Medicine (IOM) provides a more formal definition, defining quality as "the degree to which health services for individuals and populations increase the likelihood of desired health outcomes and are consistent with current professional knowledge" (IOM 1990, 5). Still, the practical meaning of quality varies depending on one's perspective and role. For example, a physician may focus on meeting prevention guidelines regarding the use of low-dose aspirin therapy to reduce the risk of heart attack. On the other hand, a nurse may be more concerned with preventing central line infections or bedsores. A manager may emphasize the bottom line, focusing on ensuring the accurate filing of insurance claims. Ultimately, quality is an inherent goal in the mission of healthcare organizations and is a responsibility of every healthcare worker.

The concept of quality also extends into the realm of patient safety. *Patient safety* refers to "freedom from accidental or preventable injuries produced by medical care" (Agency for Healthcare Research and Quality 2014). Accidents can result in errors that derail healthcare efforts or even harm patients. Accordingly, the IOM considers patient safety "indistinguishable from the delivery of quality health care" (IOM 2004, 5).

Avedis Donabedian is often identified as the individual responsible for developing a systematic framework for addressing quality in healthcare (Donabedian 1980). The Donabedian model integrates the numerous aspects of quality and the multiple perspectives of those involved in care delivery. Donabedian defines quality on the basis of three dimensions of healthcare: structure, process, and outcome. *Structure* refers to "the relatively stable characteristics of the providers of care, of the tools and resources they have at their disposal, and of the physical and organizational settings in which they work" (Donabedian 1980, 81). Elements of structure include hospitals, the healthcare workforce, financial resources, and equipment, among other things. *Process* refers to the "set of activities that go on within or between practitioners and patients" (Donabedian 1980, 80). Simply put, process consists of care delivery itself. Finally, *outcome* refers to "a change in a patient's current and future health status that can be attributed to antecedent healthcare" (Donabedian 1980, 83). Outcomes are the end result of care and can be measured at the individual level or the population level.

The Donabedian model also defines the functional relationships between the three dimensions of quality. To some degree, this relationship is linear: Structure determines process, which in turn affects outcomes. Relationships between these dimensions are, of course, more complex; outcomes, for example, often depend on factors outside of the domain of the formal healthcare system. Indeed, although quality may be assessed purely in terms of patient outcomes, from a practical standpoint an organization wishing to improve its outcomes will need to trace quality back to the more fundamental dimensions of process and structure. The current approach to improving quality involves understanding the complexity of the quality concept and its antecedents. Donabedian offers a useful framework from which care quality can be analyzed.

Quality and Quality Improvement

In the 2001 report *Crossing the Quality Chasm*, the IOM identified six key characteristics of a healthcare system that provides high-quality care: (1) It is *safe*—for everyone, all the time; (2) it is *effective*—it provides the best care based on evidence to improve outcomes; (3) it is *patient centered*—it maintains respect for patient values, preferences, and autonomy; (4) it is *timely*—patients are not subject to long waits; (5) it is *efficient*—patients receive high value for money spent; and (6) it is *equitable*—patients are treated fairly without discrimination (IOM 2001). Failure in one or more of these areas threatens care quality, limits potential benefits to patients, and can result in harm or death.

The current approach to quality has evolved from the quality assurance model, which addressed quality from a largely reactive perspective and tended to be viewed as policing and punitive in nature. Where errors or defects appeared, the central question was typically associated with blame: "Whose fault was this?" QI, by contrast, addresses quality issues both prospectively and retrospectively, with the emphasis on systems and processes. A central question in the QI era is "How can we improve our processes—the system—to improve outcomes of value to the organization?" Rather than emphasizing the individual's role in a quality issue, attention is given to the system. Systems produce outcomes, and in the words of Paul Batalden: "Every system is perfectly designed to get the results it gets" (e.g., Batalden and Davidoff 2007a, 1060).

Several key themes have emerged across all QI methodologies, notably the key role of data and evidence in analyzing problems and in designing and testing the impact of changes. Further, responsibility for quality rests with both leaders and employees. While QI efforts are top-down in the sense that management support is essential, they are bottom-up in the sense that the people with the most knowledge about a problem should be involved in designing improvement strategies. Because of the complexity of healthcare, multidisciplinary teams are frequently used to implement QI initiatives. In contrast to a quality assurance perspective, QI does not end with the solution to a particular quality issue. The healthcare environment is dynamic, and healthcare organizations face new challenges on a continuous basis. Thus, QI is often referred to as continuous quality improvement (CQI).

Key Quality Issues

Most QI efforts follow one (or more) of several formal methodologies in which the first step includes analyzing the situation and diagnosing problems. One category of quality and patient safety issues includes overuse, underuse, and misuse of care. Each of these types of problems has different causes and implications.

Overuse refers to a situation in which a patient receives a drug or treatment without medical justification. Although structure can affect overuse (you do have to pay for that fancy MRI, after all), overuse is typically a result of process issues. Examples include treating a routine ear infection with antibiotics, using an expensive MRI to make a diagnosis that could be achieved by a less expensive imaging exam, or completing a diagnostic test twice because of poor care coordination. In healthcare, more is not always better. Often less costly, equally effective solutions to many common healthcare issues are available. Overuse raises costs for patients while subjecting them to increased risk. Donald Berwick, MD, former head of the Centers for Medicare & Medicaid Services (CMS), estimates that overtreatment alone accounts for between 6 and 10 percent of all US healthcare spending (Berwick and Hackbarth 2012). Others suggest that as much as 30 percent of all healthcare provided may be unnecessary (Reilly and Evans 2009). Regardless, to provide high-quality care, a healthcare system must minimize overuse.

In contrast to overuse, underuse occurs in situations where providers fail to provide patients with medically necessary care or do not adhere to evidence-based guidelines. Examples include failure to vaccinate elderly patients against pneumonia or failure to provide beta-blockers to patients with coronary artery disease. Given the prevalence of overuse, one might not expect underuse to present as much of a challenge. However, the Agency for Healthcare Research and Quality (2013) reported that, in 2009, Americans failed to receive 30 percent of the care they needed to treat or prevent medical conditions. Failing to receive necessary care can have severe consequences, with one estimate suggesting that as many as 91,000 Americans die each year because they do not receive appropriate evidence-based care (National Committee for Quality Assurance 2007). The growth of the evidence-based medicine movement, in which providers are expected to follow specific guidelines, reflects the process nature of the underuse issue. Although process-related solutions can be highly effective, underuse can also be traced to structural issues, such as inadequate access to highly qualified healthcare providers.

Finally, *misuse* refers to incorrect diagnoses, medical errors, and other preventable conditions. In *To Err Is Human* (IOM 1999), the IOM broke the silence regarding medical errors, estimating that they cause up to 98,000 deaths each year. Examples of misuse include treating a patient with an antibiotic for which the patient has a known allergy, not taking precautions to prevent hospital-acquired infections, and operating on the wrong side of a patient. Misuse is almost always the result of a process issue. Misuse is particularly troubling because it often has serious consequences, but it is entirely preventable. Efforts to improve care coordination and increase the adoption of EHRs are designed, at least in part, to minimize the misuse of healthcare.

History of Quality Improvement

QI has been defined as the "combined and unceasing efforts of everyone—healthcare professionals, patients and their families, researchers, payers, planners and educators—to make the changes that will lead to better patient outcomes (health), better system performance (care) and better professional development" (Batalden and Davidoff 2007b, 2). QI is not simply greater vigilance for error, it is more than an emphasis on controlling processes, and it does not just refer to meetings where issues are discussed and analyzed. QI should not be considered an end goal, as it is not solely outcome oriented. Although QI may include any or all of these features, QI typically is a continuous process that includes multiple rapid cycles of improvement. Perhaps one of the most distinguishing features of QI today is that it generally includes the use of a formal methodology to achieve specified organizational goals (Health Resources and Services Administration 2014).

The QI movement in healthcare is still relatively young. In fact, the QI ideology embraced by the healthcare industry grew out of applications from the Japanese manufacturing industry. Although quality control was first emphasized in US production efforts during World War II, the quality focus deteriorated when the war ended. Disenchanted by the decision to abandon quality control programs, prominent early quality experts Joseph Juran and W. Edwards Deming accepted an invitation to help restructure Japanese production methods after World War II. Instead of relying on product inspection as a quality metric, Juran and Deming focused on improving all organizational processes. As a result, Japanese goods, once known for poor quality, made significant gains on the international market, and Japan continued to develop into a quality leader.

In the 1980s, strategies from the Japanese QI approach (a philosophy called "companywide quality control") began to infiltrate US organizations. One of the earliest such organizations, the US Naval Air Systems Command, adopted a Japanese-style management approach in the early 1980s, coining the term *total quality management* (TQM). Fortune 500 companies began to follow suit, even reaching out to quality experts trained in Japan. Congress finally brought the quality focus to the US healthcare system with the establishment of the Agency for Health Care Policy and Research (now the Agency for Healthcare Research and Quality) in 1989, but the healthcare industry progressed slowly at first. Other not-for-profit organizations arose in the years that followed to further accelerate improvement, including the Institute for Healthcare Improvement in 1991 and the National Patient Safety Foundation in 1996 (American Society for Quality 2014a). However, the IOM reports *To Err Is Human* and *Crossing the Quality Chasm* ultimately led the healthcare industry to firmly embrace the quality movement.

A bevy of policies and regulations have been enacted in an effort to achieve the change envisioned in the IOM reports. Some evidence suggests that the US healthcare industry may be moving—slowly—in the right direction, but quality remains a significant challenge. As part of the solution, healthcare organizations have a responsibility to conduct internal QI efforts to continually improve the quality of care delivered and maximize benefits to patients. The following section provides a closer look at QI, briefly describing popular methods, outlining shared themes, and identifying useful tools. Finally, the chapter provides a more detailed discussion of the role of teams in QI and what managers can do to improve team effectiveness.

Quality and Process Improvement

The overall approach to quality management adopted by the healthcare industry is often referred to as *continuous quality improvement* (CQI). CQI does not require the use of any single improvement method. Rather, CQI is an overarching strategy that includes a "structured organizational process for involving personnel in planning and executing a continuous flow of improvements to provide quality health care that meets or exceeds expectations"

(Sollecito and Johnson 2013, 4). Additionally, CQI carries with it the belief that existing operations and processes always have room for improvement and that quality gains are always possible. Organizations may adopt CQI principles for different reasons: (1) to achieve true process improvement; (2) to gain a competitive advantage in the marketplace; or (3) to conform to regulations and requirements. Regardless of the motivation, CQI supports the overall mission of healthcare organizations and offers benefits for patients as well as the organization.

Given the similarities between the definitions and principles of CQI, TQM, and QI, these terms are often used interchangeably to refer to a general strategy or focus on QI. However, numerous, distinct formal methods are designed to support QI efforts. These methods have many analogous components, often referring to a series of steps to support the development and testing of changes within an organization. In general, the methods assume that errors are preventable and that they develop as the result of poor system processes. The overall goal is to develop an understanding of how a problem develops and to use this understanding to guide improvement efforts.

Common Quality Improvement Strategies

Total Quality Management

TQM draws on behavioral science, economic theory, and process analysis and typically involves the use of both qualitative and quantitative data to guide improvements. TQM arose fairly early in the evolution of QI and does not include a formal framework. Rather, TQM consists of a set of principles that support quality. The American Society for Quality (2014b) defines TQM as a "management system for a customer-focused organization that involves all employees in continual improvement. It uses strategy, data, and effective communications to integrate the quality discipline into the culture and activities of the organization."

The principles of TQM include the following:

- *Customer focus.* The customer determines the level of quality required and thus whether QI efforts are successful and worthwhile.
- *Total employee involvement.* Organizations should encourage employee participation in QI efforts. Employee commitment depends on psychological safety, empowerment, and the proper environment.
- *Process-centered thinking.* TQM promotes process thinking in which the steps of a process are defined and performance measures are continuously monitored to detect variation.

- *Integrated system.* TQM focuses on the horizontal processes interconnecting organizational functions and roles.
- *Strategic and systematic approach.* TQM encourages the formulation of a strategic plan that integrates quality as a core component.
- *Continual improvement.* Organizations should remain analytical and creative in order to find ways to become more competitive and effective at meeting goals.
- *Fact-based decision making.* TQM requires organizations to collect and analyze data to support decision making and assess the effectiveness of improvement strategies.
- *Communication.* Communication supports employee morale and motivation.

The Model for Improvement

The Model for Improvement (MFI) consists of three fundamental questions followed by multiple Plan-Do-Study-Act (PDSA) cycles. The MFI is the preferred model of the Institute for Healthcare Improvement and is commonly used in healthcare. Many QI frameworks imply a sequence that differs from the way that most projects are completed. In contrast, the MFI derives from studies of innovation that show that discovery, learning, and intervention cannot be reduced to a linear model. The MFI encourages nonlinear learning and adaptation suggested by complexity science. As a result, the MFI calls for gradual development and testing of change in the system where it is being implemented. This process is accomplished through numerous rapid tests of small changes through PDSA cycles. Ultimately, the MFI guides improvement efforts and offers an efficient trial-and-learning methodology (Langley et al. 2009). The MFI can be divided into a planning stage and a testing stage with the following elements:

- Planning stage
  - *Goals of the effort.* Set specific, measurable aims.
  - *Ways to measure improvement.* Determine which quantitative measures will be used to evaluate changes.
  - *Changes to be made.* Select changes based on feedback from those involved with the operation, internal data, or success stories of others.
- Testing stage
  - *Plan*—Develop a plan and implement the change gradually.
  - *Do*—Implement the change and collect data for analysis.
  - *Study*—Analyze the change. Compare the results to the expectations.

– *Act*—Decide how to move forward. Determine if the change is feasible or if it needs to be altered. Either go back to the planning stage or continue with additional PDSA cycles.

Six Sigma

Six Sigma was developed by Motorola in the late 1980s. The methodology draws on TQM principles and has an added focus on identifying and eliminating the causes of errors and minimizing variation in business processes. In addition to prescribing a set of tools and methods to improve process quality, Six Sigma also creates an infrastructure of individuals with formal training in these methods ("champions," "black belts," "green belts," etc.). Over time, Six Sigma has evolved into multiple distinct methodologies for use in specific circumstances. The two most common of these methodologies are DMAIC (define, measure, analyze, improve, control) and DMADV (define, measure, analyze, design, verify). Specifically, DMAIC is intended to be used with existing processes, while DMADV should be used when implementing new processes. Although the frameworks include several steps, each step can be broken down to include additional tools and methods.

Key elements of the DMAIC framework are as follows:

- *Define* process improvement goals consistent with customer demands and organizational strategies.
- *Measure* the current process (focus on defects) and develop a baseline for future comparison.
- *Analyze* the process to identify all relevant factors and verify cause-and-effect relationships. Identify the key root cause of unacceptable variation.
- *Improve* or optimize the process on the basis of the analysis. Implement a solution and standardize the process.
- *Control* the process to sustain future gains. Create a plan to ensure that any variances are corrected before they result in defects.

The DMADV framework is as follows:

- *Define* the project goals and customer requirements.
- *Measure* and determine customer needs and specifications; benchmark against competitors and industry.
- *Analyze* the process options.
- *Design* the process to meet the customer needs.
- *Verify* the design performance and capability to meet customer needs.

Lean

Growing out of the Toyota Production System in the early 1990s, the Lean manufacturing strategy is based on a set of five production principles that encourage continuous improvement through waste reduction. Waste reduction efforts are supported by demand-flow manufacturing, a kind of "pull system" where goods and services are delivered only in direct response to a customer request. Demand-flow manufacturing practices improve the flow or smoothness of work processes. Overall, Lean aims to reduce production time, lower inventory needs, increase productivity, and allow for more efficient use of capital equipment (Langley et al. 2009). The Lean approach includes the following elements (Lean Enterprise Institute 2015):

- *Customer's perspective*. Specify value from the customer's perspective.
- *Value stream*. Identify all steps in the value stream and eliminate steps that do not create value for the customer.
- *Flow*. Ensure that value-creating steps occur in tight sequence so that the product or service flows smoothly toward the customer.
- *Pull*. Ensure that the flow of work occurs in response to customer demand.
- *Perfection*. Repeat steps 1 through 4 until a state of perfection is reached, where perfect value is created without waste.

Common Themes and Tools

The methods discussed previously are by no means the only QI methods used in healthcare or other industries. Other methods and frameworks are highly regarded. No single method has developed the reputation of being better than the others, but many QI experts have a preferred method. Additionally, although the methodologies provide a comprehensive guide to QI, many organizations use hybrid models. For example, some organizations characterize their QI approach as "Lean Six Sigma" and incorporate ideas from the Lean principles as well as Six Sigma's DMAIC framework. The MFI also incorporates Lean concepts.

The differences between the methods are often more in terms of flavor than substance. For example, some methods focus on reducing variation, while others emphasize waste reduction; some methods promote gradual change, while others promote larger changes. Regardless of the QI method used, all have the same general purpose—to provide a structured approach for evaluating processes and guiding improvement efforts.

Common features across methods can be organized into several underlying themes. First, each QI method emphasizes the importance of planning.

In the planning stage, organizations evaluate current performance, identify areas for improvement, and set specific goals for QI efforts. The second theme includes organizing and coordinating QI efforts. In this stage, organizations implement the plan developed in the previous stage. QI methods all emphasize actively managing the QI process. QI methods also examine organizations as systems and appreciate that most quality issues are a result of dysfunctional processes. Thus, QI methods all seek to understand their processes, which may initially be viewed as "black boxes." Finally, the third theme refers to sustaining change. This stage includes scaling the change up to other parts of the organization, fine-tuning and adapting the change as necessary, and ingraining QI ideologies into the organizational culture.

Another key theme is the importance of measurement and the application of measures that are valid and meaningful. Measurement may include relatively objective measures, such as patient waiting time, infection rates, and medication errors. Measures such as patient and employee satisfaction may be rather subjective but very meaningful to the organization. Furthermore, QI methods tend to value participation of relevant individuals at all organizational levels, including, at times, patients and family members. As a result, QI methods emphasize presentation in a form that is accessible and meaningful to people with different levels of methodological and quantitative skill. Examples of data and information presentation formats include run charts, fishbone diagrams, flowcharts, and Pareto charts. These methods and others are extensively described elsewhere (see, for example, Kelly 2011).

The Importance of Human Resources

The central focus of this chapter is the key role of individuals and teams in the QI process. Successful launch and initiation of QI methods clearly require support from senior management; however, successful implementation requires meaningful participation from individuals at multiple organizational levels. All QI methods emphasize both the need for data and the human capital necessary to interpret and translate data into a precise problem definition. However, the critical role of human capital and teams, while not ignored by QI experts and QI facilitators, has largely taken a back seat to the data imperative. Anecdotal evidence leads the authors of this chapter to believe that teams are taken for granted. QI initiatives frequently include a team member training and orientation component, but little in the way of ongoing monitoring and evaluation of how well the team is functioning. The team, after all, provides the brainpower for successful change efforts. If the team is dysfunctional, then whatever human capital may be present on the team will not be used to its fullest extent.

The rationale for using teams in QI efforts is clear: Employees frequently have the best insights into problem causation and the feasibility of alternative changes and interventions. Rank-and-file employees will, in most cases, be responsible for implementing the recommended changes. Because so many quality problems in healthcare are complex and have multiple causes, quality issues require a team approach, where team members can collectively share knowledge, interpret data, and generate change options. The composition of QI teams should ideally reflect the complexity and disciplinary diversity of the problems to be addressed. Membership should also include representation of individuals at multiple organizational levels because changes almost always require understanding by people at different levels in the organization.

What are the consequences of not paying attention to engaging employees and teams in QI efforts? At the most basic level, the opportunity to obtain and use the profound knowledge possessed by employees is lost. This profound knowledge includes an understanding of how a particular system operates and how multiple subsystems interact. It also includes a deep understanding of variation in system performance, and the potential reasons for such variation. All QI efforts seek to build knowledge—to learn. Absent the perspectives of those possessing profound knowledge about the system, all that remains may be observations and data that are disconnected from how the system operates.

Human Resource Practices and Team Effectiveness

As a central element in an organization's mix of strategies, QI must be supported by a set of well-aligned HR strategies. Exhibit 15.1 summarizes key questions to consider in evaluating the alignment of HR practices with QI initiatives. Each of these HR practices has implications for the success of QI efforts in the organization overall and, in particular, for the success of QI teams. Because of the importance of teams to QI methodologies, this discussion of HR practices is organized around team effectiveness.

Teams vary in their effectiveness, and a team is unlikely to naturally evolve into a well-oiled machine. In fact, teams have more reasons to fail than to succeed. Exhibit 15.2 provides a cynical list of factors that may jeopardize a well-intentioned QI effort. These recipes for failure are provided to make the point that each stage of a QI effort depends on effective teams. Teams in fact play a major role in all aspects of healthcare and are particularly central to providing safe care (Leonard, Graham, and Bonacum 2004).

The team is the primary vehicle through which problems are analyzed, solutions are generated, and change is evaluated. A team-based approach

HR Practices	Questions to Consider
Job design and job descriptions	Are team competencies and expectations included in job descriptions? Is quality addressed in the job description?
Employee recruitment and selection	Do applicants know that participation in QI activities is a key job requirement? Are job applicants appraised on their role in improving quality? Does the organization have valid methods of assessing quality-related competencies in job applicants?
Communication and culture	Is the organization sufficiently flexible to support open lines of communication, both vertically and horizontally? Do employees feel it is safe to express their views? Is teamwork an accepted means of getting the work done and communicating?
Performance management	Is participation in QI efforts part of the employee performance appraisal system? Are employees made aware of the expectations regarding their participation in QI activities?
Reward systems	Do reward systems take into consideration an employee's effectiveness as a team member and contributor to QI efforts?
Training	Do employees receive training that is directly applicable to the organization's QI methodology, such as teamwork and measurement?
Management style and organizational structure	Do managers model participatory management styles? Does the organization support decentralized decision making?
HR systems	Does the organization employ QI methodologies to improve its own HR systems?

EXHIBIT 15.1
Quality Improvement Teams and HR Practices

allows for a larger, more comprehensive, and more impactful QI effort. Although a basic understanding of common tools and methods is a requirement for any QI effort, success depends on more than just the knowledge and use of an effective method. Numerous factors affect the quality of work produced by teams (Shortell et al. 2004). The team-based approach itself introduces its own challenges, but team effectiveness is a prerequisite to a successful QI program. Managers play a key role in improving team effectiveness

EXHIBIT 15.2
Recipes for
Failure in QI

Do not have effective mechanisms to recognize individual contributions or team achievements.

Do not provide training for team members.

Don't think too much about who should be on a QI team.

Do not establish norms of psychological safety; that is, do not ensure that team members and others in the organization understand that they will suffer moderate to severe consequences if an error is made.

Do not select effective team leaders, and do not provide training to team leaders.

Do not provide adequate time for teams to meet.

Do not encourage sustained senior management support for QI efforts.

Do not provide necessary resources for QI teams.

Always assume that team members are committed to the QI mission without developing strategies to develop and assess team member engagement.

Allow a senior team member to dominate team discussions.

Do not present data in a form that is accessible to team members.

Do not provide time and a framework for teams to debrief on and improve their own team processes.

Always discount contributions of team members with lower levels of formal academic training.

---

and are therefore critical to the success of QI efforts. Accordingly, TQM and subsequent QI models reflect the importance of the manager's role in QI.

Antecedents of team effectiveness can be drawn from different levels within the organization. First, antecedents of team effectiveness can be evaluated at the individual level. As the saying goes, "The whole is only as good as the sum of its parts." A team is made of individuals. Thus, the characteristics of the individuals on the team will greatly influence the effectiveness of the team as a whole. From the HR perspective, managers should keep this fact in mind when selecting, evaluating, and training employees. Individual-level factors include job descriptions that specify that team participation is a central job function, the selection of highly qualified employees who can work effectively on teams, performance management and appraisal methods that include team work as a key job requirement, reward systems that motivate participation in team activities, and training of employees in the use of QI methods.

Second, antecedents of team effectiveness can be evaluated at the team level. One can build a car out of high-quality parts, but if the parts do not fit together well or if they are assembled incorrectly, the car may not run. Likewise, the relationships between individuals on a team will affect the effectiveness of the team as a whole. Although managers must carefully select highly qualified individuals to participate on the QI team, they must also consider team composition, including factors such as horizontal, vertical, and cultural diversity; team leadership; psychological safety; team conflict; and communication.

Finally, antecedents of team effectiveness can be evaluated at the organizational level. Even a well-made car will not work without fuel, and performance will suffer on poor roads. Similarly, higher-level organizational factors shape the environment in which a team operates. These organizational factors include the support of senior management, the availability of resources to carry out QI functions (money, time, personnel), an organizational culture that supports QI, and management training to support the QI culture. Although these features often fall under the purview of senior managers, middle managers should remain active in developing a QI culture in their own departments. Middle managers also have the responsibility to voice concerns that threaten to limit the effectiveness of QI teams. For example, if the organization does not provide sufficient resources to support QI functions, a manager has three options for recourse: (1) lobby senior management for greater resource support, (2) find a way to provide the necessary support within the department using existing resources and flexibility, or (3) do nothing and allow team performance to suffer. By understanding factors at the organizational level that support team effectiveness, managers can better inform their decisions and actions to more effectively foster team effectiveness.

Individual-Level Factors

An important first step to building an effective team is the development of job descriptions that target highly qualified team members. Here, "qualified" refers to team members who have both the technical competencies needed by the team as well as the motivation and competency to work effectively in a team environment. Of course, finding individuals with both of these sets of competencies may not always be possible. At the very least, desired team members should value and understand the importance of teamwork and demonstrate positive team citizenship behaviors and attitudes. Although revising job descriptions can help ensure the success of future QI projects, most QI team members are drawn from existing staff members. Ideally, the current cohort of employees will have been selected at least in part because of their team competencies and natural ability to work effectively on teams. Measuring team competencies in prospective employees may be challenging, but numerous methods to assess these competencies, such as behavioral interviews and the utilization of multiple interviewers in the selection process, are available. These methods are discussed more fully in Chapter 7.

Where options are available, recruiting QI team members who have both the technical qualifications and the desired team competencies is naturally desirable. Often, employees actively voice a desire to participate in QI projects. However, QI teams may also include members who do not report directly to the manager but in fact work in another part of the organization. Therefore, managers may not have the discretion to identify the best "team players" for QI team membership. Where managers do not have such discretion, they may be challenged to orient and train team members on the purpose of the QI team and expectations of team members. This process is a key part of a QI team-building process. Because of the multidisciplinary and diverse nature of QI teams, managers must also help the team work through differences in personalities, mind-sets, and professional perspectives. Although not a strict requirement, the use of a professional facilitator may be desirable in building a QI team.

QI team members and others in the organization often will not possess knowledge and skills related to QI philosophy or methods. Although some employees may have experience working on QI projects in the past, they may have used a methodology different from the one employed by the organization. Training in the organization's preferred methodology thus becomes an integral component of QI team activities. Effective training typically includes substantive knowledge (e.g., measurement, process analysis), as well as team building and discussion about how the team will use its collective knowledge and carry out its work. QI training may also at times be incorporated into an organization's overall training activities. Should an organization adopt a particular QI model, all members of the organization will need to understand the process. This understanding is important both to help organizational members implement needed changes and to address fears and uncertainties that may emerge when changes are put into place.

In addition to formal training and skill development, a large amount of meaningful learning also typically takes place as a QI project evolves. Members learn from each other and hopefully develop an improved understanding of the nature of the problems faced in their organization. For this reason, managers should ensure that QI teams include members with different levels of experience. Those with less experience often learn from and are mentored by longer-tenured employees. This variety of experience levels also helps establish continuity in the QI team, reducing the chance of having multiple team members leave the team at once.

Finally, consider the importance of employee rewards and motivation. Employees are influenced by both formal and informal motivating factors. Accordingly, managers should reward and incentivize teamwork. Numerous options are available to facilitate this strategy. Employees sometimes receive modest financial rewards for helping achieve team goals. For example, QI team members who lead a successful project to increase adherence to guidelines to reduce the incidence of bedsores may be given a gift card to a local restaurant or to an online retailer. However, although money is a strong motivator, monetary rewards are not always possible or practical. Employees can also be publicly acknowledged at staff meetings, on posters, or in organization-wide e-mail newsletters. Although QI team members are often motivated by the satisfaction of improving the way care is delivered to enhance care quality or patient safety, these kinds of reminders help support the effectiveness of the QI team and the overall mission of the organization.

In addition to rewards and recognition, employees may be motivated by the ability to gain wider recognition for their support of QI efforts. For example, as noted previously, Six Sigma has a formal system for recognizing expertise with QI methods. Supporting employee training may then provide benefits beyond skill acquisition. As employees participate in additional training and complete QI projects, they may advance in the ranking system consisting of different colored "belts." Employees with this kind of recognition may feel that they are advancing in their careers and investing in their futures.

Ultimately, when building a team, managers must consider numerous factors at the level of the individual employee. First, managers must focus on identifying the right employees or prospective employees to participate in QI teams. After membership has been decided, managers still must focus on the development of the knowledge and skills that will enable employees to be effective contributors to the overall functioning of the team.

Team-Level Factors

The success of any team endeavor depends on both the composition of the team and the manner in which the team is managed and works together. All sectors of society include examples of poorly performing teams composed of highly effective "superstars" and high-performing teams composed of "average" individuals. Team composition is thus only part of the team effectiveness equation.

Team composition refers to the size of the team as well as the backgrounds and competencies of team members. Like many teams in healthcare, QI teams have diverse memberships. The concept of diversity has multiple dimensions and includes professional background, location within the organization, level in the organization's hierarchy, demographic factors (e.g., age, gender, race), and a myriad of personality and skill factors, many of which may affect individual and team performance. Examples include communication skills, how one handles conflict, and level of assertiveness.

Diversity has the potential to improve team effectiveness and to promote support throughout the organization. From a QI perspective, diversity may generate a wider range of perspectives from which a problem can be analyzed. For example, quality and safety issues may not be apparent to individuals higher in the organization but may be glaringly visible to individuals on the front lines (Fried and Carpenter 2013). Without including lower-level staff, a QI team may not have the ability to effectively analyze processes of care. For example, an organization that limits QI team membership to clinical staff may lack key information about the patient experience. Additionally, hospital administrative clerks may have a unique perspective regarding patient admissions, for example, to which doctors and nurses are not privy. If administrative clerks are not included on the QI team, the team will not have the ability to understand how the admission process is actually carried out. The bottom line is that QI teams should include representatives from all levels of an organization. Furthermore, membership needs on the QI team may change over time, depending on the team's specific goals.

Perhaps no other area of management has received as much attention in the academic and popular literature as leadership. Multiple approaches and theories have been presented over the past 50 years, including "trait" theories, in which personal qualities and characteristics are key to effective leadership. Behavioral theories emphasize the actual actions taken by a leader, and some of these theories include the contrast between employee-oriented leadership and production-oriented leadership. Similarly, some leaders emphasize structure and formal authority, while other leaders place more emphasis on consideration and relationships. Among the most robust approaches to leadership is a contingency (i.e., situational) model, in which leadership style is matched to the situation that the leader faces. This model is an appropriate way to think about leadership in QI teams. Common across all QI models are the importance of team member participation, empowerment, and engagement, and the fact that they provide a structured approach to the work of the team. In essence, leading a QI team requires skill in systematically organizing and employing a highly structured methodology, along with attentiveness to obstacles that may hinder team success, such as conflict, dysfunctional hierarchical relationships, and professional predispositions. Note also that QI team leaders may lack formal authority over team members, and may have to rely on informal sources of influence to get work accomplished.

As the primary instruments for the implementation of QI methods, QI teams need an environment that is supportive of the philosophy and approach of QI. Among the central tenets of QI is the identification of system- and process-level problems rather than individual deficiencies. Even where individual error may have led to a medication error or another threat to patient safety, root cause analysis will often identify organizational processes that inadequately protected the organization and patients from human error. Human mistakes are thus recast in the QI culture from blaming the individual to critically evaluating the organization's processes. As the IOM titled its report on patient safety, "to err is human" (IOM 1999). This observation leads into the construct of psychological safety, defined as "a shared belief held by members of a team that the team is safe for interpersonal risk taking" (Edmondson 1999, 354). In the context of QI, interpersonal risk taking can be extended to include admitting errors, contributing to discussions of organizational processes without fear of being denigrated by others, and having the freedom to contribute information that may be contrary to the majority opinion. In fact, the need for psychological safety extends into the larger organization; that is, an organization focused on quality must establish an environment where all employees perceive the freedom to speak and be heard.

The issue of psychological safety is particularly acute in QI teams that bring together people from multiple disciplines and organizational levels. Team membership is diverse across multiple dimensions, such as hierarchy, professional status, and education. Edmondson and Roloff (2009) note the many challenges faced in creating a psychologically safe environment when so many forms of diversity are present simultaneously. In this setting, a psychologically safe environment is one in which a certified nursing assistant is comfortable expressing a view contrary to that of a physician, and where a registered nurse is comfortable suggesting a change in process that may be viewed skeptically by others. Remember also that psychological safety is a subjective phenomenon. While a manager may feel confident in having created an open and amicable environment, the employees' perceptions may be quite different—and perception is what allows for or limits openness.

Among the key features of all QI efforts is process analysis, which involves breaking down organizational processes to identify bottlenecks, blockages, inefficiencies, and waste. A fishbone diagram (also referred to as an *Ishikawa* or *cause-and-effect diagram*) is frequently employed to identify causes of defects or variation in processes and outputs. Typically, causes are grouped into such categories as people, materials, machines, and methods. The goal is to identify those causes through an iterative process of working toward root causes (sometimes referred to as the *5 Whys*). As one considers root causes, blame is commonly laid initially on individuals, but through effective leadership and direction, individuals may move from a blame-oriented perspective to one that focuses on the underlying causes of quality and safety problems.

Related to the challenge of ensuring psychological safety in a diverse setting is the issue of conflict and conflict management. The numerous sources of conflict range from interpersonal factors to differences in professional orientation and values, competition over resource allocation, and miscommunication. Conflict is inevitable in all organizations and teams, and it is particularly prevalent where changes are being developed. Such conflicts are best managed in an organization whose culture has a consistently proactive and open approach to managing conflict.

Open communication, both vertical and horizontal, is a key prerequisite of organizations wishing to engage successfully in QI activities. Communication is central to identifying quality issues, gathering information, designing change strategies, and obtaining feedback. An organization plagued by distrust and fear is unlikely to provide the climate necessary for full and timely information exchange. Furthermore, the work completed by the QI team often reflects reciprocal task interdependency, where the output of each task is the required input for other tasks. In such situations, communication becomes paramount. Ultimately, clear and open communication allows for smooth transitions in work where problems and needs can be anticipated. A team with poor communication will likely suffer, having to overcome unnecessary barriers to accomplish its goal.

Organization-Level Factors

Some of the organization-level factors that can affect team effectiveness in positive or negative manner have been mentioned previously. Indeed, these factors often limit team effectiveness by affecting the individual-level or team-level factors. One such factor is organizational culture. Organizational culture refers to the group norms and the values that support those norms. An organizational culture that supports QI establishes expectations that employees will participate in QI activities; this participation can be a source of motivation and empowerment for employees. On the other hand, in the presence of an organizational culture that does not support QI, employees may develop a collective feeling of apathy regarding QI work and, in fact, quality overall. Managers at all levels of the organization have an obligation to work to develop and promote an organizational culture for QI. Midlevel managers can work toward developing a supportive culture for QI in their own departments by emphasizing the importance of QI, recognizing successful efforts, and supporting existing efforts. Senior managers in the organization can work to establish a broader organizational culture for QI in the same way. Although efforts often spill over into other departments, affecting the rest of the organization, senior manager support is critical because it often has far-reaching effects.

Managers also have a responsibility for ensuring that QI teams have sufficient resources to carry out their work (this responsibility is also a key part of developing an organizational culture for QI). The primary resources required by a QI team are personnel and time, but teams often need other resources, such as money, equipment, training, and consultation support. Participation on a QI team may at times limit an employee's availability for other tasks. An organization that places a priority on QI will consider QI work part of the work of the organization and will accommodate these situations.

Summary

This chapter discussed the history and meaning of QI, provided a brief overview of common QI methods, and discussed HR practices related to team effectiveness. The quality movement in healthcare is in full force, and like any team-based effort, QI must be managed actively. Managers must be prepared with the knowledge and skills needed to step in and take charge and help develop a supportive environment where QI efforts can succeed.

The topics discussed in this chapter are just a small sampling of the critical elements managers must consider. Many other factors influence the success of QI efforts, either directly or indirectly. For example, the adoption of EHRs and the advancement of other health information technologies have created a rich data source. This resource can be leveraged to help support QI efforts, providing a richer understanding of processes and improving decision making. Additionally, the popularity of learning collaboratives continues to grow. Learning collaboratives are cooperatives where team members come together to learn from success (or shortcomings) of others in similar organizations working on similar QI projects. These collaboratives also represent an opportunity to spread advancements throughout the broader healthcare system. Reinventing the wheel is a waste of time and resources that delays benefits.

Finally, a few key considerations are required for the measurement of change efforts. First, QI teams may not yield the desired results right away. Developing a successful team capable of carrying out a QI effort may be success enough. Hopefully, gains will be realized as the team gains experience and matures. Second, results from change are not always immediately evident. When measuring change, one must be sure that enough time has passed for the change to have an effect. Third, target outcomes should be carefully considered and clearly defined. One surefire way to find no effect is to measure something other than what was initially intended. Finally, managers should consider the bigger picture and view QI efforts from an organization-wide or even societal perspective. Sometimes one has to take a step backward to move forward.

Discussion Questions

1. Why is the success of QI dependent on appropriate human resources management? Which HR practices do you see as most important in QI efforts?

2. What themes and methods are common across QI methodologies?

3. Why is psychological safety a prerequisite for carrying out QI activities?

4. Early in the chapter, the famous quotation is cited: "Every system is perfectly designed to get the results it gets." How is the quotation applicable to human resources management?

5. Consider a quality-oriented organization wishing to hire people

who are inclined toward working on quality issues. In addition to the technical skills required for the job, what other applicant characteristics should be examined when selecting an employee?

Experiential Exercise

Case *Note: This case was written by Jenna Green and Will Haithcock.*

About the Hospital

Prairie Regional Medical Center (PRMC), located in central Kansas, is a 245-bed hospital that offers a comprehensive range of inpatient and outpatient medical services to residents of central Kansas. The medical staff of PRMC consists of more than 125 physicians and dentists representing a number of specialties, including the following:

- Comprehensive cardiac care
- Neurosciences
- Women's health
- Emergency medicine, including a 24-hour trauma center
- Rehabilitation

Among the specialized units and facilities at PRMC are the following:

- Dedicated women's unit
- Skilled nursing facility
- Comprehensive inpatient rehabilitation unit accredited by the Commission

on Accreditation of Rehabilitation Facilities International
- Community resources center
- Laboratory accredited by the College of American Pathologists and American Association of Blood Banks
- Women's imaging center
- Wound care unit

PRMC is fully accredited for all services surveyed by The Joint Commission.

The Situation

Felix, a 68-year-old man, presented to PRMC with a peptic ulcer and underwent abdominal surgery (a diagnostic laparotomy). He was admitted to the patient tower for an anticipated four-day monitoring and recovery stay after his surgery, which was without any complications. Other than the recent operation, Felix has been in relatively good health for his age, but does have diabetes and wears hearing aids in both ears.

Renee, a registered nurse, was assigned to Felix's care during his recovery. She would be able to monitor and care for Felix for his entire recovery because she works a unique schedule of five days on, five days off, which was specifically arranged for her starting three years ago. Renee works 12-hour days from 7 am to 7 pm.

By day 3 of Felix's recovery, he began to notice that communicating with Renee had become somewhat difficult compared with the previous two days. She was short in response to his and his family's questions and noticeably yawned when she came in for routine checks. His wife also noticed that Renee had begun to take markedly longer to respond to his call lights. Later that evening before shift change, Renee took his vitals as she had done the previous two days. Everything appeared normal, so she returned to her other patients on the floor for one last check-in.

By day 4, everything had changed. Renee returned to her fourth shift at 7 am to find that Felix's status was declining. He had a temperature of 102 degrees Fahrenheit, his blood pressure was low, and he had difficulty breathing. Renee tried to quickly get caught up with all that she had missed throughout the night, but was on edge when someone mentioned that the temperature spike likely occurred during her previous shift and was missed by the nursing staff. She knew that she was the last person to sign off on Felix's chart before the night-shift transition and could not help but feel an overwhelming sense of guilt.

What Happened?

Renee now acted through a rush of pure adrenaline, as she knew she needed to quickly get to the bottom of what had happened. She retraced her steps throughout his entire course of care, and then it hit her. Amid her fatigue and constantly busy floor schedule the day before, she had forgotten to come in prior to her last vitals check to remove his hearing aids. She had taken his tympanic temperature

with both hearing aids still in when the standard recommendation is to remove hearing aids and wait 10 minutes before taking a temperature. When Renee realized her mistake, she rushed to find Pam, the new nurse manager, because she knew she had a duty to be transparent with her care. She did not know if this error was the exact cause, but Pam needed to be aware of it. After all, she thought, "I'm human, I make mistakes."

Renee was incredibly nervous to explain to Pam what had happened because she knew that Pam had never liked Renee's work schedule, which had been agreed to before Pam was hired. However, Pam had been willing to accommodate Renee's request as long as no patient complaints could be related to her long hours. Pam was hired into a nursing shortage in the hospital and was therefore in a staffing bind regardless of Renee's schedule. Also, she did not want to ruffle too many feathers since she was so new, so she was willing to try unconventional staffing rotations if her employees wanted them.

Pam then met with Bruce, the grievance coordinator, to pass along this information. Pam had simultaneously set forth an investigation to determine how the infection had been missed under their care. Once the investigation revealed that the temperature spike should have been detected under Renee's care, Pam and Bruce went to meet with Felix's wife. Felix's wife complained that Renee had been visibly drowsy, late to call lights, and unpleasant the day before, but once she knew that Renee had incorrectly taken her husband's vitals, she immediately threatened to file a formal negligence complaint with the Kansas Insurance Department and the CMS Office of the Regional Administrator in Kansas City, Missouri, if Renee was not fired immediately.

Pam returned to her office to discuss the proper course of action with Bruce. She had several considerations and a combination of possible outcomes. First, this occurrence was the first documented complaint against Renee since she had been manager, and Renee had been a very highly regarded nurse for the eight years she had been with PRMC. Since Pam liked to get to know her employees, she also knew that Renee and her husband were struggling financially and had three children to support. Her unconventional schedule had been developed to offset her husband's work schedule so that one parent could always be home with their children since they could not afford childcare. However, she too had noticed Renee coming to work midrotation looking exhausted and not as cheery as she was on the first few days of her rotation. Next, Pam had to consider the implications of the formal grievance and how it would affect her department and ultimately the hospital. Felix's increased length of stay would already

prevent the hospital from being reimbursed for his care, but Pam had to consider if firing an employee over a single mistake was at all justified to further protect the reputation of the hospital.

Questions

1. How should Pam handle the complaint by the patient? What is the danger of disregarding the patient's complaint?

2. Should Pam consider changing Renee's shift schedule? Are there any limits to the amount of shifts or hours that nurses should work? Do you think there should be?

3. How should Pam respond to Felix's wife's demand that Renee be fired?

4. Should this situation be addressed by a QI team, or is this simply an unfortunate situation arising from a troubled employee?

5. Could this situation have been avoided if the organization's human resource management systems had been different? If so, what HR systems might have played a role in this situation?

References

Agency for Healthcare Research and Quality. 2014. "Patient Safety Network Glossary." Accessed June 11. www.psnet.ahrq.gov/glossary.aspx.

———. 2013. *2012 National Healthcare Quality Report.* AHRQ Publication No. 13-0002. Rockville, MD: Agency for Healthcare Research and Quality.

American Society for Quality. 2014a. "History of Quality." Accessed June 11. http://asq.org/learn-about-quality/history-of-quality/overview/overview.html.

———. 2014b. "Total Quality Management (TQM)." Accessed June 11. http://asq.org/learn-about-quality/total-quality-management/overview/overview.html.

Batalden, P., and F. Davidoff. 2007a. "Teaching Quality Improvement: The Devil Is in the Details." *Journal of the American Medical Association* 298 (9): 1059–61.

———. 2007b. "What Is 'Quality Improvement' and How Can It Transform Healthcare?" *Quality & Safety in Health Care* 16 (1): 2–3.

Berwick, D. M., and A. D. Hackbarth. 2012. "Eliminating Waste in US Health Care." *Journal of the American Medical Association* 307 (14): 1513–16.

Donabedian, A. 1980. *Explorations in Quality Assessment and Monitoring, Volume 1: The Definition of Quality and Approaches to Its Assessment.* Chicago: Health Administration Press.

Edmondson, A. 1999. "Psychological Safety and Learning Behavior in Work Teams." *Administrative Science Quarterly* 44 (2): 350–83.

Edmondson, A., and K. Roloff. 2009. "Leveraging Diversity Through Psychological Safety." *Rotman Magazine*, September, 46.

Fried, B., and W. R. Carpenter. 2013. "Understanding and Improving Team Effectiveness in Quality Improvement." In *McLaughlin and Kaluzny's Continuous Quality Improvement in Health Care,* fourth edition, by W. A. Sollecito and J. K. Johnson, 117–54. Burlington, MA: Jones & Bartlett.

Health Resources and Services Administration. 2014. "What Is Quality Improvement?" Accessed December 16. www.hrsa.gov/quality/toolbox/methodology/qualityimprovement/index.html.

Institute of Medicine (IOM). 2004. *Patient Safety: Achieving a New Standard for Care.* Washington, DC: National Academies Press.

———. 2001. *Crossing the Quality Chasm: A New Health System for the 21st Century.* Washington, DC: National Academies Press.

———. 1999. *To Err Is Human: Building a Safer Health System.* Washington, DC: National Academies Press.

———. 1990. *Medicare: A Strategy for Quality Assurance.* Vol. 1. Edited by K. N. Lohr. Washington, DC: National Academies Press.

Kelly, D. L. 2011. *Applying Quality Management in Healthcare: A Systems Approach,* third edition. Chicago: Health Administration Press.

Langley, G. L., R. D. Moen, K. M. Nolan, T. W. Nolan, C. L. Norman, and L. P. Provost. 2009. *The Improvement Guide: A Practical Approach to Enhancing Organizational Performance,* second edition. San Francisco: Jossey-Bass.

Lean Enterprise Institute. 2015. "Principles of Lean." Accessed January 9. www.lean.org/whatslean/principles.cfm.

Leonard, M., S. Graham, and D. Bonacum. 2004. "The Human Factor: The Critical Importance of Effective Teamwork and Communication in Providing Safe Care." *Quality and Safety in Healthcare* 13 (suppl. 1): i85–i90.

National Committee for Quality Assurance. 2007. *The Essential Guide to Health Care Quality.* Washington, DC: National Committee for Quality Assurance.

Reilly, B. M., and A. T. Evans. 2009. "Much Ado About (Doing) Nothing." *Annals of Internal Medicine* 150 (4): 270–71.

Shortell, S. M., J. A. Marsteller, M. Lin, M. L. Pearson, S. Y. Wu, P. Mendel, S. Cretin, and M. Rosen. 2004. "The Role of Perceived Team Effectiveness in Improving Chronic Illness Care." *Medical Care* 42 (11): 1040–48.

Sollecito, W. A., and J. K. Johnson. 2013. "The Global Evolution of Continuous Quality Improvement: From Japanese Manufacturing to Global Health Services." In *McLaughlin and Kaluzny's Continuous Quality Improvement in Health Care*, fourth edition, by W. A. Sollecito and J. K. Johnson, 3–48. Burlington, MA: Jones & Bartlett.

Watkins, R. W. 2014. "Understanding Quality Improvement Is More Important Now Than Ever Before." *North Carolina Medical Journal* 75 (3): 220–23.

APPENDIX A: HUMAN RESOURCES METRICS

Myron D. Fottler and Bruce J. Fried

Chapter 1 discussed the role of strategic human resources (HR) management in facilitating healthcare organizations' achievement of their strategic objectives. This framework means that the organization formulates the HR policies and managerial strategies it needs to achieve its strategic goals. Being able to measure HR processes and outcomes is essential to this process. Examples might include hours of training per employee, employee productivity, and patient satisfaction. This appendix summarizes key metrics that may be used to evaluate the effectiveness and impact of HR practices.

Evaluation is important for several reasons. First, human resources represent a central component of organizational effectiveness; HR practices are linked to employee performance and organizational performance in innumerable ways. Second, in the current era, process improvement and outcomes are at center stage. For example, hospitals analyze their processes for admitting patients, and physician practices seek to reduce patient waiting time. In the same light, HR departments are responsible for analyzing and improving their own processes. Can HR processes be improved, or more fundamentally, do we even have a clear understanding of how HR processes work and what they are meant to produce? Quality improvement methodologies, like those discussed in Chapter 15, may be used to evaluate HR processes. Finally, HR departments are under continued pressure to demonstrate the value they add to the organization. What is the value proposition they offer to the organization, and what value do they add to applicants and employees? Again, articulating and measuring these issues is an essential starting point toward understanding and improvement.

Exhibit A.1 illustrates some commonly used HR metrics that fall under the categories of organizational outcomes, staffing management, organizational/employee development, and compensation. The reason such metrics have seen increased use over time is clear. Without them, organizations would have no way to know how effective a particular HR policy might be in achieving its objectives.

EXHIBIT A.1
Common HR
Metrics and
Their Formulas

Metric	Formula
Organizational outcomes	
Engagement or satisfaction ratings	Percentage of employees engaged or satisfied overall or with a given aspect of the workplace
Percentage of performance goals met or exceeded	No. of performance goals met or exceeded ÷ total no. of performance goals
Percentage receiving performance rating	No. of employees rated under a given score or rating on their performance evaluation ÷ total no. of employees
Return on investment (ROI)	(Total revenues – total costs) × 100 ÷ total costs
Revenue per employee	Revenue ÷ total no. of employees
Value added per employee	(Total revenues – total costs) ÷ total no. of full-time equivalent employees
Staffing management	
Absence rate	No. days absent in month ÷ (average no. of employees during a month × no. of workdays)
Annual turnover	No. of employees exiting the job during 12-month period ÷ average actual no. of employees during the same period
Cost per hire	(Recruitment costs + [compensation cost + benefit cost for year one]) ÷ no. of hires
Tenure	Average no. of years of service at the organization across all employees
Time to fill (average)	Total days taken to fill a job ÷ number hired
Turnover costs	Total costs of separation + vacancy + replacement + training
Yield ratio	Percentage of applicants from a recruitment source that make it to the next stage of the selection process
Organizational/employee development	
Training/ development hours	Sum of total training hours ÷ total no. of employees
Utilization percentage	Total number of employees utilizing a program/service/benefit ÷ total number of employees eligible to utilize a program/service/benefit

(continued)

Compensation	
Benefit or program costs per employee	Total cost of employee benefit/program ÷ total no. of employees
Benefits as a percent of salary	Annual benefits cost ÷ annual salary
Salary as a percentage of total compensation	Annual salary ÷ total compensation (salary + benefits + additional compensation)
Compensation or benefit–revenue ratio	Compensation or benefit cost ÷ revenue
Workers' compensation cost per employee	Total workers' compensation cost for year ÷ average no. of employees
Workers' compensation incident rate	(No. of injuries and/or illnesses per 100 full-time employees ÷ total hours worked by all employees during the calendar year) × 200,000

EXHIBIT A.1
Common HR Metrics and Their Formulas *(continued from previous page)*

Source: Adapted from Employers Resource Council (2014).

Nurse recruitment provides a good illustration of the need for metrics. A healthcare facility might spend thousands of dollars each year in nurse recruiting without ever measuring the effectiveness of different recruitment sources. Which sources produce the most or the best candidates? More fundamentally, what does "best candidates" mean? Normally, such factors as actual clinical performance, job satisfaction, and retention are considered. The solution, therefore, is to assess recruitment effectiveness using metrics. These metrics may include measurement *by recruitment source* of such factors as cost per hire, job performance in the first year, retention in first year, and so forth (Winkler 2007).

Measuring how one is doing on a given HR metric is useful; however, a manager must ask "how are we doing?" *in relation to something.* For example, are nurse retention rates rising or falling? Managers might also want to benchmark their results against those of high performers in their market niche (e.g., hospitals, physician practices, insurers). Cost per hire by itself is relatively useless unless it is presented in a form that shows whether it is trending up or down and how those costs compare to competitors' costs. The goal is to understand why costs are trending up or down and what makes competitors better recruiters. Once managers have an understanding of the meaning of their measures, they can then begin looking at processes. What aspect of the recruitment process yields the results that were observed?

Recall from Chapter 15 the well-known quotation: "Every system is perfectly designed to get the results it gets."

The Society for Human Resource Management's benchmarking service enables employers to compare their own HR metrics to those of other similar organizations on the basis of industry, size, revenue, geographic region, and so forth (www.shrm.org/research/benchmarks/). However, benchmarking alone is not a sufficient process for measuring and evaluating the impact on HR programs and strategies. While benchmarking may indicate how an HR system's performance compares to that of competitors along certain dimensions, it will not reveal the extent to which an organization's HR practices support its strategic goals. For example, if a healthcare facility had a strategic objective to move from the 50th percentile to the 30th percentile in terms of overall patient satisfaction, it might wish to know to what extent a new customer service training program has helped it achieve this goal. Benchmarking the organization's training programs against those of competitors would not answer this question.

To answer this question, managers would need to use *strategy-based metrics*, which measure HR activities that contribute to an organization's strategic goals (Becker and Huselid 2003). For the previous question, the organization might want to compare patient satisfaction scores *before and after* initiation of the customer service training. If the program has the desired effect, then patients should not only be more satisfied with the care they receive, but also plan to return as needed in the future and recommend the facility to friends and relatives.

Connecting HR practices to strategic goals often requires *data-mining techniques*. Data-mining techniques are used to sift through large amounts of employee and program data to identify correlations that employers can then use in their HR programs and practices. Data-mining systems also use other statistical analyses to sift through data looking for relationships.

Most organizations do not use HR metrics to enhance organizational performance. In one study encompassing several industries, 83 percent of executive respondents said that their HR departments regularly report HR metrics such as cost per hire to senior executives (Aon 2014). However, only 10 percent use such data to analyze their HR practices' effectiveness, and only 7 percent use it to change their HR practices. In other words, practicing managers often receive HR metric information, but most do not use it to improve their HR practices and organizational performance.

Evidence-based HR management means using data, facts, analytics, scientific rigor, and critically evaluated research or case studies to support HR proposals, decisions, practices, and conclusions. The authors of a *Harvard Business Review* article argue that managers must become more scientific in making their business decisions (Anderson and Simester 2011). They suggest implementing HR plans with an experimental group (which experiences

EXHIBIT A.2

Examples of HR Metrics Positively and Negatively Associated with High-Performance Organizations

HR Metrics	Positive Association	Negative Association
HR department productivity and expenses	• Use of HR analytics • Number of HR professionals per employee • Percentage of HR budget spent on outsourced activities • HR expense to spending expense ratio • HR expense to full-time equivalent (FTE) ratio	
Organizational outcomes	• Percentage of employees receiving a regular performance appraisal • Percentage of employees receiving regular performance feedback from multiple sources • Percentage of workforce routinely working in a self-managed, cross-functional, or project team	
Staffing management	• Number of qualified applicants per position • Percentage hired on the basis of a validated selection test • Percentage of jobs filled from within • Use of data mining to predict employee retention	• Average time to fill positions • Annual turnover rate • Cost per hire
Organizational/ employee development	• Number of hours of training for new employees (i.e., less than one year) • Number of hours of training for experienced employees • Maximum reimbursement allowed for education expenses per year • Use of data mining to predict future leadership • Greater use of self-managing work teams	• Percentage of eligible workforce covered by a common contract
Compensation	• Target percentile for total compensation when market rate equals the 50th percentile • Percentage of workforce whose merit increase or incentive pay is tied to performance • Percentage of the workforce eligible for incentive pay • Target bonuses for executives and nonexecutives	

Note: High-performance organizations are defined here as those exhibiting low employee turnover and high revenue per employee.

Sources: Becker, Huselid, and Ulrich (2001); *BNA Bulletin to Management* (2004); Dessler (2014); Frauenheim (2007); Gathrie et al. (2008); Macey et al. (2007); Messersmith (2012); Society for Human Resource Management (2014); Stevenson (2012).

new HR practices) and a control group (which does not). Then, managers can determine if the experimental group demonstrated a performance improvement relative to the control group. This process will allow a manager to predict how changing an HR program or policy might affect employee performance.

A number of research studies and case studies have demonstrated that certain HR practices are associated with higher levels of organizational performance. Examples of such practices and their metrics are shown in Exhibit A.2.

As noted in Chapter 1, no HR programs or practices are always and everywhere effective in enhancing individual and organizational performance. Rather, some HR practices are more appropriate for some industries, organizations, and strategies than others. Exhibit A.2 summarizes metric results from a variety of organizations and industries. The results show that these practices may or may not be appropriate for a given organization. Generally speaking, however, high-performing organizations select employees from a large number of qualified applicants, hire on the basis of validated criteria, provide extensive training, pay above the benchmark for each job, foster and empower a self-motivated workforce, and use HR metrics to compare themselves to past data and competitors.

References

Anderson, E., and D. Simester. 2011. "A Step-by-Step Guide to Smart Business Experiments." *Harvard Business Review*, March, 98–105.

Aon. 2014. "Executive Workplace Analytics." Accessed December 30. www.aon.com/human-capital-consulting/hrbpo/executive_workforce_analytics.jsp.

Becker, B. E., and M. Huselid. 2003. "Measuring HR? Benchmarking Is Not the Answer." *HR Magazine* 8 (12): 56–61.

Becker, B. E., M. A. Huselid, and D. Ulrich. 2001. *The HR Scorecard: Linking People, Strategy, and Performance.* Boston: Harvard Business School Press.

BNA Bulletin to Management. 2004. "Super Human Resource Practices Result in Better Overall Performance, Report Says." *BNA Bulletin to Management,* August 26, 273–74.

Dessler, G. 2014. *Human Resource Management,* fourteenth edition. Upper Saddle River, NJ: Pearson Education.

Employers Resource Council. 2014. "20 Common HR Metrics and Their Formulas." Published August 6. www.yourerc.com/blog/post/20-Common-HR-Metrics-and-their-Formulas.aspx.

Frauenheim, E. 2007. "Keeping Score with Analytics Software." *Workforce Management* 86 (10): 25–33.

Gathrie, J., W. Liu, P. Flood, and S. MacCurtain. 2008. *High Performance Work Systems, Workforce Productivity, and Innovation: A Comparison of MNCs and Indigenous Firms.* LINK Working Paper WP04-08. Dublin, Ireland: Learning, Innovation, and Knowledge Research Center, Dublin City University.

Macey, B., G. Farias, J. Rosa, and C. Moore. 2007. "Built to Change: High Performance Work Systems and Self-Directed Work Teams—A Longitudinal Field Study." In W. A. Pasmore and R. W. Woodman (eds.), *Research in Organizational Change and Development*, Volume 16, 339–418. Bingley, UK: Emerald Group Publishing.

Messersmith, J. G. 2012. "Unlocking the Black Box: Exploring the Link Between High Performance Work Systems and Performance." *Human Resource Management International Digest* 20 (3): 1118–32.

Society for Human Resource Management. 2014. "Metrics Calculators." Accessed December 30. www.shrm.org/templatetools/samples/metrics/pages/default.aspx.

Stevenson, C. 2012. "Five Ways High Performance Organizations Use HR Analytics." *TrendWatcher.* Published December 12. www.i4cp.com/trendwatchers/2012/12/12/five-ways-high-performance-organizations-use-hr-analytics.

Winkler, C. 2007. "Quality Check: Better Metrics Improve HR's Ability to Measure and Manage the Quality of Hires." *HR Magazine* 52 (5): 93–98.

APPENDIX B: CASES

Bruce J. Fried

This chapter contains six cases designed specifically to be used with the problem-based learning (PBL) methodology. This method of learning has been widely used in medicine and academic disciplines. PBL is a guided, but largely self-directed approach to learning and problem solving. The approach uses both individual investigation and research, as well as group discussion.

PBL begins with the presentation of a problem that does not have an easy answer and, frequently, does not have a perfect answer. PBL problems are complex and involve information from multiple disciplines. When the problem is presented to groups of four or five students, the first task is for the group to determine the nature of the problem and the information that group members already have about the problem. In other words, groups ask, "What do we already know about this issue?" To address any PBL problem, the group will need to obtain additional information. After discussing the problem and gaps in knowledge, the group establishes learning objectives, typically six or seven. The central question driving these learning objectives is "What do we need to know to address this problem?" The learning objectives provide the basis for the initial research to be done on the problem.

For several days after this initial group session, group members independently conduct research on their learning objectives, with each member keeping a record of information gleaned, sources of information, and any additional useful information that came to light as a result of the research efforts.

The group then reconvenes and shares information, identifying information on which the group is in consensus as well as information that may yield different conclusions. The group discusses what they have learned and attempts to resolve conflictual findings among group members. Additional research may be required to resolve outstanding issues. As information is gathered from group members, the group then produces a collaborative report, the content and length of which were specified in the problem.

Working through a problem involves group discussion in class, independent research outside of class, and a second group discussion session in class. Detailed instructions on the process follow. Prior to each discussion, the group should assign a recorder and, if desired, a group facilitator for the day.

1. **Clarify concepts.** *What are the important issues embedded in this case?* Clarify facts in the case, identify concepts lacking clarity, and attempt to reach agreement on key issues and concepts.

2. **Define the problem.** *What is the problem that needs to be addressed?* Discuss alternative definitions of the problem, and sort out which issues and aspects of the problem are worthy of further investigation. This initial analysis should yield a problem statement that serves as a starting point for the investigation. The problem statement may be revised as assumptions are questioned and new information comes to light.

3. **Identify potential explanations and share knowledge.** *What are alternative explanations for the problem? What do we already know about the problem?* Identify alternative explanations and brainstorm possibilities. Questions may be raised about matters that are unclear or inconsistent. Problems frequently have short-term causes as well as deeply embedded root causes, and group members should discuss the different ways in which the problem may be understood and explained. Groups should avoid a priori exclusion of possible explanations. Group members should also share knowledge that they have about the problem. Compiling a "What We Know (or Think We Know)" list can be helpful at this stage.

4. **Develop learning objectives.** *What additional information do we need to address the problem?* Participants will always face a gap in the information known and the information needed to address the problem. In this stage, group members identify the gaps between what the group knows and what it needs to know to address the problem. These gaps in knowledge are developed into specific learning objectives for the group. Learning objectives should be written in clear, specific language and should be submitted to the course instructor.

5. **Conduct individual research.** The learning objectives provide the basis for individual research prior to the next discussion session. Groups may discuss the kinds of sources that may be consulted, but should not discuss specific references or sources. Learning objectives are not to be divided among group members; all group members explore the same set of learning objectives. On an individual basis, group members seek information and summarize their findings in a short memo of two to three pages, including appropriate citations.

The precise form of this memo should be based on the nature of the problem and instructor preferences. For example, the memo can consist of a bulleted list, but it should be sufficiently organized so that it can be easily comprehended.

6. **Write a group response to the case questions.** During the following class session, groups synthesize the information provided by members. Discussion should focus on evaluating the validity of findings and their application to the problem, common and divergent findings, and sources consulted. Groups should also assess their success in meeting the learning objectives. During class, a final group response to the problem is constructed, and the group should begin writing the final report. After class (if necessary), each group completes work on the final response to the original problem with correctly cited supporting evidence. This final group report is submitted to the instructor.

Case 1: Implementing Comparable-Worth Legislation

In the future year 20XX, the number of women senators and congressional representatives reached a critical mass to influence legislation affecting women. Through a coalition of Republican and Democratic female legislators, a majority of male Democrats, and a small minority of Republicans, the landmark Gender Equality in the Workplace Act was narrowly passed by both houses of Congress. The law was the result of the work of the Gender Equality Workplace Task Force, cochaired by Laura Bush, wife of former president George W. Bush, and Michelle Obama, wife of former president Barack Obama. Members of the task force included former Republican senator Olympia Snowe (Maine), Facebook chief operating officer Sheryl Sandberg, and Randy Johnson, the senior vice president for labor, immigration, and employee benefits of the US Chamber of Commerce.

The wage gap between men and women has been apparent for years, and one figure continues to be cited: Women earn about 77 cents for every dollar that men earn (The White House 2014). Among the studies most often cited is a 1998 report by the Council of Economic Advisers, which estimated that between one-quarter and one-third of the wage gap cannot be explained by relevant job-related factors, and in many cases may be attributed to the dominance of males or females in the job category. Comparable worth legislation has already passed in some jurisdictions, including the state of Washington, the Canadian province of Ontario, and state government in Minnesota. While no study has denied the existence of a wage gap, its extent is subject to dispute and depends on how the figure is calculated (Kessler 2014).

The new law is intended to remedy the well-understood issue of the gap in earnings between men and women. The law goes beyond simply stating that men and women should be paid the same for doing the same work; this principle has been established for decades. The Gender Equality in the Workplace Act mandates that men and women *must be paid the same for doing work of equal value to the organization*. The idea is that women in historically female occupations have been typically paid less than men in historically male-dominated occupations. The new law was based in large part on Ontario's Pay Equity Act, which states:

> The Act requires that employers assess their pay and benefits practices to ensure that female job classes are not underpaid compared to male job classes of equal or comparable value in the same organization. Employers that are subject to the Act are required to value and compare female job classes to male job classes in their workplaces using the factors set out in the Act, and to pay female job classes at least the same as a male job class of equal or comparable value, based on the results of the job comparisons. This may require modifications to existing compensation systems or practices. (Ontario Pay Equity Commission 2012)

This new law is an amendment to the Fair Labor Standards Act and is based on the concept of comparable worth, or comparable value to the organization. Comparable worth is the idea that men and women who perform work of the same value to the organization should receive similar levels of compensation. According to this doctrine, jobs have an organizational value that can be compared across jobs of very different content. Value may be based on factors including skill requirements, effort, responsibility, educational requirements, and working conditions. The essence of the law is that women and men performing work of *equal value*—and not simply the same job as stipulated in the Equal Pay Act—should be paid approximately the same.

The law is to be implemented in stages. In the initial stages, organizations with more than 100 employees are required to put a methodology in place to assess gender equity in the organization. Although strict criteria for assessing job worth are not specified in the legislation, other jurisdictions have assessed job worth using criteria such as skills and effort, working conditions, responsibility, and educational requirements (as noted earlier). To a limited degree, the legislation permits employers to take labor market factors into consideration in assessing job worth. This stipulation was based on a demand of the Chamber of Commerce and Republican members of Congress. However, human resources (HR) directors have been warned that the Department of Labor will scrutinize carefully the use of labor market factors in assessing job worth.

Senior managers at Savant Health System are discussing with some urgency how they will comply with the new law.

Margaret, vice president of HR, stated, "We know that we are currently violating the act. Our full-time registered nurses with ten years of experience make on average $67,000 a year, while we have facilities management people earning close to $90,000. We know that 90 percent of our nurses are female, and right now, all of our facilities management people are male. I'm thinking this is just the tip of the iceberg. If we don't have a way to identify these discrepancies in the next 12 months, we'll be in violation of the Gender Equality in the Workplace Act."

Jack, president of Savant Health System, responded, "This law baffles me. You're saying that we have to identify female-dominated jobs, calculate how valuable they are to Savant, and then compare their salaries with what the act calls a male-dominated job. How in the world do we calculate value, or worth, to the organization? We value everyone and pay our employees fair wages based on their education and experience."

"That's right," responded Dorothy, VP of nursing services. "I hear complaints all the time from our nurses about salaries; they're always comparing themselves to some of the males in our organization who have much less training but are earning about the same as or even more than nurses."

"Let's not panic about this," said Margaret. "What we need in the next 12 months is not necessarily to fix any inequities, but to submit to the Department of Labor a methodology that explains how we will go about identifying inequities. Of course, down the road, we'll have to actually implement the methodology and solve any problems we might find. And keep in mind that the leadership of the Department of Labor's new Pay Equity Division is quite aggressive. The chief of the division is a former ICU nurse. She's been an active advocate for comparable worth legislation for decades, and she played no small part in the election of several key female senators in the last election. So this is not just paperwork. The Department of Labor has hired a sizeable field staff to monitor implementation of the law."

Ray, VP of finance, entered the conversation. "You know, if this pay equity exercise results in a finding that our compensation practices are out of compliance, it will wreak havoc on our budget. If we have to bump up the salaries for our female-dominated jobs, like nursing, we may face unanticipated consequences. And how do we deal with the medical technicians and nursing assistants? We all know that these two groups are unionized and represented by the Service Employees International Union. They're going to be scrutinizing this process carefully. How should we involve the union in developing this methodology?"

Margaret responded, "We haven't actually done a job evaluation exercise in years. Our salary scales have been guided largely by the labor market. So even without this legislation it is probably worth looking at our salaries in a systematic way. I'm willing to take on this project, as long as I can call on each of you to help develop the methodology. And I'd like your advice on how to involve the union. I don't want to put all this work in only to have the Department of Labor tell us we've done it all wrong."

"I think we know what the task is," said Jack. "Margaret, let's see if you can develop a schematic—an overview—of what this comparable worth methodology would look like. We'll review it at our next meeting. Where do we start? For example, how do we determine if we have male- and female-dominated jobs? How have other organizations gone about this task?"

References

Council of Economic Advisers. 1998. "Explaining Trends in the Gender Wage Gap." Published June. http://clinton4.nara.gov/WH/EOP/CEA/html/gender gap.html.

Kessler, G. 2014. "President Obama's Persistent '77-Cent' Claim on the Wage Gap Gets a New Pinocchio Rating." *The Washington Post*. Published April 9. www. washingtonpost.com/blogs/fact-checker/wp/2014/04/09/president-obamas-persistent-77-cent-claim-on-the-wage-gap-gets-a-new-pinocchio-rating/.

Ontario Pay Equity Commission. 2012. "Overview." Issued August 15. www.pay equity.gov.on.ca/en/resources/guide/ope/ope_2.php.

The White House. 2014. *The Impact of Raising the Minimum Wage on Women*. Published March. www.whitehouse.gov/sites/default/files/docs/20140325 minimumwageandwomenreportfinal.pdf.

Case 2: Physician Engagement

Copper River Community Hospital is an independent, not-for-profit 275-bed hospital located in Copper River (pop. 24,000), a rural community in the Midwest. It is located about 200 miles from a medium-sized city (pop. 130,000). It has faced problems related to decreased revenue and staff turnover.

"I don't think anyone would argue with me if I said that most of our physicians couldn't care less about this hospital. Sure, they are committed to patient care and doing what is best for the patient. In fact, some of our physicians have been known to phone and even visit patients after their discharge from the hospital. But let's face it, the average physician here would leave at the first better offer from another hospital, and we've seen our share of physicians depart over the past few years. Two other hospitals are within an hour's drive, so moving to another hospital—and taking their patients—is not much of an ordeal. Our physician retention numbers are going down, and quite frankly, I don't know what more we can do," commented Joyce, the vice president of HR, in response to the news that a leading orthopedic surgeon was leaving the hospital.

Other members of the senior management team were not so sure that their problem was unique. Beverly, VP of nursing, stated, "Listen, haven't we done all that we can really do? Our compensation is competitive, communication with physicians has improved, and we've lessened on-call time. What else is left? This is the reality of today's marketplace. We simply can't keep adding perks and hoping that physicians respond."

In fact, the problem of physician engagement ran deeper than retention. As Charles, VP of finance, noted, "Physicians can do lab work in their office. They can do EKGs in their office. They can do heart echoes, and the aggressive ones have even put CT scanners in their office—things that will generate ancillary revenue. If they're doing these procedures in their office, it hurts the hospital. We're in competition now for that revenue stream."

Joyce went on to talk about the cost of replacing a physician. "The cost is enormous. We have estimated that the cost of replacing a single physician at our hospital is $85,000—and this doesn't take into consideration the intangible costs of stress on our workforce and patients. We've got to think about recruitment, retention, and engagement at the same time. They can't be separated."

After further discussion, the team still had not established whether this hospital was unusual in its physician engagement and retention problems. In fact, some members of the team felt that Copper River was doing better than other hospitals. Others felt the hospital was about average, while still others felt it was doing worse.

Sarah, the quality improvement specialist, sought to break the deadlock. "What we need are measures. We need metrics so that we can track engagement, retention, and factors that are associated with attracting and keeping the best physicians. In fact, we should probably think about tracking these metrics with nursing staff as well."

Chris, the hospital president, agreed. "Sarah, you're absolutely right. We definitely need to do a better job of collecting and understanding data. Can you work with a team to get a handle on what data we have, and what we need?"

Sarah was excited about this possibility. "Thanks. I was hoping we'd be able to address this, because I'm seeing evidence of some quality issues that I think are related to physician engagement. Let me summarize what I think we need. First, we need a way to compare ourselves with other similar hospitals. But even before that, what measures should we use? I think we need to go beyond simple physician turnover rates or time to hire a new physician. Sorry, Joyce, I know these are the kind of metrics that HR uses, but I think we need more than just summary statistics."

Joyce responded, "That's fine, Sarah. I'm not offended in the least! But you need to understand that a lot of consulting firms out there are promising the moon. I don't think we should focus on identifying a particular vendor to measure physician satisfaction. I don't want to just hire a consulting firm to tell us what we need to do. We've got to figure out what the key drivers are, and then maybe we can design our own assessment tool or select a firm that we feel is competent to address our specific issues. You know, it's not about the money, at least in the cases I've been involved with. It's about getting the right people on board and not settling for someone who doesn't quite fit in."

James, chief of the medical staff, responded, "Well, that's easy for you to say. Do you know how hard it is to recruit an orthopedic surgeon? We can't be too picky. Sometimes, you've got to just get someone on board, treat them right, pay them right, and hope for the best."

"Yes," Joyce responded. "I know how hard it is to recruit a physician to this hospital. Unless they were brought up in this town and have family here, it's tough to convince doctors to settle here. And yes, James, I have been involved in several physician recruitment efforts. In fact, I advised against hiring Dr. Sulu. I had a feeling that coming from San Francisco, he couldn't bear the isolation of this community. Our cornfields are quite a distance from the Golden Gate Bridge."

"Okay," said Sarah. "Let me continue. As you're all saying, this is not a simple matter. If it was, we would have known the solution years ago. There are attitudinal issues and financial issues. And of course, what kind of physicians do we really need in terms of our community and changing demographics? What kind of economic relationship do we want with our physicians? How do we keep then engaged and aligned with our goals and values?"

Sarah continued, "You know, we're missing one important detail here. Physician engagement is not a one-size-fits-all proposition. What engages one physician may not be relevant or important to others. We're dealing with different specialties and different modes of practice. We have solo practitioners with admitting privileges, multispecialty and single-specialty group practices, and the emergency physician group that we contract with. And then, of course, we employ a few physicians, and spend a lot of money on locum tenens doctors. If you talk to all of these physicians, which I have, you'll hear different concerns and issues. We've got to take these into account as we think about retention and engagement."

Chris responded, "Listen, let's keep the goal in focus here. We've got to find the best physicians and get them to stay. They're our bread and butter. I don't want a lot of surveys. We've been through that too often already. Let's just do something. But I agree with Sarah. We need data. You know, this problem is infectious. First one physician leaves, then another, and before you know it, a whole bunch of physicians start thinking that they want to leave."

Sarah responded, "Thank you for your confidence in me. But I don't know if this infectiousness argument is true or not. Do the data support this? I don't know. Like you said, we need good information to help us make informed decisions. I'll come back with a report about the types of information we need, why that information is important, and how we can go about getting this information."

Looking at his watch, Chris said, "Okay, I think we've got some consensus here. Joyce and Sarah, I'd like you to work together to answer the following questions. What are the drivers of physician engagement, and to your point, Sarah, are these drivers different for different types of physicians, that is, physicians with different financial relationships with Copper River? And different specialties? Sarah, pay attention to those categories of physicians that you talked about. If the drivers are different, what kinds of strategies should we consider? Are good data available on best practices? I don't just want a consulting firm's promotional materials. Do we know what would be most effective in our environment? Listen, I think the fact that we're a relatively small hospital makes us more attuned to the community—our people know what's going on out there, how it affects the hospital, and how our choices affect the community perception. Let's see if you can come up with some answers and strategies for us. Thank you for your work on this. Now I've got to meet with that new GI doctor who wants more vegetarian options in our snack bar."

Case 3: Nurse Staffing Ratios and the State Nursing Association

Many studies have documented associations between nurse staffing levels and patient outcomes. Adequate nurse staffing is associated with a reduction in hospital readmissions, lower incidence of adverse patient events, fewer errors, reduced mortality, and other positive outcomes. In addition to empirical studies, meta-analyses and other reviews have examined nurse staffing ratios.

Given the preponderance of evidence on nurse staffing and patient safety, how should the healthcare system encourage adequate nurse staffing? California is the only state to have mandated specific nurse-to-patient ratios for different types of units. The American Nurses Association (2014) identifies three general approaches to ensure adequate staffing: (1) requiring hospitals to have a "nurse-driven staffing committee"; (2) mandating specific nurse-to-patient ratios through legislation or regulation (i.e., the California model); and (3) requiring facilities to disclose staffing levels to the public or a regulatory body.

Your state does not have any regulations regarding nurse staffing, but the public has shown strong interest in the topic. In a recent high-profile case, a pediatric patient died as a result of inadequate staffing in a community hospital.

You are a legislative assistant to the chair of the state senate's Health and Human Services subcommittee. The chair has asked you to develop a summary of the issues around different legislative approaches to nurse staffing levels. Your two- to three-page report should respond to the following issues:

- What are the alternative legislative options for addressing nurse staffing, and in which states have each of them been adopted? Does the evidence indicate that these approaches have been successful?
- How are major stakeholders likely to view each legislative strategy? Specifically focus on (1) the state nurses association, (2) the state hospital association, and (3) labor unions (almost half of the nurses in your state are unionized). Given these groups' interests, which strategies are they most and least likely to support?

Reference

American Nurses Association. 2014. "Nurse Staffing Plans and Ratios." Updated December. www.nursingworld.org/MainMenuCategories/Policy-Advocacy/State/Legislative-Agenda-Reports/State-StaffingPlansRatios.

Case 4: Is the Nurse Shortage Over for Good?

Melissa typed a furious message to her best friend from nursing school: "If I hear him say one more time that the nursing shortage is over for good, I'm going to quit this job and go someplace where my views are better respected." Melissa was the VP of nursing services at Everdeen Hospital, and she had just returned to her office from her weekly meeting with the senior management team.

As she had done for the past six months, Melissa raised the issue of the nursing labor market, stressing again that the current lull in the nursing shortage is due to short-term economic difficulties in the United States. The president of the hospital, Corie, continued to insist that nothing more needed to be done to recruit and retain nurses. "We've got nurses calling HR every day asking about employment, and we're telling them nothing is available now. They're practically demanding that we hire them! All I hear about these days is the myth of the nursing shortage. Melissa, the nursing shortage is yesterday's news. Let's move on to more important nursing issues."

Katelyn, VP of HR, concurred with the president's view. "Corie's right. But I'll tell you, my friends around the country in HR are looking at long-term shortages in lots of specialized areas. I don't want to be a naysayer, but frankly, I don't see this glut of nurses continuing. Maybe we'll start seeing shortages in specialized areas, or maybe in some geographic regions. I don't know how or when we'll see the nursing shortage return, but I am uneasy about just declaring victory."

The VP of finance, Gary, was unequivocally supportive of Corie: "All of these doomsayers in nursing schools have been telling us that the United States will be short a hundred thousand nurses—or whatever. Well, this won't be the first time that these academics are wrong. Besides, our hospital is in a very desirable location. We're in a nice suburban community about an hour from the Loop. We've been successful at recruiting nurses even though our pay rates for RNs are 10 percent lower than those in nearby hospitals. And we're getting highly qualified BSN nurses. Please don't talk about raising wages or signing bonuses, or we'll get into a needless arms race, and who knows where that will end up. I think all this talk about an impending crisis has been fabricated by the nursing school industry trying to get more faculty and increase their enrollment. And you know, in the next five years, advances in technology will probably make a lot of nursing tasks unnecessary, but are the nursing schools paying attention to robotics and artificial intelligence when they make their dire predictions? Think about it."

Melissa did her best to ignore Gary's comments, but continued making her argument about the cyclical nature of the nursing shortage. "We know that there is a relationship between the supply of nurses and the overall unemployment rate. I can get you an article from April 2012 from the *New England Journal of Medicine* warning that we're in a bubble and that the shortage will return when unemployment nationally goes down. Gary, are you ready to take this up with the editorial board of the *New England Journal*? And you know, when this shortage comes back, I'll be the one on the line. Everyone will be asking me why we didn't plan for this. And by the way, we're starting to prepare for Joint Commission accreditation. Corie, how would you like to be sitting on a 20 percent nurse vacancy rate when our good friends from The Joint Commission come to visit? And how about if nurses start writing letters to the *Chicago Tribune* about shortages and being burned out, and how patient safety is at risk at our hospital because of staff shortages? You know that reporter who writes stories for the *Trib* about healthcare in Illinois? If our nurses get vocal, he'll pounce on this, big time. Our nurse supply is a public relations disaster waiting to happen."

Corie closed his eyes and tilted his head back, exasperated and confused. Beads of sweat formed on his forehead. To his relief, his cell phone rang, and he decided to take the call, leaving the conference room for ten minutes. The VP of finance sat there mildly amused, and resumed a sudoku puzzle he had started earlier on his iPad. Katelyn, somewhat shocked by the proceedings, just stared at Melissa, wondering how Corie would react to her outburst.

Finally, Corie returned to the conference room. The phone call had given him time to collect himself. "Okay, everyone, I hear your concerns, and we need to address this in a systematic way. Melissa and Katelyn, I'd like you to do some background work. We need some questions answered, and I'd like unbiased facts about this supposed shortage situation. You may have more questions, but here are mine:

"First, has there ever really been a nursing shortage in the last 30 years? I've had people tell me that there's never a shortage of nurses, just a shortage of nurses willing to work. What's the evidence on this?

"Next, I've read about cycles of nurse shortages. It goes something like this. Nurses are dissatisfied and leave the workforce, and then we pay incentives to recruit nurses until the shortage ends. After that, we get complacent and remove the incentives, and nurses get dissatisfied again. My questions are: Do the data support this scenario? How have these cycles played out in, say, the last 30 years or so? How many years does this cycle take to work through? We've been in a surplus situation for a few years now, and if historic trends remain true, I think we should be in a shortage by now. Are we still in this cyclical pattern or what? How will we know if the cyclical pattern is over?

"I'm also concerned about what Katelyn said about the possibility of shortages in certain specialized areas of nursing. What are those areas? What should we be most concerned about? What geographic markets are most vulnerable? Is there a canary in the coal mine we should be paying attention to? And I don't know for sure, but you may find evidence that lower unemployment rates are correlated with nurse shortages. If the evidence supports this, then please: What should we be doing right now?

"Finally, what's got me really worried is what's happening nationally. We need to understand how the Affordable Care Act will affect our ability to recruit and retain nurses. Everyone's talking about primary care physicians, but how about nursing? Is there any historical precedent for large-scale policy changes affecting the supply and demand for nurses? How will the Affordable Care Act affect our ability to attract and retain nurses?

"And one more thing. As I'm sitting here in this meeting I'm starting to worry about other staff shortages. If you run across anything on, say, radiation technologists or physical therapists, let me know if we should be concerned about the Affordable Care Act and these groups. This is not essential for your report, but at some point we'll want to know about other professions and whether they show cycles similar to those of nurses. What should we be worried about?

"I'm going to put my postgraduate health administration fellow, Peter, at your disposal. He's a very committed young man, and I think he'd sacrifice his own skin to protect us. I'll ask him to put his other projects on hold, so you'll have him pretty much full-time for the next few days. He's a smart guy and knows how to get information.

"I think we all can agree that we want evidence-based answers, and not emotional responses—no offense intended, Melissa. I understand your concerns and we'll act according to what you can find out. Please send your response to me by the end of the day next Tuesday. Please keep it under three pages."

Reference

Staiger, D. O., D. I. Auerbach, and P. I. Buerhaus. 2012. "Registered Nurse Labor Supply and the Recession—Are We in a Bubble?" *New England Journal of Medicine* 366 (16): 1463–65. www.nejm.org/doi/full/10.1056/NEJMp1200641.

Case 5: A Living Wage

Methodist Hospital, a 400-bed acute care hospital, is located in a low-income community in a city in the Southwest. Like other urban hospitals, Methodist Hospital serves a large number of Medicaid patients. As a result of national legislation, the number of uninsured patients has decreased over the last three years, but the hospital remains in a chronic state of financial distress. Methodist Hospital was recently acquired by a hospital system.

The hospital has just experienced a rather bad six months. The problems started when a supervisor in the housekeeping department repeatedly violated hospital policy and federal law by tampering with time sheets for several employees. Three Latino women employees brought this violation to the attention of the local NBC affiliate. The story went viral, and within 48 hours it had been broadcast on CNN and MSNBC and published in *USA Today*. The hospital's director of public relations apologized for this "clerical error" and the supervisor's misunderstanding about procedures. The employees received back compensation for the mistake and were each given a gift certificate to a local restaurant. The supervisor received a reprimand but continued to work at the hospital. After the incident was resolved, several other employees came forward with similar complaints, indicating that they were afraid at the time to speak up. An internal investigation of the situation continues.

Less than a month later, Deborah, who earns $98,100 per year as director of information technology at Methodist Hospital, was arrested on a DUI charge after she struck and injured a mother and child at a crosswalk. The injured mother, who was a dietary aide at Methodist earning $8.50 per hour, was on her way home after picking up her child from daycare. This arrest was Deborah's third in five years for DUI, and she had in fact lost her driver's license. Her husband, a prominent orthopedic surgeon at Methodist, worked back channels with the board and the local police to reduce the charges and keep her on staff at the hospital. The hospital agreed to keep her on staff but referred her to an employee assistance program.

A week later, the *Wall Street Journal* published a story about wage discrepancies in a sample of inner-city hospitals throughout the United States. The story was based on a study conducted by a team of *Wall Street Journal* reporters working with staff at the Urban Institute. Of 50 hospitals studied, Methodist Hospital was cited as having one of the greatest wage disparities between white and minority employees (at Methodist Hospitals, minorities were mostly African Americans and Latinos). After controlling for job title and job responsibilities, tenure in the organization, experience, age, and other factors, the reporters found systematic racial bias in wages over the past ten years. Methodist Hospital, in fact, was one of only six hospitals studied exhibiting such profligate bias.

Following these incidents, the hospital continued to be a center of controversy, with repeated stories in the local newspaper, television, and social media. In the midst of this uproar, the hospital board met with the senior management team to discuss how the hospital should repair the damage caused by these incidents. A community–hospital relations team, composed of hospital staff, the vice president of HR, the director of public relations, and several community leaders, was formed. After three weeks, the team issued its report, which recommended several community outreach initiatives, diversity training for hospital employees, and the development of a stronger policy outlining expectations of hospital staff outside of the work setting. Among the team's additional recommendations was something new to the hospital, an initiative that the team highlighted as a way to get the community's attention and send a message that the hospital was truly committed to improving its relationship with the community and contributing to the city's economic development.

The report proposed that the hospital adopt a living wage policy for its employees. No other living wage policy was in place in the city. In fact, the hospital would be the largest organization in the state to adopt any form of living wage policy. The policy would likely provide a substantial benefit to the lowest-paid employees of the hospital, who were disproportionately African American and Latino.

After reviewing the report, the senior management team and board were very supportive of most of the recommendations but hesitated on the living wage policy. Because of the policy's financial implications and the uncertainty about the precise meaning of a living wage, discussion of the proposed living wage policy took up most of the meeting.

The hospital president had little familiarity with the idea of a living wage. He had heard about the concept but had no idea what its financial impact would be or how it would be implemented. In concept, he agreed that paying people more would be a popular action. But what would be the financial impact, and would it cause a ripple effect, increasing wages throughout the hospital, perhaps resulting in having to decrease staffing levels? He asked the vice president of finance and the vice president of HR to develop a two- to three-page summary report addressing the following questions:

- What is the definition of "living wage"?
- Has a living wage policy has been put into place in any jurisdictions? If so, what was the impetus for the policy? What have been the repercussions, both positive and negative?
- How is a living wage calculated? Does it vary by location, family size, and other factors? Are there different models or approaches to a living wage policy?
- What is the impact of a living wage policy on employees in the organization? Specifically, does a living wage policy raise the wages only for people who are currently paid below the living wage level? If so, how is the policy likely to affect internal equity within the organization? Alternatively, does implementing a living wage policy bump up everyone's wages?
- In comparison with other hospitals in the city, Methodist Hospital's pay structure is right in the middle, and the hospital has been pretty successful in attracting and retaining employees. How would the hospital reconcile a living wage policy with its current compensation system, which is driven mostly by market factors?
- What evidence is available on the financial impact of a living wage policy on organizations? Does such a policy have ancillary benefits that can be monetized, such as reduced turnover?

In a private conversation with the director of public relations, the hospital president said, "If we do something with this living wage idea, we've got to make it a very big deal. We'll need a press release and a press conference attended by representatives from the National Association for the Advancement of Colored People and the League of United Latin American Citizens. We've got to make it look like a very sincere effort, which of course it is."

Case 6: Same-Sex Marriage and Human Resources Policy

"Every morning when I turn on NPR I panic. It seems that every day some court is either tossing out or upholding a state's same-sex marriage ban. How in the world do we set employment policies in this environment? Our system employs people in 11 different states, and same-sex marriage laws are in a state of flux in at least half of them. What do we advise the HR directors in our facilities? They're asking us for guidance, and I simply tell them to talk to their congressional representative for advice. And from what I've heard, they're pretty much in the dark."

Thus speaks Mary, vice president of talent acquisition and people management at Sunbrook Health System, a large, not-for-profit, religiously affiliated integrated health system that includes acute care hospitals, rehabilitation hospitals, and medical groups. She is concerned with establishing a corporate policy on employee benefits that is consistent with current laws about same-sex marriage.

Mary realizes that marital status is an enormous issue that has an impact on a myriad of HR issues, as well as potent political and emotional implications. Many employee rights and benefits are dependent on marital status, and she realizes that each facility in the system, as well as the corporate office, is potentially vulnerable to a lawsuit if it is found to be in violation of state or federal law. At this time, Sunbrook Health System does not have a uniform policy on same-sex marriage, leaving each local entity to determine its own policy based on state law and community standards. Given the complexity of the issue, she has asked the system's legal department to provide guidance on a number of issues.

"With the changing environment, should Sunbrook Health System have a same-sex marriage policy that applies to all of its facilities, regardless of the legal status of same-sex marriage? That is, should we as a system see the writing on the wall and adopt a policy acknowledging same-sex marriage as a reality? What are the advantages and disadvantages of having such a systemwide policy?" She notes that Sunbrook has facilities in multiple states, including Mississippi and Minnesota.

"I assume that with a uniform policy, the Family and Medical Leave Act (FMLA) will apply to same-sex spouses," she continues. "Is this true? What happens if two men living together adopt an infant? Would they be entitled to the maternity leave currently in place in our facilities? I may be naïve, but who would be classified as the "mother"? Or do we need to overhaul our language?

"Should such a uniform policy be put into place, how should it be communicated to the local HR executive staff? Should local HR staff be involved in establishing the policy? How do we then communicate these changes to our employees in each facility? Can we allow a particular facility to opt out of the policy if it is in a state that has a law against same-sex marriage? That is, can a facility opt out if the executive staff feels that such a policy would violate community norms?

"What common questions will we need to address if we put into place a corporate policy accepting same-sex marriage? For example, for employee benefits that are not statutorily required for same-sex spouses, such as FMLA leave, will the same-sex spouse be eligible for those benefits? Would such a policy now imply that we are treating sexual preference as a protected class, even though it is not a protected class under Title VII of the Civil Rights Act? Are we creating more difficulties for ourselves by giving yet another group of employees the opportunity to take us to court?

"What IRS laws do we need to take into account in relation to this question, particularly with respect to taxes on benefits? Can you provide guidance on insurance contracts and retirement benefits that may have been put into place assuming a traditional marriage? Is the same-sex partner now to be covered?

"I know that marital status is central to so many HR policies, and I don't want to be blindsided. What other issues are likely to emerge that we can proactively respond to before we end up in court? Please provide me with a summary of your comments on these issues. Please keep the report to two to three pages so that I can share it with the hospital president and board."

INDEX

Note: Italicized page locators refer to figures or tables in exhibits.

ABOUT THE EDITORS

Bruce J. Fried, PhD, is an associate professor and director of the residential master's program in the Department of Health Policy and Management in the Gillings School of Global Public Health at the University of North Carolina at Chapel Hill. He teaches in the areas of human resources management, international and comparative health systems, and globalization and health. He has written numerous journal articles, book chapters, commentaries, and book reviews. Dr. Fried is also coeditor of and contributor to *World Health Systems: Challenges and Perspectives*, second edition (Health Administration Press, 2012). Among his research interests are the impact of organizational factors and culture on quality in healthcare settings, healthcare workforce, mental health services, and global health. Dr. Fried has conducted workshops and management training courses in Eastern Europe, Asia, Latin America, the Middle East, and the Caribbean. He received his undergraduate degree from the State University of New York at Buffalo, his master's degree from the University of Chicago, and his doctorate from the University of North Carolina at Chapel Hill.

Myron D. Fottler, PhD, is a professor of health services administration at the University of Central Florida, where he teaches courses in healthcare human resources management, service management and marketing, and health services research. He has presented more than 100 papers at profession meetings and authored more than 150 journal articles, 60 book reviews, 45 book chapters, and 28 books. His most recent coauthored books include *Achieving Service Excellence: Strategies for Healthcare*, second edition (Health Administration Press, 2010), *The Retail Revolution in Healthcare* (Praeger, 2010), *Strategic Human Resource Management in Healthcare* (Emerald, 2010), *Human Resources Management Applications*, seventh edition (South-Western Cengage, 2011), *Fundamentals of Human Resources in Healthcare* (Health Administration Press, 2011), *Advances in Healthcare Management: Biennial Review* (Emerald, 2012), and *Handbook of Healthcare Management* (Elgar, 2015). Over his career, Dr. Fottler has been active in the Health Care Management Division of the Academy of Management and the Association of University Programs in Health Administration. He was also the cofounder and coeditor of *Advances in Healthcare Management,* an annual book series featuring both empirical and review papers; served on the editorial review board for many major journals in the field; and mentored more than 50 doctoral students. He earned his MBA from Boston University and his PhD in business from Columbia University.

ABOUT THE CONTRIBUTORS

Jordan Albritton, MPH, is a doctoral student in the Department of Health Policy and Management at the University of North Carolina at Chapel Hill. He earned his master's degree in public health from East Carolina University and has several years of experience conducting implementation research in various settings. His research interests include implementation science, quality improvement, team dynamics, and global health.

Dolores G. Clement, DrPH, FACHE, is the Sentara Professor in the Department of Health Administration at Virginia Commonwealth University (VCU) and the program director of dual degree programs (MHA/MD and MHA/JD) at VCU. She has served as the American College of Healthcare Executives Regent for Virginia–Central. She holds a joint appointment in the Department of Family Medicine and Population Health in the School of Medicine at VCU. Dr. Clement earned her doctorate in health policy and administration from the University of California, Berkeley. She has investigated such areas as community health and well-being; curriculum development and assessment of competency models; distance learning; Medicare risk contracting with health management organizations (HMOs) for the elderly in the areas of quality, access, and beneficiary satisfaction; patterns of diffusion, growth, and survival of HMOs; and use of alternative payment strategies by providers.

Maria A. Curran, MA, is the chief human resources officer and vice president of human resources and community benefit at Virginia Commonwealth University (VCU) Health System. She is also an adjunct faculty member of the VCU Department of Health Administration and teaches a graduate-level course that focuses on the myriad issues facing executives when managing human capital. Ms. Curran earned a master's degree from the University of Virginia and a bachelor's degree from Rollins College.

Rupert M. Evans Sr., DHA, FACHE, is an associate professor of health administration and the chairman and director of the healthcare administration program at Governors State University. Dr. Evans is a Harvard Macy

Scholar, a fellow in the Illinois Public Health Leadership Institute (now the MidAmerica Regional Public Health Leadership Institute), and a Fellow of the American College of Healthcare Executives. He is the immediate past president of the Institute for Diversity in Health Management and the past president of the Chicago–Midwest Chapter of the National Association of Health Services Executives. He has written articles for *Hospitals & Health Networks*, *Modern Healthcare*, and the *Journal of Healthcare Management* and is the author of two textbook chapters on diversity and organizational development. He served as faculty for Rush University's Department of Health Systems Management, the Governance Institute, the American College of Healthcare Executives, the National Association of Health Services Executives, the American Organization of Nurse Executives, the American Governance and Leadership Group (now the Center for Healthcare Governance), and the International Quality and Productivity Center. He holds a doctorate in healthcare administration from Central Michigan University, a master's degree in public administration/health services management, and a bachelor of arts degree in environmental studies. Dr. Evans is a life member of Kappa Alpha Psi Fraternity Inc. and an active member of Richton Park Alumni Chapter.

Erin P. Fraher, PhD, MPP, is an assistant professor in the School of Medicine at the University of North Carolina at Chapel Hill, holding joint appointments in the Department of Family Medicine and the Department of Surgery. Her area of expertise is the collection, analysis, presentation, and dissemination of healthcare workforce data to inform policy debates. Her research focuses on the need to retool and reconfigure the healthcare workforce to meet the demands of healthcare system reform. Dr. Fraher has published extensively in peer-reviewed journals, and her well-known ability to publish policy briefs, fact sheets, data summaries, maps, and other documents that convey information in ways that reach diverse audiences has allowed her work to have broad impact.

Michael Gates, PhD, RN, is an associate professor in the School of Nursing at San Diego State University. He has a doctorate in nursing from the University of North Carolina at Chapel Hill and is an alumnus of the Robert Wood Johnson Nurse Faculty Scholar Program. He began his nursing career at the University of Tennessee in Memphis after two years as a research assistant with the health policy group at the Urban Institute and after receiving his bachelor of science degree in applied mathematics/economics from Brown University. His research interests include diversity and the nursing workforce, and he is particularly interested in the link between the healthcare workforce and outcomes of care. His work examines nurse labor market behaviors, simulation, migration, and employment trends.

John C. Hyde II, PhD, FACHE, is a professor of health services at the University of Mississippi Medical Center in the School of Health Related Professions and the School of Medicine. Additionally, he is an adjunct professor of healthcare administration at the University of Mississippi School of Business Administration. Dr. Hyde teaches graduate-level healthcare administration courses and conducts research focusing on managerial and clinical outcomes. Prior to entering academia, he served in healthcare administrative positions at the senior level. He frequently publishes and presents his research findings.

Sharon L. Jahn, MS, CEBS, CMS, is benefits director for the Virginia Commonwealth University (VCU) Health System. Previously, she was benefits manager for MCV Physicians at VCU, and she worked at Trigon Blue Cross/Blue Shield (now Anthem) in both the actuarial and third-party administration departments. Early in her career, she worked for the actuarial department of Life of Virginia and the Virginia Department of Medical Assistance Services (Medicaid). She received a bachelor's degree in mathematics from the College of William and Mary and a master's degree in risk management and insurance from VCU. She earned a Certified Employee Benefit Specialist designation in 2001 and a Compensation Management Specialist designation in 2004. She is a Fellow in the International Society of Certified Employee Benefit Specialists (ISCEBS) and serves on the board of the Richmond chapter of ISCEBS.

Cheryl B. Jones, PhD, RN, FAAN, is a professor and chair of the Division of Health Care Environments in the School of Nursing and a research fellow at the Cecil G. Sheps Center for Health Services Research at the University of North Carolina at Chapel Hill. Dr. Jones has a long-standing interest in the healthcare workforce, quality of care, and the cost of care delivery. Her work on the costs of nursing turnover is cited frequently, and she has published on the nursing workforce topic in numerous peer-reviewed journals. She has been involved in several projects examining the nursing workforce at organizational and public policy levels, and she has collaborated with others in the public and private sectors to analyze trends in the healthcare workforce and its impacts on quality of care. Dr. Jones is coauthor of *Financial Management for Nurse Managers and Executives,* fourth edition (Saunders, 2012). She obtained her bachelor's degree from the University of Florida and her master's and doctoral degrees from the University of South Carolina.

Donna L. Kaye, MA, is the director of learning and organizational development at the University of North Carolina Medical Center, where she provides leadership in the assessment of organizational needs and in the design, implementation, and evaluation of change initiatives that enhance organizational performance and health as well as individual learning. She earned a master of arts degree in liberal studies, with a concentration in organizational change, from North Carolina State University and a bachelor of science in consumer economics from Cornell University.

Donna Malvey, PhD, is an associate professor at the University of Central Florida. She received her master's degree in health services administration from George Washington University, completed an administrative residency and postgraduate fellowship in hospital administration at the Veterans Administration Medical Center in Washington, DC, and earned her doctorate in health services administration from the University of Alabama at Birmingham. Her area of specialization is strategic management. She has coauthored two books, *The Retail Revolution in Health Care* (Praeger, 2010) and *mHealth: Transforming Healthcare* (Springer, 2014). She was the recipient of a research award from the IBM Center for Healthcare Management for her study of patient flow management. Dr. Malvey is a nationally known speaker, has published extensively in the field, and has served on the editorial board of *Health Care Management Review.* She has worked as a congressional aide and served in a variety of healthcare positions, including as executive director of a national trade association that represents health professionals.

Drake Maynard, JD, retired from his position as director of employee relations and local government services for the state of North Carolina in 2011. Before holding that position, he was the senior director of human resources administration for the University of North Carolina (UNC) at Chapel Hill and personnel director for UNC Hospitals. He is on the faculty of the UNC Gillings School of Global Public Health's executive management program. He has an undergraduate degree from UNC at Chapel Hill and a law degree from the University of South Carolina. Since retiring, he has operated DMHR Services, providing human resources consulting and staff development services for state and local governments.

Marisa Morrison is a doctoral candidate in the Department of Health Policy and Management at the Gillings School of Global Public Health at the University of North Carolina (UNC) at Chapel Hill. Ms. Morrison has worked on US healthcare workforce issues as a graduate research assistant at UNC's Cecil G. Sheps Center for Health Services Research. Prior to attending UNC, Ms. Morrison worked at the Engelberg Center for Health Care

Reform at the Brookings Institution in Washington, DC. Ms. Morrison graduated from the University of Pennsylvania in 2006.

Lindsay T. Munn, MSN, RN, is a doctoral candidate in the University of North Carolina at Chapel Hill School of Nursing with a focus on healthcare systems quality and patient outcomes. The topic of her dissertation is how nursing unit dynamics influence nurses' willingness to complete error reports.

George H. Pink, PhD, is the Humana Distinguished Professor in the Department of Health Policy and Management in the Gillings School of Global Public Health at the University of North Carolina at Chapel Hill and a senior research fellow at the Cecil G. Sheps Center for Health Services Research at the university. Prior to receiving a doctorate in corporate finance, he spent ten years in health services management, planning, and consulting.

Amanda Raffenaud, MSHSA, holds bachelor's and master's degrees in health services administration and is pursuing a doctorate in public affairs. Her research interests include healthcare workforce issues, including work–family balance and recruitment and retention of employees. Ms. Raffenaud is also an instructor in the Department of Health Management and Informatics at the University of Central Florida, where she enjoys teaching and readying students for their future careers in health administration.

Howard L. Smith, PhD, is dean and professor in the College of Business at Pacific University in Forest Grove/Hillsboro, Oregon. He previously served at Boise State University as vice president for university advancement (2007–2011), dean of the College of Business and Economics (2006–2007), and professor (2011–2012). At the Anderson School of Management and School of Public Administration at the University of New Mexico, he served as dean (1994–2004), associate dean (1990–1994), and director of the Program for Creative Enterprise and the Creative Enterprise Endowed Chair (2004–2006). He received his doctorate from the University of Washington. He has published more than 230 journal articles on health services, organization theory and behavior, and strategic management. He has published seven books on prospective payment, staff development, hospital competition, healthcare financial management, strategic nursing management, reinventing medical practice, and higher education strategy. His most recent book is *Business Aha! Tips: Successful Fundraising* (CCI Press, 2014).

Kenneth R. White, PhD, APRN-BC, FACHE, FAAN, is the University of Virginia (UVA) Medical Center endowed professor of nursing and associate dean for strategic partnerships and innovation in the School of Nursing at UVA. He also holds joint appointments in the UVA Darden School of Business and McIntire School of Commerce. He has more than 40 years' experience in healthcare organizations in clinical, administrative, governance, and consulting capacities.